Vaccines:
new concepts and developments

Proceedings of the 10th International Convocation on Immunology
Buffalo, New York, 14–17 July 1986

Vaccines: new concepts and developments

Editors
Heinz Kohler and Philip T LoVerde

Editorial Assistant
Carol W Ward

The Ernest Witebsky Center for Immunology
School of Medicine
University at Buffalo
State University of New York
Buffalo, New York 14214

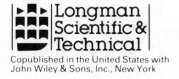
Longman
Scientific &
Technical

Copublished in the United States with
John Wiley & Sons, Inc., New York

Longman Scientific & Technical,
Longman Group UK Limited,
Longman House, Burnt Mill, Harlow,
Essex CM20 2JE, England
and Associated Companies throughout the world.

Copublished in the United States with
John Wiley & Sons, Inc., 605 Third Avenue, New York, NY 10158

© Longman Group UK Limited 1988

First published 1988

British Library Cataloguing in Publication Data

International Convocation on Immunology
  (10th: 1986: Buffalo)
  Vaccines: new concepts and developments.
  1. Vaccines
  I. Title   II. Kohler, Heinz, 1939–
  III. LoVerde, Philip T.
  615'.372   RM281

ISBN 0-582-98886-1

Library of Congress Cataloging-in-Publication Data

International Convocation on Immunology (10th: 1986:
  Buffalo, N.Y.)
  Vaccines, new concepts and developments.

  'The Ernest Witebsky Center for Immunology, School
of Medicine, University at Buffalo, State University
of New York, Buffalo, New York.'
  Includes bibliographies and index.
  1. Vaccines – Congresses.   2. Antigens – Congresses.
3. Immune response – Congresses.   I. Kohler, Heinz,
1939–   . II. LoVerde, Philip T., 1946–   .
III. Ward, Carol W.   IV. Ernest Witebsky Center for
Immunology.   V. Title.   [DNLM: 1. Vaccines – congresses.
W3 IN6856 10th 1986v / QW 805 I595 1986v]
QR189.I544   1986   615'.63   87–16882
ISBN 0–470–20888–0

Set in 10/12 Linotron 202 Times Roman

Printed and bound in Great Britain
at the Bath Press, Avon

Contents

10TH INTERNATIONAL CONVOCATION ON IMMUNOLOGY
Buffalo, New York, 14–17 July, 1986

Convocation Committee

Boris Albini
Michael A Apicella
Thomas D Flanagan
Robert J Genco
Eugene A Gorzynski
James F Mohn
Murray W Stinson
Marek B Zaleski

Heinz Kohler and
Philip T LoVerde, Co-Chairmen

Acknowledgements

The Ernest Witebsky Center for Immunology gratefully acknowledges the generous contributions in support of this convocation from

Bristol–Myers Company
Connaught Laboratories, Inc.
Hoechst–Roussel Pharmaceuticals Inc.
Hoffmann–La Roche Inc.
Lederle Laboratories, Division of American Cyanamid Company
Lilly Research Laboratories
Longman Group UK Limited
Mead Johnson, Nutritional Division
Merck Sharp & Dohme Research Laboratories
Monsanto Company
Ortho Diagnostic Systems Inc.
Pitman Moore Inc.
Reichert Scientific Instruments
Ross Laboratories
Sandoz Pharmaceuticals Corporation
Smith Kline & French Laboratories
Solvay Veterinary Inc.

Preface

It has been 190 years since Jenner introduced the concept of prevention of an infectious disease, smallpox, by active immunization with the attenuated or inactivated agent of that disease, in this case living cowpox virus, the process we now call vaccination in his honor. All of the successful vaccines developed since then for the prophylaxis of contagious diseases, which require making the vaccine with the causative agent itself, such as typhoid fever, whooping cough, poliomyelitis, etc., have always had certain defects in that they caused adverse reactions in some patients because of the extraneous materials they contained.

Consequently, the topic of vaccines with respect to new concepts and developments is a timely one because it reflects that the current demand for new vaccines that are better and safer is being met in part by major break-throughs in molecular biology and immunology.

The Tenth International Convocation on Immunology held 14–17 July 1986 in Buffalo, New York, addressed many of the practical and theoretical issues in new approaches to vaccine development as reported in this proceedings volume. The first group of papers concerns the conceptual question of what is an antigen. Papers by Lerner, Getzoff, Poljak, Margoliash and Atassi emphasize the recognition of structures which may be antigenic. These are followed by reports that address the question of antigen identification and purification. Here lipopolysaccharide (Luderitz), somatic (Apicella), fimbraial (Cisar) and carbohydrate (Linzer) antigens are discussed. Concluding this section is a presentation on epitope identification by Van Regenmortel.

A section dealing with questions regarding the biological parameters of the host response follows. Presented here is current information on the specificity and affinity of B cell triggering (Klinman); mucosal immunity (Ogra); the role of complement (Griffiss, Rice) and responses against streptococcal infections of medical (Beachey) and dental (Taubman) importance. Also in this group the role T cells play in vaccination (Mitchison) and in recognition of epitopes (Yewdell) is discussed. Benjamini and Steward each report the role of T and B cell responses against defined epitopes, and Morrison introduces the concept of chimeric antibodies that may be useful in vaccination protocols.

With the information on antigens and the host responses they elicit, the convocation turned to questions on the production and delivery of vaccines using recombinant DNA technology. The most recent information on mycobacteria (R A Young), malaria (J F Young), AIDS (Montagnier), foot-and-mouth disease (Bachrach), and cholera (Manning) is presented. The use of salmonella (Curtiss) and vaccinia virus (Paoletti and Smith) as live carriers for foreign antigens is discussed.

Questions of using idiotypes and synthetic peptides as vaccines are treated next. Roitt introduces the concepts of idiotypic vaccines and the applications of idiotype vaccines to infectious agents such as reovirus (Greene), influenza (Bona), hepatitis (Dreesman), Sendai virus (Ertl) and parasites (Lambert) and to cancer (Kohler) are reported. The use of synthetic peptides as a vaccine against influenza and cholera is demonstrated by Arnon.

Problems regarding vaccines that can cause adverse reactions are addressed by Cunningham and Stinson. Each discusses the mimicry of streptococcal antigens with heart muscle.

Two contributions provide an outlook on human (Hilleman) and animal (Murrell) vaccination.

The up-and-coming topic of immunotoxins is the subject of the paper by Jonathan Uhr as presented in an Ernest Witebsky Memorial Lecture.

Collectively, this book provides a broad survey of current and novel approaches in vaccine development. These take advantage of the newest biological and genetic techniques, thereby demonstrating that today vaccinology is in the mainstream of modern biology. The organizers of this conference hope that this book will provide an overview of this fast-moving field which is advanced by a large number of different biological and biochemical disciplines.

Heinz Kohler and Philip T LoVerde

Abbreviations

AIDS	acquired immune deficiency syndrome
APC	antigen presenting cell
bp	base pair
BSA	bovine serum albumin
CD	circular dichroism
CFA	complete Freund's adjuvant
CFU	colony forming units
CTL	cytotoxic T lymphocytes
CTP	c-terminal peptides
EBV	Epstein-Barr virus
ELISA	enzyme-linked immunosorbent assay
FITC	fluorescein isothiocyanate conjugate
GALT	gut-associated lymphoid tissue
HA	hemagglutinin
HBV	hepatitis B virus
hCG	human chorionic gonadotrophin
HIV	human immunodeficiency virus
HLA	human lymphocyte antigen
HPLC	high-pressure liquid chromatography
HSV	herpes simplex virus
HTLV	human T cell lymphotropic virus
i.p.	intraperitoneal
i.v.	intravenous
Id	idiotype
IFA	incomplete Freund's adjuvant
Ig	immunoglobulin
Ir	immune response
Iscom	immunostimulatory complex
IT	immunotoxin
kbp	kilobase pair
kD	kilodalton

KLH	keyhole limpet hemocyanin
LH	luteinizing hormone
LOS	lipooligosaccharide
LPS	lipopolysaccharide
MAb (Mab)	monoclonal antibody
MgEGTA	magnesium ethyl glycol-bis-tetraacetic acid
MHC	major histocompatibility complex
MW	molecular weight
NMR	nuclear magnetic resonance
PHA	phytohemagglutinin
SD	standard deviation
SDS–PAGE	sodium dodecyl sulfate–polyacrylamide gel electrophoresis
SEM	standard error of the mean
sIg	secretory immunoglobulin
TMVP	tobacco mosaic virus protein
TNP	trinitrophenyl
UV	ultraviolet
WHO	World Health Organization

1 Ernest Witebsky Memorial Lecture

Immunotoxins: New pharmacologic agents for the treatment of cancer and immune dysfunction

Jonathan W Uhr; R Jerrold Fulton; Ellen S Vitetta

Department of Microbiology, University of Texas Southwestern Medical School, Dallas, Texas 75235, USA

Introduction

It has been over 75 years since Paul Ehrlich suggested targeting toxic agents to microbes (Himmelweit 1960). Ehrlich visualized binding heavy metals to dyes that had affinity to parasites, thereby creating a toxic conjugate that would home to the parasites. He did not make the additional intellectual leap suggesting antibodies as the targeting vehicles. Probably the first scientist to suggest the use of antibodies as carriers was David Pressman (Pressman and Korngold 1953). Despite the vision of Ehrlich and Pressman, systematic study of such antibody–toxin conjugates did not begin until 1980 when several groups published simultaneously and independently the selective killing of cellular subsets *in vitro* using such conjugates (Krolick *et al.* 1980; Ross *et al.* 1980; Blythman *et al.* 1981; Youle and Neville 1980; Gilliland *et al.* 1980; Raso and Griffin 1980).

A cell-binding antibody conjugated to a plant or bacterial toxin has been termed an 'immunotoxin' (IT). One such toxin, ricin, like most toxic proteins produced by bacteria and plants, has a toxic polypeptide (A chain) attached to a cell-binding polypeptide (B chain) (Olsnes and Pihl 1973). The B chain is a lectin that binds to galactose-containing glycoproteins or glycolipids on the cell surface. By mechanisms that are not yet well understood, the A chain of the cell-bound ricin gains access to the cell cytoplasm presumably by receptor-mediated endocytosis and penetration of the membrane of the endocytic vesicle. There is evidence that the B chain can also facilitate the translocation of the A chain through the membrane of the endocytic vesicle (Jansen *et al.* 1982; Neville and Youle 1982; Thorpe and Ross 1982; Houston 1982). In the cytoplasm, the A chain of ricin inhibits protein synthesis by enzymatically inactivating the EF-2 binding portion of the 60 S ribosomal subunit. It is thought that one molecule of A chain in the cytoplasm of a susceptible cell can kill it (Olsnes and Pihl 1981).

The A and B chains of ricin can be separated, purified and covalently linked

3

to antibodies derivatized with the thiol-containing cross-linker, SPDP. In the case of A chain-containing immunotoxins, the antibody portion substitutes for the lectin portion (B chain), thus allowing the specific targeting of the toxic A chain to the relevant target cells.

The Murine BCL₁ Model

This disease bears a close resemblance to the prolymphocytic form of chronic lymphocytic leukemia in the human, i.e. splenomegaly and severe leukemia (Slavin and Strober 1977; Muirhead *et al.* 1981). Injection of one BCL_1 cell into a normal BALB/c mouse results in leukemia in approximately one-half of the recipients 12 weeks later (Vitetta *et al.* 1982). Tumor-bearing mice usually survive for 3–4 months after receiving 10^5–10^6 tumor cells. The BCL_1 tumor cells bear large amounts of cell surface IgMλ and traces of IgDλ, both of which have the same idiotype.

Elimination of BCL₁ cells from bone marrow

The efficacy of immunotoxins in specifically killing subsets of cells *in vitro* has led to their application to deletion of particular cell types from suspensions of bone marrow cells. The ultimate objective is to facilitate bone marrow transplantation in the human as an approach to treatment of cancer and diseases of the hematopoietic system. Autologous bone marrow transplantation is used as an adjunct to treatment for certain types of cancer that are highly susceptible to X-irradiation and/or chemotherapy. The approach is to obtain bone marrow from a patient in remission (preferably in the first remission) and to freeze it. If the patient subsequently relapses, the patient is then subjected to 'supralethal' therapy with X-irradiation and/or chemotherapy in order to eradicate the tumor. The patient is then rescued from death by infusion of his own bone marrow.

It would, of course, be highly desirable to purge such bone marrow of cancer cells by a cancer cell-reactive immunotoxin. The only requirement of such an immunotoxin is that it should not damage the stem cells which are needed to reconstitute the patient's hematopoietic system.

In initial experiments, immunotoxins containing anti-idiotypic antibody directed against the tumor-derived Ig were incubated with populations of BCL_1 tumor cells and control cells. The specific immunotoxin decreased protein synthesis in the populations containing tumor cells by 70–80%; the percentage of tumor cells in these populations was also 70–80%. Control immunotoxins containing irrelevant antibodies had no effect on BCL_1 cells, nor did specific immunotoxins have an effect on normal splenocytes, on T cell tumors, or on another B cell tumor bearing a different idiotype. Anti-idiotype antibody by itself did not affect protein synthesis in BCL_1 cells. These results indicate that immunotoxin-mediated killing of neoplastic B cells in a mixed population is specific (Krolick *et al.* 1980).

Similar studies were performed using a tumor-infiltrated bone marrow (Krolick *et al.* 1982a) (containing 15% BCL_1 cells) because of the clinical implications of removing tumor cells from marrow. In addition, it was possible to evaluate the nonspecific killing of stem cells by adoptively transferring the treated cells into lethally irradiated recipients. In these studies, anti-Ig immunotoxin was used since the only requirement for the specificity of the immunotoxin was that it kill all the tumor cells but *not* the stem cells. Thus, it was possible to use a polyvalent antibody against Ig rather than an anti-idiotypic antibody. The results of these experiments (Fig. 1) indicate that: (1) the hematopoietic system of all the animals was reconstituted because all lethally irradiated mice survived; (2) 15 of 20 mice treated with tumor-reactive immunotoxin did not develop tumors over a period of 25 weeks of observation. Of the five animals that relapsed, all had idiotype-positive cells that were susceptible to the *in vitro* lethal effect of anti-Ig containing

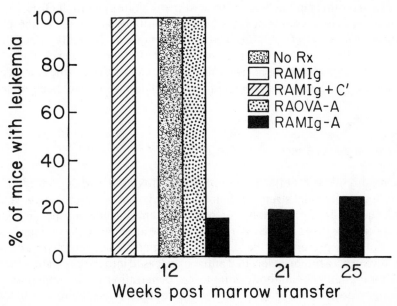

Figure 1. Adoptive transfer into lethally irradiated recipients of BCL_1-containing bone marrow cells treated with rabbit antibody to mouse Ig conjugated with A chain. Bone marrow cells containing 10 to 15% tumor cells were injected into groups of 20 mice at 10^6 marrow cells/mouse. Every two weeks after adoptive transfer the mice were examined for leukemia. At 25 weeks, all surviving mice were killed and 10^6 spleen cells were adoptively transferred into normal recipients. The spleen cells from one of the mice caused a tumor in these recipients 10 weeks later. Thus, this mouse is scored as leukemic at 25 weeks.

immunotoxins. Hence, no evidence was obtained for the emergence of an immunotoxin-resistant variant. Rather, the results of immunotoxin treatment in these studies was consistent with the survival of one cell per 1×10^6 cells injected. Results similar to ours have been obtained by Thorpe *et al.* (1982) using antibody–ricin conjugates in the presence of lactose to delete tumor cells from rat bone marrow. We extended this approach to the removal of neoplastic B cells from human bone marrow and demonstrated that the tumor cells are killed but that the CFU_{GM} BFU_E are not (Muirhead *et al.* 1983).

Another approach to facilitating the bone marrow transplantation problems using immunotoxins is the elimination of T cells from HLA-matched bone marrow. The elimination of T cells is necessary to prevent the graft-versus-host disease (GVHD) that frequently accompanies such allogeneic transplantation (Thomas, 1982). Prior studies have shown that a combination of antibody and complement is a highly effective maneuver to remove T cells and prevent GVHD (Prentice *et al.* 1984). Studies by Kersey and his co-workers (Filipovich *et al.* 1984; Vallera *et al.* 1982) over the past several years have shown the feasibility of using antibodies to T cells conjugated to intact ricin in the presence of 0.1 M-galactose. This is a highly effective approach. Similar studies have been performed by E Vitetta in collaboration with Paul Martin and others in the Seattle Bone Marrow Transplantation Group using antibody–A chain conjugates in which the antibody is specific to the CD3 antigen (Martin *et al.*, unpublished). This conjugate is highly effective at killing T cells in human bone marrow (Press *et al.* 1986). However, there are other problems with the use of such allogeneic marrow, such as the emergence of late graft rejection and B cell lymphoma, that have not yet been solved.

In-vivo therapy of BCL₁

The requirements for effective use of immunotoxins *in vivo* are considerably more formidable and stringent than their *ex vivo* use as described above for bone marrow transplantation. Potential problems include nonspecific toxicity, specific toxicity due to cross-reactivity of the antibody in the immunotoxin with antigens present on life-supporting normal tissue, interaction of immunotoxin with tumor-associated antigens released into the circulation thereby forming antigen–antibody complexes, penetration of the immunotoxin into neoplastic tissue or into body compartments where there is a blood–tissue barrier, and immune responses to the immunotoxin.

For the initial experiments (Krolick *et al.* 1982b), mice bearing massive tumor burdens (20% of body weight or approximately 10^{10} tumor cells) were employed. The strategy was to reduce the tumor burden by at least 95% using nonspecific cytoreduction and to eliminate the remaining tumor cells with immunotoxins directed against either the idiotype or the δ chain of sIgD on the BCL₁ cells. The rationale for using anti-δ is that sIgD is present on a large proportion of B cell tumors and, therefore, would present a more practical reagent for clinical therapy. Furthermore, after cytoreductive therapy, there are virtually no sIgD-positive normal B cells or serum IgD to bind the immunotoxin. Normal B cells can also be regenerated from sIgD⁻ cells. In these experiments, nonspecific cytoreduction was accomplished with a combination of splenectomy and fractionated total lymphoid irradiation (TLI). Animals receiving no further treatment other than TLI and splenectomy were dead within eight weeks (Fig. 2). The injection of these cytoreduced mice with control immunotoxins or antibody alone did not prolong their survival. In contrast, animals receiving anti-δ immunotoxins appeared disease-free as judged by the absence of detectable idiotype-positive cells 10 to 18 weeks later in three of four experiments. In one experiment, treated mice relapsed at 8–10 weeks after immunotoxin therapy. It should also be noted that 14 weeks after such immunotoxin treatment, mice in remission had normal or

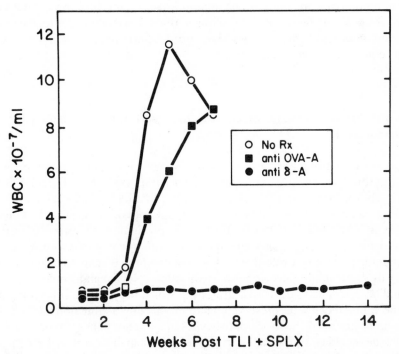

Figure 2. Effect of TLI, splenectomy and administration of immunotoxin on leukemic relapse of BCL₁-bearing mice. After nine doses of TLI and splenectomy, mice were injected with two doses of 20 μg of anti-δ or control immunotoxin or were not injected. There were nine mice per group. Leukemic relapse was monitored by determining the number of white cells in the blood of the treated mice. The control mice were all dead at seven weeks after TLI. The rabbit anti-mouse δ-A chain-treated group was monitored for a period of 14 weeks post-TLI, at which point the experiment was terminated. ○, No treatment; ■, anti-OVA-A; ●, anti-δ-A.

above-normal levels of sIgD-bearing B lymphocytes. Hence, stem cells, pre-B cells or sIgD⁻ lymphocytes had fully restored the virgin B cell compartment.

These results suggest that: (1) either remaining tumor cells had been eradicated in the animals that appeared tumor-free or that some viable tumor cells remained but were 'held in check' by host resistance mechanisms; (2) immunotoxin specific to a normal tissue component, in this case sIgD, can be used to render animals disease-free and the host can survive the effects of such cross-reactivity and can reconstitute the B cell compartment. To determine whether the animals were disease-free, tissues were then transferred from disease-free animals 25 weeks after treatments. All animals adoptively transferred tumor into normal mice, indicating that the animals were not tumor-free and suggesting that host resistance had developed.

The partial success of these experiments was probably due to the fact that nonspecific cytoreduction was successful in reducing the number of remaining tumor cells to a level which could be effectively killed by a nonlethal dose of the immunotoxin. In addition, the immunotoxins in this instance did not kill all the remaining tumor cells yet prolonged remissions occurred. Presumably, the remaining viable tumor cells did not produce progressive disease because of a tumor-specific immune response.

Use of B chain-containing immunotoxins to potentiate A chain-containing immunotoxins

It is known that in many cases ricin conjugates are significantly more toxic than antibody–A chain conjugates (Jansen *et al.* 1982; Neville and Youle 1982; Thorpe and Ross 1982; Houston 1982). In addition, free B chains can synergize *in vitro* with A chain-containing immunotoxins in specifically killing target cells (Neville and Youle, 1982). It is postulated, therefore, that the greater toxicity of ricin-containing immunotoxins as compared with A chain-containing immunotoxins is due to the capacity of the B chain to facilitate the entry of A chain into the cytoplasm (reviewed in Neville and Youle 1982). It would be desirable to develop a strategy in which the putative transport role of the B chain could be preserved while minimizing its function as a lectin. One approach would be to utilize two types of immunotoxins. Tumor-reactive antibodies could be conjugated to either ricin A chain or ricin B chain. Affinity purification of the immunotoxins on their respective antigens would be used to remove free A and B chains. Using the two immunotoxins, the two subunits of the ricin toxin could, thereby, be delivered independently to the same target cell.

To test this approach, a human neoplastic B cell line (Daudi) was treated with a low concentration of RAHIg-A that did not inhibit its protein synthesis. A goat anti-rabbit Ig–B chain conjugate also did not affect Daudi cells. However, when the cells were treated with RAHIg–A, washed, and then treated with different concentrations of GARIg–B, there was significant potentiation of cytotoxicity (Vitetta *et al.* 1983, 1984). When GARIg alone was used or when GARIg was mixed with 1% free B chains (the maximum estimate contamination of the secondary IT), no potentiation of the killing by RAHIg–A was observed. These experiments demonstrate that the potentiation of killing is dependent upon the covalent attachment of the B chain to the secondary antibody.

An irrelevant secondary IT (GA-OVA-B) was ineffective at potentiating killing by the RAHIg–A. In addition, an irrelevant primary IT (RA-OVA-A) or antibody (RAHIg) followed by the GARIg–B did not inhibit protein synthesis (data not shown).

We can only speculate on the subcellular events that underlie the synergy. It is likely that a portion of the two immunotoxins that bind to the same target cell are endocytosed together and are present in the same endosome. Therein, interchain disulfide bonds may be split and free A and B chains may be released into the endocytic vesicle. The B chain would then facilitate translocation of the A chain into the cytoplasm with resultant cell death. These results represent a new strategy for utilizing the toxic property of the A chain and the translocating ability of the B chain in a way that retains the *specificity* conferred by the antibody of A chain immunotoxin.

Additional strategies to optimize the use of A chain immunotoxins

There are four problems with the use of A chain immunotoxins that have been studied and in which progress has been made:

1. Lack of specific target cell toxicity of some A chain immunotoxins. So-called lysosomotropic agents that raise the pH of endocytic vesicles have been shown to potentiate A chain immunotoxins (Casellas *et al.* 1984; Ramakrishnan and Houston 1984). These agents include ammonium chloride, chloroquine and monensin. The above studies have been carried out *in vitro*. It remains to be determined whether such agents can be used successfully *in vivo* and, in particular, if they potentiate target cell toxicity, whether they potentiate nonspecific toxicity to the host as well.
2. Rapid uptake of A chain- and B chain-containing immunotoxins by the liver due to their mannose-containing carbohydrates. It is known that Kupffer cells have receptors for mannose (Stahl *et al.* 1978) and these undoubtedly account in large measure for the rapid uptake of immunotoxins by the liver and their consequent divergence from target cells. Thorpe and colleagues (Thorpe *et al.* 1985) have developed a chemical procedure to destroy the majority of mannose residues from ricin. Such partially

deglycosylated molecules are not taken up rapidly by the liver and, hence, have a longer half-life in the circulation. It has been shown that such partially deglycosylated A and B chains function quite effectively as immunotoxins (Vitetta and Thorpe 1985). A chain immunotoxins appear unaffected by the deglycosylation whereas B chain immunotoxins are reduced 3–5-fold in effectiveness. It may be helpful to use such deglycosylated immunotoxins *in vivo*, but further studies will be needed to determine the effect of deglycosylation on therapeutic index.

3. The lectin binding site on the B chain may affect the specificity of B chain immunotoxins *in vivo*. It has been shown biochemically that inactivation of the lectin binding activity of the B chain can be achieved by chloramine-T-mediated iodination with virtually full retention of the capacity of B chain as an immunotoxin to potentiate A chain immunotoxin killing (Vitetta 1986). It should be possible, therefore, to generate B chains by recombinant DNA techniques in which the lectin binding site has been inactivated by site-directed mutagenesis and the potentiating activity retained.

4. Stability of the disulfide bond *in vivo*. There is conflicting evidence regarding the stability of the SPDP linkage of A chain to antibody *in vivo*. Our own studies (Fulton *et al.*, unpublished) suggest that there is some instability *in vivo*. The problem of reduction of this bond *in vivo* is that not only is some of the immunotoxin inactivated, but the free antibody generated from such immunotoxins then competes with the immunotoxin for antigenic sites on the target cell. Hence, even a modest instability can result in a significant reduction of specific target cell toxicity. We have recently made immunotoxins using the Fab fragment of monoclonal or polyvalent antibody directed against particular immunoglobulin isotypes such as IgD. A chains can be directly bound to the cysteine on the heavy chain that forms the inter H chain disulfide bond on the intact molecule. Thus, using Ellman's reagent, one can bind the sulfhydryl group on the A chain to the cysteine in question resulting in a disulfide bond without an amino acid spacer. This bond appears to be more stable *in vivo*. In addition, it has recently been shown that Fab antibody directed against the immunoglobulin of B lymphocytes has a different intracellular fate than intact antibody of the same specificity (Metezeau *et al.* 1984). The Fab fragment after binding to surface Ig and endocytosis of the complex does *not* go directly to lysosomes. In contrast, intact antibody and its bound surface Ig do go to lysosomes. Hence, this different intracellular pathway could allow Fab–A chain immunotoxins to translocate the A chain into the cytosol before destruction by lysosomal enzymes.

In-vivo therapy of the BCL₁ tumor with univalent versus divalent anti-δ A chain IT

We have compared the effectiveness of the IgG–A and F(ab)–A ITs in mice bearing the BCL_1 tumor. The original model of the *in vivo* BCL_1 tumor has been modified in order to obtain results more rapidly. We have shown that 1–3 weeks after the injection of 10^6–10^7 BCL_1 cells into normal BALB/c mice, approximately 40% or $(4–8) \times 10^7$ cells in the spleens of these mice bear the BCL_1 idiotype. Since the spleen is the primary site of early tumor growth, an enumeration of the number of idiotype-positive spleen cells represents a fairly accurate measurement of the tumor burden in these animals. These mice were injected with different doses of the IgG–A or F(ab)–A chain. The antibody was a monoclonal rat anti-mouse δ chain of the IgG_{2b} isotype. Twenty-four to forty-eight hours after injection of the IT, the spleens were removed and analyzed for the presence of idiotype-positive cells. As shown in Fig. 3, as determined by the number of idiotype-positive cells remaining in the spleen, both univalent and divalent ITs eliminated the majority of the tumor cells in a

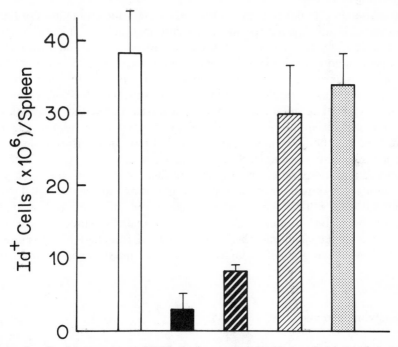

Figure 3. *In vivo* treatment of BCL_1 leukemia with JA12-A or Fab′–JA12-A. Mice were injected, i.p., with 5×10^6 BCL_1 tumor cells. Three weeks after injection of tumor cells, groups of four mice were treated with a single i.v. injection of PBS (□) or 0.5 mg of JA12-A (▨), Fab′–JA12-A (■), JA12 (▨) or Fab′–JA12 (▨). Twenty-four hours after treatment, spleens were removed and tumor cells were quantified by FACS analysis after staining with rabbit anti-idiotype and FITC-goat anti-rabbit antibody.

period of 24 hours following injection of a single dose of 0.5 mg IT. The F(ab)–IT–A appeared more effective than the divalent IT–A and this difference has been observed in additional experiments. Tumor cell number did not decrease further after another 24 hours. Antibody alone or a control IT (RtIg–A chain) did not induce killing (data not shown). This dose of IT gave maximal killing with both ITs. Although the observed killing represents only 80–90% of the initial tumor cells, the total number of tumor cells killed was $(3–3.5) \times 10^7$. It should also be noted that the status of the remaining BCL_1 cells is not known. These cells could be programmed for death. Adoptive transfer assays will be necessary to quantify the number of *viable* tumor cells present in the remaining population of idiotype-positive cells. There was no evidence of liver or kidney damage in these animals. Further work will be aimed at optimizing the killing of BCL_1 cells by the F(ab)–A anti-δ IT.

Future prospects

Our own plan is to develop an optimal regimen for the elimination of BCL_1 cells in mice utilizing the recent model described above. This will require study of repeated treatments, use of lysosomotropic agents, and the injection of B chain immunotoxins in the piggyback approach. These experiments will determine our strategy for treating patients with B cell tumors in Phase I trials. It remains to be determined whether anti-δ F(ab)–IT–A chain immunotoxins will be suitable reagents for such trials or whether antibodies to other B cell differentiation antigens would be better candidates. Clearly, combinatorial therapy will be required in the future in an effort to deal with the heterogeneity of tumor cells.

In addition, preparation of recombinant DNA-derived A and B chains is taking place in a number of laboratories, including our own. DNA-derived immunotoxins will be important when sufficient information is available regarding structure–function relationships to plan desired alterations in these molecules. In the meantime, there is much to learn from native materials with regard to the generation of optimal immunotoxins and strategies for their use.

Acknowledgements

We thank our colleagues Drs Krolick, Villemez, Isakson and Cushley who collaborated with us on these studies, our technicians Ms C Bockhold, Mr Y Chinn, Ms S Gorman, Ms R Nisi, Mr J Hudson, Ms L Trahan and Mr T Tucker, and Ms F Hall and Ms C Baselski for secretarial assistance. These studies were supported by NIH grant CA-28149

References

Blythman H E, Casellas P, Gros O, Gros P, Jansen F K, Paolucci F, Pau B, Vidal H 1981. Immunotoxins: hybrid molecules of monoclonal antibodies and a toxin subunit specifically kill tumor cells, *Nature (London)* **290**: 145–6

Casellas P, Bourrie B J P, Gros P, Jansen F 1984. Kinetics of cytotoxicity induced by immuno-toxins: enhancement by lysosomotropic amines and carboxylic ionophores, *Journal of Bio-logical Chemistry* **259**: 9359–64

Filipovich A H, Youle R J, Neville D M Jr, Vallera R, Quinones R, Kersey J H 1984. *Ex vivo* treatment of donor bone marrow with anti-T-cell immunotoxins for prevention of graft-versus-host disease, *The Lancet* **8375**: 469–72

Fulton R J, Uhr, J W, Vitetta E S 1986. The effect of antibody valency and lysosomotropic amines on the synergy between ricin A chain- and ricin B chain-containing immunotoxins, *Journal of Immunology* **136**: 3103–9

Gilliland D G, Steplewski Z, Collier R J, Mitchell K F, Chang T H, Koprowski H 1980. Antibody-directed cytotoxic agents: use of monoclonal antibody to direct the action of toxin A chains to colorectal carcinoma cells, *Proceedings of the National Academy of Sciences USA* **77**: 4539–53

Himmelweit F 1960. *The Collected Papers of Paul Ehrlich*, Pergamon, New York, vol 3

Houston L L 1982. Transport of ricin A chain after prior treatment of mouse leukemia cells with ricin B chain, *Journal of Biological Chemistry* **257**: 1532–7

Jansen F K, Blythman H E, Carriere D, Casellas P, Gros O, Gros P, Laurent J C, Paolucci F, Pau B, Poncelet P, Richer G, Vidal H, Voison G A 1982. Immunotoxins: hybrid molecules combining high specificity and potent cytotoxicity, *Immunological Reviews* **62**: 185–216

Krolick, K A, Villemez C, Isakson P, Uhr, J W, Vitetta E S 1980. Selective killing of normal or neoplastic B cells by antibodies coupled to the A chain of ricin, *Proceedings of the National Academy of Sciences USA* **77**: 5419–23

Krolick K A, Uhr, J W, Slavin S, Vitetta E S 1982a. *In-vivo* therapy of a murine B cell tumor (BCL$_1$) using antibody-ricin A chain immunotoxins, *Journal of Experimental Medicine* **155**: 1797–1809

Krolick K A, Uhr J W, Vitetta E S 1982b. Selective killing of leukemia cells by antibody–toxin conjugates; implications for autologous bone marrow transplantation in the treatment of cancer, *Nature (London)* **295**: 604–5

Metezeau P, Elguindi I, Goldberg M 1984. Endocytosis of the membrane immunoglobulins of mouse spleen B cells: a quantitative study of its rate, amount and sensitivity to physiological, physical and crosslinking agents, *EMBO Journal* **3**: 2235–42

Muirhead M J, Holbert M H, Uhr J W, Vitetta E S 1981. BCL$_1$, a murine model of prolympho-cytic leukemia, *American Journal of Pathology* **105**: 306–15

Muirhead M J, Martin P J, Torok-Storb B, Uhr J W, Vitetta E S 1983. Use of an antibody-ricin A chain conjugate to delete neoplastic B cells from human bone marrow, *Blood* **62**: 327–32

Neville D M Jr, Youle R J 1982. Monoclonal antibody ricin or ricin A chain hybrids: kinetic analysis of cell killing for tumor therapy, *Immunological Reviews* **62**: 75–91

Olsnes S, Pihl A 1973. Different biological properties of the two constituent peptide chains of ricin. A toxic protein inhibiting protein synthesis, *Biochemistry* **12**: 3121–6

Olsnes S, Pihl A 1981. Chimeric toxins, in J Drews, F Dornes (eds) *Pharmacology of Bacterial Toxins*. Pergamon Press, New York

Prentice H G, *et al.* 1984. Depletion of T lymphocytes in donor marrow prevents significant graft-versus-host disease in matched allogeneic leukaemic marrow transplant recipients, *The Lancet* **8375**: 472–6

Press O, Vitetta E, Farr A, Hansen J, Martin P 1986. Efficacy of ricin A chain immunotoxins directed against human T cells, *Cellular Immunology* **102**: 10–20

Pressman D, Korngold L 1953. The *in vivo* localization of anti-Wagner-osteogenic-sarcoma antibodies, *Cancer* **6**: 619–23

Ramakrishnan S, Houston L L 1984. Inhibition of human acute lymphoblastic leukemia cells by immunotoxins: potentiation by chloroquine, *Science* **223**: 58–61

Raso V, Griffin T 1980. Specific cytotoxicity of a human immunoglobulin-directed Fab′–ricin A chain conjugate, *Journal of Immunology* **125**: 2610–16

Ross W C J, Thorpe P E, Cumber A J, Edwards D C, Hinson C A, Davies A J S 1980. Increased toxicity of diphtheria toxin for human lymphoblastoid cells following covalent linkage to anti-(human lymphocyte) globulin or its F(ab′)₂ fragment, *European Journal of Biochemistry* **104**: 381–90

Slavin S, Strober S 1977. Spontaneous murine B cell leukemia, *Nature (London)* **272**: 624–6

Stahl P D, Rodman J S, Miller M J, Schlesinger P H 1978. Evidence for receptor-mediated binding of glycoproteins, glycoconjugates, and lysosomal glycosidases by alveolar macrophages, *Proceedings of the National Academy of Sciences USA* **75**: 1399–1403

Thomas E D 1982. The role of marrow transplantation in the eradication of malignant disease, *Cancer* **49**: 1963–9

Thorpe P E, Ross W C J 1982. The preparation and cytotoxic properties of antibody toxin conjugates, *Immunological Reviews* **62**: 119–58

Thorpe P E, Mason D W, Brown A N F, Simmonds S J, Ross W C J, Cumber A J, Forrester J A 1982. Selective killing of malignant cells in a leukemic rat bone marrow using an antibody ricin conjugate, *Nature (London)* **297**: 594–6

Thorpe P E, Detre S I, Foxwell B M J, Brown A N F, Skilleter D N, Wilson G, Forrester J A, Stirpe F 1985. Modification of the carbohydrate in ricin with metaperiodate–cyanoborohydride mixtures: effects on toxicity and *in vivo* distribution, *European Journal of Biochemistry* **147**: 197–206

Vallera D A, Youle R J, Neville D M Jr, Kersey J H 1982. Bone marrow transplantation across major histocompatibility barriers. V. Protection of mice from lethal graft-vs-host disease by pretreatment of donor cells with monoclonal anti-Thy 1.2 coupled to the toxin ricin, *Journal of Experimental Medicine* **155**: 949–54

Vitetta E S 1986. Synergy between immunotoxins prepared with native ricin A chains and chemically-modified ricin B chains, *Journal of Immunology* **136**: 1880–7

Vitetta E S, Thorpe P E 1985. Immunotoxins containing ricin A or B chains with modified carbohydrate residues act synergistically in killing neoplastic B cells *in vitro*, *Cancer Drug Delivery* **2**: 191–8

Vitetta E S, Krolick K A, Uhr J W 1982. Neoplastic B cells as targets for antibody–ricin A chain, *Immunological Reviews* **62**: 159–83

Vitetta E S, Cushley W, Uhr J W 1983. Synergy of ricin A chain-containing immunotoxins and ricin B chain-containing immunotoxins in *in vitro* killing of neoplasic human B cells, *Proceedings of the National Academy of Sciences USA* **80**: 6332–5

Vitetta E S, Fulton R J, Uhr J W 1984. The cytotoxicity of cell-reactive immunotoxin containing ricin A chain is potentiated with an anti-immunotoxin containing ricin B chain, *Journal of Experimental Medicine* **160**: 341–6

Youle R J, Neville D M Jr 1980. Anti-Thy-1.2 monoclonal antibody linked to ricin is a potent cell-type-specific toxin, *Proceedings of the National Academy of Sciences USA* **77**: 5483–6

2 Conceptual basis of antigens

The chemistry of antigen–antibody union

Alfonso Tramontano; Kim D Janda; Richard A Lerner

Department of Molecular Biology, The Research Institute of Scripps Clinic, 10666 North Torrey Pines Road, La Jolla, California 92037, USA

The immune system is unique among biological processes. It assembles and employs a variety of immunoglobulins that exhibit binding specificities to practically any substance perceived as an antigen. Unlike other receptor-mediated processes, the binding phenomena of an immunological response can be literally dissected from the rest of the system simply by harvesting these immunoglobulins from a serum. The simplicity of antibody binding is reflected in the evolution of various accessory functions, such as the complement cascade or opsinization for the neutralization of antigenic matter. Likewise, antibody–antigen binding is exploited in artificial systems by associating toxins or other functional molecules with the antibody by some physical method.

This characteristic of antibodies prompts the question – how does this simple binding differ from the complex binding interactions of enzymes or other receptors which directly effect morphological or chemical changes? The passive recognition of antigenic structures is often characterized by very high affinity constants, whereas binding of enzymes to their substrates, an active process, does not necessarily express tight binding. It would appear that the functional expression of binding has been sacrificed in immune proteins so that high affinity may be achieved. Conversely, one may say that enzymes redirect their intrinsic binding affinity to perform an active process. This idea was first formulated by Pauling when he recognized that the catalytic function of enzymes may be due to the maximal binding between the enzyme and the reacting ligand in its transition state structure, resulting in a reduced activation energy for the reaction (Pauling 1946, 1948). The classical binding of antibody to antigen is described as binding interactions directed to stable structures. The notion of enzyme–transition state complementarity as the appropriate 'lock and key' for catalysis provokes the thought that an antibody might similarly behave as a catalyst if it were directed to a stable analog of a chemical transition state (Jencks 1969). The transition state analog concept has been successfully applied to the design of enzyme inhibitors. In the immunological experiment these substances might be used as immunogens to elicit unusual, catalytic antibodies. By correspondence, an antibody–hapten pair which defines a catalyst would become an enzyme–inhibitor system through the transition state–hapten relationship. The design we have implemented applies what has been learned from inhibition of proteolytic enzymes by transition state analogs (Tramontano *et al.* 1986a). Initially, experiments were devised to treat the mechanism of ester hydrolysis, a facile example of enzyme-catalyzed transacylation, in a protocol for deriving catalytically active antibodies. We shall describe here how antibodies elicited to suitable transition state analogs can exhibit many of the chemical attributes of enzymes. This study would also serve to emphasize the principles for correlating binding site structure with function.

The combining sites of antibodies have been considered as potential templates for simulating the environment of an enzyme active site (Kohen *et al.* 1980a, 1980b; Raso and Stollar 1975; Royer 1980). Only recently, with the advent of monoclonal antibodies, has it become feasible to investigate the chemical properties of antibodies of uniform specificities. We have approached this problem equipped with the monoclonal antibody technology and the benefit of enzymological precedent in the design of transition state analogs for application as immunological haptens.

Transition state of esterolysis and hapten design

The formation and cleavage of the peptide bond is of obvious importance in biology. This is a special example of transacylation processes, which are characterized by carbonyl addition–elimination mechanisms. The acyl group

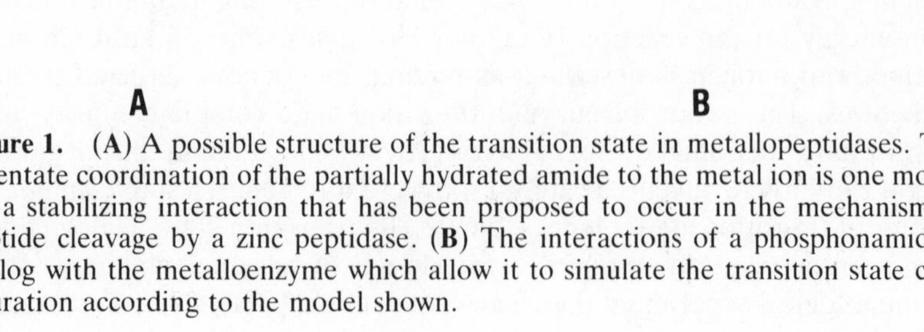

A   **B**

Figure 1. (A) A possible structure of the transition state in metallopeptidases. The bidentate coordination of the partially hydrated amide to the metal ion is one model for a stabilizing interaction that has been proposed to occur in the mechanism of peptide cleavage by a zinc peptidase. (B) The interactions of a phosphonamide analog with the metalloenzyme which allow it to simulate the transition state configuration according to the model shown.

may, therefore, possess varying degrees of tetrahedral character in the transition state. The enzymes which catalyze transacylation reactions might be expected to bind well those analogs of the substrate having a tetrahedral configuration about the acyl center (Bernhard and Orge 1959; Jencks 1975). This is true for serine proteases, where a covalent bond between the ligand and the enzyme is formed temporarily (Imperiali and Abeles 1986; Westerlik and Wolfenden 1972; Thompson 1973), as well as for metalloenzymes, which catalyze the direct hydration of amides or esters.

Enzymes in the latter category are inhibited by compounds with a tetrahedral configuration bestowed by a phosphoryl or phosphonyl group in place of the scissile amide unit (Galardy *et al.* 1983; Jacobsen and Bartlett 1981; Weaver *et al.* 1977). A proposed mechanism of peptide bond hydrolysis in metalloenzymes employs the metal ion either to polarize the amide carbonyl by coordination, or to deliver a coordinated hydroxide to that group (Lipscomb 1982). Both of these functions might operate as in Fig. 1A. Recent structural studies show that the transition state analogs have the phosphono group as a ligand to the metal ion in the active site (Fig. 1B), (Weaver *et al.* 1977; Christianson and Lipscomb 1986). The hydrolysis of carboxylic esters is a simple example of transacylation, which should also be approximated by a phosphonate-containing analog of the transition state. The binding of the

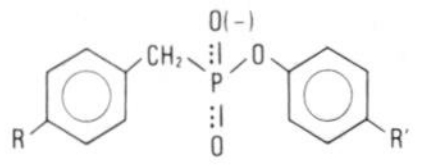

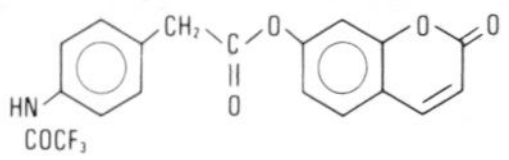

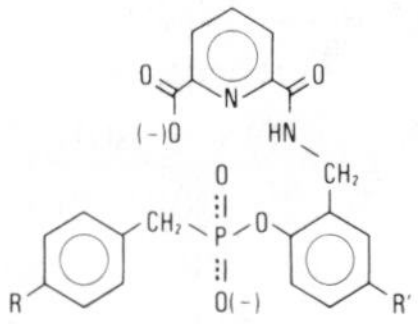

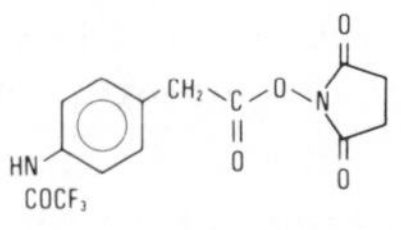

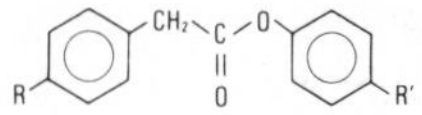

Figure 2. Haptens and substrates used in the production and assay of monoclonal antibodies with esterolytic properties. The procedures for the synthesis of these and analytical data will be reported elsewhere. The identity of substituents R and R′ are as follows. Structure **1**, **3** and **7**: R = NHCOCF$_3$, R′ = NHCOCH$_3$; structures **2** and **4**: R = NHCOCF$_3$, R′ = NHCO(CH$_2$)$_4$COON(COCH$_2$)$_2$; structure **8**: R = NHCOCF$_3$, R′ = NHCO(CH$_2$)$_2$COOH; structure **9**: R,R′ = NHCOCH$_3$; structure **10**: R = NHCOCF$_3$. R′ = H; structure **11**: R = NHCOCH$_3$, R′ = NHCOCF$_3$.

charged phosphonate group might well describe a stabilizing interaction in the transition state which would lead to catalysis. Ester hydrolysis reactions generally proceed at convenient spontaneous rates under physiological conditions that are tolerable for antibodies. Therefore, any small rate acceleration would be easily detected.

The structure we chose to elaborate was selected according to certain criteria. These included the availability and stability of the organophosphorus precursors, as well as the corresponding carboxylic acid substrate, the convenience of the chemical synthesis for its prepartion, and the adaptability to diverse schemes for immunological presentation. A basic molecular unit which provides the necessary features is the substituted aryl phenylacetic acid structure. By including amino substituents in the aromatic rings, simple chemical modification would introduce an appendage for coupling to immunogenic carrier proteins for haptenic presentation. Accordingly, we constructed phosphonate esters 1–4 (Fig. 2) to mimic an activated state in ester hydrolysis. The dipicolinic acid containing ligands 3 and 4 were designed to include a metal ion coordination site for analogy with the metalloenzyme model. Such structures might be recognized immunologically as chelates (Reardan *et al.* 1985). Initially, substance 4 was utilized as a non-chelated hapten along with the simpler phosphonate 2 to obtain specific monoclonal antibodies. Though the role of the picolinyl appendage is not fully understood, only hapten 4 has yielded catalytic antibodies.

Monoclonal antibodies selected by immunoassay and esterolytic assay

The monoclonal antibody technology provides a continuous source of uniform immunoglobulin of any desired specificity. Without this methodology these efforts would meet insurmountable obstacles, if only because the variability of an immune response, even within the same animal species, would make it very difficult to reproduce results (Milstein 1985).

Our strategy was to generate as many unique clonal specificities as was practical from a given immunization protocol and to select initially among these for immunoreactivity (Niman and Elder 1982). All hybridoma clones producing antibodies of significant titer were considered for esterolytic assay. Furthermore, IgGs were preferred for their facile purification by ion exchange chromotography. Careful purification is essential for the removal of trace impurities with nonspecific esterolytic activity. Thus, approximately 50–100 clones secreting anti-hapten antibody were initially identified in a particular fusion experiment. About two-thirds of these are not viable in cultures. The remainder were subcloned and their isotype was determined. The hybridomas, producing IgG with titer above 1:64, were propagated in ascites tumors to produce the antibody in large quantity. The IgG fraction was isolated from ascites fluid in greater than 90% purity.

The substrate designed for the esterolysis assay was based on the large difference in fluorescence of 7-hydroxycoumarin and its acylated derivatives. The fluorescence change upon hydrolysis of coumarin esters is easily detectable at nanomolar concentrations. The phenolic character of the coumarin ring should allow it to be accommodated into the hapten binding site. The trifluoroacetamidophenylacetyl ester **5** behaved accordingly, showing fluorescence intensities at 455 nm (excitation at 355 nm) proportional to the extent of hydrolysis. The fluorescence intensity of 7-hydroxycoumarin is pH-dependent, increasing sharply above pH 7.0. The practical range of pH for the assay is limited by the fast spontaneous rate of hydrolysis of the ester above pH 8.0. Initially, the concentration of ester was set to about four-fold greater than the protein concentration and the mixture was incubated at pH 7.2 for 10 minutes, noting any change in fluorescence above background.

We have assayed 28 monoclonal antibodies to phosphonate **2** from two separate immunization/fusion experiments. None of these demonstrated ability to hydrolyze substrate **5**. Similarly, 12 antibodies to **4** were assayed. Two of these showed measurable fluorescence change occurring in 5–10 minutes at pH 7.0, 23 °C. The reaction then ceased and the background rate of hydrolysis was reestablished. The fluorescence change corresponded to about 50% of that for complete hydrolysis.

Combining site directed transacylation of activated esters

We have described in detail the nature of this antibody-mediated esterolysis, including the specificity and the kinetics of the reaction. The stoichiometry of the reaction and the chemical behavior of the products led to the hypothesis that a stable acylated antibody is formed from the transacylation of the ester to a nucleophilic group in the combining site (Tramontano *et al.* 1986a).

The antibody-enhanced production of 7-hydroxycoumarin by esterolysis of acylated derivatives is unique for the trifluoroacetamidophenylacetyl ester. The process is not detected with a coumarin ester having the apparently minor structural variation of a methyl group replacing the trifluoromethyl group of **5**. The reaction is presumably not defined by this leaving group since the reactive *N*-hydroxysuccinimide ester **6** will also specifically combine with the antibodies to produce an inactive product. The termination of the reaction is noted by the return of the rate of fluoresence increase to the background level. The net change in fluorescence is proportional to the amount of protein added. When this concentration is known independently from Lowry assay and the average molecular weight of an IgG is assumed to be 150000, the stoichiometry is consistent with the reaction of one mole of ester per mole of combining sites. The reaction proceeds according to second order kinetics and the initial rate shows enzyme-like saturation.

Our preliminary observations also included indications of pH-dependence of the rate. The modest rate increase at pH 8.0 versus pH 7.0 suggested the ionization of an active base for nucleophile. Since an active protein was recovered by exposure of the inactive product to high pH or hydroxylamine, this product was formulated as a chemically modified protein in which a specific residue of the combining site is acylated. The ability of the haptenic phosphonates to block this reaction is shown in terms of their inhibition constants. Furthermore, the inactivation of the protein by tyrosine- and histidine-specific reagents was noted. The haptens are also able to block these inactivation reactions. It is not possible to distinguish between the existence of an acylimidazole or an acyltyrosine by treatment of the transacylation product with either tetranitromethane or diethylpyrocarbonate followed by deacylation at pH 9.0. The acylated protein is protected from irreversible inactivation by either reagent. This may simply mean that the covalent and noncovalent interactions of the acyl group are sufficient to impede both carboethoxylation of histidine and nitration of tyrosine in the combining site.

The original intent behind the use of the dipicolinic acid-containing hapten was to determine if that ligand would be recognized immunologically as a metal chelate. Though we made no attempt to impose metal ion coordination upon the hapten–carrier conjugate as an immunogen, the possibility remained that an anti-hapten antibody might accept the chelate form. We tested the effect of added picolinic acid and added zinc on the antibody-enhanced esterolysis with the coumarin reagent. No effect on the primary reaction was observed with up to 100 μM added zinc and picolinic acid. The involvment of trace metal ions was excluded by the failure of added EDTA to affect the reaction.

Catalytic esterolysis

The reaction occuring in the antibody combining site appears to result in acyl transfer to an essential residue of the combining site, forming a stable acylated antibody. This result was unexpected since a covalent mechanism is not suggested by the phosphonate ester. However, we believe that the binding interaction directed to the phosphonate moiety helps to stabilize the transition state or tetrahedral intermediate leading to this reaction. The observed mechanism could represent a deviation from the expected pathway which is a result of the particular choice of substrate used to study the activity. The labile esters were employed primarily because they are useful in the assay to detect low levels of esterolytic activity.

Since histidine is implicated as a crucial residue in the combining site, we reasoned that the imidazole group may participate in either nucleophilic or general base catalysis. This is known to occur in the catalysis of ester hydrolysis by imidazole (Bender *et al.* 1984). In the context of an active site, where the imidazole group is provided by the protein structure, this alternative would be manifested as covalent or noncovalent catalysis by the enzyme. We proposed that the functional groups in the active site allow two alternate mechanisms for transacylation to compete and that the prevailing pathway would change with the choice of substrate.

Indeed, an investigation of substrate specificity has revealed that these same antibodies are true enzymic catalysts when the appropriate substrates are identified (Tramontano *et al.* 1986b). These new esters are distinguished by the structural congruence of both the acyl group and the leaving group with fragments of the haptenic ligand. In addition, the leaving group basicity precludes acylation of the imidazole of histidine, as is possible with the labile esters **5** and **6**. The leaving group structure suggested by the hapten is the disubstituted phenolate with some abbreviated *para*-substituent to occupy the site of the coupling appendage. The acetamide group was used to replace this linkage in the free haptenic inhibitors **1** and **3**. The analogous substrate would have the 2-picolinylcarboxamidomethyl-4-acetamidophenol as the alcohol portion of the ester. As a first approximation of this, we prepared the 4-acetamidophenyl ester **7** which is analogous to the phosphonate **1**. The absence of the structurally significant *ortho*-substituent might diminish the potential binding of the ligand, but should not drastically affect the chemical reactivity of the ester bond.

When a mixture of this ester and the antibody from hybridoma 6D4 in a molar ratio of 50:1 is analyzed over time by liquid chromotography (HPLC), the accelerated hydrolysis of the ester was apparent from the decrease of its peak and the concurrent increase in two new peaks which correspond with the expected products. Under these conditions the ester is completely consumed in 60–80 minutes, during which time the background rate accounts for about 12–16% hydrolysis (Fig. 3). The chromatographic profile is the same as that produced by treatment with hog liver esterase. Nonspecific antibodies or antihapten antibodies, which were inactive in the stoichiometric reaction with coumarin ester **5** do not have this ability. The succinylated ester **8**, which is also highly congruous to the haptens, is hydrolyzed by the antibody at a somewhat slower rate than the corresponding acetamide **7**. This rate difference is also seen with hog liver esterase (Table 1). It may represent the unfavorable electrostatics of the charged succinate interacting with the protein, or the disadvantage of a hydrophilic ligand binding to a hydrophobic active site. Similar esters that are not accepted as substrates include **9** which demonstrates the absolute requirement of the trifluoromethyl group, as was also observed in the stoichiometric reaction. More remarkable is the specificity imparted by the acetamide group of the phenol. The phenyl ester **10** is of approximately the same reactivity as 4-acetamidophenyl ester **7** and is more congruous with the haptenic structure than the coumarin ester **5**; yet here again the antibody has no effect on the hydrolytic rate. Ester **11**, in which the trifluoroacetyl and the acetyl groups of structure **7** are interchanged, presents a unique option for inverted orientation of the ester bond in the binding site, if the similarities of the phenolic and benzylic moieties allow this kind of

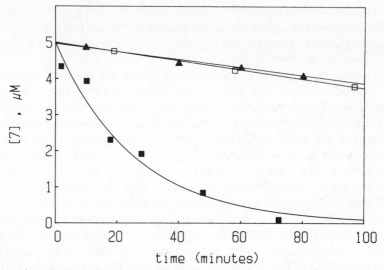

Figure 3. Rate of hydrolysis of carboxylic ester **7** determined by HPLC under the conditions described in Table 1 (50 mM-phosphate buffer pH 8.0, 23 °C). ▲, Uncatalyzed (background) rate of hydrolysis; □, effect of 0.5 μM nonspecific monoclonal IgG; ■, 0.1 μM anti-**4** monoclonal antibody from hybridoma 6D4. The superimposed curve represents a theoretical exponential decay which fits the data points.

Table 1 Hydrolysis of carboxylic esters by monoclonal antibody (from hybridoma 6D4) and by hog liver esterase (Sigma; EC 3.1.1.1) determined by HPLC on an analytical RP-C18 column (Vydac 218TP54) with isocratic elution (65:35 water:acetonitrile; 0.1% trifluoroacetic acid) at a flow rate of $1.0 \, ml \, min^{-1}$ and detector set to 245 nm. The initial substrate concentration was 5 μM and that of internal standard (acetophenone) was 10 μM in 50 mM phosphate buffer at pH 8.0. The retention times (minutes) were as follows: acetophone, 5.0; **7** 8.3; **8** 6.7; **9** 4.1; **10** 11.1 (40% acetonitrile elution); **11** 8.2. The antibody concentration was 15 μg/ml (0.1 μM) and that of esterase was 5.5 μg/ml. The reaction mixtures were kept at 23 °C and aliquots were analyzed at intervals of 2 to 20 minutes. Three or more determinations were used to plot a curve from which the half-life of the reaction is estimated (see Fig. 3)

Substrate	$t_{\frac{1}{2}}$ (min)		k_{uncat}‡
	Antibody (6D4)	Esterase	$(\times 10^5 \, s^{-1})$
7	16 ± 3	4 ± 1	2.8
8	55 ± 5	52 ± 5	3.8
9	*	4 ± 1	0.25
10	*	<2†	1.63
11	*	5 ± 1	6.10

* The ester was not consumed faster than the background rate of hydrolysis.
† The reaction is too rapid to be measured accurately by HPLC.
‡ The rate constants were determined spectrophotometrically (at 245 nm) by measuring initial rates of five concentrations of ester.

Table 2 Kinetic parameters for hydrolysis of esters **7** and **8** by monoclonal antibody. A Perkin–Elmer lambda 4B spectrophotometer, equipped with thermostated cell holder, was used to measure absorption changes at 245 nm. Cells containing the substrate at concentrations of 0.5 to 50 μM in phosphate buffer (50 mM, pH 8.0) were pre-equilibriated at 25 °C. The concentration of active IgG in a stock solution was found by reacting with coumarin ester **5** and measuring the yield of hydroxycoumarin by fluorescence. The kinetic run was initiated by addition of an aliquot of the antibody stock solution (in 50 mM phosphate buffer, pH 8.0) calculated to give 100 nM–IgG. The mixture was allowed to equilibrate for 2 to 3 minutes and the rate was then measured during the subsequent 10 minutes. The absorption change for complete hydrolysis ($\Delta\epsilon_{245}$ 4500 M^{-1} cm^{-1}) was determined by treatment with esterase. Kinetic parameters were obtained from Lineweaver–Burk plots. Inhibition constants were determined from a plot of the slopes with at least four inhibitor concentrations. The data were analyzed by linear regression.

Substrate	K_m ($\times 10^6$ M)	K_i ($\times 10^7$ M)	V_{max} ($\times 10^9$ MS^{-1})	k_{cat} ($\times 10^2$ s^{-1})	k_{cat}/k_{uncat}
7	1.90 ± 0.20	1.60 ± 0.40	2.2 ± 0.2	2.7 ± 0.2	960
8	0.62 ± 0.05	0.65 ± 0.25	1.0 ± 0.1	0.8 ± 0.1	210

interchange. Nevertheless, this possibility is not manifested by the accelerated hydrolysis of this ester. On the other hand, the hydrolysis of all these esters is accelerated by the indiscriminate esterase from hog liver. Chemical selectivity is a distinguishing feature of the catalytic antibody and may be considered a reflection of the exquisite binding specificity of immunological recognition.

Reaction kinetics were measured spectrophotometrically by following the absorption change at 245 nm. The pseudo first-order rate shows enzyme-like saturation, and the phosphonate ligands behave as competitive inhibitors in Lineweaver–Burk analysis. Kinetic parameters obtained with these substrates are tabulated along with the inhibition constants found with phosphonate **3** (Table 2). Under these conditions the acceleration above the background rate is about 1000-fold for substrate **7** and about 200-fold for substrate **8** (corrected for the background hydrolysis rate). The pH at which these measurements were made are most likely not optimal. Preliminary indications suggest that this reaction is more sensitive to pH than the transacylation with coumarin ester. The catalytic reaction is nearly undetectable at pH 7.0.

Nucleophilic versus general base mechanism and catalysis

Indications that a histidine is critical to the activities of the esterolytic antibodies provided the earliest clue regarding the mechanism of transacylation. The nucleophilic character of imidazole is well established. However, there is no evidence that enzymes employ the imidazole group of histidine for nucleophilic catalysis. On the other hand, the function of the imidazole group of histidine in general acid–base catalysis is widely appreciated in enzyme mechanism (Walsh 1979). The dual role of imidazole as a nucleophilic and general base catalyst in ester hydrolysis is well understood (Bender *et al.* 1984). The transition between these mechanisms is determined by the relative rates of formation and breakdown of the two possible tetrahedral intermediates: that derived from addition of imidazole to the acyl group versus that from hydroxide addition. The relatively labile coumarin ester **5** forms an imidazole adduct which can readily collapse to the acyl imidazole intermediate by loss of the coumarin alkoxide. This step becomes more difficult with poor leaving groups that form less stable alkoxides. The 7-hydroxycoumarin ($pK_a \sim 8.3$) is a substantially better leaving group than 4-acetamidophenol ($pK_a\,9.9$). The 4-acetamidophenyl ester **7** may, therefore, form a tetrahedral adduct with water or hydroxide and the breakdown of this is presumably catalyzed (Fig. 4). As evidence for the existence of separate mechanisms, we find that the product of the reaction of the antibody with ester **5** is not an intermediate in the catalytic reaction with **7**. Indeed, **5** acts as a specific inactivator of the catalyst when it is added to a mixture of the antibody and ester **7**. The two esters are differentiated with considerable fidelity, as the

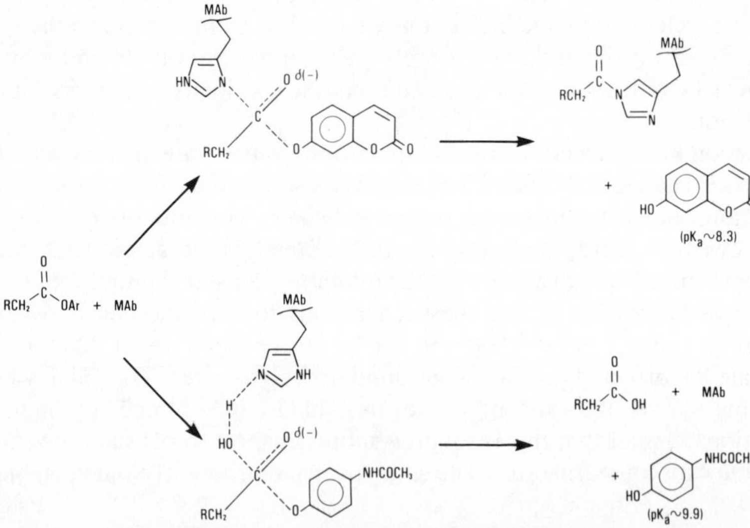

Figure 4. A proposed scheme to account for the divergent chemistry observed in the reaction of an anti-**4** monoclonal antibody with carboxylic esters **5** and **7**. A histidine residue in the combining site is presumed to act as a nucleophilic (upper pathway) or general-base (lower pathway) catalyst during the formation and breakdown of a tetrahedral intermediate. The ester with a good leaving group reacts by the upper pathway since the rate-limiting step, formation of the intermediate, is facile. This pathway is precluded for the ester with a poor leaving group since the rate-limiting step, breakdown of the intermediate, is not catalyzed relative to the analogous step in the lower pathway, which may be general-base catalyzed.

antibody is observed to turn over several hundred-fold with substrate **7** without noticeable inactivation. Catalysis by the antibody through both mechanisms implies that the binding interactions can stabilize either transition state in these two-step processes. However, only the general base process (rate-limiting breakdown to products) is relevant to the intention of the experimental design.

The contribution of binding to catalysis via this general base mechanism is illustrated best by the different behavior of 4-acetamidophenyl ester **7** and phenyl ester **10**. Phenol as a leaving group (pK_a 9.89) is equivalent to 4-acetamidophenol, yet the hydrolysis of **10**, is not catalyzed by these antibodies. Neither is a stoichiometric reaction apparent, although **10** has the correct structure for the acyl group. Therefore, though this ligand may bind to the protein, the interaction is not proper for the expression of the inherent esterase function. The effect of binding to the acetamide group of **7** is sufficient to stabilize the rate-limiting transition state. Further refinement of the substrate structure, as in the addition of the picolinate substituent, will reveal the full extent of the binding interactions in catalysis.

Conclusions and prospects

The success of this basic inquiry demonstrates a fundamental relationship between immunological binding and enzymic binding. The generation of artificial enzymes by eliciting an antibody which can stabilize a transition state has long been expected as a corollary to Pauling principle catalysis. Efforts to derive antibodies with other catalytic activities are in progress in our laboratories and elsewhere (Pollack *et al.* 1986). Proteins which exhibit the properties of both antibodies and enzymes may deserve a special designation. We suggest the term 'abzyme' for this class of molecules.

The direction of future research in this area will no doubt merge with ongoing efforts for artificial enzyme design. For example, the ability to impart hydrolytic activity to antibodies of predetermined specificity suggests that site-specific reagents or catalysts can be created at will. Aside from the fundamental interest of that prospect, it can have enormous practical benefit to protein chemistry. In addition, there remains the intriguing question of what effect antibodies with specific catalytic activities might have on an immune response directed toward proteins which display an epitope for this activity. We hope that this work will inspire renewed interest in the possibilities of antibody–ligand interaction which transcend the simple role in binding antigen.

This is Contribution No. 8495MB from the Department of Molecular Biology, The Research Institute of Scripps Clinic, La Jolla, California.

References

Bender M L, Bergeron R J, Komiyama M 1984. In *The Bioorganic Chemistry of Enzymatic Catalysis*. Wiley, New York, pp. 150–2

Bernhard S A, Orgel L E 1959. Mechanism of enzyme inhibition by phosphate esters, *Science* **130**: 625–6

Christianson D W, Lipscomb W N 1986. Structure of the complex between an unexpectedly hydrolyzed phosphonamidate inhibitor and carboxypeptidase A, *Journal of the American Chemical Society* **108**: 545–6

Galardy R E, Kontoyiannidou-Ostrem V, Kortylewicz Z P 1983. Inhibition of angiotensin converting enzyme by phosphonic amides and phosphonic acids, *Biochemistry* **22**: 1990–5

Imperiali B, Abeles R H 1986. Inibition of serine proteases by peptidyl fluoromethyl ketones, *Biochemistry* **25**: 3760–7

Jacobsen N E, Barlett P A 1981. A phosphonamidate dipeptide analogue as an inhibitor of carboxypeptidase A, *Journal of the American Chemical Society* **103**: 654–7

Jencks W P 1969. In *Catalysis in Chemistry and Enzymology*. McGraw–Hill, New York, p 288

Jencks W P 1975. Binding energy, specificity and enzymic catalysis – the Circe effect, in A Meister (ed) *Advances in Enzymology* **43**: 219–410

Kohen F, Kim J B, Barnard G, Lindner H R 1980a. Antibody-enhanced hydrolysis of steroid esters, *Biochimica et Biophysics Acta* **629**: 328–37

Kohen F, Kim J B, Lindner H R, Eshhar Z, Green B 1980b. Monoclonal immunoglobulin G augments hydrolysis of an ester of the homologous hapten, *Federation of European Biochemical Societies Letters* **111**: 427–31

Lipscomb W N 1982. Acceleration of reactions by enzymes, *Accounts of Chemical Research* **15**: 232–8

Milstein C 1985. From antibody structure to immunological diversification of immune response, *Science* **231**: 1261–8

Niman H L, Elder J H 1982. mAbs as probes of protein structure: Molecular diversity among the envelope glycoproteins (gP70s) of the murine retroviruses, in D H Katz (ed) *Monoclonal Antibodies and T-Cell Products*. CRC, Boca Raton, Florida, pp. 23–51

Pauling L 1946. Molecular architecture and biological reactions, *Chemistry and Engineering News* **24**: 1375–7

Pauling L 1948. Chemical achievement and hope for the future, *American Scientist* **36**: 51–8

Pollack S J, Jacobs J W, Schultz P G 1986. Selective chemical catalysis by an antibody, *Science* **234**: 1570–3

Raso V, Stollar B D 1975. The antibody–enzyme analogy. Comparison of enzymes and antibodies specific for phosphopyridoxyltyrosine, *Biochemistry* **14**: 584–99

Reardan D T, Meares C F, Goodwin D A, McTigue M, David G S, Stone M R, Leung J P, Bartholomew R M, Frincke J M 1985. Antibodies against metal chelates, *Nature (London)* **316**: 265–8

Royer G P. Enzyme-like synthetic catalysts (Synzmes), *Advances in Catalysis* **29**: 197–227

Thompson R C 1973. Use of peptide aldehydes to generate transition-state analogs of elastase, *Biochemistry* **12**: 47–52

Tramontano A, Janda K D, Lerner R A 1986a. Chemical reactivity at an antibody combining site elicited by mechanistic design of a synthetic antigen, *Proceedings of the National Academy of Sciences USA* **83**: 6736–40

Tramontano A, Janda K D, Lerner R A 1986b. Catalytic antibodies, *Science* **234**: 1566–70

Walsh C 1979. In *Enzymatic Reaction Mechanisms*. Freeman, San Francisco, California, p. 43

Weaver L H, Kester W R, Matthews B W 1977. A crystallographic study of the complex of phosphoramidon with thermolysin. A model for the presumed catalytic transition state and for the binding of extended substrates, *Journal of Molecular Biology* **114**: 119–32

Westerlik J O, Wolfenden R 1972. Aldehyde inhibitors of papain, *Journal of Biological Chemistry* **247**: 8195–7

Structural implications for antigenic recognition

Elizabeth D Getzoff; Duncan E McRee; Hans E Parge; Michael A Capozza; Susan L Bernstein; John A Tainer

Department of Molecular Biology, Research Institute of Scripps Clinic, La Jolla, California 92037, USA

Introduction

Bacterial pilins represent an interesting class of molecules that incorporate structural questions on several levels of organization. Starting with the primary sequence, the protein must fold into the proper secondary and tertiary structure and then self-assemble into the filamentous quaternary structure of the pilus. Also needed for this assembly are processing of the pilin leader sequence, any protein modification (including methylation of the amino terminus), transport of the molecule across the bacterial membrane and possibly specific interaction and assembly on the cell surface. Finally, the resulting macromolecular assembly must perform a number of important biological functions apart from those associated with folding, processing, and assembly.

The pilus serves as one of the major surface antigens on the gonococcal cell. To evade the host immune response, pilin undergoes antigenic variation (Hagblom *et al.* 1985), generating a wide repertoire of serotypes. Antibodies to these individual serotypes react only minimally with heterologous serotypes (Brinton *et al.* 1978; Buchanan 1975) even though the amino terminal portion of the molecule is conserved among the serotypes (Hagblom *et al.* 1985). This gives rise to a situation in which the antigenic diversity in the molecule must be generated while maintaining the other aspects of pilus function and structure.

The development of synthetic peptide vaccines requires a knowledge of the structural basis for protein antigenicity at a molecular level. The development of techniques using anti-peptide antibodies (Lerner 1982) and monoclonal antibodies to whole proteins (Köhler and Milstein 1975) makes it possible to examine the antigenicity of specific protein sites. As a result, recent studies, using both anti-peptide antibodies corresponding to protein sites and monoclonal antibodies that are directed against proteins of known three-dimensional structure, have produced new information concerning the relationship between antigenicity and protein structure (Getzoff *et al.* 1987; Geysen *et al.* 1987; Berzofsky 1985; Benjamin *et al.* 1984).

Unfortunately, the proteins whose structures have been determined are generally not the proteins of interest to immunologists designing antibodies and vaccines against human pathogens. Despite enormous advances in methodology and theoretical understanding in biochemistry, molecular biology, protein structure and immunology, the design and development of vaccines have not for the most part seen significant advances from the approach used by Pasteur. Below, we outline our approach to tapping the detailed information present in the three-dimensional structures of proteins determined by X-ray crystallography to increase understanding of the antigenicity of pathogens and thus aid the design of effective vaccines. Although this approach is presented for gonococcal pilin, we expect it to have general application to other protein antigens of unknown structure.

We show that gonococcal pilin has structural and sequence similarity to the 4-α-helix bundle protein, tobacco mosaic virus coat protein (TMVcp), which self-assembles to form the virus coat. The observed similarity with TMVcp has been used for the design of experiments on assembly and crystallization. For antigenicity studies, TMVcp has the disadvantage of aggregating to form self-assemblies unlike those of pilin. Myohemerythrin (MHr), another protein with a 4-α-helix bundle fold, is monomeric, and has been used to identify structural correlations for sequential antigenic determinants of 4-α-helix bundle domains. Experiments on MHr suggest that the correlated structural parameters of surface exposure, protruding shape and mobility represent an antigenic bias for sequential sites appropriate for peptide vaccine design (Geysen *et al.* 1987).

A structural model for pilin

One of the major achievements of X-ray crystallography has been the discovery that protein structures occur in a small number of distinct folding domains (e.g. Richardson 1981). For a protein of known sequence and unknown structure, examination of the overall pattern of predicted secondary structural elements and sequence similarity to conserved regions of proteins with known three-dimensional structures can be used to develop rational models for possible folding topologies. Building such possible models for the structure of antigens provides information allowing the choice of specific sequence areas for raising anti-peptide antibodies that are likely to react with the native protein antigen.

Using a data bank of known structures (Bernstein *et al.* 1977), our basic approach is as follows: (1) identification of the probable secondary structural elements; (2) selection of possible tertiary structural motifs based upon the identity and placement of the secondary structural elements; (3) detailed search of sequences of the proteins known to fall in the same structural class(es) to find limited levels of sequence–structure homology; and (4) construction of a model consistent with the identified probable secondary structure, tertiary motif and similarity to a given known structure within that class. Since the level of sequence homology identified may not be statistically significant for a single pairwise matching, it is important to perform the alignment in a way that gives a higher weight to the conserved and invariant sequence positions in both the known protein structure and the protein being modeled. In our approach, the development of a specific model is dependent upon step 3 and is not attempted without the identification of a similar known structure. Once a tertiary structural model is obtained from this procedure, specific experimental questions regarding structure and function can be addressed. Details of these methods and results will be published elsewhere; here we will outline our results for their application to gonococcal pilin.

The position of individual secondary structural elements in a polypeptide sequence can be predicted with about 60% accuracy from empirically deter-mined parameters (Kabsch and Sander 1983; Sternberg and Thornton 1978) that reflect the preferred occurrence of each amino acid in each type of secondary structure. Application of these parameters to the primary amino acid sequence for the *Neisseria gonorrhoeae* pilin (Meyer *et al.* 1984; School-nick *et al.* 1984) results in the structure predictions shown in Fig. 1. Analysis of

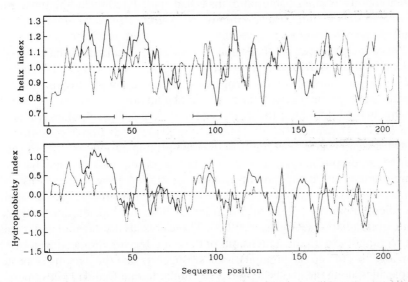

Figure 1. α-Helix conformational prediction and hydrophobicity profiles for MS11 gonococcal pilin (solid line) and TMVcp (strain *vulgare*, dotted line). Empirical parameters (Chou and Fasman 1978; Eisenberg *et al.* 1982) were averaged over five residues and plotted versus position in the alignment of the pilin and TMVcp se-quences. Breaks in each curve indicate deletions relative to the other sequence. α-Helical values above 1.0 (dashed line) indicate probable α-helical secondary struc-ture; horizontal bars indicate α-helices in TMVcp.

these predictions (Parge *et al.* 1987; Deal *et al.* 1985) suggests that of the known three-dimensional structural motifs, the best-fit structural pattern would be that of an up-and-down 4-α-helix bundle. Within the class of up-and-down 4-α-helix bundle proteins, the similar pattern and match of sequence-conserved regions in gonococcal pilin occurs for TMVcp (Parge *et al.* 1987; Deal *et al.* 1985). Five TMVcp sequences (Barker *et al.* 1984) were aligned with sequences of gonococcal pilin by pattern matching of amino acid parameters critical to stability or function, such as hydrophobicity, charge, side-chain branching, ability to hydrogen bond, etc, rather than absolute amino acid identity. When the predicted α-helical and hydrophobicity profiles for TMVcp are superimposed with those of the gonococcal pilin according to this alignment, the similarity is apparent (Fig. 1).

Another source of information concerning pilin protein structure and antigenic sites comes from the observed sequence variation resulting from immune pressure (Fig. 2). The *N*-terminal portion of the gonococcal pilin sequence is highly conserved; whereas antigenic variation occurs predominantly in the *C*-terminal region and is the result of insertions and deletions of two to five amino acid residues as well as single amino acid changes (Hagblom *et al.* 1985). The region of greatest variability occurs between the two cysteines located at positions 121 and 151. The conserved *N*-terminal sequence of gonococcal pilin, beginning with the unusual *N*-methylphenylalanine, is homologous to other bacterial pilins (Deal *et al.* 1985) including those from *Neisseria meningitidis*, *Pseudomonas aeruginosa*, *Moraxella nonliquefaciens* and *Bacteroides nodosus*.

Since the proposed 4-α-helical model for gonococcal pilin is based upon a theoretical similarity to the known protein structure of TMVcp (Bloomer *et al.* 1978), an analysis of the properties of TMVcp might prove useful for predicting experiments with the gonococcal pilin protein. Preliminary experiments suggest that this is the case (Deal *et al.* 1985). The solubility conditions for TMVcp (Durham *et al.* 1971) have allowed the prediction of conditions for the disassembly and reassembly of the pilin protein into fibers. Identification of the conditions necessary to dissociate the protein into subunits has been important in the development of X-ray crystallography studies. From the dissociated state, we have been able to grow small protein crystals with a needle-like morphology, which diffract to about 2.8 Å resolution using synchrotron radiation (Parge *et al.* 1987). These crystals display molecular packing compatible with the dimensions of the pilin structure model developed by analogy to TMVcp. Preliminary analysis suggests that the packing of protein molecules along the needle axis may be similar to that found in pilus fibers. A diffraction data set to 3.5 Å has been collected and the structure solution is in progress. Currently, both CD and X-ray diffraction results confirm the 4-α-helix bundle model (Parge *et al.* 1987).

These studies on pili are still ongoing; however, we have been doing parallel studies on the model protein antigen MHr which is a monomeric protein of known three-dimensional structure with a similar 4-α-helix bundle

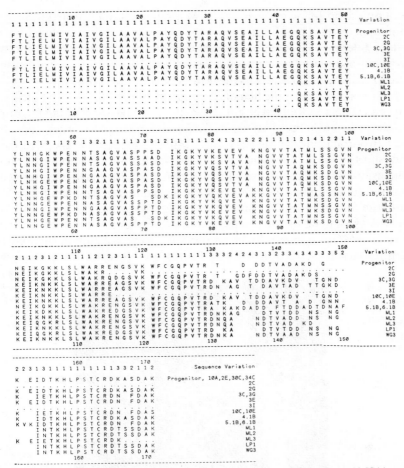

Figure 2. Alignment of gonococcal pilin protein sequences. The original MS11 strain is labeled Progenitor; MS11 variants appearing after phase variation (piliation/non-piliation cycle; Segal *et al.* 1985) are labeled with a number followed by a letter; other strains are labeled with two letters followed by a number. Dots indicate unsequenced regions. Sequence variation (given by a single digit) is tabulated by the number of different amino acid residues identified for a given sequence position (numbered top and bottom), with deletions (blanks) counted as an additional residue. (Sequence data from Hagblom *et al.* 1985.)

topology. The work on MHr summarized below suggests that intrinsic structural features of this fold may bias immune recognition of sequential antigenic determinants.

Myohemerythrin: a protein model for antigenicity

Myohemerythrin was selected as a good model protein for detailed experimental study of structure and antigenicity (Tainer *et al.* 1984, 1985b) because of the following features: a well-refined atomic structure with information on local mobility (temperature factors); non-mammalian origin to reduce tolerance in experimental animals; the presence of the iron center providing an internal spectroscopic check for native structure; and a disaggregated monomeric state at very high protein concentrations.

MHr is a member of the hemerythrin family of proteins, which function as oxygen carriers in four invertebrate phyla. The MHr fold is an antiparallel bundle of four α-helices (named A, B, C and D in sequence order) surrounding a two-iron center at the active site, with a loop region at the *N*-terminus and shorter loops between the helices and at the *C*-terminus. Three-dimensional crystal structures with temperature factors have been refined at high resolution for two members of the hemerythrin family: monomeric MHr from the marine worm *Themiste zostericola* (S Sheriff, J L Smith and W A Hendrickson, unpublished results) and octameric hemerythrin from *Themiste dyscritum* (Stenkamp *et al.* 1983). A rigorous analysis of mobility in these two high-resolution crystal structures by Sheriff and Hendrickson together with

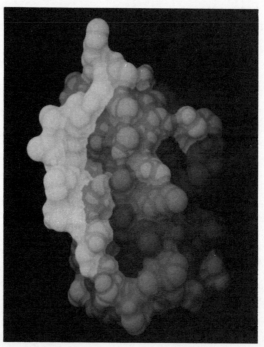

Figure 3. Patterns of mobility on the molecular surface of MHr. The solid external molecular surface is color-coded by the average main-chain temperature factors using a radiating-body gray scale. The molecule is oriented with the helices vertical and the two-iron center toward the top. The darkest colors (lowest temperature factors) are associated with the A helix (lower right) and the brightest colors (highest temperature factors) with the C helix (upper left). This raster graphics representation was calculated using M L Connolly's program RAMS (Connolly 1985) and displayed on an AED raster graphics display. (Modified from Tainer *et al.* 1984, Fig. 1a.)

their collaborators at the University of Washington (Sheriff *et al.* 1985) allowed the determination of consistent temperature factors after correction for crystal contacts.

The differential mobility of MHr (Fig. 3) is typical of the patterns seen in high-resolution protein structures: different intra-domain structural elements show significant variation in their mobility. In the temperature factors before adjustment for the effects of crystal contacts, the A and D helices are relatively highly ordered, the C helix is highly mobile and the B helix varies from being relatively well ordered at the *N*-terminal end to relatively mobile at the *C*-terminal end. Regions involving residues 1–17 (*N*-terminal loop), 38–50 (*N*-terminus of the B helix), and 85–94 (C–D loop) show the greatest increase in relative mobility when corrected for crystal contacts. Examination by residue of the exposed molecular surface and corrected average main-chain temperature factors indicates that a large portion (over 80%) of the molecular surface is relatively mobile. This corrected pattern of mobility is consistent with a qualitative analysis of the local and underlying stereochemical interactions (Tainer *et al.* 1984). As seen in Fig. 3, mobility is highly correlated with surface topography (Tainer *et al.* 1985c) with the most highly protruding convex regions having the fewest intramolecular packing interactions and hence the most flexibility.

Myohemerythrin peptides

The selection of peptides from the myohemerythrin sequence was based on the main-chain temperature factors averaged by residue, since the main-chain mobility reflects the global conformational variability of the protein. Both helical and non-helical peptide regions were selected for synthesis. The 12 peptides synthesized include 83 of myohemerythrin's 118 residues (70% of the sequence). Of the exposed molecular surface area of myohemerythrin (5846 Å^2), the peptides synthesized account for 4005 Å^2 (69%). The four peptides synthesized for each of three categories encompass roughly equal parts of the protein surface area: 'hot' or mobile (23.0%), 'cold' or ordered (19.3%), and 'hot/contact' (mobile after correction for crystal contacts, 26.2%). Three of the hot peptides were chosen to include residues liganding the irons; in native protein the mobility of these sequences is limited to conformations which do not disrupt the metal ligand geometry. All the peptides chosen have large areas of exposed molecular surface available for interaction with antibodies. Of course, highly exposed amino acid residues tend to be less hydrophobic and, due to their external, relatively unconstrained position, more highly mobile than internal residues.

Regions of high mobility and protruding shape are most antigenic

To define the possible role of molecular surface mobility in the antigenic recognition of the native protein by anti-peptide antibodies, polyclonal antibodies to each selected sequence were raised against synthetic peptides in pairs of rabbits (Tainer *et al.* 1984). The anti-peptide antisera were originally assayed for reactivity against the homologous immunizing peptide by enzyme-linked immunosorbent assay (ELISA; Table 1). All but one of the synthetic peptides were immunogenic; their relative immunogenicity is not correlated with their mobility. The anti-peptide antisera were next assayed for reactivity with myohemerythrin (Table 1). The same results were obtained when the ELISA was performed under less denaturing conditions (the protein was not dried or methanol-fixed to the plate). All anti-peptide antisera raised against cold peptides (22–35, 26–35, 96–109 and 100–109) gave negative or low reactivity with the protein, while all anti-peptide antisera raised against hot peptides (excluding peptide 42–51, which did not raise any anti-peptide antibodies) gave higher reactivity against the protein. Of the antisera against hot peptides, those with the lowest reactivity to myohemerythrin (57–66 and 63–72) also had the lowest reactivity against their respective homologous immunizing peptides. The relative averaged avidity of the anti-peptide antisera against the protein (peptides 3–16 > 7–16 > 37–46, > 57–66 > 63–72, 69–82, 73–82, 96–109) matched the pattern of relative antigenicity; antisera with higher titers generally showed greater avidity.

Table 1 Reactivity of MHr anti-peptide antisera

Sequence position	ELISA titers*		Immunoprecipitation	
	αPeptide vs peptide	αPeptide vs MHr	^{125}I-MHr (cpm)†	Inhibition by peptide (%)‡
Hot/contact				
3–16	640–1280	12800	14849	97.1
7–16	640–1280	3200	7384	92.6
37–46	640–1280	9500	4026	100.0
42–51	—	—	0	0.0
Hot				
57–66	160–320	600	7277	80.0
63–72	160–320	375	2543	77.6
69–82	>2560	1050	3774	91.3
73–82	>2560	1400	2154	62.0
Cold				
22–35	1280–2560	—	180	0.0
26–35	320–640	60	0	0.0
96–109	1280–2560	200	2617	22.5
100–109	320–640	—	0	0.0

Source: Data from Tainer *et al.* (1984).
* ELISA titers are expressed as the reciprocal of antibody dilution extrapolated to bind 50% of 50 pmol antigen per well.
† Average of two independent experiments, after correction for nonspecific binding.
‡ 100.0% minus percentage of activity remaining in the presence of the peptide.

Antigenicity studies were repeated in immunoprecipitation assays under conditions preserving the native structure of myohemerythrin (Tainer *et al.* 1984). Retention of the characteristic visible spectrum with a 338 nm peak due to the iron center verified that the ligand environment remained unchanged, indicating that the protein was largely in its native conformation under the assay conditions. The results of these immunoprecipitation studies (Fig. 4;

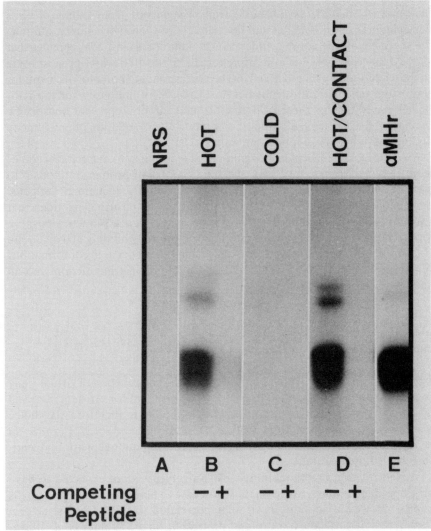

Figure 4. Comparison of the anti-protein reactivities of antibodies raised against hot, cold, and hot/contact peptides. Lanes are representative polyacrylamide gel electrophoreses of the immunoprecipitates in the presence (+) and absence (−) of competing peptide. Lane A, control normal rabbit serum; lane B, hot peptide 57–66; lane C, cold peptide 26–35; lane D, hot/contact peptide 3–16; lane E, intact MHr. (From Tainer *et al.* 1984, Fig. 3.)

Table 1) were consistent with the ELISA analyses: antisera against hot peptides react more strongly with myohemerythrin, than do antisera against cold peptides. To confirm the specificity of the anti-peptide antisera, immunoprecipitation was also done in the presence of homologous and heterologous peptides. The anti-myohemerythrin reactivity of antisera raised against the hot peptides was strongly inhibited by incubation with the corresponding homologous peptide, whereas incubation with the irrelevant heterologous peptide (synthesized from a sequence from influenza virus hemaglutinin) did not inhibit anti-myohemerythrin reactivity, thus confirming the specificity of the antisera. Interestingly, antisera against cold peptides that showed low reactivity with the protein (22–35, 96–109) were, at most, only slightly inhibited by incubation with the corresponding homologous peptides suggesting that the anti-myohemerythrin reactivity measured for the antibodies raised against these cold peptides may largely represent nonspecific binding. All of these results appear to support the correlation of antigenicity and mobility for anti-peptide antibodies.

Evidence for the mechanistic significance of mobility to antigenicity comes from detailed studies involving the binding of anti-protein antibodies to peptide analogs of the protein sequence to identify sequential antigenic determinants (Geysen *et al.* 1987). Further screening using peptides that encompassed substitutions of all 20 amino acids in each sequence position localized the specific side chains essential for antibody binding at a given site (Getzoff *et al.* 1987). These essential side chains often occur in conformations requiring side-chain movements (induced fit) for direct interaction with an antibody combining site.

Implications to the design of vaccines

Improved methods of peptide synthesis make the construction of virtually any sequential polypeptide antigen possible. The problem for efficient, rational design of vaccines based upon anti-peptide antibodies is, therefore, the choice of appropriate sequences from proteins to synthesize and study. For this, an increased theoretical understanding of protein immunogenicity and antigenicity is fundamental.

The correlation of site mobility with antigenicity is not expected to have direct predictive value, except in those few cases where the atomic structure is known. However, mobility is strongly correlated to the related structural parameters of surface exposure and protruding shape (Tainer *et al.* 1985a, 1985b, 1985c; Novotny *et al.* 1986; Thornton *et al.* 1986) as well as to hydrophilicity and sequence variability (Tainer *et al.* 1985b), so the choice of peptides for a synthetic vaccine can make use of all of these parameters. Based upon their studies on TMVcp, Westhof *et al.* (1984) pointed out that the reactivity of anti-peptide antibodies with the parent protein is related to the mobility of contiguous determinants within the protein, and that this local flexibility is in turn associated with the bends, turns and loops. Different types of protein secondary structure may indeed have different behavior with regard to mobility: for example, loops tend to be most flexible in the middle of their sequence, while β strands tend to be more flexible at the ends. However, the type of secondary structure alone does not determine the antigenicity of protein sites.

Furthermore, certain sites on a molecule may not elicit an immune response even though they are flexible, if B cells reactive to these regions are not present as a result of tolerance or possible evolutionary effects on the germ line repertoire. Still, in some instances, a combination of parameters correlated with mobility may be useful in predicting potential antigenic sites; a structure prediction of turns and other nonrepetitive secondary structure could be combined with hydrophilicity profiles and sequence variation data to select sequences likely to be more mobile and antigenic. Based upon the arguments presented here, the most highly variable regions of pilin are likely to be most reactive toward anti-peptide antibodies. Detailed structural and antigenicity studies for pilin are in progress, including work to crystallize a pilin–antibody complex and electron microscopy studies of the binding of pilus fibers by anti-peptide antibodies encompassing the entire sequence. The result of this work may well produce some surprises about the structural basis for antigenic recognition.

References

Barker W C, Hunt L T, Orcutt B C, George D G, Yeh L S, Chen H R, Blomquist, M C, Johnson G C, Seibel-Ross E I, Ledley R S 1984. *Protein Sequence Database of the Protein Identification Resource*, National Biomedical Research Foundation, Washington, DC

Benjamin D C, Berzofsky J A, East I J, Gurd F R N, Hannum C et al. 1984. The antigenic structure of proteins: a reappraisal, *Annual Review of Immunology* 2: 67–101

Bernstein F C, Koetzle T F, Williams G J B, Meyer E F, Brice M D, et al. 1977. The protein data bank: a computer-based archival file for macromolecular structures, *Journal of Molecular Biology* 112: 535–42

Berzofsky J A 1985. Intrinsic and extrinsic factors in protein antigenic structure, *Science* 229: 932–40

Bloomer A C, Champness J N, Bricogne G, Staden R, Klug A 1978. Protein disk of tobacco mosaic virus at 2.8 Å resolution showing the interactions within and between subunits, *Nature (London)* 276: 362–8

Brinton C C, Bryan J, Dillon J, Guerina N, Jacobson L J, Labik A, Lee S, Levine A, Lim S, McMichael J, Polen S, Rogers K, To A C C, To S C M 1978. Uses of pili in gonorrhea control: role of bacterial pili in disease, purification and properties of gonococcal pili, and progess in the development of a gonococcal pilus vaccine for gonorrhea, in G F Brooks, E C Gotschlich, K K Holmes, W D Sawyer, F E Young (eds) *Immunobiology of Neisseria gonorrhoeae*. American Society of Microbiology, Washington, DC, pp 155–78

Buchanan T M 1975. Antigenic heterogeneity of gonococcali pili, *Journal of Experimental Medicine* 141: 1470–5

Chou P Y, Fasman G D 1978. Prediction of secondary structure of proteins from their amino acid sequence, *Advances in Enzymology* 47: 45–148

Connolly M L 1985. Depth-buffer algorithms for molecular modelling, *Journal of Molecular Graphics* **3**: 19–24

Deal C D, Tainer J A, So M, Getzoff E D 1985. Identification of a common structural class for *Neisseria gonorrheae* and other bacterial pilins, in G K Schoolnik (ed) *The Pathogenic Neisseriae*. American Society for Microbiology, Washington, DC, pp 302–8

Durham A C H, Finch J T, Klug A 1971. States of aggregation of tobacco mosaic virus protein, *Nature New Biology* **229**: 37–50

Eisenberg D, Weiss R M, Terwilliger T C, Wilcox W 1982. Hydrophobic moments and protein structure, *Faraday Symposium of the Chemical Society* **17**: 109–20

Getzoff E D, Geysen H M, Rodda S J, Alexander H, Tainer J A, Lerner R A 1987. Mechanisms of antibody binding to a protein, *Science* **235**: 1191–6

Geysen H M, Tainer J A, Rodda S J, Mason T J, Alexander H, Getzoff E D, Lerner R A 1987. Chemistry of antibody binding to a protein, *Science* **235**: 1184–90

Hagblom, P, Segal E, Billyard E, So M 1985. Intragenic recombination leads to pilus antigenic variation in *Neisseria gonhorrhoeae*, *Nature* (*London*) **315**: 156–8

Kabsch W, Sander C 1983. How good are predictions of protein secondary stucture? *FEBS Letters* **155**: 179–82

Köhler G, Milstein C 1975. Continuous cultures of fused cells secreting antibody of predefined specificity, *Nature* (*London*) **256**: 495

Lerner R A 1982. Tapping the immunological repertoire to produce antibodies of predetermined specificity, *Nature* (*London*) **299**: 592–6

Meyer T F, Billyard E, Haas R, Storzbach S, So M 1984. Pilus genes of *Neisseria gonorrhoeae*: chromosomal organization and DNA sequence, *Proceedings of the National Academy of Sciences USA* **81**: 6110–14

Novotny J, Handschumacher M, Haber E, Bruccoleri R E, Carlson W B, Fanning D W, Smith J A, Rose G D 1986. Antigenic determinants in proteins coincide with surface regions accessible to large probes (antibody domains), *Proceedings of the National Academy of Sciences USA* **83**: 226–30

Parge H E, McRee D E, Deal C D, So M, Capozza M A, Getzoff E D, Tainer J A 1987. Crystallization and structural model for *Neisseria gonorrheae* pilin, *Nature* (*London*) (in preparation)

Richardson J S 1981. The anatomy and taxonomy of protein structure, in C B Anfinsen, J T Edsall, F M Richards (eds) *Advances in Protein Chemistry*. Academic Press, New York, pp 167–339

Schoolnik G K, Fernandez R, Tai J Y, Rothbard J, Gotschlich E C 1984. Gonococcal Pili: primary structure and receptor binding domain, *Journal of Experimental Medicine* **159**: 1351–70

Segal E, Billyard E, So M, Storzbach S, Meyer T F 1985. Role of chromosomal rearrangement in *N. gonorrhoeae* pilus phase variation, *Cell* **40**: 293–300

Sheriff S, Hendrickson W A, Stenkamp R E, Sieker L C, Jensen L H 1985. Influence of solvent accessibility and intermolecular contacts on atomic mobilities in hemerythrins, *Proceedings of the National Academy of Sciences USA* **82**: 1104–7

Stenkamp R E, Sieker L C, Jensen L H 1983. Adjustment of restraints in the refinement of methemerythrin and azidomethemerythrin at 2.0 Å resolution, *Acta Crystallographica* **B39**: 697–703

Sternberg M J E, Thornton J M 1978. Prediction of protein structure from amino acid sequence. *Nature* (*London*) **271**: 15–20

Tainer J A, Getzoff E D, Alexander H, Houghten R A, Olson A J, Lerner R A, Hendrickson W A 1984. The reactivity of anti-peptide antibodies is a function of the atomic mobility of sites in a protein, *Nature* (*London*) **312**–: 127–33

Tainer J A, Getzoff E D, Olson A J 1985a. Topography and mobility of molecular surfaces: implications for macromolecular recognition and antigenicity, in J Hermans (ed) *Molecular Dynamics and Protein Structure*. University of North Carolina, Chapel Hill, North Carolina, pp 110–15

Tainer J A, Getzoff E D, Paterson Y, Olson A J, Lerner R A 1985b. The atomic mobility component of protein antigenicity, *Annual Review of Immunology* **3**: 501–35

Tainer J A, Getzoff E D, Sayre J, Olson A J 1985c. Modeling intermolecular interactions: topography, mobility, and electrostatic recognition, *Journal of Molecular Graphics* **3**: 103–5

Thornton J M, Edwards M S, Taylor, W R and Barlow D J 1986. Location of 'continuous' antigenic determinants in the protruding regions of proteins, *EMBO Journal* **5**: 409–13

Westhof E, Altschuh D, Moras D, Bloomer A C, Mondragon A, Klug A, Van Regenmortel M H V 1984. Correlation between segmental mobility and the location of antigenic determinants in proteins, *Nature (London)* **311**: 123–6

Structure and specificity of monoclonal anti-lysozyme antibodies

A G Amit*; G Boulot*; V Guillon*; M Harper*; F Lema*; R A Mariuzza*;
R J Poljak*; S E V Phillips†

* Department d'Immunologie, Institut Pasteur, 75724 Paris Cedex 15, France
† The Astbury Department, University of Leeds, Leeds, United Kingdom

Introduction

Protein molecules are among the most frequent and diverse antigens confronting the immune system. Several proteins, such as hen egg-white lysozyme (HEL), have been used in different laboratories to explore the precise interactions between antigens and antibodies, as reviewed by Benjamin *et al.* (1984).

The definition of specific antigen–antibody interactions and the obtention of a three-dimensional model describing them is the object of the research presented here. HEL was chosen as a model antigen for this work because it is a small, well characterized protein, very immunogenic in several strains of mice, and because its three-dimensional structure is known to high resolution (Blake *et al.* 1967). Natural variants of HEL occur in the eggs of other species of gallinaceous birds with antigenic differences scattered all along their amino acid sequences.

In this study, 27 murine (BALB/c) monoclonal anti-HEL antibodies were obtained and characterized. The complexes between the Fab fragments of two of the monoclonal antibodies (MAbs) and HEL in one case, and pheasant lysozyme (PHL) in another case, have been crystallized and studied by X-ray diffraction techniques. The results of those studies are presented here.

Monoclonal anti-HEL antibodies

Two separate cell fusions were performed using BALB/c mice immunized with HEL. Seven clones were obtained from a first fusion (one animal), 20 clones from a second fusion (one animal) (Harper *et al.* 1987). All clones secreted IgG1 (κ) anti-HEL MAbs, the product of secondary responses. The binding of the MAbs to eight avian lysozymes and human lysozyme, as determined by an enzyme-linked immunosorbent assay (ELISA) is shown in

Fig. 1. Binding to the heterologous lysozymes is shown as a percentage of the homologous binding. This test allowed us to classify the 27 monoclonal anti-HEL antibodies into 10 groups. The MAbs within each group share lack of binding capacity to one or more of the lysozymes of the test panel (Fig. 1). These observations allow the location of some of the HEL antigenic determinants recognized by the MAbs. Thus, antibodies D1.2 and D1.3 recognize epitopes that include position 121, since the avian lysozymes that are not bound by those antibodies have sequence variations at position 121. MAbs

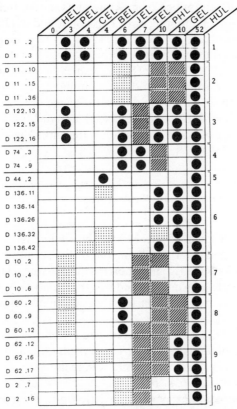

Figure 1. Binding tests (ELISA) of the anti-HEL MAbs to a panel of lysozymes. Eight egg-white lysozymes were used from the following species: HEL, chicken; PEL, partridge; CEL, California quail; BEL, bobwhite quail; JEL, Japanese quail; TEL, turkey; PHL, pheasant; GEL, guinea-hen. HUL is human lysozyme. The number of amino acid differences in their sequences, from 0 to 52, are indicated at the top. The 27 MAbs are listed at the left side of the figure. The relative binding of the MAbs to the different lysozymes is shown as a percentage of the binding to the homologous antigen, HEL. Heteroclitic binding (≥125%) is shown by diagonal lines; equivalent binding (68 to 125%) is shown by a white rectangle; intermediate binding (26 to 67%) by dots; weak (or no) binding by black circles. This test allows to divide the MAbs into ten groups, listed at right.

D1.2 and D1.3, as well as other MAbs included within one group, differ in their properties, indicating that they are not repeat isolates of the same clone.

Some of the antibodies characterized in Fig. 1 are heteroclitic since they bind heterologous antigens with apparent association constants (estimated from competition binding assays) which are higher than those determined by the method of Friguet *et al.* (1985) for the homologous antigen (see below). Thus for example, the antibodies of group 2 bind pheasant lysozyme (PHL) and guinea-fowl lysozyme with (about four-fold) higher apparent association constants than HEL.

The equilibrium dissociation constants of some of the antibodies listed in Fig. 1 have been determined from Klotz plots, at different HEL concentrations. The fraction of antibody or of Fab not bound to HEL was determined by ELISA as described by Friguet *et al.* (1985). The association constant (K_A) of Fab D1.3 was thus determined to be $4.5 \pm 0.6 \times 10^7 \, \text{M}^{-1}$. That of IgG D11.10 is $1.7 \pm 0.5 \times 10^7 \, \text{M}^{-1}$. The K_A values of other antibodies of Fig. 1, determined by the same method, were found to be from $8 \times 10^6 \, \text{M}^{-1}$ to $5.3 \times 10^7 \, \text{M}^{-1}$. These values are within the range of those observed in other laboratories for anti-HEL antibodies (Sakato *et al.* 1971; Pecht *et al.* 1971; Kobayashi *et al.* 1982) and for anti-protein antibodies in general (Karush 1978).

Crystallization and preliminary X-ray diffraction study of Fab–lysozyme complexes

Fab fragments of each of the MAbs shown in Fig. 1 were obtained as previously described (Mariuzza *et al.* 1983). Lysozyme–Fab complexes were prepared by incubating a 1.25 molar excess of lysozyme relative to Fab for 12 hr at 4 °C. The complexes were purified by HPLC and/or by chromatofocusing, and submitted to crystallization trials as described before (Mariuzza *et al.* 1983).

The complex HEL–Fab D1.3 crystallized from 15–20% polyethylene glycol (PEG) 6000 solutions at pH 6.0. The crystals grow as bipyramids, reaching dimensions of up to 1.5 mm × 0.6 mm × 0.4 mm. They are monoclinic, space group $P2_1$ with $a = 55.6 \, \text{Å}$, $b = 143.4 \, \text{Å}$, $c = 49.1 \, \text{Å}$, $\beta = 120.5°$ and one molecule of the complex per asymmetric unit. Their diffraction patterns extend to beyond 2.5 Å resolution using synchrotron radiation.

The complex between the heteroclitic Fab D11.15 and the heterologous antigen PHL has also been crystallized using 15% PEG 8000 solutions, pH 5.5. The crystals grow as rectangular prisms of up to 0.6 mm × 0.2 mm × 0.15 mm. They are monoclonic, space group $C2$, with $a = 159.0 \, \text{Å}$, $b = 49.0 \, \text{Å}$, $c = 178.2 \, \text{Å}$, $\beta = 92.2°$. Their diffraction pattern extends to about 3.0 Å resolution using an X-ray beam from a synchrotron source ($\lambda = 1.41 \, \text{Å}$).

Three-dimensional structure of a lysozyme–Fab complex

The crystalline Fab D1.3–HEL complex was chosen for detailed X-ray diffraction investigations (Fig. 2). X-ray intensities were measured using a four-circle automated diffractometer. The phases of the reflexions were determined by the multiple isomorphous replacement method using three heavy atom derivatives: $(NH_4)_2PtCl_4$, p-OH-mercuribenzene sulfonate and $K_3F_5UO_2$. A Fourier map of the electron density was calculated at 2.8 Å resolution and a model, using the amino acid sequences of V_H and V_L (Verhoeyen *et al.* 1986), was fitted to it on an interactive graphics system using the program FRODO (Jones 1985). The atomic coordinates were refined by alternate cycles of crystallographic least-squares refinement and model building (Amit *et al.* 1986); the final R-factor is 0.28, excluding solvent molecules.

The Fab moiety of the complex appears in an extended conformation (Fig. 2). Comparison of its structure with those of other Fabs determined by X-ray diffraction (reviewed by Amzel and Poljak 1979; Davies and Metzger 1983) indicates no appreciable change in the relative arrangement of the V_H–V_L regions.

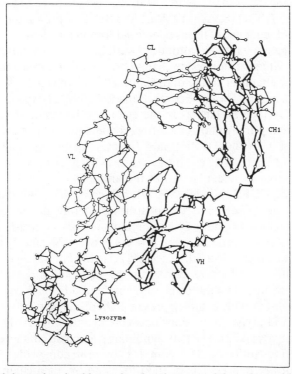

Figure 2. Alpha-carbon backbone showing the trace of the polypeptide chains in the HEL–Fab D1.3 complex. The C_L and V_L regions of the light chain (thinner trace) as well as the C_H1 and V_H regions of the heavy chain (thicker trace) of Fab are shown. The label for lysozyme is placed at the substrate-binding cavity of the enzyme.

A comparison of the positions of the Cα of the complexed lysozyme with those of the free crystalline lysozyme in its tetragonal form gives a root mean square deviation of 0.64 Å, comparable to the error of the atomic coordinates in the complex, which is estimated to be ±0.6 Å. Differences in side-chain conformation are more difficult to assess but on the average they also appear to be very small. In conclusion, there is no distortion of the structure of the bound antigen within the resolution limits of the present analysis.

The interface between antigen and antibody is a large area. About 700 Å^2 of the solvent-accessible area of the antibody combining site are buried after complex formation. About 750 Å^2, equivalent to 11% of the lysozyme total solvent-accessible area, are buried by complex formation with the antibody.

Seventeen antibody residues make close contacts with the antigen. Seven of those residues belong to the V_L region: His30, Tyr32, Tyr49, Tyr50, Phe91, Trp92, Ser93. Ten V_H residues closely contact the antigen: Thr30, Gly31, Tyr32, Trp52, Gly53, Asp54, Arg96, Asp97, Tyr98 and Arg99 [sequence positions are numbered as in Kabat *et al.* (1983)]. Note that V_L Tyr49 and V_H Thr30 are included in 'framework' segments of those regions.

Sixteen lysozyme residues contact the 17 antibody residues listed above. They are: Asp18, Asn19, Arg21, Gly22, Tyr23, Ser24, Leu25, Asn27, Lys116, Gly117, Thr118, Asp119, Val120, Gln121, Ile124 and Leu129. Thus, the amino acid sequence of the antigenic determinant is clearly discontinuous.

The contacting antigen–antibody surfaces are irregular and complementary, with protruding side chains of one lying in surface depressions of the other. The chemical nature of the interactions is of van der Waals contacts and hydrogen bonds. The close contacts made by Gln121 explain why replacement of this residue by His, as in the egg-white lysozymes from partridge, California quail, turkey and guinea-fowl renders the antigen unrecognizable by antibody D1.3 (Fig. 1). PHL and Japanese quail lysozyme also have a substitution at position 121 (Gln → Asn) as well as in other parts of the sequence making close contacts with the antibody.

The four V_H CDR3 residues (96–99) making contact with the antigen are encoded by the D segment, demonstrating its role in the generation of *functional* diversity in antibody combining sites. By contrast, the junction point of the somatic recombination process between V_L and J_L (position 96) does not contact the antigen (distance > 6 Å) in the Fab D1.3–HEL complex. This observation can be extended to the D–J_H junction point in V_H which does not contribute directly to the antigen–antibody D1.3 contacts.

The antigen–antibody complex presented here can be taken as a model for idiotype, anti-idiotype interactions between an antibody (Ab1) and an anti-idiotypic antibody (Ab2). The two combining sites could contact each other as in the lysozyme–antibody D1.3 complex, by protruding side chains of one that fit in surface depressions of the other and by main-chain–main-chain contacts. The comformation of the contacting residues of the second antibody (Ab2) could thus mimic that of the antigen without necessarily constituting a precise replica of it.

Acknowledgements

We thank: M Verhoeyen for making the amino acid sequences of V_H and V_L D1.3 available to us before publication; C Wilmot for solvent-accessible surface calculations; F Gauthier for expert secretarial help; and the Laboratoire d'Utilisation du Rayonnement Synchrotron, CNRS, for the use of a graphics system. This research was supported by grants from the Institut Pasteur, CNRS, INSERM and a short-term EMBO fellowship (ASTF 4777) to SEV Phillips.

References

Amit A G, Mariuzza R A, Phillips S E V, Poljak R J 1986. Three-dimensional structure of an antigen-antibody complex at 2.8 Å resolution, *Science* **233**: 747–53

Amzel L M, Poljak R J 1979. Three-dimensional structure of immunoglobulins *Annual Review of Biochemistry* **48**: 961–97

Benjamin D C, Berzofsky J A, East I J, Gurd F R N, Hannum C, Leach S J, Margoliash E, Michael J G, Miller A, Prager E M, Reichlin M, Sercarz E E, Smith-Gill S J, Todd P E, Wilson A C 1984. The antigenic structure of proteins: a reappraisal, *Annual Review of Immunology* **2**: 67–101

Blake C C F, Mair G A, North A C T, Phillip D C, Sarma V R 1967. On the conformation of the hen egg-white lysozyme molecule, *Proceedings of the Royal Society of London B* **167**: 365–77

Davies D R, Metzger H 1983. Structural basis of antibody function, *Annual Review of Immunology* **1**: 87–117

Friguet B, Chaffotte A F, Djavadi-Ohaniance L, Goldberg M 1985. Measurements of the true affinity constant in solution of antigen–antibody complexes by enzyme-linked immunosorbent assay, *Journal of Immunological Methods* **77**: 305–19

Harper M, Lema F, Boulot G, Poljak R J 1987. Antigen specificity and cross-reactivity of monoclonal anti-lysozyme antibodies, *Molecular Immunology* **2**: 97–108

Jones T A 1985. Interactive computer graphics: FRODO, in H Wyckoff, C H W Hirs, S N Timasheff (eds) *Methods in Enzymology*. Academic Press, New York, vol. 115, part B, pp 157–70

Kabat E A, Wu T Y, Bilofsky H, Reid-Milner M, Perry H 1983. *Sequences of Proteins of Immunological Interest*. Public Health Service, National Institutes of Health, Washington, DC

Karush F 1978. The affinity of antibody: range, variability and the role of multivalence, in G W Litman, A Good (eds) *Comprehensive Immunology: Immunoglobulins*. Plenum Medical Book Company, New York and London, vol 5

Kobayashi T, Fujio H, Kondo K, Dohi Y, Hirayama A, Takagaki Y, Kosaki G, Amano T 1982. A monoclonal antibody specific for a distinct region of hen egg-white lysozyme, *Molecular Immunology* **19**: 619–30

Mariuzza R A, Jankovic D Lj, Boulot G, Amit A G, Saludjian P, Le Guern A, Mazié J C, Poljak R J 1983. Preliminary crystallographic study of the complex between the Fab fragment of a monoclonal anti-lysozyme antibody and its antigen, *Journal of Molecular Biology* **170**: 1055–8

Pecht I, Maron E, Arnon R, Sela M 1971. Specific excitation energy transfer from antibodies to dansyl-labeled antigen: studies with the 'loop' peptide of hen-egg-white lysozyme. *European Journal of Biochemistry* **19**: 368–71

Sakato N, Fujio H, Amano T 1971. The electric charges of antibodies directed to unique regions of hen egg-white lysozyme, *Biken Journal* **14**: 405–11.

Verhoeyen M, Berek C, Jarvis J M, Winter G 1986. Personal communication

A hypothesis on the requirement of T cells for effective self–non-self discrimination of protein antigens

E Margoliash; Ellen K Lakey; Lisa Casten; Susan K Pierce

Department of Biochemistry, Molecular Biology and Cell Biology, Northwestern University, Evanston, Illinois 60201, USA

The humoral immune system is endowed with the remarkable capacity to recognize and respond to a vast array of foreign antigenic substances and to maintain an unresponsive state to self. The underlying cellular and molecular mechanisms which ensure self–non-self discrimination remain largely unknown. In particular it is not clear whether the B cell antigen receptor alone is capable of such discrimination. For studying the antigenic behavior of proteins there are obvious advantages to a small protein, of known primary and tertiary structures, for which a very large number of structural variants are known, both natural and obtained by chemical modification, and which can be readily manipulated chemically in a controlled fashion. Eukaryotic or mitochondrial cytochromes c, having all these characteristics, have been extensively used as model antigens since the mid-1960s (Reichlin *et al.* 1966, 1970; Nisonoff *et al.* 1967, 1970; Margoliash *et al.* 1967, 1970), following the introduction of immunization techniques that allowed the reproducible eliciting of antibodies directed against this relatively poor immunogen. One of the most important of its advantages is that all maintain the same polypeptide backbone spatial structure, termed the 'cytochrome c fold' (Margoliash 1972) so that differences in amino acid sequence among eukaryotic cytochromes c of different species are reflected only in local differences in surface topography where the residue side chains vary, making it a paticularly suitable object for the study of topographic antigenic determinants. A succinct review of these studies is given by Benjamin *et al.* (1984). An early observation was that antisera obtained against one cytochrome c cross-reacted with all others tested, even when amino acid sequence differences approached 50% (Margoliash *et al.* 1970). A representative set of such observations is shown in Table 1 in which competition between ^{125}I-labeled and unlabeled antigens, as well as complement fixation tests, were employed to measure the extent of cross-reactivity. Somewhat different values were exhibited by different antisera, but the trends remained the same.

In apparent contradistinction to this quasi-universal reactivity of anti-cytochrome c antisera were the results of studies aimed at defining what

Table 1 Correlation between complement fixation, antibody binding competition and primary structure variations for various cytochromes c employing a rabbit anti-horse cytochrome c antiserum*

Cytochrome c	Percentage homologous reaction at maximum in complement fixation	Percentage homologous labeled antigen displaced in binding competition	Number of variant residues from horse cytochrome c
Horse	100	93	0
Donkey	100	91	1
Cow, sheep, pig	60	70	3
Finback whale	45		5
Kangaroo	38	55	7
Rabbit	35	50	6
Rhesus monkey	25		11
Chicken	19	50	11
Human, chimpanzee	16	53	12
Pekin duck	13	45	14
Tuna	27	40	17
Screw worm fly	0	55	24
S. cynthia	0	30	29
Yeast iso-1	5	6	45

Source: Margoliash et al. (1970)

* Rabbit anti-horse cytochrome c antiserum 7B3,4 was employed. Horse cytochrome c fixed 70 C'$_{H50}$ units out of a total of 100 added to the complement fixation reaction mixture. In the competition experiments, ^{125}I-labelled horse cytochrome c (4 μg) was used as a test antigen and 75 μg of unlabeled cytochromes c added.

sections of the protein's surface bound to these antibodies, i.e. what constituted the antigenic determinants that presumably had given rise to these antibodies (Urbanski and Margoliash 1977; Eng and Reichlin 1979; Jemmerson and Margoliash 1979; Berman and Harbury 1980; Hannum et al. 1985; Hannum and Margoliash 1985). Indeed, with the unraveling of the partial or complete so-called antigenic structures of several cytochromes c it became evident that antigenic determinants on heterologous cytochromes c always contained residues that differed from the corresponding residues in the host's cytochrome c, whether the antiserum was produced in rabbits or mice, and that wherever such residue differences occurred corresponding antibody populations could be elicited (see review by Benjamin et al. 1984). The single exception to this rule was ascribed to cross-reactivity of B cell clones directed towards an immunodominant glutamic acid side chain with a corresponding aspartyl residue (Urbanski and Margoliash 1977). Nevertheless, not only did the antibodies raised against a heterologous cytochrome c cross-react, sometimes extensively, with the host's own protein, as indicated above, but one could in fact elicit antibodies against the host protein, by injecting rabbits with rabbit cytochrome c conjugated to acetylated γ-globulin or polymerized by reaction with glutaraldehyde (Nisonoff et al. 1967; Jemmerson and Margoliash 1979a). The amount of antibody thus produced was low, averaging only about 10% of the response to a typical heterologous cytochrome *c*. Interestingly, these rabbit-anti-rabbit cytochrome *c* antibodies were shown to be entirely directed to the three areas of the protein that had varied most recently in the course of the evolutionary descent of mammalian cytochromes *c* (Jemmerson and Margoliash 1979a). This prompted the hypothesis that such self immunogen specificities represented a stimulation of cross-reactive clones, the repertoire for which had not yet been eliminated by evolutionary selection operating against the retention of potential autoimmune responses.

The protein structural background for all these observations did not become clear until the recent study of the rabbit and mouse antibody responses to pigeon cytochrome *c* (Hannum *et al.* 1985; Hannum and Margoliash 1985). Not only was it shown that antibodies were directed to four sites on the antigens which among them contained all seven residue differences between immunogen and host proteins, but also that the majority of the antibody, 80% or more, was directed toward an assembled topographic determinant composed of three amino acids from the carboxyl-terminal α-helix of the protein,

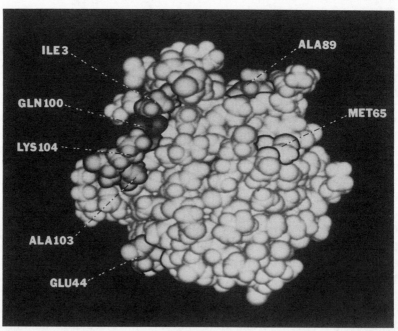

Figure 1. Back view of a computer-generated space-filling model of pigeon cytochrome *c*. The positions visible from this side of the molecule at which pigeon cytochrome *c* differs from the mouse protein are indicated by lines following the contours of the atoms representing each residue. Methionine residue 65 is also indicated. The authors are grateful to Mr Richard Feldman, National Institutes of Health, for providing the computer graphics model. According to Hannum *et al.* 1982.

glutamine-100, alanine-103 and lysine-104, and a single residue from the spatially overlapping amino-terminal α-helix, isoleucyl-3. It had earlier been shown that the same area constituted the major T cell determinant of pigeon cytochrome *c*, with respect to mice, that the T cell antigen was a peptide fragment containing the carboxyl-terminal end of the protein chain, and that tobacco hornworm moth cytochrome *c* or its peptide fragment having a very similar but not identical carboxyl-terminal sequence, was an even better T cell antigen than pigeon cytochrome *c* for mice primed with or T cell hybrids directed against pigeon cytochrome *c* (Solinger *et al.* 1979; Ultee *et al.* 1980; Hannum *et al.* 1982; Lakey *et al.* 1986a, 1986b). Employing a plate binding assay, it was shown that the host protein, rabbit or mouse cytochrome *c*, could fully compete against antibodies elicited by pigeon cytochrome *c*, and that all the antibodies raised bound the host protein but with considerably lower affinity than to the immunogen. This indicated that the antigen–antibody interaction involves not only the so-called immunodominant residues, namely those which differed between pigeon and host proteins, but also the surrounding surface of the protein which is identical in the pigeon, mouse and rabbit proteins (Hannum *et al.* 1985; Hannum and Margoliash 1985). Further, it was possible to estimate what proportion of the total energy of interaction between antibody and antigen was due to interaction with the pigeon-specific side chains, and what proportion therefore resulted from interaction with the surrounding surface of the antigen. At 50% antibody bound and using the same amount of antibody for the plate binding assays, with pigeon and mouse or rabbit cytochrome *c*, the difference in binding energy contributed by the pigeon specific side chains is given by:

$$\Delta\Delta G = -R\,T \ln \frac{[\text{mouse or rabbit cytochrome } c]_{50\%}}{[\text{pigeon cytochrome } c]_{50\%}}$$

The results of such calculations, given in Table 2, demonstrate that in every case a large proportion of the energy of interaction was provided not by the immunodominant residues but by the surrounding protein surface. This then is the obvious basis for the extensive cross-reactivity between different

Table 2 Binding energies of anti-pigeon cytochrome *c* antibodies to pigeon and mouse cytochromes *c*

Anti-pigeon cytochrome *c* antibody	$\Delta\Delta G$ of binding to immunodominant residues (kcal mol^{-1})	Binding energy not due to immunodominant residues* (%)
Mouse primary	−2.9	65–81
Mouse secondary	−3.8	54–75
Rabbit hyperimmune	−6.0	27–60

Source: According to Hannum amd Margoliash (1985) and Hannum *et al.* (1985).
* For a total of $\Delta\Delta G$ of −8.2 to −14.9 kcal mol^{-1} ($K_a = 10^5 \text{M}^{-1}$ to 10^{10}M^{-1}).

cytochromes *c* with antibodies raised against any one of them, and also presumably for the weak self-immunogenic properties of cytochrome *c*. In this connection, it should be noted that because of these binding energy relationships one cannot interpret the binding of antibodies to a self protein, or to a segment of a self protein, as necessarily representing an autoimmune phenomenon. Because of the size of antibody combining sites, an antibody, evoked by the influence of a residue at which the immunogen differs from the corresponding host protein, could very well bind to a structure shared by the immunogen and host proteins, as far as 15 Å away on the protein surface. Furthermore, from the point of view of the distinction between potential self antigens and non-self antigens, the few calories of binding energy which are provided by the immunodominant residues are clearly much too weak a basis for a safe separation of self and non-self at the level of antibodies, making a second tier of regulation essential to prevent the ubiquitous formation of anti-self antibodies and the resultant autoimmune phenomena.

Specifically, in the present case, our results suggest that the ability of antibodies elicited in mice or rabbits by pigeon cytochrome *c* to discriminate between pigeon and mouse or rabbit cytochrome *c* is insufficient to account for the relative ineffectiveness of a cytochrome *c* to elicit antibodies in the species from which it was prepared. If this is indeed the case, the distinction between self and non-self in the humoral response must reside in another major aspect of the stimulatory mechanism, namely in the antigen-specific activation of T cells to provide a helper function for B cells. It would seem that to be most effective, the second level of regulation would best be designed to depend on a different form of the antigen than the first level. This would be true even if the T and B cell immunodominant residues are the same, as occurs for the major T cell and B cell determinants in pigeon cytochrome *c* with respect to mice as discussed above. This would seem to be the case, since while B lymphocyte antigen receptors are often exquisitely specific for the conformation of the antigenic determinant on the surface of the native antigen, T cells appears to have very little ability to recognize their antigenic determinants in the native protein (Benjamin *et al.* 1984). Rather, the helper T cells studied to date, specific for such globular proteins antigens as cytochrome *c* (Casten *et al.* 1985; Kovak and Schwartz 1985), myoglobin (Bush *et al.* 1984), ovalbumin (Shimonkevitz *et al.* 1983) and lysozyme (Allen *et al.* 1984) require that the protein first be denatured, generally by being broken up into peptide fragments, and presented to the T cell in association with the class II gene products present on the surface of an antigen presenting cell (APC). Presentation of the antigen to the T cell is believed to require the uptake of the native protein by the APC, its transport to a cytoplasmic acid compartment where proteolytic cleavage occurs and the subsequent transport of the released peptides to the plasma membrane where these can be recognized by the T cell in association with Ia [reviewed in Unanue (1984)].

As has been demonstrated for several other systems, the ability of APC to activate cytochrome-*c* specific T cells is blocked by inhibitors which interfere with either the uptake of cytochrome c from solution, the function of acid vesicles, or of the proteases they contain (Casten *et al.* 1985; Kovac and Schwartz 1985). Thus, the stimulation of a T cell hybrid, specific for pigeon cytochrome c, is blocked by paraformaldehyde fixation of APC or preincubation of APC with chloroquine, ammonium chloride or the protease inhibitor leupeptin (Fig. 2). In contrast, such treatments have no effect on the APC's ability to stimulate a cytochrome c-specific T cell when provided with a 'processed' form of the antigen, namely the carboxyl-terminal peptide of pigeon cytochrome c, residues 81–104, which contains the T cell anigenic determinant.

A role for antigen processing in T-cell-dependent B cell activation has been suggested by the demonstration that in the spleen in addition to macrophages and dendritic cells, B cells function as APCs for helper T cells (Chestnut *et al.* 1982; Kakiuchi *et al.* 1983; Ashwell *et al.* 1984; Jelachich *et al.* 1986). In addition, B cells which express surface Ig that binds antigen appear to be very efficient in the presentation of their specific antigen, requiring far less antigen and fewer B cells to maximally activate T cells as compared to nonspecific B cells. The evidence suggests that binding the antigen to the surface Ig may serve either to signal the B cell to enhanced processing and/or presentation (Casten *et al.* 1985), or to concentrate antigen for subsequent processing and presentation (Rock *et al.* 1984; Lanzavecchia 1985). Results from this labora-

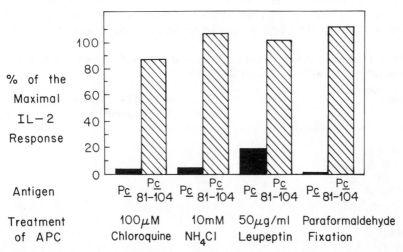

Figure 2. Native pigeon cytochrome c (Pc) requires antigen processing to be presented to a Pc-specific T cell hybrid, TPc9.1, while a C-terminal peptide fragment, residues 81–104 (Pc 81–104), does not. In the first three experiments splenic B cells were washed and paraformaldehyde-fixed after incubation for 4 hr with antigen (26 μM) either Pc (solid bars) or Pc 81–104 (hatched bars) and inhibitors then plated (5 × 10⁵ cells/0.2 ml) with 5 × 10⁴ TPc9.1 cells. In the fourth experiment cells were paraformaldehyde-fixed prior to culture with the antigens Pc or Pc 81–104 and TPc9.1 cells. In all cases supernatants were removed after 24 hr and tested for IL-2 content as described (Casten *et al.* 1985).

tory indicate that both these mechanisms may be at play and that while the surface Ig may be unique in its ability to transduce a signal for enhanced processing, several other B cell surface proteins may suffice to concentrate antigen for subsequent processing and presentation. Fab fragments of rabbit anti-mouse Ig antibodies, either monovalent or divalent, augment the ability of B cells to process and present native pigeon cytochrome c or the peptide fragment, Pc 81–104, in that maximal T cell activation is achieved using 10-fold less antigen or 10-fold fewer B cells as APC than in the absence of anti-Ig (Table 3) (Casten *et al.* 1985). Augmentation appears to be independent of receptor-mediated internalization of the antigen, because B cells treated with anti-Ig and subsequently paraformaldehyde-fixed are enhanced in their presentation of the peptide fragment. This augmentation does not appear to be due to a measurable increase in surface Ia expression, as estimated by using fluoresceinated antibody to Ia. The Ig antigen receptor appears to be unique in signalling the B cells in this fashion, as similar augmentation is not achieved by treatment of B cells with antibodies directed towards other surface proteins such as Ia which have been suggested by others to transduce activating signals (Corley *et al.* 1985).

In addition to its ability to signal B cells to enhanced presentation, surface Ig may also serve to concentrate antigen for subsequent processing, as indicated by the results of other investigators (Rock *et al.* 1984; Lanzavecchia 1985). To examine this possibility, cytochrome c was conjugated to anti-Ig antibodies, creating a universal antigen capable of binding to all splenic B cells expressing surface Ig. This conjugate is presented approximately 100- to

Table 3 Pigeon cytochrome c coupled to antibodies directed against various B cell surface proteins are effective T cell antigens*

Antigen	Concentration of Pc antigen required for 50% maximal IL-2 response (M)
Pc	1.2
Pc 81–104	1.0
Pc + (Fab')$_2$ anti-Ig	0.10
Pc + Fab' anti-Ig	0.20
Pc 81–104 + (Fab')$_2$ anti-Ig	0.10
Pc + anti-I-A^k	1.0
Pc-(anti-Ig)	0.012
Pc-(anti-K^k)	0.041
Pc-(anti-I-A^k)	0.035
Pc-(anti-I-A^s)	2.2

* Pigeon cytochrome c specific T cells (5×10^4 cells/0.2 ml) were cultured with purified H-2^k splenic CBA/J B cells (5×10^5 cells/0.2 ml) and the antigens shown. The monovalent and divalent Fab fragments of rabbit anti-mouse Ig [Fab' anti-Ig and F(ab')$_2$ anti-Ig, respectively] were added to cultures in concentrations of 1–5 μg/ml (Casten *et al.* 1985). The conjugates of pigeon cytochrome c (Pc) and monoclonal antibodies directed against Ig, K^k, I-A^k and I-A^s were synthesized using a bifunctional cross-linking reagent.

1000-fold more efficiently than either cytochrome *c* alone, cytochrome *c* with unconjugated anti-Ig or cytochrome *c* coupled to an antibody of an irrelevant specificity which does not bind to B cells of the haplotype used in these studies (Table 3). The cytochrome *c*–anti-Ig antibody conjugates are not unique in their ability to be efficiently processed and presented by B cells because cytochrome *c* conjugated to antibodies specific for the B cell surface class I (anti-K^k) or class II (anti-I-A^k) gene products are also very efficiently presented. These results indicate that binding of the native antigen to any one of several B cell surface structures is sufficient to enhance processing. However, under physiological conditions presumably only the surface Ig binds antigen and consequently serves an antigen concentrating function. These results suggest that under limiting antigen concentrations, such as may occur *in vivo*, only those B cells which bind antigen may be capable of producing sufficient quantities of the T cell anigenic peptide to attract helper T cells to their surface so that they can be activated to release the necessary B cell growth and differentiation factors. Thus, the ability to process and present antigen has a central role in the antigen-specific activation of B cells.

In summary, the question as to how the requirement for antigen processing and presentation might ensure a suitably specific humoral response, is central to the mechanisms of self–non-self recognition. Even though the B cell receptor does not appear to be capable of a very high degree of specificity, the superimposed mechanism for producing an effective T cell antigen will necessarily compound the discriminating ability of the overall system. This would be the case even if the T cell receptor were no better able to distinguish between self and non-self antigens than the B cell receptor. This concept leads to a testable hypothesis that self-reactive antibodies should be more readily induced in naive B cell populations when the requirement for antigen processing and presentation is bypassed by artificially providing directly the T cell elaborated growth and differentiation factors. Future studies designed to elucidate the mechanisms underlying antigen-receptor mediated B cell antigen presentation and the development of the antigen-specific T cell repertoire with particular regard to the development of tolerance to intracellular self proteins such as the mitochondrial cytochrome *c*, should yield further insight into the process of self–non-self discrimination.

References

Allen P M, Strydom D J, Unanue E R 1984. Processing of lysozyme by macrophages: identification of the determinant recognized by two T cell hybridomas, *Proceedings of the National Academy of Sciences USA* **81**: 2489–93

Ashwell J D, DeFranco A L, Paul W E, Schwartz R H 1984. Antigen presentation by resting B cells: radiosensitivity of the antigen presentation function and the distinct pathways of T cell activation, *Journal of Experimental Medicine* **159**: 881–905

Benjamin D C, Berzofsky J A, East I J, Gurd F R N, Hannum C H, Leach S J, Margoliash E,

Michael J G, Miller A, Prager E M, Reichlin M, Sercarz E E, Smith-Gill S J, Todd P E, Wilson C 1984. The antigenic structure of proteins: a reappraisal, in *Annual Review of Immunology*. Academic Press, New York, vol 2, pp 67–101

Berman P W, Harbury H A 1980. Immunochemistry of cytochrome *c*. Identification of antigenic determinants through the study of hybrid molecules, *Journal of Biological Chemistry* **255**: 6133–42

Bush M, Gurd F R N, Streicher H Z, Berkower I J, Berzofsky J A 1984. The role of antigen conformation in determining requirements for antigen processing for T-cell activation, in E Secarz, L Chess, H Cantor (eds) *Regulation of the immune system*. Alan R Liss Inc., New York, pp 135–42

Casten L A, Lakey E K, Jelachich M L, Margoliash E, Pierce S K 1985. Anti-immunoglobin augments the B cell antigen presentation function independently of internalization of a receptor–antigen complex, *Proceedings of the National Academy of Sciences USA* **82**: 5890–4

Chestnut R W, Colon S M, Grey H M 1982. Antigen presentation by normal B cells, B cell tumors, and macrophages: functional and biochemical comparisons, *Journal of Immunology* **128**: 1764–8

Corley R B, LoCascio N J, Ovnic M, Haughton G 1985. Two separate functions of Class II (Ia) molecules: T cell stimulation and B cell excitation, *Proceedings of the National Academy of Sciences USA* **82**: 516–20

Eng J, Reichlin M 1979. Fractionation of rabbit anti-horse cytochrome *c* – I. Specificity of the isolated fractions, *Molecular Immunology* **16**: 225–32

Hannum C H, Margoliash 1985. Assembled topographic antigenic determinants of pigeon cytochrome *c*, *Journal of Immunology* **132**: 3303–13

Hannum C, Ultee M, Matis L A, Schwartz R H, Margoliash E 1982. The major B and T cell determinant on pigeon cytochrome *c* in B10.A mice, in M Z Atassi (ed) *Immunobiology of Proteins and Peptides – II*. Plenum Publishing Corp., New York, pp 37–52

Hannum C H, Matis L A, Schwartz R H, Margoliash E 1985. The B10.A mouse B cell response to pigeon cytochrome *c* is directed against the same area of the protein that is recognized by B10.A T cells in association with the E^k:E^k Ia molecule, *Journal of Immunology* **132**: 3314–22

Jelachich M L, Lakey E K, Casten L, Pierce S K 1986. Antigen presentation is a function of all B cell subpopulation separated on the basis of size, *European Journal of Immunology* **16**: 411–16

Jemmerson R, Margoliash E 1979a. Specificity of the antibody response of rabbits to a self-antigen, *Nature (London)* **282**: 468–71

Jemmerson R, Margoliash E 1979b. Topographic antigenic determinants on cytochrome *c*. Immunoadsorbent separation of the rabbit antibody populations directed against cytochrome *c*, *Journal of Biological Chemistry* **254**: 12706–16

Kakiuchi T, Chestnut R W, Grey H M 1983. B cells as antigen presenting cells: the requirement for B cell activation, *Journal of Immunology* **131**: 109–14

Kovac Z, Schwartz R H 1985. The molecular basis of the requirement for antigen processing of pigeon cytochrome *c* prior to T cell activation, *Journal of Immunology* **134**: 3233–40

Lakey E K, Margoliash E, Fitch F W, Pierce S K 1986a. Role of L3T4 and Ia in the heteroclitic response of T cells to cytochrome *c*, *Journal of Immunology* **136**: 3933–8

Lakey E K, Margoliash E, Flouret G, Pierce S K 1986b. Peptides related to the antigenic determinant block T cell recognition of the native protein as processed by antigen presenting cells, *European Journal of Immunology* **16**: 721–7

Lanzavecchia A 1985. Antigen-specific interacting between T cells and B cells, *Nature (London)* **314**: 537–9

Margoliash E 1972. The molecular variation of cytochrome *c* as a function of the evolution of species, *Harvey Lecture Series* **66**: 177–247

Margoliash E, Reichlin M, Nisonoff A 1967. The antigenic behaviour of cytochrome *c*, *Science* **158**: 531

Margoliash E, Nisonoff A, Reichlin M 1970. Immunological activity of cytochrome *c*. I. Precipitating antibodies to monomeric vertebrate cytochrome *c*, *Journal of Biological Chemistry* **245**: 931–9

Nisonoff A, Margoliash E, Reichlin M 1967. Antibodies to rabbit cytochrome *c* arising in rabbits, *Science* **155**: 1273–5

Nisonoff A, Reichlin M, Margoliash E 1970. Immunological activity of cytochrome *c*. II. Localization of a major antigenic determinant of human cytochrome *c*, *Journal of Biological Chemistry* **245**: 940–6

Reichlin M, Fogel S, Nisonoff A, Margoliash E 1966. Antibodies against cytochrome *c* from vertebrates. *Journal of Biological Chemistry* **241**: 251–3

Reichlin M, Nisonoff A, Margoliash E 1970. Immunological activity of cytochrome *c*. III. Enhancement of antibody detection and immune response initiation by cytochrome *c* polymers, *Journal of Biological Chemistry* **245**: 947–54

Rock K L, Benacerraf B, Abbas, A K 1984. Antigen presentation by hapten-specific B lymphocytes I. Role of surface immunoglobulin receptors. *Journal of Experimental Medicine* **160**: 1102–13

Shimonkevitz R, Kappler R, Marrack P, Grey H 1983. Antigen recognition by H-2 restricted T cells. I. Cell-free antigen processing, *Journal of Experimental Medicine* **158**: 303–16

Solinger A M, Ultee M E, Margoliash E, Schwartz R H 1979. T-lymphocyte response to cytochrome *c*. I. Demonstration of a T-cell heteroclitic proliferative response and identification of a topographic antigenic determinant on pigeon cytochrome *c* whose immune recognition requires two complementing major histocompatibility complex-linked immune response genes, *Journal of Experimental Medicine* **150**: 830–48.

Ultee M E, Margoliash E, Lipkowski A, Flouret G, Solinger A M, Lobwohl D, Matis L A, Chen C, Schwartz R H 1980. The T lymphocyte response to cytochrome *c*. II. Molecular characterization of a pigeon cytochrome *c* determinant recognized by proliferating T lymphocytes of the B10.A mouse, *Molecular Immunology* **17**: 809–22

Unanue E R 1984. Antigen-presenting function of the macrophage, *Annual Review of Immunology* **2**: 395–429

Urbanski G J, Margoliash E 1977. Topographic determinants on cytochrome *c*. I. The complete antigenic structures of rabbit, mouse, and guanaco cytochromes *c* in rabbits and mice. *Journal of Immunology* **118**: 1170–80

Comparison of the submolecular recognition of proteins by T and B cells

M Zouhair Atassi; Garvin S Bixler Jr

Verna and Marrs McLean Department of Biochemistry, Baylor College of Medicine, Houston, Texas 77030, USA

Introduction

The importance of localization of the molecular features on protein molecules that are recognized by the immune system was appreciated quite early (LaPresle 1955; Porter 1957). Localization of the antigenic regions on viral antigens was also recognized over 20 years ago as a possible route for vaccines based on sythetic peptides (Anderer 1963; Anderer and Schlumberger 1965). However, it was felt that the complexity of protein structure made this goal beyond reach at that time (Anderer 1963). In fact, it was not until the antigenic structure of myoglobin (Mb) was determined 12 years later (Atassi 1975) that the first full antigenic structure of a protein was known. This was followed three years later (Atassi 1978) by the determination of the second complete antigenic structure of a protein, i.e. lysozyme. Determination of these and other antigenic structures provided for the first time fascinating insights of what antibodies recognize on a protein (i.e. the antigenic sites) and formulated the foundation for our present concepts of this recognition.

It is, however, well known that the immune responses to protein antigens involve recognition by T cells as well as antibodies. In fact it was shown over seven years ago (Okuda *et al.* 1979) that the synthetic antigenic sites of Mb that are the target of antibody recognition are also recognized by T cells. But, generally, in contrast to our extensive knowledge on antibody recognition of proteins, the submolecular details of T-cell recognition have not until recently been defined for a protein. Now the entire polypeptide chains of several protein molecules have been screened and for each protein the full sub-molecular profile of its T-cell recognition determined. The localization of the regions that are recognized by T cells on a protein, for which the antigenic structure (i.e. the regions recognized by antibodies) is also known, has enabled the first comparisons of immune recognition at the submolecular level by T cells and B cells. Since only a few multi-determinant proteins have been examined in such detail, it is necessary to caution against hasty and premature generalizations.

General features of antibody (B-cell) recognition

From the studies on Mb (Atassi 1975), lysozyme (Atassi 1978) and subsequently on several other protein antigens including hemoglobin (Hb) (Kazim and Atassi 1980, 1982; Yoshioka and Atassi 1983, 1986); ragweed allergen Ra3 (Atassi and Atassi 1985, 1986) and influenza virus hemagglutinin (HA) (Atassi and Kurisaki 1984; Atassi and Webster 1983), several conclusions were made (Atassi 1975, 1978) and have since been substantiated by many workers with a variety of protein systems. Since these studies have already been extensively reviewed (Atassi 1975, 1978, 1984), only the highlights will be mentioned here. The relationship of the antigenic (antibody binding) sites to the sites of T cell recognition, however, will be discussed in more detail in the subsequent sections.

Antigenic sites of proteins are architecturally of two types. They may comprise residues that are on a continuous segment of the protein chain (Atassi, 1975), or are distant in sequence, but, due to the folding of the polypeptide chain, come into close proximity (Atassi 1978). The attributes of antigenic sites include: small size and well defined boundaries; presence in limited number; surface location; conformational sensitivity; sensitivity to environmental changes (amino acid substitutions); and variation of the immunodominancy with the antiserum (for detailed discussions, see Atassi 1975, 1977, 1978, 1980, 1984). The factors which determine the architecture of the site cannot be defined unequivocally at this stage. However, it has been tentatively concluded that stabilization of the structure by internal disulfide cross-links is important to the maintenance of discontinuous sites (Lee and Atassi 1976). The location of an antigenic site for a given protein is structurally inherent and is independent of the immunized species. However, the responses to the sites are regulated by intersite cellular interactions and the recognition of and responses to each antigenic site are under separate genetic control (Okuda *et al.* 1979; David and Atassi 1982).

T-cell recognition of proteins

Definition of the submolecular features involved in antibody recognition of proteins has rendered a wealth of information on the molecular basis of B-cell recognition and factors affecting this recognition (for reviews, see Atassi 1975, 1978, 1980, 1984; David and Atassi 1982). In contrast, until recently, very little has been known about T-cell recognition of proteins. The molecular localization of the full T-cell recognition profile of a complex multideterminant protein antigen has not previously been accomplished.

Recently, by applying the comprehensive synthetic overlapping peptide approach introduced by Kazim and Atassi (1980), the full profiles of T-cell recognition for several proteins have been determined. In localizing the sites, we applied the procedures previously described for the delineation of the continuous antigenic sites of Hb (Kazim and Atassi 1980, 1982) and considered the activities of individual peptides as well as activities residing in the overlap regions of adjacent peptides. It should be noted, however, that the overlapping peptide strategy is not designed to give the precise boundaries of the sites nor is it implied that each of the T sites comprises the entire region specified. Rather, the T sites will reside within those regions. Indeed, the regions containing T sites were made intentionally larger than the expected size of the site in order to avoid assignment errors stemming from close delineation at this early stage.

Myoglobin

In earlier studies (Okuda *et al.* 1978, 1979) it was shown that the immune response to sperm-whale myoglobin is controlled by genes in the I region of mouse H-2. The synthetic antigenic sites were found (Okuda *et al.* 1979) to stimulate T-cell responses, with the responses to each site being under separate genetic control. Although these studies revealed that the sites recognized by antibodies were also recognized by T cells, they could not give any information on whether there were additional sites on the protein that were recognized only by T cells and for which no antibody responses could be detected.

By application of the overlapping peptide strategy to Mb, the continuous sites of T-cell recognition of Mb in three high-responder mouse strains have been delineated (Bixler and Atassi 1983, 1984b). Thirteen 17-residue peptides, having five-residue overlaps, were examined *in vitro* for their ability to stimulate lymph cells from Mb-primed DBA/2 (H-2^d), BALB/c (H-2^d) and SJL (H-2^s) mice as well as long-term cultures of Mb-specific T cells. This strategy has enabled the localization of the full profile of dominant sites of T-cell recognition in Mb for these mouse strains (Fig. 1). Several regions of the molecule (T sites) were found to stimulate Mb-primed lymph node cells and

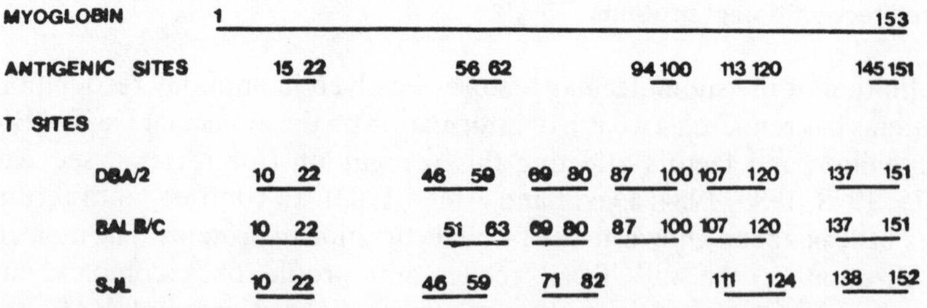

MYOGLOBIN	1					153
ANTIGENIC SITES	15 22	56 62	94 100	113 120		145 151
T SITES						
DBA/2	10 22	46 59	69 80	87 100	107 120	137 151
BALB/C	10 22	51 63	69 80	87 100	107 120	137 151
SJL	10 22	46 59	71 82	111 124		138 152

Figure 1. Schematic diagram showing the full profile of the regions of sperm-whale myoglobin that carry the continuous sites of T-cell recognition (T sites) in three mouse strains. It is not implied that the entire regions shown comprise the T site, rather that the sites reside within these regions. (From Bixler and Atassi 1983, 1984b.)

Mb-specific long-term T-cell cultures. Of these T sites, one region, residues 107–125, was clearly immunodominant in these strains and was found to coincide with the previously defined antigenic (i.e. antibody binding) site 4 of Mb (Atassi 1975). Also, other regions stimulated T cells and appeared to coincide with previously known antigenic sites (see Fig. 1). It is noteworthy that, in addition to sites recognized by both T and B cells, the protein has other sites which are recognized exclusively by T cells and to which no detectable antibody response is directed.

To define precisely the boundaries of the immunodominant T site residing within region 107–120, a new approach was introduced (Bixler *et al.* 1986). Two sets of peptides were synthesized. One set represented a stepwise elongation by one-residue increments of the Mb sequence. In the other set, the peptides were similarly elongated by stepwise single residue increments and then, in addition, brought to a uniform size of 14 residues by nonsense (a randomly selected sequence of residues bearing no homology to the Mb sequence) residues (Fig. 2). The longer peptides (nonsense extended) usually

---

A. MB PEPTIDES HAVING INCREASING SIZE OF NATURAL SEQUENCE

```
107-120    ILE-SER-GLU-ALA-ILE-ILE-HIS-VAL-LEU-HIS-SER-ARG-HIS-PRO
108-120        SER-GLU-ALA-ILE-ILE-HIS-VAL-LEU-HIS-SER-ARG-HIS-PRO
109-120            GLU-ALA-ILE-ILE-HIS-VAL-LEU-HIS-SER-ARG-HIS-PRO
110-120                ALA-ILE-ILE-HIS-VAL-LEU-HIS-SER-ARG-HIS-PRO
111-120                    ILE-ILE-HIS-VAL-LEU-HIS-SER-ARG-HIS-PRO
112-120                        ILE-HIS-VAL-LEU-HIS-SER-ARG-HIS-PRO
113-120                            HIS-VAL-LEU-HIS-SER-ARG-HIS-PRO
```

B. NATURAL MB SEQUENCES EXTENDED BY NONSENSE SEQUENCE TO A UNIFORM SIZE

```
N(108-120)    GLY-SER-GLU-ALA-ILE-ILE-HIS-VAL-LEU-HIS-SER-ARG-HIS-PRO
N(109-120)    GLY-ALA-GLU-ALA-ILE-ILE-HIS-VAL-LEU-HIS-SER-ARG-HIS-PRO
N(110-120)    GLY-ALA-SER-ALA-ILE-ILE-HIS-VAL-LEU-HIS-SER-ARG-HIS-PRO
N(111-120)    GLY-ALA-SER-GLY-ILE-ILE-HIS-VAL-LEU-HIS-SER-ARG-HIS-PRO
N(112-120)    GLY-ALA-SER-GLY-THR-ILE-HIS-VAL-LEU-HIS-SER-ARG-HIS-PRO
N(113-120)    GLY-ALA-SER-GLY-THR-GLY-HIS-VAL-LEU-HIS-SER-ARG-HIS-PRO
```

Figure 2. The primary structure of the synthetic peptides employed for the definition of the T site, previously found to localize within region 107–120 of sperm whale Mb (9). (A) Peptides representing stepwise extensions by one residue of the natural Mb sequence from His-113 to Pro-120. Peptide 113–120 coincidentally corresponds to the previously defined antigenic (antibody binding) site 4 of Mb. (B) Peptides in which the structures shown in (A) are extended by a 'nonsense' sequence to a uniform size of 14 residues by addition of an appropriate segment of the 'nonsense' sequence. (From Bixler *et al.* 1986.)

gave higher proliferative responses than their shorter counterparts having the same Mb region (Fig. 3). Thus, a minimum peptide size is required for optimal T-cell stimulation (Bixler *et al.* 1986). The T site subtends, in three high-responder mouse strains, residues 109–119 or 110–120 depending on strain and, in three low-responder strains, maps to residues 108–120 (Fig. 4). Thus, in this case, the T site coincides with the site of B-cell recognition, previously mapped to reidues 113–120 (Atassi 1975), and resides in a small, discrete surface region of the protein chain.

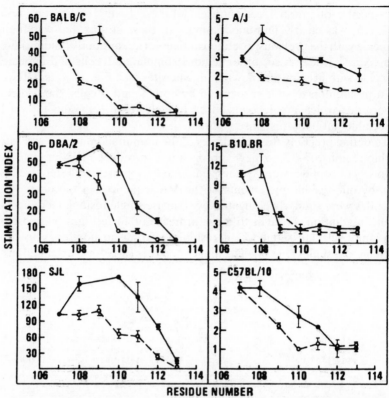

Figure 3. Summary of proliferative responses of lymph node cells obtained from six mouse strains to *in vitro* challenge with peptides of the natural sequence (○) or peptides extended by 'nonsense' sequence to a uniform size (●). The maximum proliferative responses obtained are plotted against the corresponding residue added. Mouse strains were characterized as either high (BALB/c, DBA/2 and SJL) or low (A/J, B10.BR and C57BL/10) responders to Mb. Background responses for the unstimulated cells range from 1094 cpm to 4680 cpm. (From Bixler *et al.* 1986.)

Lysozyme

The localization of the 'continuous' T-cell recognition sites of hen egg lysozyme was also approached by the overlapping synthetic peptide strategy. Eight overlapping peptides encompassing the entire protein chain of lysozyme were synthesized and examined for their ability to stimulate *in vitro* proliferation of T cells from several mouse strains (A/J, H-2^a; BALB/c and DBA/2, H-2^d; B10.BR, H-2^k; DBA/1, H-2^q; SJL, H-2^s) that had been primed with native lysozyme. This approach enabled the identification of a full profile of *in vitro* active lysozyme peptides and the localization of four major T-cell recognition sites (Fig. 5), three of which were subject to individual genetic control (Bixler *et al.* 1984a, 1984b).

STRAINS   H-2

HIGH RESPONDERS

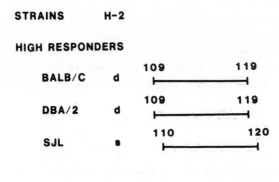

LOW RESPONDERS

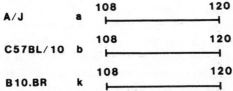

Figure 4. Summary of the precise boundaries of the T side within region 107–120 of sperm-whale Mb as defined in six mouse strains which were either high or low responders to Mb. (From Bixler *et al.* 1986.)

Lysozyme	1					129

Strain	Haplotype				
A/J	a	16 27	34 47	49 62	96 110
BALB/C	d	16 27		49 62	96 110
DBA/2	d	16 27		49 62	96 110
B10.BR	k	17 29		49 62	
DBA/1	q	16 27	34 47	49 62	96 110
SJL	s	17 29		49 62	106 116
T SITES		1	2	3	4

Figure 5. Schematic diagram showing the regions on hen egg lysozyme that have been shown to carry the continuous sites of T-cell recognition (T sites) with several mouse strains. Note that each T site shown falls within but may not necessarily include all the region indicated. In addition to the four T sites shown in this diagram, long-term cultures of lysozyme-primed T cells were found to mount a proliferative response to the three surface-simulation synthetic sites. (From Bixler *et al.* 1984a, 1984b.)

In previous studies from this laboratory, the antigenic (i.e. antibody binding) sites of lysozyme were found to have a discontinuous architecture. The sites could be mimicked by 'surface-simulation' synthesis (Atassi 1978). The recognition of the surface-simulation synthetic antigenic sites by T cells has been explored in a mouse strain (B10.BR) that is a high responder to lysozyme. The discontinuous antigenic sites of lysozyme also had the capacity to stimulate proliferation of T cells driven by native lysozyme in long-term cultures (Bixler and Atassi 1984a). Thus, in addition to the four continuous T sites, T-cell recognition of lysozyme also involves discontinuous sites. This is the first clear demonstration that, contrary to a long-held impression, T-cell recognition is not restricted only to sequence features, but can also be directed to protein discontinuous surface areas of high conformational dependency.

Hemoglobin

Fourteen overlapping peptides encompassing the entire beta chain of adult human hemoglobin were examined *in vitro* for their ability to stimulate lymph node cells from Hb-primed B10.D2 (H-2^d) and SJL (H-2^s) mice. Several regions of the molecule (T sites) were found to stimulate Hb-primed lymph node cells and thus enabled the localization of the full profile of T-cell recognition (Fig. 6) of the beta chain by these mouse strains (Yoshioka *et al.* 1986). Some of the regions that stimulated T cells appeared to coincide with those shown to be recognized by antibodies (i.e. B cells) (Yoshioka and Atassi 1986). In addition to sites recognized by both T and B cells, the protein has other sites that are recognized exclusively by T cells and to which no detectable antibody response is directed.

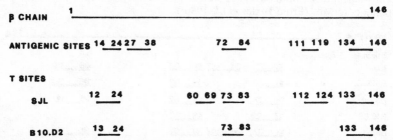

Figure 6. Schematic diagram showing the full profile of the regions of the β chain of HbA that carry the continuous sites of T-cell recognition (T sites) in two mouse strains. The T-cell recognition sites are also compared with the sites of mouse antibody (B cell) recognition. It is not implied that the entire regions shown comprise the T site, rather that the sites reside within these regions. (From Yoshioka *et al.* 1986.)

Ragweed allergen Ra3

Using a comprehensive synthetic strategy has recently enabled (Kurisaki *et al.* 1986) the localization of the continuous regions of Ra3 that are recognized by T cells from mice immunized with Ra3. Ten overlapping peptides encompassing the entire Ra3 molecule were examined *in vitro* for their ability to stimulate lymph node cells from Ra3-primed BALB/c (H-2^d), C3H/HE (H-2^k), SWR (H-2^q) and SJL (H-2^s) mice. Several regions of the molecule (T sites) were found to stimulate Ra3-primed lymph node cells (Fig. 7). Three of the regions recognized by T cells coincided with regions previously shown to be recognized by antibodies (i.e. B cells) (Atassi and Atassi 1985, 1986). In addition to sites recognized by both T and B cells the protein has at least one site which is recognized exclusively by T cells and to which no detectable antibody response is directed (Fig. 7).

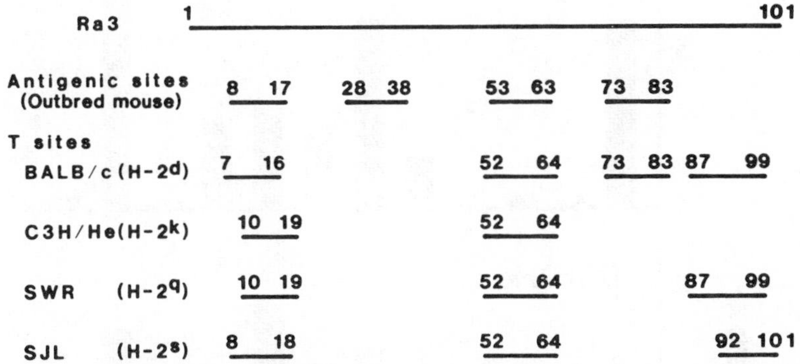

Ra3 1					101
Antigenic sites (Outbred mouse)	8 17	28 38	53 63	73 83	
T sites					
BALB/c (H-2^d)	7 16		52 64	73 83	87 99
C3H/He (H-2^k)	10 19		52 64		
SWR (H-2^q)	10 19		52 64		87 99
SJL (H-2^s)	8 18		52 64		92 101

Figure 7. Schematic diagram showing the full profile of the regions of Ra3 that carry the continuous sites of T-cell recognition (T sites) in four mouse strains. The T-cell recognition sites are also compared with the sites of outbred mouse antibody (B-cell) recognition. It is not implied that the entire regions shown comprise the T site, rather that the sites reside within these regions. (From Kurisaki *et al.* 1986.)

Influenza virus hemagglutinin

Protein antigenic sites occupy invariably surface areas. Thus, when the three-dimensional structure of a protein is known, its surface can be readily screened for the continuous antigenic sites by the systematic synthesis and examination of the immunochemical activities of all its exposed segments. This approach was applied to influenza A virus hemagglutinin. Twelve peptides, representing continuous surface segments of HA, have been found to bind anti-viral antibodies raised in outbred mice and antibodies in human sera obtained from subjects after influenza A virus infection (Atassi and Webster 1983; Atassi and Kurisaki 1984). Antisera to the peptides raised in mice were found to bind to intact virus. In most cases, these antibodies did not bind to disrupted virus. In the various mouse strains, several of the peptides stimulated *in vitro* proliferative responses of T cells from virus(X31)-primed mice (Fig. 8) (Atassi and Kurisaki 1984, in press). Priming with the peptides, individually or in equimolar mixture, produced in many cases T cells that recognized, *in vitro*, only the peptide or the peptide as well as intact virus. However, the pattern of peptide recognition was not necessarily related to that obtained after priming with virus. These studies have shown that: (a) 'Continuous' antigenic sites of proteins can be localized by systematic synthetic scanning of the surface; (b) T-cell recognition of submolecular regions of the

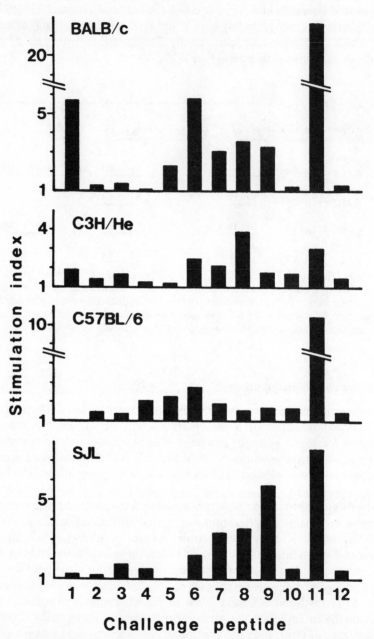

Figure 8. The peptide T-cell recognition profile in four mouse strains that had been immunized with an optimum dose of X31 virus. The results, which are expressed in stimulation index (cpm of stimulated cells/cpm of unstimulated cells), summarize the values of maximum responses at the optimum *in vitro* challenge dose for each peptide. (From Atassi and Kurisaki 1986.)

HA is important in immune responses to the infecting virus; (c) T cells which recognized the virus can be generated only in a few cases by priming with peptide in appropriate mouse strains; and (d) the antibody and T-cell responses to the individual sites of HA are under Ir gene control.

Concluding remarks

The delineation of the profiles of T- and B-cell reognition of these proteins has enabled us to compare, at the submolecular level, the regions involved in immune recognition and has led us to several conclusions. The sites which are reognized by anti-protein antibodies are in most cases recognized by T cells. However, T cells recognize, in addition, areas to which no antibody response is detectable. T cells are not restricted to recognition of a particular antigenic architecture, but like B cells, T cells recognize both continuous and discontinuous sites. Both the antigenic (antibody binding) sites and the T sites are present in limited number. Although the boundaries of all of the T sites in the above proteins have not yet been precisely defined, it is apparent that the T sites comprise discrete regions of the molecule and are similar in this regard to the antibody binding sites. Contrary to recently revived postulates (Benjamin *et al.* 1984), the fine specificity of T cells is neither limited in number nor different from that of B cells. In addition, the popular view that T cells recognize only sequential features (i.e. continuous sites) can now be dismissed.

The regions of T-cell recognition which have been localized probably reflect the responses of numerous T-cell subpopulations, each of which perceives the T site somewhat differently. Thus, various T-cell clones may recognize different overlapping parts of a site (i.e. shifting to the right or to the left). The average of all of these reactivities, or the maximal effective response, would be defined as the T site. This would be consistent with the heterogeneous nature of the T-cell response at the clonal level with regard to the fine submolecular specificities, as has been demonstrated during B-cell recognition (Atassi 1975, 1978, 1980, 1984).

The T sites, like the antigenic sites, are under H-2 gene control, with each site being under separate genetic control (Okuda *et al.* 1979; Twining *et al.* 1981; David and Atassi 1982; Bixler and Atassi 1984b). In addition, the responses to the sites are regulated by intersite cellular influences which could either be help or suppression (Atassi *et al.* 1981).

In order to take full advantage of the technological developments of defining and synthesizing antigenic sites and to apply these new technologies to the introduction of new vaccines or to the delineation of new methods to manipulate the immune response as a means of clinical intervention, it is necessary to understand and appreciate in the smallest detail the interaction of the immune system with antigens. The studies reviewed here have systematically examined several molecules for the submolecular regions involved in immune recognition of proteins at both the B- and T-cell levels. Further, these studies have provided strategies for the localization of the full profiles of T- and B-cell recognition of proteins. The benefits derived from the application of precise chemical and synthetic methods in the rapid delineation of regions of recognition were clearly and unambiguously demonstrated.

Attempts to develop effective anti-viral vaccines using small synthetic peptides have so far met with little success. Such studies have relied entirely on the production of anti-peptide antibodies, ignoring the fact that the immune recognition by T cells plays an important role in the responses to protein antigens (Okuda *et al.* 1979; Young and Atassi 1982; Bixler and Atassi 1983, 1984b; Bixler *et al.* 1984a, 1984b; Yoshioka *et al.* 1986) and the regulation of these responses due to critical intersite influences exerted by T cells (Krco *et al.* 1981; David and Atassi 1982). Although it is encouraging that our anti-peptide antibodies bind to intact virus, attempts at protection by peptide immunization will aim at achieving T-cell memory. They will, therefore, be based on designs derived from the full unraveling of the submolecular profiles of both B- and T-cell recognition on the virus and better understanding of the genetic control and regulatory influences of these site-specific responses.

References

Anderer F A 1963. Preparation and properties of an artificial antigen immunologically related to tobacco mosaic virus, *Biochimica et Biophysica Acta* **71**: 246–8

Anderer F A, Schlumberger H D 1965. Properties of different artificial antigens immunologically related to tobacco mosaic virus, *Biochimica et Biophysica Acta* **97**: 503–9

Atassi H, Atassi M Z 1985. Localization of the continuous allergenic sites of ragweed allergen Ra3 by a comprehensive synthetic strategy, *FEBS Letters* **188**: 96–100

Atassi H, Atassi M Z 1986. Antibody recognition of ragweed allergen Ra3: Localization of the full profile of the continuous antigenic sites by synthetic overlapping peptides representing the entire protein chain, *European Journal of Immunology* **16**: 229–35

Atassi M Z 1975. Antigenic structure of myoglobin. The complete immunochemical anatomy of a protein and conclusions relating to antigenic structures of proteins, *Immunochemistry* **12**: 423–38

Atassi M Z 1977. The complete antigenic structure of myoglobin: Approaches and conclusions for antigenic structures of proteins, in M Z Atassi (ed) *Immunochemistry of Proteins*. Plenum Press, New York, vol 2, pp 77–176

Atassi M Z 1978. Precise determination of the entire antigenic structure of lysozyme: Molecular features of protein antigenic structures and potential of 'surface-simulation' synthesis, a powerful new concept for protein binding sites, *Immunochemistry* **15**: 909–36

Atassi M Z 1980. Precise determination of protein antigenic sites has unravelled the molecular immune recognition of proteins and provided a prototype for synthetic mimicking of other protein binding sites, *Molecular and Cellular Biochemistry* **32**: 21–44

Atassi M Z 1984. Antigenic structures of proteins. Their determination has revealed important aspects of immune recognition and generated strategies for synthetic mimicking of protein binding sites, *European Journal of Biochemistry* **145**: 1–20

Atassi M Z, Kurisaki J 1984. A novel approach for localization of the continuous protein antigenic sites by comprehensive synthetic surface scanning: Antibody and T-cell activity to several influenza hemagglutinin synthetic sites, *Immunological Communications* **13**: 539–51

Atassi M Z, Kurisaki J 1986. Synthetic localization of T- and B-cell recognition sites of influenza virus hemagglutinin and the antibody and the T-cell responses to the sites, *Protides of the Biological Fluids* **34**: 157–60

Atassi M Z, Webster R G 1983. Localization, synthesis and activity of an antigenic site on influenza virus hemagglutinin, *Proceedings of the National Academy of Sciences USA* **80**: 840–4

Atassi M Z, Yokota S, Twining S S, Lehmann H, David C S 1981. Genetic control of the immune response to myoglobin. VI. Inter-site influences in T-lymphocyte proliferative response from the analysis of cross-reactions of ten myoglobin in terms of substitutions in the antigenic sites and in environmental residues of the sites, *Molecular Immunology* **18**: 945–8

Benjamin D C, Berzofsky J A, East I J, Gurd F R N, Hannum C, Leach S J, Margoliash E, Michael J G, Miller A, Prager E M, Reichlin M, Sercarz E E, Smith-Gill S J, Todd P E, Wilson A C 1984. The antigenic structure of proteins: A reappraisal, *Annual Reviews of Immunology* **2**: 67–101

Bixler G S, Atassi M Z 1983. Molecular localization of the full profile of the continuous regions recognized by myoglobin primed T-cells using synthetic overlapping peptides encompassing the entire molecule, *Immunological Communications* **12**: 593–603

Bixler G S, Atassi M Z 1984a. T-cell recognition of lysozyme. III. Recognition of the 'surface-simulation' synthetic antigenic sites, *Journal of Immunogenetics* **11**: 245–50

Bixler G S, Atassi M Z 1984b. T-cell recognition of myoglobin. Localization of the sites stimulating T-cell proliferative responses by synthetic overlapping peptides encompassing the entire molecule. *Journal of Immunogenetics* **11**: 339–53

Bixler G S, Yoshida T, Atassi M Z 1984a. T-cell recognition of lysozyme. I. Localization of regions stimulating T-cell proliferative response by synthetic overlapping peptides encompassing the entire molecule, *Experimental and Clinical Immunogenetics* **1**: 99–111

Bixler G S. Yoshida T, Atassi M Z 1984b. Localization and genetic control of the continuous T-cell recognition sites of lysozyme by synthetic overlapping peptides representing the full profile of the protein chain, *Journal of Immunogenetics* **11**: 327–38

Bixler G S, Bean M, Atassi M Z 1986. Site recognition by protein-primed T cells shows a non-specific size requirement beyond the essential residues on the site: demonstration by defining an immunodominant T site in myoglobin, *Biochemical Journal* **240**: 139–46

David C S, Atassi M Z 1982. Genetic control and intersite influences on the immune response to sperm whale myoglobin, *Advances in Experimental Medicine and Biology* **150**: 97–126

Kazim A L. Atassi M Z 1980. A novel and comprehensive synthetic approach for the elucidation of protein antigenic structures: determination of the full antigenic profile of the alpha chain of human hemoglobin, *Biochemical Journal* **191**: 261–4

Kazim, A L, Atassi M Z 1982. Structurally inherent antigenic sites. Localization of the antigenic sites of the alpha chain of human hemoglobin in three host species by a comprehesive synthetic approach, *Biochemical Journal* **203**: 201–8

Krco C J, Kazim A L, Atassi M Z, David C S 1981. Genetic control of the immune response to hemoglobin. I. Separate genetic control of the A and B subunits of human hemoglobin and the influence of the H-2D end by *in vitro* lymphocyte proliferative response, *Journal of Immunogenetics* **8**: 315–22

Kurisaki J, Atassi H, Atassi M Z 1986. T cell recognition of Ragweed allergen Ra3: Localization of the full T-cell profile by synthetic overlapping peptides representing the entire protein chain, *European Journal of Immunology* **16**: 236–40

LaPresle C 1955. Etude de la degradation de la serum-albumine humaine par un extrait de rate de lapin. I. Conditions optimum d'activite et mode d'action des proteases de la rate du lapin, *Bulletin de la Société de Chemie Biologique (Paris)* **37**: 969–75

Lee C L, Atassi M Z 1976. Enzymic and immunochemical properties of lysozyme. XVII. Delineation of the third antigenic site of lysozyme by application of a novel 'surface-simulation'

69

synthetic approach directly linking the conformationally-adjacent residues forming the site, *Biochemical Journal* **159**: 89–93

Okuda K, Christadoss P, Twining S S, Atassi M Z, David C S 1978. Genetic control of the immune response to sperm whale myoglobin in mice. I. T-lymphocyte proliferative response under H-2-linked Ir gene control, *Journal of Immunology* **121**: 866–8

Okuda K, Twining S S, David C S, Atassi M Z 1979. Genetic control of the immune response to sperm-whale myoglobin in mice. II. T-lymphocyte proliferative response to the synthetic antigenic sites, *Journal of Immunology* **123**: 182–8

Porter R R 1957. The isolation and properties of a fragment of bovine-serum albumin which retains the ability to combine with rabbit antiserum, *Biochemical Journal* **66**: 677–86

Twining S S, David C S, Atassi M Z 1981. Genetic control of the immune response to myoglobin. IV. Mouse antibodies in outbred and congenic strains against sperm whale myoglobin recognize the same antigenic sites that are recognized by antibodies raised in other species. *Molecular Immunology* **18**: 447–50

Yoshioka N, Atassi M Z 1983. Localization of the antigenic sites on the beta chain of human hemoglobin by a comprehensive synthetic peptide approach, *Abstracts 5th International Congress of Immunology, Kyoto, Japan* **232**: 0023

Yoshioka N, Atassi M Z 1986. Antigenic structure of human haemoglobin: Localization of the antigenic sites of the beta chain in three host species by synthetic overlapping peptides representing the entire chain, *Biochemical Journal* **234**: 441–7

Yoshioka M, Yoshioka N, Atassi M Z 1986. T-cell recognition of human haemoglobin: Localization of the full T-cell recognition profile of the beta chain by a comprehensive synthetic strategy, *Biochemical Journal* **234**: 449–52

Young C R, Atassi M Z 1982. Dissection of the molecular parameters for T cell recognition of a myoglobin antigenic site, *Advances in Experimental Medicine* **150**: 79–93

3 Antigen identification and purification

Lipopolysaccharides, the O antigens and endotoxins of Gram-negative bacteria: Relationships of chemical structure and biological activity

Otto Lüderitz; Chris Galanos; Hubert Mayer; Ernst Th Rietschel

Max-Planck-Institut für Immunbiologie, Stübeweg 51, D-78 Freiburg, and Forschungsinstitut Borstel, D-2061 Borstel, Federal Republic of Germany

Introduction

Lipopolysaccharide (LPS) is an amphipathic macromolecule forming an essential constituent of the outer membrane of the Gram-negative bacterial cell. Interest in this compound originated many decades ago when it was recognized that it represents the main heat-stable antigen, the O antigen, of Gram-negative bacteria and is, at the same time, the endotoxin of these bacteria. As such it is an important factor in pathogenicity, being responsible for many pathophysiological effects accompanying Gram-negative infection.

LPSs of different Gram-negative bacteria are constructed according to a common general architecture. They consist of a hydrophilic polysaccharide region and a hydrophobic lipid, the lipid A. The polysaccharide can be subdivided into the O-specific polysaccharide and the core oligosaccharide (Fig. 1).

The present review will discuss structural features of the LPS molecule, its

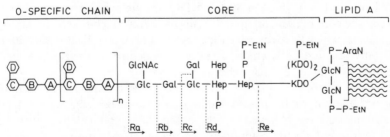

Figure 1. General structure of a *Salmonella* LPS. Key: A–D, sugar residues; Gal, D-galactose; Glc, D-glucose; GlcN, D-glucosamine; GlcNAc, N-acetyl-D-glucosamine; Hep, L-glycero-D-*manno*-heptose; KDO, 2-keto-3-deoxy-D-*manno*-octonate; AraN, 4-amino-L-arabinose; P, phosphate; EtN, ethanolamine; ~, hydroxy and nonhydroxy fatty acids; Ra to Re, incomplete R-form LPS.

antigenic properties, and first insights into the structure/activity relationships of lipid A.

Structure of lipopolysaccharides

The O-specific chains of LPS consist, in general, of repeating units of identical oligosaccharides (Lüderitz *et al.* 1982). The number of repeating units, and consequently the length of the chains in an LPS preparation, express great variability (from 0 to more than 30 repeating units) (Tsai and Frash 1982). In some bacteria O chains may be formed by a homopolysaccharide (*E. coli* O8 and O9, *Citrobacter*, *Yersinia*), in others very short O chains comprising not more than a few sugar units may be present, or, in some cases, O chains are lacking (Jann and Jann 1984; Hitchcock *et al.* 1986). These latter lipopolysaccharides resemble R mutant LPSs which are discussed below.

The O chains contain the immunodeterminant structures which define the immunological O specificity of LPSs and the parental bacterial strain. The great advances in the technology of carbohydrate analysis have led to the elucidation of more than 100 O chain structures including many from clinically relevant Gram-negative pathogens (see Lüderitz *et al.* 1983). Increasing numbers of new sugar classes are being identified as well as unusual sugar combinations.

In contrast to the O chains, the core structures of Enterobacteriaceae exhibit a lower degree of diversity. They are more uniform in composition and structure (Jann and Jann 1984). The outer core region usually contains hexoses (e.g. *N*-acetyl-D-glucosamine, D-glucose, and D-galactose) while the inner region consists of unusual sugars which are specific for many core types, i.e. L-*glycero*-D-*manno*-heptose (Hep) and 2-keto-3-deoxy-D-*manno*-octonoate (KDO), both being constituents widely found among serotypes of Gram-negative bacteria (see Fig. 1). However, core types with quite different composition and structural features have also been identified (Lüderitz *et al.* 1982; Kotelko 1986). Even in these a KDO residue appears to form the link between the core region and lipid A. This has been concluded from methylation analyses which have revealed the presence of KDO or KDO-like material in all reinvestigated LPSs which had previously been described as lacking this constituent (Brade 1985; Rietschel *et al.* 1985).

In the inner core ionic groups, such as the amino groups of ethanolamine, phosphoryl and pyrophosphoryl residues and the carboxyl groups of KDO, are accumulated. It is believed that these, together with bivalent cations, play a role in interlinking the components of the outer membrane.

For structural and biological studies the so-called R mutants proved to be of great value. These mutants have a defect in the biosynthesis of LPS and, therefore, synthesize incomplete LPS. Depending on the defective biosynthetic step, they lack the O chains (Ra-form LPSs) or the O chains and parts of the core (Rb- through Re-form LPSs). The most defective R-form LPSs are synthesized by Re mutants; they contain only KDO and lipid A (see Fig. 1). With the aid of such defective LPSs, core structures have been successfully evaluated. It is, however, only very recently that the linkages of the KDO oligosaccharide in the core of enterobacteria have been definitely determined as those shown in Fig. 1 (H Brade *et al.* 1985; Rietschel *et al.* 1985).

Structural investigations of lipid A have been preferentially performed on Re-form LPSs because of their high content of lipid A. Lipid A has been found to represent an unusual phospholipid. It contains a central hydrophilic backbone of a bisphosphorylated β-1,6-linked D-glucosamine disaccharide (Fig. 2). One phosphate group is ester-linked to the hydroxyl group at C4' of the non-reducing glucosamine (GlcNII), the other one is linked to C1 of GlcNI by an α-glycosidic linkage (Gmeiner *et al.* 1969). In *Salmonella*, these phosphate groups are substituted in submolar amounts by 4-amino-L-arabino-β-pyranose (Batley *et al.* 1982) and phosphorylethanolamine, respectively (Fig. 2) (Strain *et al.* 1985). The backbone carries fatty acyl residues which confer the lipophilic properties to the molecule. The amino groups of GlcNI and GlcNII are substituted by (*R*)-3-hydroxytetradecanoic acid (3-OH-14:0), that of GlcNII carrying dodecanoic (12:0), that of GlcNI is partly substituted by hexadecanoic acid (16:0). The two hydroxyl groups at C3 and C3' of the backbone are also substituted by 3-OH-14:0 residues with that at C3' carrying tetradecanoic acid (14:0) which is partly oxidized to (S)-2-OH-14:0. The hydroxyl group at C4 is free and that at C6' represents the attachment point of the core (Rietschel *et al.* 1983, 1984; Strain *et al.* 1983; Takayama *et al.* 1983).

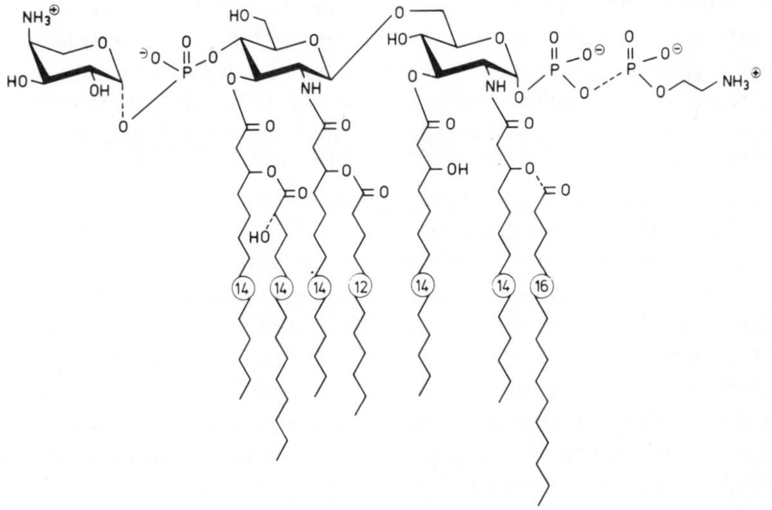

Figure 2. Structure of lipid A of *Salmonella minnesota* Re mutant (Rietschel *et al.* 1984). Broken lines indicate incomplete substitution. KDO is linked to the primary hydroxyl group in position 6'. Numbers in circles indicate the number of carbon atoms in the acyl chains.

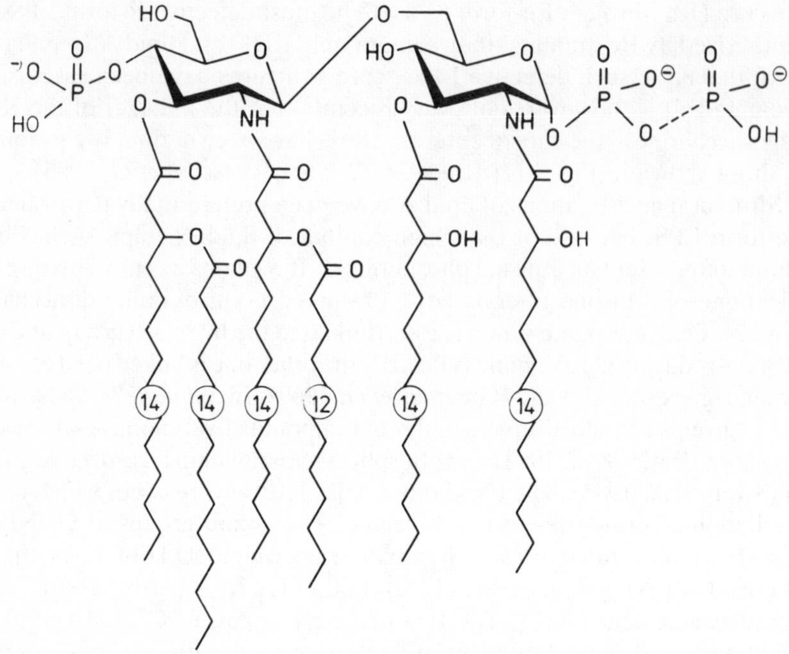

Figure 3. Structure of lipid A of *E. coli* O8 Re. (see Rietschel *et al.* 1984). For explanations see Fig. 2.

Similarly to O chains and core, lipid A also exhibits microheterogeneity due to incomplete substitutions of the backbone. In the mixture of structurally related compounds, the hepta-acyl compound of Fig. 4d probably represents a most completed species and a main fraction for most cultivation batches.

In recent years a number of lipid As from different enterobacteria and other bacterial families have been investigated. The most simple structure has been found in the lipid A of *E. coli* (Fig. 3; Rosner *et al.* 1979). The backbone is partially substituted by a phosphate group and by six acyl residues, i.e. four moles of 3-OH-14:0 and one mole each of 12:0 and 14:0 (Rietschel *et al.* 1984). This lipid A represents a hexa-acyl compound.

Structural studies on lipid A received great impulses when temperature-dependent KDO mutants were isolated from *Salmonella*. These mutants were found to stop LPS synthesis when shifted to the non-permissive temperature. They still underwent one or two divisions in the absence of KDO synthesis, but then terminated growth (Walenga and Osborn 1980; Galanos *et al.* 1985a). Analysis of such cells revealed the presence of incomplete lipid A molecules. Lipid A precursor Ia contains the bisphosphorylated glucosamine disaccharide backbone substituted by four 3-OH-14:0 residues in the same positions as in complete lipid A (C2, C3, C2′, C3′); it lacks KDO and the non-hydroxylated acyl residues. Lipid A precursor Ib has the same basal structure, but contains an additional mole of 16:0 linked to the 3-OH of

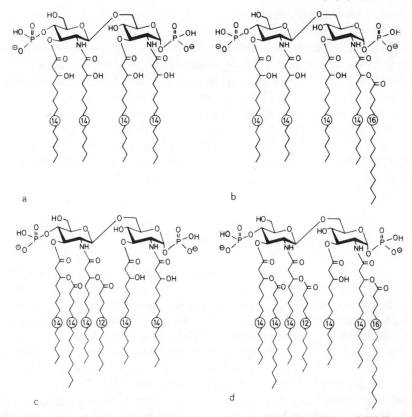

Figure 4. Compounds whose chemical synthesis has been performed (Shiba and Kusumoto 1984): a and b, lipid A precursors Ia and Ib, respectively; c, hexa-acyl compound of *E. coli* lipid A; d, hepta-acyl compound of *Salmonella* lipid A. For explanations see Fig. 2.

the hydroxy fatty acid at C2 (Fig. 4). Lipid A precursor II molecules are related to precursor Ia and Ib, and contain additional polar head groups, phosphorylethanolamine, or 4-aminoarabinose, or both (Raetz *et al.* 1985).

Finally, mutants defective in early steps of lipid A biosynthesis have been isolated. They make monomeric incomplete lipid A molecules representing di- and tri-acylglucosamine-1-phosphates, lipid X and lipid Y (Raetz 1984).

Similarly to the R mutants, the KDO- and lipid A-defective mutants have provided the basis for an understanding of the biosynthetic pathways of the early steps in LPS and lipid A biosynthesis (Raetz 1984; Walenga and Osborn 1980; Lehmann and Hansen-Hagge 1984).

From the results of studies on various endotoxic entero- and non-enterobacterial lipid As, general architectural principles regarding many lipid A structures have become obvious. These common structural features include the bisphosphorylated β-1,6-linked D-glucosamine disaccharide, its frequent substitutions at the phosphoryl residues by polar head groups, and the presence of ester- and amide-linked (R)-3-hydroxyacyl or (R)-3-acyloxyacyl residues. The lipid As may differ in the amount and identity of polar head groups, and in the number, chain length and type of acyl residues.

The molecules of Fig. 4 are main fractions in the heterogenous mixtures of the natural preparations. They represent tetra-, penta-, hexa-, and hepta-acyl compounds of the same basic structure, and hence express increasing lipophilic properties. Recently, their total chemical synthesis has been performed. In all respects (TLC, IR, NMR), the synthetic and natural products proved to be identical, thus confirming the elaborated structures (Shiba and Kusumoto 1984).

Antigen determinants of lipopolysaccharides

In wild-type S-form LPS all three regions, i.e. the O chains, the core and lipid A, contain immunodeterminant structures, but only those present on the O chains are fully expressed. These O chain determinants specify the O factors which characterize each serotype and which form the basis of immunological classifications, e.g. the Kauffmann–White scheme of *Salmonella*.

For a number of clinically relevant Gram-negative bacteria and pathogens, the O factor determining structures or the immunodominant substructures have been identified (Jann and Jann 1984). Recently, O factors or part structures thereof have been chemically synthesized. Thus, O-specific artificial antigens and immunogens have been constructed which make available highly specific antisera valuable for use in clinical diagnosis (Lüderitz *et al.* 1983).

The immunodetermining structures residing in the core are essentially cryptic as long as they are present in internal positions of the sugar chain. They are fully expressed, however, in the R-form LPSs (Ra to Re). These R-form LPSs contain different core sugars as non-reducing end groups; these function as immunodeterminants and confer the respective R specificities (Lüderitz *et al.* 1983).

Only limited cross-reactivity exists between LPSs belonging to different R-types or the corresponding R mutants. Nevertheless, it is often useful to purify R antibodies; this can be achieved with the aid of immunoadsorbents which have been prepared from hydrazine-treated R-form LPSs. Marked cross-reactions are often seen between R LPSs (or R mutants) belonging to the same R-type but deriving from different bacterial genera or families. This is due to the fact that core types of different bacteria often contain closely related structures, particularly in the inner core region (Jann and Jann 1984). In this context, a recent observation of interest is that *Chlamydia trachomatis* LPS resembles Re mutant LPS in composition by containing KDO and lipid A (Nurminen *et al.* 1985) as well as in the ability to exhibit pronounced cross-reactivity with Re-form LPSs of enterobacteria, in addition to a unique *Chlamydia* specificity (L Brade *et al.* 1985).

Recently, a new antigenic determinant has been discovered to be present in LPS of all Gram-negative bacteria tested so far with the exception of Re-form LPS (Brade and Brade 1985b). In some LPSs this new common specificity is cryptic, in others it is well expressed. Thus, *Acinetobacter calcoaceticus* anti-serum was the first source of antibodies against the new antigenic deter-minant. In LPS where the new specificity is cryptic, it becomes unmasked and reactive with the *Acinetobacter* antiserum after controlled hydrolysis with mild acid. This treatment liberates the KDO disaccharide of the core side chain but leaves intact the linkages of the main core oligosaccharide chain. At this stage, lipid A antigenicity is still hidden. It is assumed that the new specificity is determined by the KDO residue in the main chain substituted in position 5. Human and animal sera naturally contain a protein which exhibits specificity for the new antigen. The biological significance of this protein is at present not known.

The cryptic antigenic determinants of lipid A, as present in LPS, are unmasked in the free lipid A obtained from LPS after mild acid hydrolysis. Free lipid A is immunogenic, especially when combined with a suitable carrier, such as the bacterial cell or erythrocytes, or when incorporated into liposomes, or as a conjugate containing active lipid A fragments coupled to a protein. Anti-lipid A antibodies are estimated by the passive hemolysis test or by enzyme-linked immunosorbent assays (ELISA) (Galanos *et al.* 1984b).

Due to the close structural relationships among lipid As of Enterobacter-iaceae and other families, pronounced antigenic cross-reactions are seen. The antibodies do not generally react with LPS-bound lipid A (but see Kasai *et al.* 1985).

At least two antigenic specificities are exposed in free lipid A (Brade and Brade 1985a). They are related to the phosphate groups of the backbone. Ester-linked fatty acids do not play a role in specificity, but at least one amide-bound fatty acid as well as the free primary hydroxyl group at position 6' seem to be important structural elements required for antigenicity. Cer-tainly, synthetic lipid A immunogens and antigens will soon reveal further prerequisites for lipid A antigenicity.

It is noteworthy that anti-lipid A antibodies occur naturally in animals and humans. Their increased levels in patients with certain Gram-negative infec-tions indicate that under special natural conditions lipid A determinants become sufficiently exposed to express immunogenicity. This is also true for R-form antibodies which are found in normal sera.

Under defined conditions, anti-lipid A antisera suppress pyrogenicity and inhibit the local Shwartzman reaction in rabbits, and protect mice from the abortive effects of endotoxin. Active or passive immunization failed to pro-tect mice from the lethal effects of endotoxin (Galanos *et al.* 1984b).

Anti-R and anti-lipid A antibodies are directed against structures common

Table 1 Biological activities of lipid A and natural and synthetic lipid A precursors Ia

Preparation	Biological test systems									
	Lethal toxicity	Pyrotoxicity	Endotoxin tolerance	Local Schwartzman reaction	Anti-tumor activity	Limulus gelation activity	Mitogenicity (B cells)	Induction of prostaglandin synthesis	Anti C' activity	Antigenicity
Precursor Ia										
Natural	++	+	++	–	++	++	++	++	–	++
Synthetic	++	+	++	–	++	++	++	++	–	++
E. coli lipid A	++	++	++	++	++	++	++	++	++	++

Source: Galanos *et al.* (1984a).

to most LPSs and seem to react with them at least to some extent *in vivo*. Thus rabbit and human antisera against *E. coli* Rc and Re LPSs are capable of cross-protecting mice infected with *E. coli*, *Klebsiella* or *Pseudomonas* bacteria (Braude *et al.* 1977; McCabe *et al.* 1977). Clinical trials have also been made (Baumgartner *et al.* 1985).

Structure/activity relationships: studies with synthetic compounds

The first lipid A analogs were synthesized about four years ago, when the exact positions of the ester-linked fatty acids on the backbone had not yet been identified (Shiba and Kusumoto 1984). These preparations, therefore, contained acyl or acyloxyacyl residues at arbitrary positions (at positions 2, 3, 4, 2' and 6'). All the preparations, after alkali treatment, exhibited pronounced lipid A antigenicity, and some of them displayed typical endotoxic effects, especially those containing acyloxyacyl groups. The effective doses, however, were about 100 to 1000 times higher than natural lipid A. Some preparations were found to be toxic, but devoid of pyrogenicity, and vice versa. *Limulus* activity was absent from all preparations. In contrast to natural lipid A, most synthetic preparations were insoluble in water and, under these conditions, inactive. After the introduction of carboxyl groups into the molecule by succinylation, they became soluble and some of them more active, including preparations devoid of phosphate (Tanamoto *et al.* 1984).

Lipid A precursor Ia represents an incomplete lipid A of relatively simple structure (tetra-acyl compound; see Fig. 4a). Since it exhibits endotoxic activities, it was chosen as the first target for chemical synthesis. Natural and synthetic precursors Ia were tested in parallel in a number of biological test systems and were found to exhibit identical activities (Table 1). Compared to lipid A, they were of similar antigenicity, toxicity, mitogenicity and effectiveness in inducing endotoxin cross-tolerance and prostaglandin synthesis. They were, however, of low pyrogenicity, devoid of anticomplementary activity and unable to induce or provoke the local Shwartzman phenomenon (Galanos *et al.* 1984a).

In one biological assay synthetic and natural precursors Ia differed. While the synthetic preparation did not express mitogenicity with spleen cells derived from the LPS-nonresponder mouse strain C3H/HeJ, natural precursor Ia proved to be highly effective. It could be shown that the natural precursor was contaminated by a product whose removal by thin-layer chromatography abolished this activity. The contaminant, if it is a bacterial protein, must be a very effective mitogen, at least in combination with precursor Ia, since preparations containing less than 1 % protein were still highly active (Galanos *et al.* 1986).

Precursor Ib represents a penta-acyl compound and, thus, holds a position between precursor Ia and *E. coli* lipid A (see Fig. 4). It was found that natural and synthetic precursors Ib were strongly active in expressing local Shwartzman reactivity (Galanos *et al.* 1985a). A synthetic isomer of precursor Ib which contained the 3-O(16:0)-14:0 residue linked to the amino group of GlcNII also exhibited strong Shwartzman reactivity (Galanos *et al.* 1986). It is concluded that not a specific position of 16:0 but rather the increase in hydrophobicity renders the molecule Shwartzman-reactive.

Finally, the chemical syntheses of *E. coli* and *Salmonella* lipid A have been achieved (Fig. 4). Table 2 shows the results of biological tests performed with the synthetic and natural preparations. Synthetic *E. coli* lipid A presents itself as a potent endotoxin indistinguishable from natural *E. coli* and *Salmonella* lipid A. The synthetic hepta-acyl compound, expressing the structure of a main fraction in natural *Salmonella* lipid A, is less active (pyrogenicity, Shwartzman reactivity), although in some tests it exhibits strong activity (lethality in GalN mice, *Limulus* gelation activity, mitogenicity), thus resembling the tetra-acyl compound (Galanos *et al.* 1985b, 1986).

Compounds corresponding to those of Fig. 4 but lacking one or both phosphate groups were also synthesized and tested for their biological activity. The synthetic compounds corresponding to precursor Ia lacking a phosphoryl group at either position 1 or position 4' proved to express, according to the test system, similar or diminished activities compared to the bisphosphoryl compound. In the case of the more lipophilic synthetic *E. coli* preparation, the monophosphoryl compounds were less soluble and these preparations showed significantly reduced endotoxic activities. Synthetic precursor Ia and *E. coli* lipid A lacking both phosphoryl groups were insoluble in water and biologically inactive (Galanos *et al.* 1984a; Kotani *et al.* 1985; Homma *et al.* 1985).

Analogs corresponding to the monomeric lipid A precursors X and Y have also been synthesized and tested for biological activities. Such compounds were found to exhibit lethal toxicity in GalN mice, *Limulus* gelation, tumor-necrotizing activities and low pyrogenicity (Matsuura *et al.* 1985).

As far as we know today, all Gram-negative bacteria contain LPS. Not every LPS, however, is an endotoxin. Especially in the group of photosynthetic bacteria, increasing numbers of LPSs are being identified which contain stucturally 'unusual' lipid A devoid of endotoxicity (Weckesser *et al.* 1979; Mayer and Weckesser 1984).

From the available data initial concepts concerning structure/activity relationships can be anticipated:

1. The polar head groups of lipid A do not contribute directly to activity, although they may increase solubility.
2. The role of phosphoryl groups is not clear, though through decreasing hydrophobicity they render the molecule water-soluble. Whether there is also a direct influence of phosphate on activity cannot be decided at this time.

Table 2 Biological activities of synthetic and natural *E. coli* and *Salmonella* lipid A

Preparation	Biological test systems								
	Lethality	Pyrogenicity	Local Shwartzman reaction	Limulus gelation activity	Anti-tumor activity	Endotoxin tolerance	Mitogenicity (B cells)	Induction of prostaglandin synthesis	Antigenicity
E. coli lipid A.									
Natural	++	++	++	++	++	++	++	++	++
Synthetic*	++	++	++	++	++	++	++	++	++
Salmonella lipid A									
Natural	++	++	++	++	++	++	++	++	++
Synthetic†	+	+	–	++	n.t.	n.t.	++	+	++

Source: Galanos *et al.* 1985b, 1986.
* Hexa-acyl compound.
† Hepta-acyl compound.
n.t. not tested.

83

3. The acylated backbone is important for activity and the smallest structure retaining activity is the tetra-acylated backbone represented by lipid A precursor Ia, which exhibits lethality, *Limulus* activity, mitogenicity, antigenicity, weak pyrogenicity, but no Shwartzman activity.

4. Loss of ester-linked fatty acids results in inactivity. The nature and location of the fatty acids on the backbone seem to be critical prerequisites for activity.

5. From results obtained with synthetic analogs and with *Rhodocyclus tenuis* LPS it is concluded that position 4 of GlcNI should be free. Whether 3-hydroxy fatty acids and their natural (*R*) configuration are important has not yet been investigated.

6. For pyrogenicity and Shwartzman reactivity at least one acyloxyacyl residue, but not more than two, seem to be important in order to create the critical lipophilic properties of the molecule.

7. Lipid A antigenicity is retained in preparations deprived of phosphate and ester-linked fatty acids. Recently, two distinct specificities have been identified with the aid of polyclonal anti-lipid A antibodies; their determinant structure is still unknown, but phosphate groups are clearly involved.

8. Certain biological lipid A effects seem to be separable as natural and synthetic preparations have been encountered which do not express the whole spectrum of activities. Thus, an independent expression of toxicity, Shwartzman reactivity, pyrogenicity, *Limulus* activity and mitogenicity has occasionally been found.

A number of nontoxic LPS containing lipid A of unusual structure have been identified. These nontoxic lipid As have been grouped tentatively as follows (Mayer and Weckesser 1984): lipid A may contain a sugar substituent glycosidically linked to position 4 of GlcNI or 4' of GlcNII (*Rhodocyclus tenuis, Rhodomicrobium vannielii*); the usual amide-bound 3-hydroxy fatty acid is partly or completely replaced by a 3-oxo fatty acid (*Rhodobacter sphaeroides, Rh. capsulata*); the lipid A backbone is devoid of phosphate groups (*Rhodomicrobium vannielii, Rhodopseudomonas acidophila, Chromatium vinosum, Thiocapsa roseopersicina*); the usual lipid A backbone is replaced by a diaminohexose, 2,3-diamino-D-glucose (*Rhodopseudomonas viridis, Rh. sulfoviridis, Rh. palustris, Pseudomonas diminuta, Ps. vesicularis, Nitrobacter hamburgensis, N. winogradskyi*).

Perspectives

Old endotoxin is still attractive, feared and beloved, with ever-new attributes being discovered, iridescent in unexpected different copies expressing different properties. The fantasy of the bacteria to work out a common architectural principle for endotoxin, to accept it, and to modulate it to an almost unbelievable diversity of stuctures, to use old and to invent new pathways for synthesizing usual and very unusual building blocks and to arrange them to very complicated molecules which fulfill the physiological function for the cell – this will continue to fascinate scientists of many disciplines and occupy them for years to come.

In many respects, the direction of future endotoxin research will be determined by the efforts made in research and industry on the chemical synthesis of lipid A, its partial structures and analogs, thus utilizing the harvest of analytical work of the past and future. As a result, pure, uniform determinants should be placed at the disposal of the researchers in biology, immunology and medicine. These studies will lead to a recognition of minimal essential structures of lipid A responsible for distinct activities.

Many open questions and interesting problems for future endotoxin research have been discussed in the numerous reviews of the past; some have been resolved (see Westphal *et al.* 1986). Protection against Gram-negative infections with specific antibodies against common LPS determinants (core, lipid A), the molecular basis of endotoxin/cell interaction and the mechanisms of cell stimulation, the fate of endotoxin in the higher organism, its role in infection, the search for lipid A substructures or derivatives which express beneficial and are devoid of fatal endotoxic effects – these are some of the old goals. But as more synthetic compounds become available the approaches of tomorrow will probably change. New fields of endotoxin research will then be entered.

Acknowledgement

We would like to thank H Kochanowski, L Lay and R Brugger for the preparation of the manuscript.

References

Batley M, Packer N H, Redmond J W 1982. Configurations of glycosidic phosphates of lipopolysaccharide from *S. minnesota* R595, *Biochemistry* **22**: 6580–6

Baumgartner J D, Glauser M P, McCutchan J A, Ziegler E J, van Melle G, Kaluber M R, Vogt M, Miehl Muehlen E, Leuthy R, Chiolero R, Geroulanos S 1985. Prevention of Gram-negative shock and death in surgical patients by antibody to endotoxin core glycolipid, *The Lancet* **8446**: 59–63

Brade H 1985. The occurrence of 2-keto-3-deoxyoctonic acid-5-phosphate in lipopolysaccharide of *Vibrio cholerae Ogawa* and *Inaba*, *Journal of Bacteriology* **161**: 795–8

Brade H, Moll H, Rietschel E Th 1985. Structural investigations on the inner core region of lipopolysaccharides from *Salmonella minnesota* rough mutants. *Biomedical Mass Spectrometry* **12**: 602–9

Brade L, Brade H 1985a. Characterization of two different antibody specificities recognizing distinct antigenic determinants in free lipid A of *Escherichia coli*, *Infection and Immunity* **48**: 776–81

Brade L, Brade H 1985b. A 28 000-Dalton protein of normal mouse serum binds specifically to the inner core region of bacterial lipopolysaccharide, *Infection and Immunity* **50**: 687–94

Brade L, Nurminen M, Mäkelä P H, Brade H 1985. Antigenic properties of *Chlamydia trachomatis* lipopolysaccharide, *Infection and Immunity* **48**: 569–72

Braude A I, Ziegler E J, Douglas H, McCutchan J A 1977. Protective properties of antisera to R core, *Microbiology* **1977**: 253–6

Galanos C, Lehmann V, Lüderitz O, Rietschel E Th, Westphal O, Brade H, Brade L, Freudenberg M A, Hansen-Hagge T, Lüderitz Th, McKenzie G, Schade U, Strittmater W, Yamamoto M, Shimamoto T, Kusumoto S, Shiba T 1984a. Endotoxic properties of chemically synthesized lipid A part structures. Comparison of synthetic lipid A precursor and synthetic analogues with biosynthetic lipid A precursor and free lipid A. *European Journal of Biochemistry* **140**: 221–7

Galanos C, Freudenberg M A, Jay F, Nerkar D, Veleva K, Brade H, Strittmatter W 1984b. Immunogenic properties of lipid A, *Review of Infectious Diseases* **6**: 546–52

Galanos C, Hansen-Hagge T, Lehmann V, Lüderitz O 1985a. Comparison of the capacity of two lipid A precursor molecules to express the local Shwatzman phenomenon, *Infection and Immunity* **48**: 355–8

Galanos C, Lüderitz O, Rietschel E Th, Westphal O, Brade H, Brade L, Freudenberg M, Schade U, Imoto M, Yoshimura H, Kusumoto S, Shiba T 1985b. Synthetic and natural *Escherichia coli* free lipid A express identical endotoxic activities, *European Journal of Biochemistry* **148**: 1–5

Galanos C, Lüderitz O, Freudenberg M, Brade L, Schade U, Rietschel E Th, Kusumoto S, Shiba T 1986. Biological activity of synthetic heptaacyl lipid A representing a component of *Salmonella minnesota* R595 lipid A, *European Journal of Biochemistry* **160**: 55–9

Gmeiner J, Lüderitz O, Westphal O 1969. Biochemical studies on lipopolysaccharides of *Salmonella* R mutants 6. Investigations on the structure of the lipid A component, *European Journal of Biochemistry* **7**: 370–9

Hitchcock P J, Leive L, Mäkelä P H, Rietschel E Th, Strittmatter W, Morrison D C A 1986. Review of lipopolysaccharide nomenclature past, present and future, *Journal of Bacteriology* **166**: 699–705

Homma J, Matsuura M, Kanegasaki S, Kawakubo Y, Kojima Y, Shibukawa N, Kumazawa Y, Yamamoto A, Tanamotot K, Yasuda T, Imoto M, Yoshimura H, Kusumoto S, Shiba T 1985. Structural requirements of lipid A responsible for the functions: A study with chemically synthesized lipid A and its analogues, *Journal of Biochemistry* **98**: 395–406

Jann K, Jann B 1984. Structure and biosynthesis of O-antigens, in E Th Rietschel (ed) *Handbook of Endotoxin: Chemistry of endotoxin*. Elsevier Science Publishers, Amsterdam, vol 1, pp 138–86

Kasai N, Arata S, Mashimo J, Okuda K, Aihara Y, Kotani S, Takada H, Shiba T, Kusumoto S 1985. *In vitro* antigenic reactivity of synthetic lipid A analogues as determined by monoclonal and conventional antibodies, *Biochemical and Biophysical Research Communications* **128**: 607–12

Kotani S, Takada H, Tsujimoto M, Ogawa T, Takahashi I, Ikeda T, Otsuka K, Shimauchi H, Kasai N, Mashimo J, Nagao S, Tanaka A, Tanaka S, Harada K, Shiba T, Kusumoto S, Imoto M, Yoshimura H 1985. Synthetic lipid A with endotoxic and related biological activities, comparable to a natural lipid A from *Escherichia coli* Re-mutant, *Infection and Immunity* **49**: 225–37

Kotelko K 1986. *Proteus mirabilis*: Taxonomic position, peculiarities of growth, components of the cell envelope, in *Current Topics in Microbiology and Immunology* **129**: 181–215

Lehmann V, Hansen-Hagge T 1984. Late steps in lipid A synthesis–structure and properties of lipid A intermediates isolated from lipid A mutants, in E Th Rietschel (ed) *Handbook of Endotoxin: Chemistry of endotoxin*. Elsevier Science Publishers, Amsterdam, vol 1, pp 269–83

Lüderitz O, Freudenberg M A, Galanos C, Lehmann V, Rietschel E Th, Shaw D H 1982.

Lipopolysaccharides of Gram-negative Bacteria, in S Razin, S Rottem (eds) *Membrane Lipids of Prokaryotes* (*Current Topics in Membranes and Transport*). Academic Press Inc., New York, vol 17, pp 79–151

Lüderitz O, Tanamoto K, Galanos C, Westphal O, Zähringer U, Rietschel E Th, Kusumoto S, Shiba T 1983. Structural principles of lipopolysaccharides and biological properties of synthetic partial structures, *ACS Symposium Series* **231**: 3–17

Matsuura M, Yamamoto A, Kojima Y, Homma J Y, Kiso M, Hasegawa A 1985. Bilogical activities of chemically synthesized partial structure analogues of lipid A, *Journal of Biochemistry* **98**: 1229–37

Mayer, H, Weckesser J 1984. 'Unusual' lipid As: Structure, taxonomical relevance and potential value for endotoxin research, in E Th Rietschel (ed) *Handbook of Endotoxin: Chemistry of endotoxin*. Elsevier Science Publishers, Amsterdam, vol 1, pp 221–47

McCabe W R, Johns M A, Craven D E, Bruins S C 1977. Clinical implications of enterobacterial antigens, *Microbiology – 1977*: 293–7

Nurminen M, Rietschel E Th, Brade H 1985. Chemical characterization of *Chlamydia trachomatis* lipopolysaccharide, *Infection and Immunity* **48**: 573–5

Raetz C R H 1984. *Escherichia coli* mutants that allow elucidation of the precursors and biosynthesis of lipid A, in E Th Rietschel (ed) *Handbook of Endotoxin: Chemistry of endotoxin*. Elsevier Science Publishers, Amsterdam, vol 1, pp 248–68

Raetz C R H, Purcell S, Meyer M V, Qureshi N, Takayama K 1985. Isolation and characterization of eight lipid A precursors from a 3-deoxy-D-*manno*-octulosonic acid-deficient mutant of *Salmonella typhimurium*, *Journal of Biological Chemistry* **260**: 16080–8

Rietschel E Th, Sidorczyk Z, Zähringer U, Wollenweber H W, Lüderitz O 1983. Analysis of the primary structure of lipid A, in *Bacterial Lipopolysaccharides, Structure, Synthesis, and Biological Activities. ACS Symposium Series* **231**: 195–218

Rietschel E Th, Wollenweber H W, Brade H, Zähringer U, Lindner B, Seydel U, Bradaczek H, Barnickel G, Labischinski H, Giesbrecht P 1984. Structure and conformation of the lipid A component of lipopolysaccharides, in E Th Rietschel (ed) *Handbook of Endotoxin: Chemistry of endotoxin*. Elsevier Science Publishers, Amsterdam, vol 1, pp 187–220

Rietschel E Th, Brade H, Brade L, Kaca W, Kawahara K, Lindner B, Lüderitz T, Tomita T, Schade U, Seydel U, Zähringer U 1985. Newer Aspects of the chemical structure and biological activity of bacterial endotoxins, in J W Ten Cate, H R Bühler, A Stark, J Levin (eds) *Bacterial Endotoxins: Structure, biomedical significance and detection with the Limulus amoebocyte lysate test*. A R Liss Inc., New York, pp 31–50

Rosner M R, Khorana H G, Satterthwait A C 1979. The structure of lipopolysaccharide from a heptoseless mutant of *Escherichia coli* K12. II The application of ^{31}P NMR spectroscopy, *Journal of Biological Chemistry* **254**: 5918–25

Shiba T, Kusumoto S 1984. Chemical synthesis and biological activity of lipid A analogs, in E Th Rietschel (ed) *Handbook of Endotoxin: Chemistry of endotoxin*. Elsevier Science Publishers, Amsterdam, vol 1, pp 284–306

Strain S M, Fesik S W, Armitage I M 1983. Characterization of lipopolysaccharide from a heptoseless mutant of *Escherichia coli* by carbon 13 nuclear magnetic resonance, *Journal of Bilogical Chemistry* **258**: 2906–10

Strain S M, Armitage I M, Anderson L, Takayama K, Qureshi N, Raetz C R H 1985. Location of polar substituents and fatty acyl chains on lipid A precursors from a 3-deoxy-D-*manno*-octulosonic acid-deficient mutant of *Salmonella typhimurium*, *Journal of Biological Chemistry* **260**: 16089–98

Takayama K, Qureshi N, Mascagni P 1983. Complete structure of lipid A obtained from the lipopolysaccharide of the heptoseless mutant of *Salmonella typhimurium*, *Journal of Biological Chemistry* **258**: 12801–3

Tanamoto K, Zähringer U, McKenzie G R, Galanos C, Rietschel E Th, Lüderitz O, Kusumoto S, Shiba T 1984. Biological activities of synthetic lipid A analogs: pyrogenicity, lethal toxicity, anticomplement activity, and induction of gelation of *Limulus* amoebocyte lysate, *Infection and Immunity* **44**: 421–6

Tsai C M, Frasch C E 1982. A sensitive silver stain for detecting lipopolysaccharides in polyacrylamide gels, *Analytical Biochemistry* **119**: 115–19

Walenga R W, Osborn M J 1980. Biosynthesis of Lipid A. Formation of acyl-deficient lipopolysaccharide in *Salmonella typhimurium* and *Escherichia coli*, *Journal of Biological Chemistry* **255**: 4257–63

Weckesser J, Drews G, Mayer H 1979. Lipopolysaccharides of photosynthetic prokaryotes, *Annual Review of Microbiology* **33**: 215–39

Westphal O, Lüderitz O, Galanos C, Mayer H, Rietschel E Th 1986. The story of bacterial endotoxin, *Advances in Immunopharmacology* **3**: 13–34

Nontypable *Haemophilus influenzae*: A model for the development of vaccines to bacterial somatic antigens

Timothy F Murphy*†; M Bud Nelson*†; Kathleen C Dudas*; Linda C Bartos*; Michael A Apicella*·†

* *Division of Infectious Diseases, Department of Medicine and the*
† *Department of Microbiology School of Medicine, State University of New York at Buffalo, Buffalo, New York 14214, USA*

Introduction

Haemophilus influenzae type b is the most common cause of meningitis and acquired mental retardation in the United States. Prevention by vaccination has been the goal of public health authorities since Fothergill and Wright demonstrated the importance of bactericidal antibody in offering protection against the microbe. Since 1970 efforts have been directed at the development of a vaccine composed of the capsular b polysaccharide. Like meningococcal capsular polysaccharides, the *H. influenzae* type b polysaccharide is poorly immunogenic in the age group at greatest risk for infection, children between two months and two years of age. To circumvent this lack of immunogenicity recent efforts have focused on the development of a conjugate vaccine consisting of the b polysaccharide conjugated to protein carriers such as tetanus or diphtheria toxoid. These materials are now in the process of being tested in field trials to define immunogenicity and efficacy in this susceptible pediatric population.

The impetus to seek new antigens for vaccine application for *Haemophilus* infections has prompted investigators to search for other noncapsular surface antigens which might be potential targets for bactericidal antibody and be capable of generation of such antibody in young children. In addition, the recent observation that nontypable *H. influenzae* is a significant human pathogen with the potential to cause middle ear disease has extended this search to seek potential immunogens which might be effective in prevention of this frequent childhood illness as well as the most serious meningeal consequences of infection with encapsulated type b strains (Murphy and Apicella 1987).

When considering a bacterial antigen as a vaccine candidate, three major considerations must be raised: (1) it must be conserved among strains of the bacterial species whose disease one wishes to prevent; (2) it must be the 'right' antigen in that antibody generated to it will prevent the disease; and (3) it must be a 'good' immunogen in that these protective antibodies will be elicited in the population at risk and that these antibodies will persist for sufficient time to provide protection throughout the risk period. Using these criteria as aims, we have undertaken a study of the surface antigens of *H. influenzae* for a potential vaccine candidate with these characteristics.

Surface antigens of *H. influenzae*

Somatic antigens on the surface of *H. influenzae* include lipo-oligosaccharide (LOS), fimbriae and outer membrane proteins (OMPs). LOS is a complex macromolecule which likely plays an important role in pathogenesis. Although not yet excluded as a vaccine candidate, two lines of evidence suggest that LOS is not an optimal antigen for a vaccine. First, infants who suffer meningitis due to *H. influenzae* type b have antibodies to LOS at the time of infection, suggesting that antibody to LOS is not protective (Shenep *et al.* 1982). Second, LOS of *H. influenzae* shows antigenic heterogeneity indicating that antibody to LOS of one strain may not protect from infection by other strains (Apicella *et al.* 1985; Campagnari *et al.* 1987). Since antibody to LOS is important in protection from infection by numerous other Gram-negative bacteria, this observation with *H. influenzae* is somewhat surprising and therefore needs additional testing. Further study will clarify the role of LOS in the human immune response to infection and determine whether LOS antigens will be useful as vaccine components.

Fimbriae are hair-like extensions from the bacterial surface and are present in both type b and nontypable strains of *H. influenzae* (Apicella *et al.* 1984). Fimbriae function as adherence factors resulting in enhanced bacterial colonization of mucosal surfaces (Beachey 1981). Antibody to fimbriae can inhibit bacterial adherence, thereby preventing infection. Accordingly, fimbrial antigens can be considered as a possible vaccine candidate. Fimbriae from type b strains have been purified and characterized (Guerina *et al.* 1985; Stull *et al.* 1984). However, the role of fimbriae in the pathogenesis of *H. influenzae* is unclear (Kaplan *et al.* 1983; Sable *et al.* 1985). In order for fimbriae to be useful as a vaccine component, it will be necessary to identify common fimbrial antigens and determine whether such antigens will induce antibody which is protective.

Studies of the OMPs of *H. influenzae* have only recently been undertaken and in the last five years considerable understanding of the function, isolation and antigenicity of these proteins has been reached. Three major OMPs (P1, P2 and P5) are heterogeneous among strains and can be used as a basis of typing systems (Barenkamp *et al.* 1981; Murphy *et al.* 1983; Murphy and Apicella 1985). Antibodies to P2 of type b strains are protective in an infant rat model of meningitis (Munson *et al.* 1983). However, these protective antigens appear to be strain-specific. An OMP called P6 has been identified in strains of *H. influenzae*. P6 has a molecular weight of 16,600 daltons and possesses many characteristics which indicate it might be an effective vaccine.

Antigenic conservation of P6

The presence of P6 in the outer membrane of *H. influenzae* has been noted by several groups of investigators and has been the subject of recent investigation. P6 is present in all isolates of *H. influenzae* tested thus far, including typable and nontypable strains (Barenkamp *et al.* 1981; Loeb & Smith 1980; Murphy *et al.* 1983). The protein comprises a relatively small proportion of the total protein content of the outer membrane; estimates range from 1 to 5% of the outer membrane by weight (Munson and Granoff 1985; Murphy *et al.* 1986b).

Surface exposure is an important characteristic of a vaccine component because the antigen must be accessible to protective antibody. Several lines of evidence indicate that a portion of P6 is exposed on the surface of the bacterium: (1) monoclonal and polyclonal antibodies to P6 stain the whole organism by immunofluorescence (Munson and Granoff 1985); (2) absorbed antiserum immunoprecipitates the protein (Munson and Granoff 1985); (3) P6 is accessible to bactericidal antibody (Murphy *et al.* 1986b); and (4) antibody to P6 can be eluted from the surface of the intact bacterium (unpublished observation).

The protein is present in all strains and exposed on the surface of the organism. The next question one must address is whether the protein is antigenically conserved. For example, will immunizing with P6 from one strain produce strain-specific antibody, serotype-specific antibody, or antibody to all strains of *H. influenzae*? By monoclonal antibody analysis, we have demonstrated that P6 contains an epitope which is common to all strains of *H. influenzae* (Murphy *et al.* 1985). However, analysis with a monoclonal antibody allows one to draw conclusions only regarding the single determinant recognized by that antibody and not about the antigenic characteristics of the protein as a whole. Therefore, a series of experiments was designed to characterize the degree of antigenic heterogeneity or antigenic conservation of P6 among strains of *H. influenzae* (Murphy *et al.* 1986a).

First, individual rabbits were immunized with P6 isolated from two nontypable strains. These antisera were assayed by Western blot against 25 clinical isolates of nontypable *H. influenzae*. Both antisera contained antibodies to P6 of all 25 strains tested. The titer of antibody to the homologous P6 was similar in titer to P6 of the other strains. Second, two antisera raised to whole cells of two additional strains of nontypable *H. influenzae* contained antibody to P6 of all 25 strains by Western blot assay. Third, three monoclonal antibodies were developed from individual mice immunized with whole cells of three additional strains of nontypable *H. influenzae*. All three monoclonal antibodies recognized a determinant on all 25 strains. The isolates used in these experiments were recovered from a broad range of patients in diverse clinical settings from several cities in the United States. Prototype strains of all eight OMP subtypes (Murphy *et al.* 1983) and all six OMP serotypes (Murphy and Apicella 1985) were included among the 25 strains. These data indicate that P6 is a highly conserved antigen on the outer membrane of nontypable *H. influenzae*. The protein might be composed of multiple antigenic determinants which are common to many strains. Alternatively, P6 might contain an immunodominant determinant which is present on P6 of all strains.

P6 as a target for protective human antibody

Since the presence of bactericidal antibodies in serum is related to protection from infection due to *H. influenzae* type b (Fothergill and Wright 1933) and encapsulated meningococci (Goldschneider *et al.* 1969), there has been interest in studying bactericidal antibody to nontypable *H. influenzae* in serum. Indeed, there is evidence that bactericidal antibody is related to protection from otitis media caused by the bacterium. The absence of bactericidal antibody to a strain of nontypable *H. influenzae* in the sera of children is associated with susceptibility to otitis media due to nontypable *H. influenzae* (Shurin *et al.* 1980). Identifying surface structures which are targets of human bactericidal antibody would therefore direct efforts in vaccine development because such a structure might present a protective antigen.

Pooled normal human serum contains antibody to P6 of all 25 strains of nontypable *H. influenzae* described above (Murphy *et al.* 1986a). To assess the role of the protein as a target for human bactericidal antibody, P6 was isolated and coupled to an affinity column. Depleting normal human serum of antibodies to P6 by affinity chromatography resulted in reduced bactericidal activity of that serum for nontypable *H. influenzae*. Immunopurified antibodies to P6 from human serum were bactericidal. Finally, preincubation of bacteria with a monoclonal antibody which recognizes a surface epitope on P6 inhibited human serum bactericidal killing. Taken together, these experiments establish that P6 is a target for human bactericidal antibodies (Murphy *et al.* 1986b).

This observation provides evidence that P6 plays an important role in human immunity to infection by nontypable *H. influenzae* and might represent a protective antigen. Additional data implicating P6 as a potentially protective antigen comes from the observation that antibody to P6 protects infant rats from meningitis due to *H. influenzae* type b (Munson and Granoff 1985). It will be important to determine whether antibodies to P6 are indeed protective and, if so, whether the determinants on P6 to which protective antibodies are directed are conserved among strains. Once these determinants are identified, it would be feasible to develop a protein vaccine to prevent infections due to nontypable *H. influenzae*. In addition, a conjugate vaccine which includes P6 might be effective in preventing infections caused by strains of *H. influenzae* type b.

Cloning the P6 gene

To assess further the potential of P6 as a vaccine, it would be useful to have a large amount of the protein to study. In addition, if P6 proves to be effective as a vaccine component, a practical method for producing large amounts of the protein will be necessary. Since P6 comprises only 1–5% of the outer membrane, purification of the protein from the organism is inefficient and these P6 preparations might contain other contaminating bacterial components. Recombinant DNA technology offers an effective strategy to produce large quantities of a protein vaccine molecule. *H. influenzae* genomic DNA fragments can be inserted in an expression vector that expresses the foreign DNA insert in *Escherichia coli*. The strategy has proven feasible for three higher molecular weight OMPs of *H. influenzae* (Thomas and Rossi 1986). Therefore, the method was employed to clone the gene which codes for P6 in *E. coli* using a lambda phage.

A phage library was constructed by isolating DNA from a strain of *H. influenzae*, mechanically shearing the DNA and packaging into λ gt 11 (Young *et al.* 1985). The phage were allowed to infect *E. coli* and the resulting plaques were immunologically screened using monoclonal and polyclonal antibodies to P6. After screening approximately 10^5 plaques, four clones were identified as expressing the P6 gene. A Western blot assay of one of the clones (clone 0) shows a band with characteristics identical to those of P6 in *H. influenzae*. The molecular weight is 16,600 daltons and the protein contains determinants recognized by two monoclonal antibodies which are highly specific for *H. influenzae*. The DNA insert in clone 0 is between two and three kilobases in size. Work is underway to sequence the P6 gene and to clone the gene into a suitable vector to express large quantities of the protein.

Summary

An outer membrane protein of *H. influenzae* referred to as P6 has been identified and characterized. The protein possesses several characteristics which indicate it may represent an effective vaccine: (1) the protein is present in all strains of *H. influenzae*; (2) P6 is surface-exposed; (3) it is antigenically conserved among strains; (4) P6 is a target for human bactericidal antibodies suggesting it is a protective antigen; (5) a protein is likely to be immunogenic in infants, the population at highest risk for *H. influenzae* meningitis; (6) the gene that codes for P6 can be cloned into lambda phage.

This will allow hyperexpression of the protein in *E. coli*. Future work will be directed at identifying the potentially protective determinants on P6.

Acknowledgements

The work detailed in this paper has been supported by NIAID grant AI19641. The authors wish to acknowledge the secretarial assistance of Ms Phyllis Rosenberg.

References

Apicella M A, Shero M, Dudas K C, Stack R R, Klohs W, LaScolea L J, Murphy T F, Mylotte J M 1984. Fimbriation of *Haemophilus* species isolated from the respiratory tract of adults, *Journal of Infectious Diseases* **150**: 40–3

Apicella M A, Dudas K C, Campagnari A, Rice P, Mylotte J M, Murphy T F 1985. Antigenic heterogeneity of lipid A of *Haemophilus influenzae*, *Infection and Immunity* **50**: 9–14

Barenkamp S J, Munson R S, Granoff D M 1981. Subtyping isolates of *Haemophilus influenzae* type b by outer-membrane protein profiles, *Journal of Infectious Diseases* **143**: 668–76

Beachey E H 1981. Bacterial adherence: Adhesion receptor interactions mediating the attachment of bacteria to mucosal surfaces, *Journal of Infectious Diseases* **143**: 325–45

Campagnari A A, Gupta M R, Dudas K C, Murphy T F, Apicella M A 1987. Antigenic diversity of lipo-oligosaccharides of nontypable *Haemophilus influenzae*, *Infection and Immunity* **55**: 882–7

Fothergill L D, Wright J 1933. Influenzal meningitis: Relation of age incidence to bactericidal power of blood against causal organism 1933, *Journal of Immunology* **24**: 273–84

Goldschneider I, Gotschlich E C, Artenstein M S 1969. Human immunity to the meningococcus. I. The role of humoral antibodies, *Journal of Experimental Medicine* **129**: 1307–26

Guerina N G, Langerman S, Schoolnik G K, Kessler T W, Goldmann D A 1985. Purification and characterization of *Haemophilus influenzae* pili, and their structural and serological relatedness to *Escherichia coli* and mannose-sensitive pili, *Journal of Experimental Medicine* **161**: 145–59

Kaplan S L, Mason E O Jr, Wiedermann B L 1983. Role of adherence in the pathogenesis of *Haemophilus influenzae* type b infection in infant rats, *Infection and Immunity* **42**: 612–17

Loeb M R, Smith D H 1980. Outer membrane protein composition in disease isolates of *Haemophilus influenzae*: Pathogenic and epidemiological implications, *Infection and Immunity* **30**: 709–17

Munson R S Jr, Granoff D M 1985. Purification and partial characterization of outer membrane proteins P5 and P6 from *Haemophilus influenzae* type b, *Infection and Immunity* **49**: 544–9

Munson R S Jr, Shenep J L, Barenkamp S J, Granoff D M 1983. Purification and comparison of outer membrane protein P2 from *Haemophilus influenzae* type b isolates, *Journal of Clinical Investigation* **72**: 677–84

Murphy T F, Apicella M A 1985. Antigenic heterogeneity of outer membrane proteins of nontypable *Haemophilus influenzae* is a basis for a serotyping system, *Infection and Immunity* **50**: 15–21

Murphy T F, Apicella M A 1987. Nontypable *Haemophilus influenzae*: A review of clinical aspects, surface antigens and the human immune response to infection, *Reviews of Infectious Diseases* **9**(1): 1–15

Murphy T F, Dudas K C, Mylotte J M, Apicella M A 1983 A subtyping system for nontypable *Haemophilus influenzae* based on outer membrane proteins, *Journal of Infectious Diseases* **147**: 838–46

Murphy T F, Nelson M B, Dudas K C, Mylotte J M, Apicella M A 1985. Identification of a specific epitope of *Haemophilus influenzae* on a 16 600 dalton outer membrane protein, *Journal of Infectious Diseases* **152**: 1300–7

Murphy T F, Bartos L C, Campagnari A A, Nelson M B, Apicella M A 1986a. Antigenic characterization of the P6 protein of nontypable *Haemophilus influenzae*, *Infection and Immunity* **54**(3): 774–9

Murphy T F, Bartos L C, Rice P A, Nelson M B, Dudas K C, Apicella M A 1986b. Identification of a 16 600 dalton outer membrane protein on nontypable *Haemophilus influenzae* as a target for human serum bactericidal antibody, *Journal of Clinical Investigation* **78**(4): 1020–7

Sable N A, Connor E M, Hall C B, Loeb M R 1985. Variable adherence of fimbriated *Haemophilus influenzae* type b to human cells, *Infection and Immunity* **48**: 119–23

Shenep J L, Munson R S Jr, Granoff D M 1982. Human antibody responses to lipopolysaccharide after meningitis due to *Haemophilus influenzae* type b, *Journal of Infectious Diseases* **145**: 181–90

Shurin P A, Pelton S I, Tager I B, Kasper D L 1980. Bactericidal antibody and susceptibility to otitis media caused by nontypable strains of *Haemophilus influenzae*, *Journal of Pediatrics* **97**: 364–9

Stull T L, Mendelman P M, Haas J E, Schoenborn M A, Mack K D, Smith A L 1984. Characterization of *Haemophilus influenzae* type b fimbriae, *Infection and Immunity* **47**: 787–96

Thomas W R, Rossi A A 1986. Molecular cloning of DNA coding for outer membrane proteins of *Haemophilus influenzae* type b, *Infection and Immunity* **52**: 812–17

Young R A, Bloom B R, Grosskinsky C M, Ivanyi J, Thomas D, Davis R W 1985. Dissection of *Mycobacterium tuberculosis* antigens using recombinant DNA, *Proceedings of the National Academy of Sciences USA* **82**: 2583–7

Identification, characterization and functional properties of antigenically distinct fimbriae on *Actinomyces*

John O Cisar; Ann L Sandberg; Maria K Yeung; Jacob A Donkersloot; Bruce M Chassy; Michael J Brennan; Stephan E Mergenhagen

The Laboratory of Microbiology and Immunology, National Institute of Dental Research, National Institutes of Health, Bethesda, Maryland 20892, USA

Introduction

The adherence of bacteria to mucosal surfaces is recognized as an important event in microbial colonization and the subsequent initiation of disease. Thus, the adhesins of pathogenic bacteria can be considered as virulence factors and potential antigens for the development of vaccines. Bacterial adherence frequently involves fimbriae or pili which bind to specific receptors on mucosal surfaces. The fimbriae on several Gram-negative bacteria such as enterotoxigenic and uropathogenic strains of *Escherichia coli* and *Neisseria gonorrhea* have been extensively studied and characterized (Gaastra and de Graaf 1982; Normark *et al.* 1986; Schoolnik *et al.* 1986; Sharon and Ofek 1986). Fimbriae also occur on various Gram-positive species including some which contribute to the pathogenesis of oral infections. *Actinomyces viscosus* and strains of *Streptococcus sanguis* and *S. mitis* are primary colonizers of teeth. Their establishment may initiate inflammation and provide a microenvironment which favors further colonization by various Gram-negative bacteria associated with advancing periodontal lesions. Early events in this process include the attachment of actinomyces and streptococci to the tooth surface, the interaction of these bacteria with each other and their adherence to various host cells.

The identification of two antigenic types of fimbriae (type 1 and type 2) on certain oral actinomyces has provided a basis for investigating the potential involvement of these surface structures in a variety of interactions including bacterial adherence to tooth and epithelial surfaces, coaggregation with other oral bacteria and phagocytosis by polymorphonuclear leukocytes. It is becoming increasingly apparent that these events are probably all mediated by fimbriae. The following discussion summarizes the functional properties of actinomyces fimbriae and current investigations of the structure of these adhesins.

96

Antigenically distinct fimbrial adhesins of *Actinomyces*

The presence of antigenically distinct fimbriae on *A. viscosus* strain T14V has been firmly established (Cisar 1986). Isolated fimbriae react as two unrelated antigens in cross-immunoelectrophoresis and monoclonal as well as specific polyclonal antibodies against either type 1 or type 2 fimbriae react with some but not all of the fimbriae observed on bacteria by immunoelectron microscopy. Moreover, fimbriae have been observed on mutants that are type 1^+2^- and type 1^-2^+ but not on those that are type 1^-2^- (Cisar *et al.* 1987b). In contrast to the fimbriae of strain T14V, those of *A. naeslundii* WVU45 react as a single antigenic component which is cross-reactive with the type 2 but not with the type 1 fimbriae of *A. viscosus* T14V. The presence of different fimbriae on these bacteria appears to correlate with their selective colonization of different oral tissue surfaces. Actinomyces with both type 1 and type 2 fimbriae such as *A. viscosus* T14V colonize the teeth of adults and are abundant in dental plaque whereas strains with only type 2 fimbriae similar to those of *A. naeslundii* WVU45 are preferentially found on epithelial surfaces (Cisar *et al.* 1985).

Actinomyces type 1 fimbriae are the principal adhesins for the tooth surface as indicated experimentally by studies of bacterial adsorption to saliva-treated hydroxyapatite (SHA). Specific rabbit antibodies or Fab fragments against type 1 but not against type 2 fimbriae inhibit this interaction (Clark *et al.* 1984) and mutant cells that are type 1^+2^- adhere well to SHA while cells that are type 1^-2^+ adhere poorly (Cisar *et al.* 1987b). The acidic proline-rich proteins found in saliva and as constituents of the acquired salivary pellicle coating the tooth surface appear to be the receptors for type 1 mediated adsorption (Gibbons *et al.* 1986). While the actinomyces attach to proline-rich protein-coated surfaces, direct binding of the soluble protein to these bacteria has not been demonstrated. This may indicate exposure of the receptor by a conformational change that occurs when the soluble protein becomes surface-associated or alternatively, a low affinity of actinomyces type 1 fimbriae for the receptor. In either case, type 1 mediated adherence appears to involve protein–protein interactions since the acidic proline-rich proteins are not glycosylated.

Unlike type 1, the type 2 fimbriae of *A. viscosus* and *A. naeslundii* strains are associated with a lectin activity for certain galactose- and *N*-acetylgalactosamine-containing receptors (Cisar 1986). This activity was initially detected by the coaggregation of actinomyces with certain streptococci and subsequently by bacterial interactions with various sialidase treated mammalian cells including erythrocytes, epithelial cells and polymorphonuclear leukocytes (Sandberg *et al.* 1986). The latter interaction is of particular interest because it results in phagocytosis and killing of the actinomyces and presumably in the release of lysosomal enzymes which contribute to inflammation. In addition to the inhibition of these various interactions by free galactose and *N*-acetylgalactosamine, methyl β-D-galactoside and certain β-linked galactosides such as lactose (Galβ1→4Glc) also inhibit whereas methyl α-D-galactoside does not. Studies with more complex saccharides have identified Galβ1→3GalNAc as the most potent inhibitor of the actinomyces lectin and have shown that GalNAcβ1→3Gal is also quite active. The former structure occurs commonly in the O-linked oligosaccharide chains of mammalian membrane glycoproteins and is frequently linked to terminal sialic acid whereas the latter is present in globoside, a membrane glycolipid. The specificity of the actinomyces lectin is further defined by the lack of inhibition observed with Galβ1→4GlcNAc, a sequence commonly found in N-linked chains of glycoproteins. While receptors for the actinomyces on mammalian cells appear to be the O-linked oligosaccharide chains of glycoproteins (Brennan *et al.* 1986) and possibly certain glycolipids (Brennan *et al.* 1987) those on streptococci are polysaccharides. Recently, the receptor-associated polysaccharide of *S. sanguis* 34 has been purified and shown to be composed of a repeating hexasaccharide unit with N-acetylgalactosamine at the nonreducing end in α1→3 linkage to L-rhamnose (McIntire *et al.* 1987). Thus, the actinomyces lectin appears to interact with receptors on different surfaces that are structurally related but not identical.

The association of lectin activity with type 2 fimbriae of actinomyces is supported by various findings (Cisar 1986). Fab fragments prepared from rabbit anti-type 2 but not from anti-type 1 antibody block the lactose sensitive coaggregation of *A. viscosus* T14V with *S. sanguis* 34. Moreover, mutants of strain T14V and of *A. naeslundii* WVU45 that specifically lack type 2 fimbriae fail to participate in lactose sensitive interactions with *S. sanguis* 34, as well as with epithelial cells and polymorphonuclear leukocytes (Sandberg *et al.* 1986). A somewhat unexpected property of isolated type 2 fimbriae is their lack of agglutinating activity and inability to bind with measurable affinity to receptor-bearing cells (Cisar 1986). However, when aggregated by specific monoclonal antibodies or when coated on latex beads, purified type 2 fimbriae mediate lactose-sensitive hemagglutination of sialidase-treated erythrocytes. Related observations include the demonstration that actinomyces aggregate with asialofetuin-coated latex beads but exhibit no detectable binding of the soluble glycoprotein. Thus, lectin-mediated adherence clearly depends on a cooperative effect of multivalent binding that magnifies the strength of many low-affinity lectin sites. Moreover, the sites appear to be spatially distributed on fimbriae in a way that permits bacterial attachment to surface-associated receptors with minimal binding of soluble receptor-bearing macromolecules. This preference may be an important consideration in explaining lectin-mediated microbial adherence in secretions such as saliva which contain asialoglycoproteins that are potential inhibitors of attachment.

Molecular cloning of *Actinomyces viscosus* genes in *Escherichia coli* and expression of fimbrial subunits

While the functional properties of each fimbrial antigen have been identified, efforts to determine the structure of these adhesins have been limited by the failure to identify conditions that result in complete dissociation of the isolated fimbriae. This is illustrated by the complex electrophoretic patterns of purified type 1 and type 2 fimbriae in SDS–polyacrylamide gels (Fig. 1, A

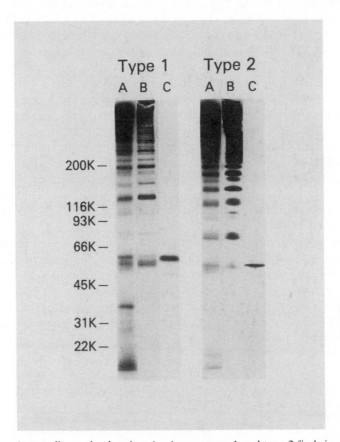

Figure 1. Autoradiographs showing *A. viscosus* type 1 and type 2 fimbriae partially dissociated by SDS–polyacrylamide gel electrophoresis and the reactions of specific mouse monoclonal antibodies with the separated protein bands and with the respective fimbrial subunits from clones of *E. coli* expressing *A. viscosus* genes: A, ^{125}I-labeled type 1 or type 2 fimbriae; B, type 1 or type 2 fimbriae transferred to nitrocellulose; C, type 1 or type 2 fimbrial subunits from clones of *E. coli* carrying plasmids pMY3833 or pAV3463 respectively, transferred to nitrocellulose. Gels (labeled A) were fixed and dried prior to autoradiography. Nitrocellulose transfers (labeled B and C) were overlaid with anti-type 1 monoclonal antibody 8A or anti-type 2 monoclonal antibody 5A as indicated followed by ^{35}S-labeled goat anti-mouse IgG prior to autoradiography.

lanes). Significantly, all proteins which migrate as bands with molecular weights of approximately 60×10^3 and greater are reactive with several specific monoclonal antibodies directed against different repeating epitopes of type 1 or type 2 fimbriae (Fig. 1, B lanes). To identify the respective subunits, cloning of actinomyces genes in *E. coli* was initiated.

The gene encoding the 65 kilodalton (kD) type 1 fimbrial subunit was cloned as a 4–6 kilobase (kb) insert of *A. viscosus* T14V chromosomal DNA and further localized on a 1.9 kb PstI–BamHI fragment using pUC19 as an expression vector (Yeung *et al.* 1987). Expression of a 59 kD type 2 subunit was detected from a 48 kb insert of *A. viscosus* T14V DNA using the cosmid vector pHC79 (Donkersloot *et al.* 1985). Upon subcloning, the gene has been identified on a 2.5 kb SmaI fragment using the expression vector pKK223–3. In addition, plasmids carrying portions of each fimbrial gene have been found to express truncated proteins. Subclones containing the 1.4 kb fragment obtained by SalI digestion of the type 1 gene express the *N*-terminal 47 kD region of the subunit (Fig. 2), while subclones carrying the 0.5 kb *C*-terminal portion of this gene do not produce an immunoreactive product. Other plasmids which carry fragments of the type 2 gene express the *N*-terminal 22 kD region or the *C*-terminal 35kD region of the subunit (Fig. 2).

Various findings indicate that the cloned proteins are unassembled fimbrial subunits. They comigrate in SDS gel electrophoresis with antigenically similar proteins released from partially dissociated fimbriae (Fig. 1, C lanes) and are also present in cytoplasmic extracts of *A. viscosus*. In addition to the reactions with specific rabbit antibody, the intact type 1 subunit as well as the 47 kD *N*-terminal polypeptide react with each of five monoclonal antibodies directed against three different repeating type 1 epitopes. Moreover, rabbit antibody prepared against the cloned type 1 subunit reacts in Western blotting with partially dissociated type 1 fimbriae to give a pattern that is indistinguishable from that obtained with anti-fimbrial antibody (Yeung *et al.* 1987). In studies of type 2 fimbriae, nine monoclonal antibodies have been produced

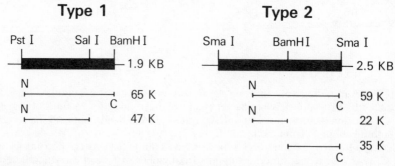

Figure 2. *A. viscosus* T14V chromosomal DNA inserts (▬▬) carried by plasmids pMY3833 and pAV3463 which encode the subunits of actinomyces type 1 and type 2 fimbriae respectively. The fimbrial subunits (———) as well as the *N*- and *C*-terminal polypeptides produced by subclones carrying fragments of each fimbrial gene are aligned with the respective DNA coding region.

against different epitopes. As shown by ELISA, eight of these antibodies react with the cloned 59 kD subunit and of these, one reacts with the N-terminal 22 kD region and two with the C-terminal 35 kD region. The reaction of five different anti-type 2 antibodies with the intact subunit but not with either fragment suggests that the subunit conformation depends on the presence of both fragments. This suggestion is consistent with the finding that the intact subunit is a heat-modifiable protein whereas the N- and C-terminal fragments are not. Thus, the unheated subunit isolated from *E. coli* as well as that from *A. viscosus* migrates as a 45 kD protein and as a 59 kD protein when boiled in the presence of SDS. In contrast, the apparent molecular weights of the N- and C-terminal regions are not altered by heating. Similar results have been obtained in studies of the 65 kD type 1 subunit which is heat-modifiable and with its 47 kD N-terminal segment which is not (Yeung *et al.* 1987). Affinity columns prepared with specific monoclonal antibodies have proven highly useful for the purification of each cloned subunit. Based on results from gel filtration experiments, the isolated subunits exist as monomers or possibly dimers under nondenaturing conditions and exhibit no tendency to aggregate or self-assemble into larger structures. It is not yet known whether the subunits possess functional activities like those of fimbriae.

Further progress in defining the structural basis of fimbriae-mediated bacterial adherence will depend upon identification and characterization of the receptor binding sites. In this regard, the ability of specific rabbit antibodies and their Fab fragments to inhibit bacterial adherence has not been observed with any of five monoclonal antibodies that react with three different epitopes on the type 1 fimbriae and with the cloned 65 kD subunit. Even when assayed together, the different monoclonal antibodies fail to block bacterial adsorption to SHA (Cisar *et al.* 1987a). Inhibition of lectin-mediated adherence has been observed with monoclonal antibodies that react with

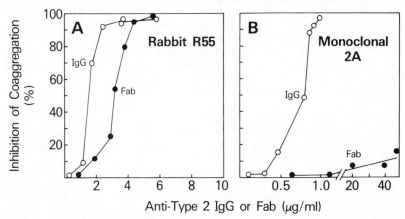

Figure 3.   Inhibition of the lactose-sensitive coaggregation between *A. viscosus* T14V and *S. sanguis* 34 by: A, anti-type 2 rabbit immune IgG and Fab fragments; B, anti-type 2 mouse monoclonal antibody 2A(γG1) and Fab fragments prepared from this protein.

different epitopes of type 2 fimbriae and with the cloned 59 kD subunit, but monoclonal Fab fragments fail to inhibit (Fig. 3). The latter result implies that the epitopes recognized are not directly involved in lectin binding. In studies of gonococcal pili, receptor binding has been attributed to an immunorecessive region of the pilin subunit and is not blocked by antibodies directed against various immunodominant epitopes (Rothbard *et al.* 1985; Schoolnik *et al.* 1986). An analogous separation of antigenic and functional domains within the fimbrial subunits of actinomyces could account for the inabilities of certain monoclonal antibodies and Fab fragments to block adherence. An additional possibility is raised by recent genetic evidence suggesting that the lectin activity of digalactoside-binding pili of *E. coli* depends on the presence of a minor subunit in this structure (Lindberg *et al.* 1986). The association of functional activities with minor structural components of the actinomyces fimbriae could account for the failure of the various monoclonal antibodies to block adherence. A precise definition of the structure and distribution of binding sites on fimbriae would contribute to the basic understanding of bacterial attachment and might also suggest effective strategies for the induction of antibodies that block this event and thereby prevent the initial step in the establishment of an infectious process.

References

Brennan M J, Cisar J O, Sandberg A L 1986. A 160-kilodalton epithelial cell surface glycoprotein recognized by plant lectins that inhibit the adherence of *Actinomyces naeslundii*, *Infection and Immunity* **52**(3): 840–5

Brennan M J, Joralmon R A, Cisar J O, Sandberg A L 1987. Binding of *Actinomyces naeslundii* to glycosphingolipids, *Infection and Immunity* **57**(2): 487–9

Cisar J O 1986. Fimbrial lectins of the oral actinomyces, in D Mirelman (ed) *Microbial Lectins and Agglutinins: Properties and biological activity*. Wiley, New York, ch 8 pp 183–96 (Wiley series in ecological and applied microbiology)

Cisar J O, Brennan M J, Sandberg A L 1985. Lectin-specific interaction of *Actinomyces* fimbriae with oral streptococci, in S E Mergenhagen, B Rosan (eds) *Molecular Basis of Oral Microbial Adhesion*. American Society for Microbiology, Washington, DC, pp 159–63

Cisar J O, Barsumian E L, Siraganian R P, Yeung M K, Hsu S D, Curl S H, Clark W B, Vatter A E, Sandberg A L 1987a. Monoclonal antibodies against the type 1 fimbrial antigen of *Actinomyces viscosus* T14V (in preparation)

Cisar J O, Vatter A E, Sandberg A L, Curl S H, Hurst-Calderone S, Clark W B 1987b. Mutants of *Actinomyces viscosus* T14V lacking type 1, type 2 or both fimbrial adhesins (in preparation)

Clark W B, Wheeler T T, Cisar J O 1984. Specific inhibition of adsorption of *Actinomyces viscosus* T14V to saliva-treated hydroxyapatite by antibody against type 1 fimbriae, *Infection and Immunity* **43**(2): 497–501

Donkersloot J A, Cisar J O, Wax M E, Harr R J, Chassy B M 1985. Expression of *Actinomyces viscosus* antigens in *Escherichia coli*: cloning of a structural gene (fim A) for type 2 fimbriae, *Journal of Bacteriology* **162**(3): 1075–8

Gaastra W, de Graaf F K 1982. Host-specific fimbrial adhesins of noninvasive enterotoxigenic *Escherichia coli* strains, *Microbiological Reviews* **46**(2): 129–61

Gibbons R J, Hay D I, Schluckebier S K 1986. Proline-rich proteins are pellicle receptors for type

1 fimbriae of *A. viscosus*, *Journal of Dental Research* **65** (Special Issue): 179 (Abstract 84)

Lindberg F, Lund B, Normark S 1986. Gene products specifying adhesion of uropathogenic *Escherichia coli* are minor components of pili, *Proceedings of the National Adacemy of Sciences USA* **83**(6): 1891–5

McIntire F C, Bush C A, Wu S S, Li S C, Li Y T, McNeil M, Tjoa S S, Fennessey P V 1987. Structure of a new hexasaccharide from the coaggregation polysaccharide of *Streptococcus sanguis* 34, *Carbohydrate Research* (in press)

Normark S, Båga M, Göransson M, Lindberg F P, Lund B, Norgren M, Uhlin B E 1986. Genetics and biogenesis of *Escherichia coli* adhesins, in D Mirelman (ed) *Microbial Lectins and Agglutinins: Properties and biological activity*. Wiley, New York, ch 5 pp 113–43 (Wiley series in ecological and applied microbiology)

Rothbard J B, Fernandez R, Wang L, Teng N N H, Schoolnik G K 1985. Antibodies to peptides corresponding to a conserved sequence of gonococcal pilins block bacterial adhesion, *Proceedings of the National Academy of Sciences USA* **82**(3): 915–19

Sandberg A L, Mudrick L L, Cisar J O, Brennan M J, Mergenhagen S E, Vatter A E 1986. Type 2 fimbrial lectin mediated phagocytosis of oral *Actinomyces* spp. by polymorphonuclear leukocytes *Infection and Immunity* **54**(2): 472–6

Schoolnik G K, Rothbard J B, Gotschlich E C 1986. Structure–function analysis of gonococcal pili, in D Mirelman (ed) *Microbial Lectins and Agglutinins: Properties and biological activity*. Wiley, New York, ch 6 pp 145–68 (Wiley series in ecological and applied microbiology)

Sharon N, Ofek I 1986. Mannose specific bacterial surface lectins, in D Mirelman (ed) *Microbial Lectins and Agglutinins: Properties and biological activity*. Wiley, New York, ch 3 pp 55–81 (Wiley series in ecological and applied microbiology)

Yeung M K, Chassy B M, Cisar J O 1987. Cloning and expression of a type 1 fimbrial subunit of *Actinomyces viscosus* T14V, *Journal of Bacteriology* **169**(4): 1678–83

Structural characterization of the serotype carbohydrate antigens of *Streptococcus mutans*

Rosemary Linzer; M Sreenivasulu Reddy; Michael J Levine

School of Dental Medicine, State University of New York at Buffalo, Buffalo N 14214, USA

Introduction

Streptococcus mutans is regarded as a prime etiologic agent in the development of dental caries – or in laymen's terms, tooth decay. *Streptococcus mutans* does not appear in the oral flora until after tooth eruption. When it is present, it selectively colonizes the tooth surface. Establishment on the tooth surface is a multifaceted process. Initial adherence is not to the tooth directly but to a layer of salivary components which form a pellicle on the enamel surface. Although nonspecific, low-affinity ion interactions may contribute to this attachment, evidence for high-affinity reactions between *S. mutans* and specific salivary components has been presented. Levine *et al.* (1978) reported that the interaction of purified salivary components with *S. mutans* is inhibited by treatment of the salivary components with α-galactosidase. In related experiments, Gibbons and Qureshi (1979) noted that certain galactosides and amines inhibit the attachment of *S. mutans* to experimental pellicles. Other investigators have identified and purified salivary reactive proteins or adhesins from the *S. mutans* cell wall (Ogier *et al.* 1984).

Once initial adherence has occurred, accumulation takes place with the bacterial plaque growing in size and complexity. *Streptococcus mutans* produces extracellular glucosyltransferase enzymes which appear to play a key role in this process. Glucosyltransferases produce water insoluble glucans which form the plaque matrix, promote cohesion between *S. mutans* cells, and contribute to the entrapment of other bacteria, bacterial products, and oral constituents in the developing plaque (for a review of this topic, see Doyle and Ciardi 1983). The glucans also appear to act as a diffusion barrier, keeping the acid products of bacterial metabolism in close proximity to the enamel surface. *Streptococcus mutans* is both acidogenic and the most aciduric of the oral streptococci, a fact which contributes to its role in dental decay.

Can immunological means aid in interrupting this caries process? Antibodies to the serotype antigens and glucosyltransferase enzymes of *S. mutans* have been shown to interfere with adherence and accumulation of the bacteria *in vitro* (Hamada and Slade 1976a; Linzer and Slade 1976). *In vivo* studies have shown that immunization with whole cells, surface proteins and glucosyl-transferase can protect animals from development of dental decay in laboratory infections with *S. mutans* (for review, see McGhee and Michalek 1981). Therefore, several laboratories around the world are actively pursuing the development of potential anti-caries vaccines (see papers by Taubman and Smith and by Curtiss in this convocation).

Because of their possible role in future caries vaccines and because of their diagnostic value, the serotype polysaccharide antigens of *S. mutans* have been studied extensively. This paper will review the identification and chemical characterization of the serotype antigens. It will also present recent work on the structural characterization of the serotype polysaccharides utilizing methylation analysis.

Chemical and serological characterization of the serotype antigens

In 1924, Clarke isolated and described a streptococcus from deep carious lesions which he believed to be the causative agent of decay (Clarke 1924). Clarke named the isolate *Streptococcus mutans*. It was not until 1960 that Fitzgerald and his coworks demonstrated the cariogenic properties of *S. mutans* in gnotobiotic rats (Fitzgerald *et al.* 1960). Slight differences were noted among the strains designated as *S. mutans*, and serotyping was undertaken in the 1970s by Bratthall (1970) and Perch *et al.* (1974). DNA base homology and DNA–DNA hybridization studies were also initiated in the 1970s resulting in the reclassification of *Streptococcus mutans* into five species (Coykendall 1977). The serotypes corresponded well with the genetic classification. *Streptococcus mutans*, comprising serotypes *c*, *e*, and *f*, and *S. sobrinus*, comprising serotypes *d* and *g*, are the most frequently isolated species from human carious lesions (Perch *et al.* 1974). *Streptococcus cricetus*, serotype a, and *S. rattus*, serotype *b*, are infrequently identified in humans. *Streptococcus mutans* is the only species that has been isolated from the blood of patients with subacute endocarditis (Perch *et al.* 1974). Strains of *S. mutans*, *S. cricetus*, *S. sobrinus* and *S. rattus* have been shown to be cariogenic in animals fed diets high in readily fermentable carbohydrates. A fifth species, *S. ferus*, was isolated from wild rats and appears to be limited to wild rat populations. *Streptococcus sobrinus* serotype *h* and an additional species, *S. macacae*, were more recently identified in monkeys (Beighton and Russell 1981; Beighton *et al.* 1984).

A variety of methods have been used to solubilize the serotype antigens beginning with Lancefield-type extracts of whole cells. The antigens have since been solubilized from purified cell wall preparations by muramidase digestion of the walls (Knox *et al.* 1983). This confirmed that the serotype polysaccharides are cell wall components and covalently linked to peptidoglycan.

Table 1 Chemical composition of the serotype antigens of the '*mutans*' group of streptococci

Genetic group	Serotype	Strain	Composition (wt %)			Reference
			Rhamnose	**Glucose**	**Galactose**	
S. mutans	c	Ingbritt	69	29	—	Linzer *et al.* 1976
	c	GS5	43	29	—	Wetherell and Bleiweis 1975
	e	MT703	56	37	—	Hamada and Slade 1976b
	e	V-100	52	24	—	Wetherell and Bleiweis 1978
	e	LM7	48	24	—	Linzer *et al.* 1986
	f	OMZ175	43	22	—	*Vide infra*
	f	MT557	59	39	—	Hamada *et al.* 1976
S. cricetus	a	HS6	—	10	54	Mukasa and Slade 1973a
S. sobrinus	d	B13	—	33	62	Linzer and Slade 1974
	g	6715	—	10	61	Iacono *et al.* 1975
	h	MFe28	3	16	75	Okahashi *et al.* 1984
S. rattus	b	FA1	47	—	27	Mukasa and Slade 1973b

Table 1 summarizes the carbohydrate compositions for the '*mutans*' group of streptococci. The serotype *b* carbohydrate of *S. rattus* is unique in being composed of galactose and rhamnose. It is the only serotype carbohydrate that demonstrates a negative charge on immunoelectrophoresis. Hapten inhibition studies suggest that a terminal galactose unit contributes to the specificity of its immunological determinant. The serotype *a*, *d*, *g* and *h* antigens are neutral polymers of galactose and glucose. They demonstrate strong serological cross-reactions. Intensive studies with the *a*, *d* and *g* antigens have demonstrated that multiple determinants are present on these polysaccharides (Linzer *et al.* 1975; Takada *et al.* 1984).

Strains of *S. cricetus and S. sobrinus* also possess high concentrations of rhamnose in their cell walls. Rhamnose:glucose polysaccharides (RGPs) have been purified and characterized from strains of serotypes *d* and *g* (Prakobphol *et al.* 1980; Prakobphol and Linzer 1980). The serotype *d* and *g* antigens and RGPs are both chemically and serologically distinct. Several mutants have been identified that lack the serotype *g* antigen, but none has been found to lack the rhamnose polymer. Antisera raised to the mutant strains have high titers of antibodies to the rhamnose polymer; however, antisera to a strain possessing the serotype polysaccharide will have high titers to the serotype antigen and low or negligible titers to the RGP antigen. This apparent suppression of the immunogenicity of the rhamnose:glucose polysaccharide exists even though the RGP antigen comprises 40–50% of the dry weight of the serotype *d* and *g* cell walls.

In quantitative percipitin assays, the serotype *d* antigen appears to demonstrate higher affinity for its antibody than does the RGP antigen (Fig. 1). By comparing the linear portions of the precipitin curves, it can be noted that on a weight basis five times as much RGP as serotype *d* polysaccharide is required to precipitate the same amount of antibody protein. This phenomenon may be due to one or both of the following: a higher concentration or greater multiplicity of determinants on the serotype polysaccharide or a more open structure that allows greater access of antibodies to the serotype polysaccharide than to the RGP antigen. In their structural studies of the serotype *d* antigen, Brown and Bleiweis (1979) reported that the polysaccharide contains units of 1,6-linked glucose, 1,6-linked galactose and 1,3-linked glucose and small amounts of a 1,6-linked galactofuranoside unit. Branching appeared limited to approximately every sixth unit. Although the exact structure could not be determined, the serotype *d* antigen appeared to have a very open configuration. In contrast, our studies with the RGP polymer suggested a

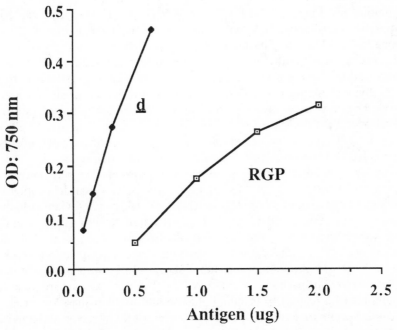

Figure 1. Quantitative precipitin assay of *S. sobrinus* serotype *d* antigen and RGP antigen with their respective antisera.

backbone of alternating 1,2- and 1,3-linked rhamnose units with glucose side chains at the 2-position of the 1,3-linked rhamnose (Linzer *et al.* 1985). The presence of 1,2-linkages would have a profound effect on the shape of the RGP antigen and on the availability of the determinants. These structural differences may explain the apparent differences in antibody affinity.

The serotype *c*, *e* and *f* antigens of *S. mutans* are polymers of rhamnose and glucose which chemically appear very similar although they are serologically distinct (Table 1). Hapten inhibition studies have suggested that terminal α-galactose units contribute specificity to the serotype *c* and *f* antigens. A terminal β-glucose unit appears to contribute specificity to the serotype *e* antigen.

Structural studies of the serotype antigens of *Streptococcus mutans*

In studies reporting the original purification of the serotype *c*, *e* and *f* antigens, the polysaccharides were solubilized using techniques involving hot acid, hot concentrated formamide, or high temperature and pressure. For structural studies, an enzyme digestion technique was chosen to avoid random hydrolysis and thereby to preserve the structure of the polysaccharide. Mutanolysin, an M-1 *N*-acetylmuramidase from *Streptomyces globisporus* 1829 was used to produce cell lysis and antigen solubilization (for details of the technique, see Linzer *et al.* 1985). Clarified cell digests were fractionated by sequential chromatography on columns of DEAE-Sephadex A-25 and Sephadex G-100 resin (Pharmacia Fine Chemicals, Piscataway, NJ, USA). The chromatographically purified samples were examined for carbohydrate and peptidoglycan constituents using colorimetric assays, gas–liquid chromatography, and amino acid analysis (for details of techniques, see Linzer *et al.* 1985). The polysaccharides appeared to remain covalently linked with fragments of the peptidoglycan polymer. All contained a rhamnose-to-glucose ratio of 2:1. Hapten inhibition studies were used to confirm earlier reports of the nature and configuration of the terminal saccharide units.

The serotype antigens were examined by gas chromatography–mass spectroscopy (GC/MS) analysis. Methylation of the polysaccharide samples was carried out by the method of Hakomori (1964). The permethylated oligosaccharides were converted to partially methylated hexitol acetates and 6-deoxyhexitol acetates by the acetolysis–hydrolysis procedure described by Stellner *et al.* (1973). The derivatives were identified using a Hewlett–Packard model 5992 gas chromatograph–mass spectrometer with a glass column (0.2 cm × 200 cm) packed with 3% OV-225. The derivatives were identified by elution with respect to terminal glucose and by their mass spectrum.

Table 2 summarizes the proposed structures for the serotype antigens of *S. mutans* and also presents the structure proposed for the rhamnose:glucose antigen of *S. sobrinus*. Although the serotype *c*, *e* and *f* polysaccharides of *S.*

Table 2 Proposed structures for the *Streptococcus mutans* serotype antigens and the RGP antigen of *Streptococcus sobrinus*

Strain	Serotype	Proposed structure	Reference
S. mutans			
Ingbritt	*c*	Rhal-3Rhal-2Rhal-3Rhal-> $\quad$|α-1,2$\quad\quad$|α-1,2 $\quad$Glc$\quad\quad\quad$Glc	Linzer *et al.* 1986
LM7	*e*	Rhal-3Rhal-2Rhal-3Rhal-> $\quad$|β-1,2$\quad\quad$|β-1,2 $\quad$Glc$\quad\quad\quad$Glc	Linzer *et al.* 1986
OMZ175	*f*	Rhal-2Rhal-3Rhal-2Rhal-> $\quad$|α-1,3$\quad\quad$|α-1,3 $\quad$Glc$\quad\quad\quad$Glc	*Vide infra*
S. sobrinus			
6715-T$_2$	—	Rhal-3Rhal-2Rhal-3Rhal-> $\quad$|1,2 $\quad$Glc $\quad$|1,2 $\quad$Glc $\quad$|α-1,6 $\quad$Glc	Linzer *et al.* 1985

mutans contain rhamnose and glucose in approximately a 2:1 ratio, they are serologically distinct. The proposed structures for these antigens aid in elucidating the basis for their serological specificity. The serotype *c* and *e* antigens are distinguished from the serotype *f* antigen by their backbone structure. The *c* and *e* antigens have a backbone of alternating 1,2- and 1,2,3-linked rhamnose units with branching at the 2-position of the 1,2,3-linked rhamnose. In contrast, the serotype *f* antigen has a backbone of alternating 1,3- and 1,2,3-linked rhamnose units with branching at the 3-position of the 1,2,3-linked rhamnose. The serotype *c* antigen is distinguished from the serotype *e* antigen by having terminal α-linked glucose units in contrast to the β-linked units of serotype *e* antigen.

The backbone structure of the serotype *f* antigen was confirmed by periodate oxidation studies. Coligan *et al.* (1975) described a backbone structure similar to that of the *f* antigen for the Lancefield group A, AV, and C polysaccharides. The A and C antigens had side chains of amino sugars consisting of β-1,3-linked *N*-acetylglucosamine in the A antigen and α-1,3-linked di-*N*-acetylgalactosamine in the C antigen. The AV antigen was unbranched.

RGP antigens were characterized from strains of serotype *d* and *g* of *S. sobrinus* and appear to be chemically and serologically identical. The terminal α-1,6-diglucose unit contributes significantly to the specificity of the RGP antigen, and antisera to the RGP antigen do not cross-react with the serotype *c* antigen. In contrast, antisera to serotype *c* polysaccharide showed weak cross-reactivity with the RGP antigen. In continuous culture studies, RGP antigen from cells grown at pH 7.5 had a 65% decrease in recovery of 1,6- and 1,2-linked glucose units versus antigen from cells grown at pH 6.5. This decrease in recovery of RGP determinants was accompanied by an increase in cross-reactivity with anti-serotype *c* serum, confirming the close structural relatedness of these two antigens (Linzer *et al.* 1986).

Future directions

Although the polysaccharide antigens are highly specific for *S. mutans*, the purified antigens are poorly immunogenic. Thus their incorporation in a caries vaccine would require the use of appropriate adjuvants. As with other carbohydrate antigens, the immunogenicity of the serotype antigens of *S. mutans* may be increased by complexing the polysaccharides with lipids and proteins (Grossi *et al.* 1983). Also, the immunogenicity of antigens presented orally may be potentiated by administration in liposomes. In rat immunization studies by Genco *et al.* (1983), antigen-containing liposomes appeared to stimulate IgA production specifically by the mucosal immune system when presented orally.

Recently, Wachsmann *et al.* (1986) reported the preparation of a bivalent vaccine consisting of the purified polysaccharide antigen from *S. mutans* strain OMZ175 covalently coupled to a cell wall protein. The cell wall protein was one of several proteins the investigators had characterized as interacting with saliva proteins. Wachsmann and coworkers reported that the oral administration of their conjugate in liposomes induced a local salivary IgA response directed against both the polysaccharide antigen and the cell surface protein. Development of similar bivalent vaccines with the serotype *c* or *d* polysaccharides may significantly broaden the spectrum of these potential agents. Consideration should be given to the question of whether or not the *d* antigen might suppress the immunogenicity of the *c* antigen in a multivalent vaccine. Such inhibition appears to occur on the bacterial surface between the *d* antigen and the RGP polysaccharide. Alternatively, synthetic carbohydrates based on the structures reported here might contribute to the development of safe and effective multivalent anticaries vaccines.

Acknowledgements

This work was supported in part by Public Health Services grant DE 05017 from the National Institute of Dental Research.

References

Beighton D, Russell R R B 1981. The isolation and characterization of *Streptococcus mutans* serotype *h* from dental plaque of monkeys (*Macaca fascicularis*), *Journal of General Microbiology* **124**: 271–9

Beighton D, Hayday H, Russell R R B, Whiley R A 1984, *Streptococcus macacae* sp. nov. from dental plaque of monkeys (*Macca fascicularis*), *International Journal of Systematic Bacteriology* **34**: 332–5

Bratthall D 1970. Demonstration of five serological groups of streptococcal strains resembling *Streptococcus mutans*, *Odontologisk Revy* **21**: 143–52

Brown T A, Bleiweis A S 1979. Chemical, immunochemical, and structural studies of the cross-reactive antigens of *Streptococcus mutans* AHT and B13, *Infection and Immunity* **24**: 326–36

Clarke J K 1924. On the bacterial factor in the aetiology of dental caries, *British Journal of Experimental Pathology* **5**: 141–7

Coligan J E, Schnute W C, Kindt T J 1975. Immunochemical and chemical studies on streptococcal group-specific carbohydrates, *Journal of Immunology* **114**: 1654–8

Coykendall A L 1977. Proposal to elevate the subspecies of *Streptococcus mutans* to species status, based on their molecular composition. *International Journal of Systematic Bacteriology* **27**: 26–30

Doyle R J, Ciardi J E (eds) 1983. *Proceedings: Glucosyltransferases, glucans, sucrose, and dental caries*, Sp. Supp. *Chemical Senses*. IRL Press, Oxford

Fitzgerald R J, Jordan H V, Stanley H R 1960. Experimental caries and gingival pathologic changes in the gnotobiotic rat, *Journal of Dental Research* **39**: 923–35

Genco R J, Linzer R, Evans R T 1983. Effects of adjuvants on orally administered antigens, *Annals of the New York Academy of Science* **409**: 650–88

Gibbons R J, Qureshi J V 1979. Inhibition of adsorption of *Streptococcus mutans* strains to saliva-treated hydroxyapatite by galactose and certain amines, *Infection and Immunity* **26**: 1214–17

Grossi S, Prakobphol A, Linzer R, Campbell L K, Knox K W 1983. Characterization of serological cross-reactivity between polysaccharide antigens of *Streptococcus mutans* serotypes *c* and *d*, *Infection and Immunity* **39**: 1473–6

Hakomori S 1964. A rapid permethylation of glycolipid and polysaccharide catalyzed by methylsulfinyl carbanion in dimethyl sulfoxide, *Journal of Biochemistry (Tokyo)* **55**: 205–8

Hamada S, Slade H D 1976a. Adherence of serotype *e* *Streptococcus mutans* and the inhibitory effect of Lancefield group E and *S. mutans* type *e* antiserum, *Journal of Dental Research* **55**: 65C–74C

Hamada S, Slade H D 1976b. Purification and immunochemical characterization of the type *e* polysaccharide antigen of *Streptococcus mutans*, *Infection and Immunity* **14**: 68–76

Hamada S, Gill K, Slade H D 1976. Chemical and immunological properties of the type *f* polysaccharide antigen of *Streptococcus mutans*, *Infection and Immunity* **14**: 203–11

Iacono V J, Taubman M A, Smith D J, Levine M J 1975. Isolation and immunochemical characterization of the group-specific antigen of *Streptococcus mutans* 6715, *Infection and Immunity* **11**: 117–28

Knox K W, Campbell L K, Bratthall D 1983. Detection of antigens in enzymic lysates of cell wall from *Streptococcus mutans* strains, *Journal of Dental Research* **62**: 1033–7

Levine M J, Herzberg M C, Levine M S, Ellison S A, Stinson M W, Li H C, Van Dyke T 1978. Specificity of salivary-bacterial interactions: role of terminal sialic acid residues in the interaction of salivary glycoproteins with *Streptococcus sanguis* and *Streptococcus mutans*, *Infection and Immunity* **19**: 107–15

Linzer R, Slade H D 1974. Purification and characterization of *Streptococcus mutans* group *d* cell wall polysaccharide antigen, *Infection and Immunity* **10**: 361–8

Linzer R, Slade H D 1976. Characterization of an anti-glucosyltransferase serum specific for insoluble glucan synthesis by *Streptococcus mutans*, *Infection and Immunity* **13**: 494–500

111

Linzer R, Mukasa H, Slade H D 1975. Serological purification of polysaccharide antigens from *Streptococcus mutans* serotypes *a* and *d*: characterization of multiple antigenic determinants, *Infection and Immunity* **12**: 791–8

Linzer R, Gill K, Slade H D 1976. Chemical composition of *Streptococcus mutans* type *c* antigen: comparison to type *a*, *b*, and *d* antigens, *Journal of Dental Research* **55**: 109A–15A

Linzer R, Reddy M S, Levine M J 1985. Structural studies of the rhamnose–glucose polysaccharide antigen from *Streptococcus sobrinus* B13 and 6715-T$_2$, *Infection and Immunity* **50**: 583–5

Linzer R, Reddy M S, Levine M J 1986. Immunochemical aspects of serotype carbohydrate antigens of *Streptococcus mutans*, in S Hamada, S M Michalek, H Kiyono, L Menaker, J R McGhee (eds) *Molecular Microbiology and Immunobiology of Streptococcus mutans*. Elsevier, Amsterdam, pp 29–38

McGhee J R, Michalek S M 1981. Immunobiology of dental caries: microbial aspects and local immunity, *Annual Reviews of Microbiology* **35**: 595–638

Mukasa H, Slade H D 1973a. Extraction, purification and chemical and immunological properties of the *Streptococcus mutans* group 'a' polysaccharide cell wall antigen, *Infection and Immunity* **8**: 190–8

Mukasa H, Slade H D 1973b. Structure and immunological specificity of the *Streptococcus mutans* group b cell wall antigen, *Infection and Immunity* **7**: 578–85

Okahashi N, Nishida Y, Koga T, Hamada S 1984. Immunochemical characteristics of *Streptococcus mutans* serotype *h* carbohydrate antigen, *Microbiology and Immunology* **28**: 407–13

Ogier J A, Klein J P, Sommer P, Frank R M 1984. Identification and preliminary characterization of saliva-interacting surface antigens of *Streptococcus mutans* by immunoblotting, ligand blotting and immunoprecipitation, *Infection and Immunity* **45**: 107–12

Perch B, Kjems E, Ravn T 1974. Biochemical and serological properties of *Streptococcus mutans* from various human and animal sources, *Acta Pathologica et Microbiologica Scandinavica* **82B**: 357–70

Prakobphol A, Linzer R 1980. Purification and immunological characterization of a rhamnose–glucose antigen from *Streptococcus mutans* 6715-T$_2$ (serotype *g*), *Infection and Immunity* **30**: 140–6

Prakobphol A, Linzer R, Genco R J 1980. Purification and characterization of a rhamnose-containing cell wall antigen of *Streptococcus mutans* B13 (serotype *d*), *Infection and Immunity* **27**: 150–7

Stellner K, Saito K, Hakomori S 1973. Determination of amino sugar linkages in glycolipids by methylation, *Archives of Biochemistry and Biophysics* **155**: 464–72

Takada K, Wyszomirska J, Shiota T 1984. Serological characterization of *Streptococcus mutans* serotype polysaccharide and its different molecular weight forms, *Infection and Immunity* **45**: 464–9

Wachsmann D, Klein J P, Scholler M, Ogier J, Ackermans F, Frank R M 1986. Serum and salivary antibody responses in rats orally immunized with *Streptococcus mutans* carbohydrate protein conjugate associated with liposomes, *Infection and Immunity* **52**: 408–13

Wetherell J R Jr, Bleiweis A S 1975. Antigens of *Streptococcus mutans*: characterization of a polysaccharide antigen from walls of strain GS-5, *Infection and Immunity* **12**: 341–8

Wetherell J R Jr, Bleiweis A S 1978. Antigens of *Streptococcus mutans*: isolation of a serotype-specific and a cross-reactive antigen from walls of strain V-100 (serotype *e*), *Infection and Immunity* **19**: 160–9

Operational aspects of epitope identification: structural features of proteins recognized by antibodies

M H V Van Regenmortel; S Muller; V F Quesniaux; D Altschuh; J P Briand

Laboratoire d'Immunochimie, Institut de Biologie Moléculaire et Cellulaire du CNRS, 15 rue Descartes, 67084 Strasbourg Cédex, France

Introduction

The antigenic reactivity of a protein refers to its capacity to bind specifically to the functional binding sites or paratopes of certain immunoglobulin molecules. When such a binding is observed experimentally, the particular immunoglobulin molecule becomes known as an antibody specific for the protein. The paratopes of antibody molecules are made up of six highly accessible loops of hypervariable sequence that interact to varying degrees with the protein antigen. That portion of the antigen which during the binding reaction comes into contact with the paratope of the antibody is called an antigenic determinant or epitope. According to this definition of epitope, the source and origin of the antibody used to identify a particular epitope on a protein are irrelevant. Although the antibody is most commonly obtained from an animal immunized with the protein antigen in question, it could also originate from an animal immunized with a related antigen possessing either the same epitope or a cross-reacting one. For example, such a related antigen could be a peptide fragment of the protein which is able to elicit antibodies that recognize the whole protein. The peptide may correspond to a region of the protein that appears not to be immunogenic when the whole protein is used for immunization. Such an apparent lack of immunogenicity could be due to the fact that the corresponding epitope is not immunodominant in the complete protein molecule; as a result the level of antibodies in the anti-protein serum that are specific for the epitope may be insufficient for detection by some immunoassays.

The antibody used to identify a particular protein epitope may also be derived from a non-immunized animal or from an animal for which the immunizing stimulus is unknown. An example of this is the monoclonal antibodies which are specific for epitopes in DNA (Lafer *et al.* 1981), RNA (Eilat *et al.* 1982) and histones (Laskov *et al.* 1984) and which are derived from autoimmune mice.

The concept of epitope

It is customary to distinguish the antigenicity of a protein, i.e. its ability to react with antibodies, from its immunogenicity or ability to induce an immune response. A self-antigen, for instance, possesses antigenic reactivity although it may be nonimmunogenic in the autologous host. The same distinction between antigenicity and immunogenicity applies to epitopes which may or may not show immunogenicity depending on host factors such as the immunoglobulin gene repertoire, self-tolerance and various regulatory mechanisms. Some authors consider that the concept of epitope necessarily involves both properties of antigenic reactivity and immunogenicity, a viewpoint which makes the existence of epitopes in a protein depend on immunogenetic and immunoregulatory mechanisms. In the case of myoglobin, for instance, Atassi (1984) argued that the regions consisting of residues 1–6 and 121–127 were not epitopes of the protein, although the corresponding peptides 1–6 and 121–127, when injected as free or conjugated peptides, were able to induce antibodies that recognized the complete myoglobin molecule (Atassi and Young 1985). These two regions are highly accessible at the surface of myoglobin (Thornton *et al.* 1986) but seem, at least in some systems, to induce fewer antibodies in animals immunized with native myoglobin than some other antigenic regions of the molecule (Atassi 1984; Benjamin *et al.* 1984).

Another difficulty in defining epitopes arises from the fact that the antigenic reactivity of a native protein and that of its denatured counterpart are usually very different. This means that it is necessary to ascertain whether an epitope is actually present in the native or denatured form of the protein. This problem has become particularly relevant in recent years because of the popularity of solid-phase immunoassays. There is considerable evidence that proteins may undergo some denaturation or physical distortion when they are adsorbed to plastic in solid-phase immunoassays. This is particularly noticeable with monoclonal antibodies, since many of them bind to antigen adsorbed to plates but not to antigen in solution, or vice versa (Mierendorf and Dimond 1983; Friguet *et al.* 1984; Al Moudallal *et al.* 1984; Altschuh *et al.* 1985; Vaidya *et al.* 1985; McCullough *et al.* 1985). When protein antigens are adsorbed on to a solid phase, it is thus questionable whether the epitopes corresponding to the native state are preserved. In order to ascertain if antibodies elicited by peptides of a given protein truly recognize the 'native' form of the protein, as is often claimed (Green *et al.* 1982; Luka *et al.* 1983), it is necessary to test these antibodies in a liquid-phase type of assay. This is of considerable importance for evaluating potential peptide vaccines since the neutralization epitopes may be preserved only in antigens with an intact tertiary structure.

The fact that antibodies raised by immunization with denatured proteins or peptides often do not react with the corresponding native molecule can be linked to the concept of cryptotope. This has been defined (Jerne 1960) as an epitope that becomes antigenically reactive only after breakage, depolymerization or denaturation of the antigen. In virus particles, cryptotopes are also found on the surfaces of coat protein monomers that become buried after polymerization (Al Moudallal *et al.* 1985). There is also evidence that polymerized proteins possess epitopes that are not present in the constituent protein monomers. Such epitopes, which have been called neotopes (Van Regenmortel 1966) are found in most viruses (Neurath and Rubin 1971; Van Regenmortel 1982) and may be of relevance in neutralization.

Finally, it should be stressed that the exact delineation of epitopes is only possible by X-ray crystallography of antigen–antibody complexes, since this is the only method which allows all the contact residues of both epitope and paratope to be identified. Until now, only one epitope of lysozyme has been delineated in this fashion. Most protein epitopes described in the literature correspond actually to cross-reactive structures in the form of short linear peptides, and these are unlikely to reproduce exactly the three-dimensional cluster of residues to which antibodies bind in the native protein. Even the distinction between continuous and discontinuous epitopes (Atassi and Smith 1978) may be difficult to apply in practice, since short fragments that are antigenically active and are therefore labeled continuous epitopes could actually correspond to small subregions of larger discontinuous epitopes.

Operational aspects of antigenicity

In a world devoid of immunoglobulins, the concept of epitope would not have arisen in human minds. Clearly, epitopes are relational entities which require complementary paratopes for their operational definition.

The number of epitopes present on any antigen has been a fertile source of controversy. Some authors consider this number to be relatively small (Atassi 1984), a conclusion that could have been influenced by the fact that certain immunogenic regions are immunodominant. A more widely held view states that the entire accessible surface of a protein consists of a large number of overlapping epitopes (Benjamin *et al.* 1984). The advent of hybridoma technology has provided a means to estimate roughly the number of different epitopes that can be distinguished on an antigen. This is done by assuming that a protein possesses as many epitopes as the number of different monoclonal antibodies that can be raised against it. In the case of insulin, this number has been estimated to be around 100 (Schroer *et al.* 1983). However, classical immunoassays cannot establish whether two monoclonal antibodies recognize exactly the same set of residues in an antigen but with different affinities, or whether they recognize two slightly different or overlapping sets of residues. At this level of analysis, the elucidation of antigenic structure becomes transformed into a study of the immune repertoire specific for the antigen. When the analysis of antibody specificity is restricted to the immunogen only, certain differences in fine specificity of individual monoclonal antibodies may go unnoticed. A recent study of the immunosuppressive drug, cyclosporin (Cs) may be taken as an example (Quesniaux *et al.* 1986).

The rigid ring structure of Cs (Fig. 1) represents a highly constrained peptide which is a good model for studying the structural and conformational parameters that govern epitope–paratope interactions. A panel of 180 monoclonal antibodies specific for Cs were analyzed for their ability to discriminate between more than 100 synthetic analogs modified at each of the 11 residues of Cs. Some of the antibodies, for instance, were particularly sensitive to substitutions on residues 1–6 while others recognized mainly residues 6, 8 and 9 (Fig. 1). NMR and X-ray crystallographic studies of conformationally modified Cs analogs showed that epitope recognition by antibody was influenced by small structural and conformational variations in the Cs molecule. However, some of the antibodies also recognized the linear form of the molecule in which the ring structure is interrupted between residues 7 and 8. Some of the differences in fine specificity of individual Cs monoclonal antibodies were only discernible because of the availability of a large number of Cs analogs. The results of this study showed that it may be feasible to distinguish Cs from inactive Cs metabolites by means of monoclonal antibodies.

The operational nature of epitope identification is also demonstrated by the influence of different immunoassays on the apparent antigenic reactivity of peptides. This is illustrated in Table 1 with five continuous epitopes of histone H2A tested by means of four H2A rabbit antisera. Several peptides were found to react with H2A antibodies in only some of the immunoassays presumably because the peptide conformation was not the same in all assay

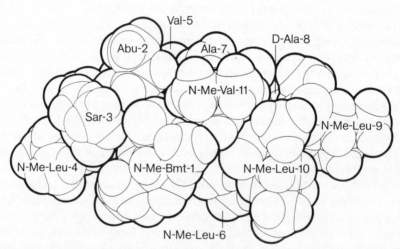

Figure 1. Space-filling model of cyclosporin. N-Me-Bmt, *N*-methyl-(4*R*)-4-[(*E*)-2-butenyl]-4-methyl-ʟ-threonine; Abu, α-aminobutyric acid; Sar, sarcosine. Some Cs monoclonal antibodies recognize mainly residues 1–6; others recognize mainly groups of residues such as 6 + 8 + 9, or 3 + 5 + 7 + 9 + 11 or 1 + 3 + 4 + 6 + 11, etc.

Table 1 Antigenic activity of synthetic peptides of H2A in different immunoassays

Sequence of peptide	H2A antiserum	Binding assay (ELISA) with antigen adsorbed to plastic		Inhibition of reaction between H2A antiserum and:	
		Peptide	Peptide conjugate	H2A	H2A fragment 1–89 or 91–129
1–15	1	−	−	+	+
	3	+	−	+	−
12–26	1	−	−	−	−
	2	−	−	−	+
65–85	1	+	+	+	ND
	4	+	−	+	ND
85–100	1	+	+	+	ND
	2	−	+	+	ND
116–129	1	−	ND	−	−
	2	−	ND	−	+

Source: From Muller *et al.* 1986.
ND – Not determined.

formats (Muller *et al.* 1986). For instance, in the direct binding assay using unconjugated peptide 1–15, only antiserum 3 revealed antigenic activity in the peptide bound to the solid phase (Table 1). Conjugation of this peptide to albumin rendered it inactive. In inhibition assays where the peptide was free in solution, both antisera 1 and 3 showed that peptide 1–15 possessed antigenic activity. The results obtained with peptides 12–26 and 116–129 (Table 1) show that the antigenic activity of some peptides becomes apparent only in inhibition assays probably because in this test format the epitope is in a more appropriate conformation than when the peptide is conjugated to a carrier or adsorbed to the solid phase. These results underline the danger of drawing generalizations about the antigenicity of peptides (or lack thereof) from only one type of assay, for instance using a test where peptides are coupled to plastic rods (Geysen 1985; Geysen *et al.* 1985) or to resins (Shi *et al.* 1984).

Which structural features of antigens do antibodies recognize?

Attempts to correlate the position of epitopes in proteins with certain features of their primary, secondary and tertiary structures have been mainly concerned with continuous epitopes (Berzofsky 1985; Van Regenmortel 1986a). Unfortunately the antigenicity data base is limited to a small number of continuous epitopes whose approximate locations were established by antigenic cross-reactivity studies (Van Regenmortel 1986b).

Antibodies bind to the surface of native proteins and it is thus to be expected that epitopes of native proteins will consist of residues exposed at the surface of the molecule. Recently this expectation was verified by two independent groups (Thornton *et al.* 1986; Novotny *et al.* 1986). Most linear segments that were highly accessible in the proteins under study were found also to possess a high segmental mobility. A correlation between the location of continuous epitopes and mobile segments of proteins has previously been established (Westhof *et al.* 1984; Tainer *et al.* 1985) and since mobility often coincides with the position of surface loops (Rose *et al.* 1985), both properties of accessibility and mobility are interconnected. It is noteworthy that the complementarity-determining regions of antibody molecules (i.e. the paratopes) also consist of protruding loops with a high segmental mobility. Algorithms have been developed to predict regions of high accessibility and mobility from the primary structure of proteins (Hopp 1985; Karplus and Schulz 1985). Furthermore, local maxima in protein hydrophilicity plots (Hopp and Woods 1981; Hopp 1986) also tend to correspond to exposed residues and to reverse turns, indicating that hydrophilicity is also linked to mobility. This is illustrated in Fig. 2 for the four histones H2A, H2B, H3 and H4. These plots clearly show that in this case there is a general agreement between the location of maxima in hydrophilicity plots and regions predicted to have a high segmental mobility, and that the great majority of these regions are also antigenic (Muller *et al.* 1982, 1983, 1985, 1986). One major exception concerns the epitope located in residues 44–61 of H2A. In the case of tobacco mosaic virus protein and myoglobin, the correlation between the positions of peaks of hydrophilicity and segmental mobility was much poorer than with the histones (Westhof *et al.* 1984; Thornton *et al.* 1986).

Seven of the eight chain termini of the four histones were found to correspond to epitopes. *N* and *C*-termini of proteins often correspond to epitopes presumably because they are located at the surface of the molecule and have a high relative segmental mobility (Thornton and Sibanda 1983; Westhof *et al.* 1984).

When short, flexible peptides are used as probes to locate antigenic regions in proteins, it is the regions corresponding to mobile segments of the polypeptide chain that tend to be identified as epitopes. However, when longer peptides possessing a specific conformation are used as probes, regions that are structured and possess a low mobility may also reveal themselves to be antigenic (Al Moudallal *et al.* 1985). When monoclonal antibodies are used for antigenic analysis, it is mainly discontinuous epitopes that are revealed. Antigenicity and the types of epitopes observed clearly depend on the probes and on the methods used to define them.

Most of our knowledge concerning the location of epitopes in proteins was obtained by analyzing cross-reactive antigenicity (Van Regenmortel 1986b). In view of the multispecific and heterospecific nature of antibodies (Richards

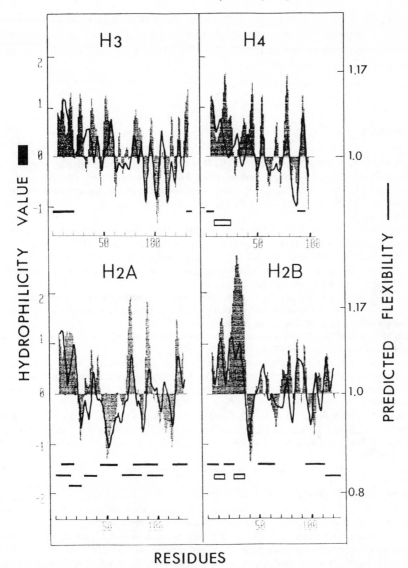

Figure 2. Hydrophilicity and mobility profiles of histones H3, H4, H2A and H2B calculated according to Hopp and Woods (1981) and Karplus and Schulz (1985), respectively. Bars represent the positions of epitopes localized with polyclonal antibodies specific for the corresponding histones. Boxes correspond to epitopes identified with monoclonal antibodies from autoimmune mice (H2B) or from mice immunized with H4. The precise location of epitopes is as follows: H3, residues 1–21, 130–135; H4, residues 1–8, 9–23, 88–96; H2A, residues 1–15, 5–18, 12–26, 28–42, 44–61, 65–85, 85–100, 90–105, 116–129; H2B, residues 1–11, 6–18, 15–25, 26–35, 50–65, 94–113, 114–125.

et al. 1975; Al Moudallal *et al.* 1982; Underwood 1985) it is futile to search for the 'true' antigenic structure to which a paratope is supposed to fit perfectly. Cross-reactive fit rather than absolute fit is the rule underlying epitope–paratope interactions.

References

Al Moudallal Z, Briand J P, Van Regenmortel M H V 1982. Monoclonal antibodies as probes of the antigenic structure of tobacco mosaic virus, *EMBO Journal* 1: 1005–10

Al Moudallal Z, Altschuh D, Briand J P, Van Regenmortel M H V 1984. Comparative sensitivity of different ELISA procedures for detecting monoclonal antibodies, *Journal of Immunological Methods* 68: 35–43

Al Moudallal Z, Briand J P, Van Regenmortel M H V 1985. A major part of the polypeptide chain of tobacco mosaic virus protein is antigenic, *EMBO Journal* 4: 1231–5

Altschuh D, Al Moudallal Z, Briand J P, Van Regenmortel M H V 1985. Immunochemical studies of tobacco mosaic virus. VI. Attempts to localize viral epitopes with monoclonal antibodies, *Molecular Immunology* 22: 329–37

Atassi M Z 1984. Antigenic structures of proteins. Their determination has revealed important aspects of immune recognition and generated strategies for synthetic mimicking of protein binding sites, *European Journal of Biochemistry* 145: 1–20

Atassi M Z, Smith J A 1978. A proposal for the nomenclature of antigenic sites in peptides and proteins, *Immunochemistry* 15: 609–10

Atassi M Z, Young C R 1985. Discovery and implications of the immunogenicity of free small synthetic peptides: powerful tools for manipulating the immune system and for production of antibodies and T cells of preselected submolecular specificities, *CRC Critical Reviews in Immunology* 5: 387–409

Benjamin D C, Berzofsky J A, East I J, Gurd F R N, Hannum C, Leach S J, Margoliash E, Michael J G, Miller A, Prager E M, Reichlin M, Sercarz E E, Smith-Gill S J, Todd P A, Wilson A C 1984. The antigenic structure of proteins: a reappraisal, *Annual Review of Immunology* 2: 67–110

Berzofsky J A 1985. Intrinsic and extrinsic factors in protein antigenic structure, *Science* 229: 932–40

Eilat D, Hochberg M, Fischel R, Laskov R 1982. Antibodies to RNA from autoimmune NZB/NZW mice recognize a similar antigenic determinant and show a large idiotypic diversity, *Proceedings of the National Academy of Sciences USA* 79: 3818–22

Friguet B, Djavadi-Ohaniance L, Goldberg M E 1984. Some monoclonal antibodies raised with a native protein bind preferentially to the denatured antigen, *Molecular Immunology* 21: 673–7

Geysen H M 1985. Antigen–antibody interactions at the molecular level: adventures in peptide synthesis, *Immunology Today* 6: 364–9

Geysen H M, Mason T J, Rodda S J, Meloen R H, Barteling S J 1985. Amino acid composition of antigenic determinants: implications for antigen processing by the immune system of animals, in R A Lerner, R M Channock, F Brown (eds) *Vaccines 85*. Cold Spring Harbor Laboratory, pp 133–7

Green N, Alexander H, Olson A, Alexander S, Shinnick T M, Sutcliffe J G, Lerner R A 1982. Immunogenic structure of the influenza virus hemagglutinin, *Cell* 28: 477–87

Hopp T P 1985. Prediction of protein surfaces and interaction sites from amino acid sequences, in K Alitalo, P Partanen, A Vaheri (eds) *Synthetic Peptides in Biology and Medicine*. Elsevier, Amsterdam, pp 3–12

Hopp T P 1986. Protein surface analysis. Methods for identifying antigenic determinants and other interaction sites, *Journal of Immunological Methods* 88: 1–18

Hopp T P, Woods K R 1981. Prediction of protein antigenic determinants from amino acid sequence, *Proceedings of the National Academy of Sciences USA* **78**: 3824–8

Jerne N K 1960. Immunological speculations, *Annual Review of Microbiology* **14**: 341–58

Karplus P A, Schulz G E 1985. Prediction of chain flexibility in proteins. A tool for the selection of peptide antigens, *Naturwissenschaften* **72**: 212

Lafer E M, Rauch J, Andrzejewski C Jr, Mudd D, Furie B, Furie B, Schwartz R S, Stollar B D 1981. Polyspecific monoclonal lupus autoantibodies reactive with both polynucleotides and phospholipids, *Journal of Experimental Medicine* **153**: 897–909

Laskov R, Muller S, Hochberg M, Giloh H, Van Regenmortel M H V, Eilat D 1984. Monoclonal antibodies to histones from autoimmune NZB/NZW F1 mice, *European Journal of Immunology* **14**: 74–81

Luka J, Sternas L, Jornvall H, Klein G, Lerner R 1983. Antibodies of predetermined specificity for the NH$_2$ terminus of a cellular protein p53 react with the native molecule: evidence for the presence of different p53s. *Proceedings of the National Academy of Sciences USA* **80**: 1199–203

McCullough K C, Crowther J R, Butcher R N 1985. Alteration in antibody reactivity with foot-and-mouth disease virus (FMDV) 146S antigen before and after binding to a solid phase or complexing with specific antibody, *Journal of Immunological Methods* **82**: 91–100

Mierendorf R C Jr, Dimond R L 1983. Functional heterogeneity of monoclonal antibodies obtained using different screening assays, *Analytical Biochemistry* **135**: 221–9

Muller S, Himmelspach K, Van Regenmortel M H V 1982. Immunochemical localization of the C-terminal hexapeptide of histone H3 at the surface of chromatin subunits, *EMBO Journal* **1**: 421–5

Muller S, Soussanieh A, Bouley J P, Reinbolt J, Van Regenmortel M H V 1983. Localization of two antigenic determinants in histone H4, *Biochimica et Biophysica Acta* **747**: 100–6

Muller S, Couppez M, Briand J P, Gordon J, Sautière P, Van Regenmortel M H V 1985. Antigenic structure of histone H2B, *Biochimica et Biophysica Acta* **827**: 235–46

Muller S, Plaue S, Couppez M, Van Regenmortel M H V 1986. Comparison of different methods for localizing antigenic regions in histone H2A, *Molecular Immunology* **23**: 593–601

Neurath A R, Rubin B A 1971. *Viral Structural Components as Immunogens of Prophylatic Value*. Karger, Basel

Novotny J, Handschumacher M, Haber E, Bruccoleri R E, Carlson W B, Fanning D W, Smith J A, Rose G D 1986. Antigenic determinants in proteins coincide with surface regions accessible to large probes (antibody domains), *Proceedings of the National Academy of Sciences USA* **83**: 226–30

Quesniaux V, Tees R, Schreier M H, Wenger R M, Donatsch P, Van Regenmortel M H V 1986. Monoclonal antibodies to cyclosporin, in J F Borel (ed) *Progress in Allergy*. Karger, Basel, vol. 38: pp 108–22

Richards F F, Konigsberg W H, Rosenstein R W, Varga J M 1975. On the specificity of antibodies. Biochemical and biophysical evidence indicates the existence of polyfunctional antibody combining regions, *Science* **187**: 130–7

Rose G D, Gierasch L M, Smith J A 1985. Turns in peptides and proteins, *Advances in Protein Chemistry* **37**: 1–109

Schroer J A, Bender T, Feldmann R J, Kim K J 1983. Mapping epitopes on the insulin molecule using monoclonal antibodies, *European Journal of Immunology* **13**: 693–700

Shi P T, Riehm J P, Todd P E E, Leach S J 1984. The antigenicity of myoglobin-related peptides synthesised on polyacrylamide and polystyrene resin supports, *Molecular Immunology* **21**: 489–96

Tainer J A, Getzoff E D, Paterson Y, Olson A J, Lerner R A 1985. The atomic mobility component of protein antigenicity, *Annual Review of Immunology* **3**: 501–35

Thornton J M, Sibanda B L 1983. Amino and carboxy-terminal regions in globular proteins, *Journal of Molecular Biology* **167**: 443–60

Thornton J M, Edwards M S, Taylor W R, Barlow D J 1986. Location of 'continuous' antigenic determinants in the protruding ends of proteins, *EMBO Journal* **5**: 409–13

Underwood P A 1985. Theoretical considerations of the ability of monoclonal antibodies to detect antigenic differences between closely related variants, with particular reference to heterospecific reactions, *Journal of Immunological Methods* **85**: 295–307

Vaidya H C, Dietzler D N, Ladenson J H 1985. Inadequacy of traditional ELISA for screening hybridoma supernatants for murine monoclonal antibodies, *Hybridoma* **4**: 271–6

Van Regenmortel M H V 1966. Plant virus serology, *Advances in Virus Research* **12**: 207–71

Van Regenmortel M H V 1982. *Serology and Immunochemistry of Plant Viruses*. Academic Press, New York

Van Regenmortel M H V 1986a. Which structural features determine protein antigenicity? *Trends in Biochemical Sciences* **11**: 36–9

Van Regenmortel M H V 1986b. Definition of antigenicity in proteins and peptides, in H Peeters (ed) *Protides of the Biological Fluids*. Pergamon Press, Oxford, vol. 34: 81–6

Westhof E, Altschuh D, Moras D, Bloomer A C, Mondragon A, Klug A, Van Regenmortel M H V 1984. Correlation between segmental mobility and the location of antigenic determinants in proteins, *Nature (London)* **311**: 123–6

4 Host response

The specificity and affinity of B cell triggering

Norman R Klinman; Phyllis-Jean Linton

Department of Immunology, Scripps Clinic & Research Foundation, La Jolla, California 92037, USA

Introduction

The efficacy of any approach to enhancing immune responses to pathogens or neoplasias is dependent on developing appropriate immunogens as well as maximizing the utilization of the host's immune mechanism. Appropriately, the bulk of this symposium addresses the current status of various approaches to the former issue. In this paper, we will attempt to summarize the current state of knowledge concerning the latter issue, particularly with respect to B cell repertoire expression and the mechanism by which the affinity of antigen–B cell receptor interaction serves to insure selective B cell stimulation while minimizing reactivity to self. Since high affinity and highly specific responses would seem ideal, our discussion will include potential limitations inherent in the expressed B cell repertoire *per se* particularly with respect to the ability to access appropriate cells and how these limitations may be overcome.

Genetically determined limitations in B cell repertoire expression

Underlying any approach to manufacturing an ideal vaccine is the faith that the B cell repertoire is 'unlimited' and, therefore, with an appropriate immunogen an antibody response should be obtained. There are, however, substantial limitations on the expressed B cell repertoire including those imposed during B cell maturation within an environment replete with self antigens and anti-idiotypic recognition as well as limitations imposed by the genetic capacity of a given individual to generate specificities.

Over the years, the perception has grown that because of the vastness of the B cell repertoire, multiple, and redundant, specificities should be available for any given antigenic determinant. This perception was initially fostered by the finding that responses to single haptenic determinants can be extremely diverse (Kreth and Williamson 1973) and was later reinforced by early estimates that the murine B cell repertoire exceeded 10^7 specificities (Klinman and Press 1975b) and the ultimate identification of molecular mechanisms that could account for the generation of at least 10^8–10^{10} specificities (Seidman *et al.* 1978; Max *et al.* 1979; Early *et al.* 1980). Added to this, B cells can rapidly accumulate somatic mutations after immunization (Griffiths *et al.* 1984; McKean *et al.* 1984; Gearhart *et al.* 1981) so that the B cell repertoire could be essentially limitless.

However, findings from studies of the diversities of responses to protein antigen determinants, which, in contrast to most haptens, would likely differ from self determinants by slight nuances, belie this conclusion, since such responses can be extremely restricted (Cancro *et al.* 1978). This is particularly true of primary responses which probably antecede any substantial accumulation of somatic mutations. Thus, in an examination of the response to the influenza hemagglutinin, although more than 10^3 distinct antigenic determinants clustered around a handful of regions within the molecule can be discriminated by monoclonal antibodies, relatively few can be recognized by the B cell repertoire in any given individual mouse (Cancro *et al.* 1978). These findings were the first indication that, although the primary B cell repertoire of a murine strain is exceedingly diverse, there are likely to be antigenic determinants on important immunogens such as viruses that cannot be recognized by a given mouse and may not be recognized by the strain as a whole.

Such a conclusion is even more apparent when very young mice (two to three weeks of age) are examined (Cancro *et al.* 1979). In young mice, the repertoire has not fully developed and therefore is much less extensive. Since genetically identical mice express essentially the same repertoire at this stage of development, more than 90% of the recognizable determinants on the influenza hemagglutinin are not recognized by the strain as a whole.

Because the determination of the upper limit of diversity of any set that includes more than 10^7 to 10^8 members is exceedingly difficult, the exact size of the primary murine B cell repertoire is not yet known. However, several findings indicate that, even though the genetic mechanism responsible for generating variable regions may be capable of generating greater than 10^{10} specificities (assuming all possible permutations of V_H, D and J, as well as junctional diversity) (Seidman *et al.* 1978; Max *et al.* 1979; Early *et al.* 1980), the repertoire which is actually generated is not a random representation of all possible V-region segment combinations. In every instance wherein clonotypes can be identified by sequence, specificity, or idiotype, all individuals of a given strain appear to express reproducibly the same clonotypes (reviewed in Sigal and Klinman 1978). This is true not only for clonotypes expressed at unusually high frequency (predominant clonotypes) but also for clonotypes expressed at substantially lower frequencies (Sigal *et al.* 1977; Manser *et al.* 1985). Thus, there is fidelity in the hierarchy of variable region combinations which are chosen for expression within genetically identical individuals. This serves as a clear indication that V-region combinatorial association is not a totally random or stochastic process. Such a conclusion is supported by the findings of reproducible differences in repertoire expression of neonates versus adults versus aged individuals (Klinman and Press, 1975a; Sigal *et al.* 1977; Fung and Kohler 1980; Denis and Klinman 1983; Riley *et al.* 1986; Yancopoulos *et al.* 1984; Perlmutter *et al.* 1985; Zharhary and Klinman 1986).

Importantly, each of the aforementioned characteristics of the repertoire of mature primary B cells (i.e. extensive diversity and nonrandomness) are equally characteristic of cells of the B cell lineage prior to surface immunoglobulin (sIg) expression (Riley *et al.* 1983; Riley and Klinman 1985; Klinman and Stone 1983; Froscher and Klinman 1985; Nishikawa *et al.* 1983; Juy *et al.* 1983). Thus, interaction with the antigenic or idiotypic environment is essential neither for the generation of a diverse repertoire nor for the inequality of clonotype expressions. Studies at the sIg^- B cell precursor level have also indicated that B cells are expressed as clones of multiple (10^1-10^3) identical sister cells (Klinman and Stone 1983). Given the findings that approximately 5 $\times$ 10^7 B cells are generated within the murine marrow per day (Osmond and Owens 1984), and that B cells are expressed as expanded clones, then fewer than 10^5 specificities would be expressed from within the bone marrow per day, thereby limiting repertoire expression during the first two or three months of life to 10^7-10^8 specificities.

Taken together, these findings would indicate that mice of a given V-region haplotype will reproducibly express only a subset of all the 'potential' V-region combinations. Since mice differing in their heavy- and light-chain V-region haplotypes reproducibly express different repertoires, one might expect that, to the extent that repertoire expression is nonrandom and is determined by inherited V-region genes, evolutionary selection could play a substantial role in repertoire determination.

Environmentally imposed limitations on B cell repertoire expression

Although, as discussed above, studies of sIg^- bone marrow precursor cells indicate that environmental selection does not appear to be essential for repertoire diversification or predominant clonotype expression, we now have several examples of environmentally induced clonotype elimination during B cell maturation (Riley and Klinman 1985; Klinman and Stone 1983; Froscher and Klinman 1985; Morrow *et al.* 1987). There is a substantial amount of information indicating that B cells pass through a developmental stage during which they are susceptible to inactivation by contact with tolerogens or anti-immunoglobulin (including anti-idiotype) (Metcalf and Klinman 1976, 1977; Nossal 1987). Recently, a comparison of the repertoire as expressed in precursor cells just prior to sIg expression versus mature bone marrow versus splenic B cells has identified numerous examples of clonotypes that are present prior to sIg receptor expression and absent, or greatly reduced in representation, after sIg expression (Riley and Klinman 1985; Klinman and

Stone 1983; Froscher and Klinman 1985; Morrow *et al.* 1987). These examples cover a broad range of antigens including murine cytochrome *c*, phosphoryl-choline (PC), (4-hydroxy-3-nitrophenyl)acetyl (NP), and α(1–3)-dextran. The latter case is particularly interesting in that precursors to lambda bearing α(1–3)-dextran-specific B cells in Igh^b mice are present in lower frequency in mature B cell populations than would be anticipated by their representation in the sIg$^-$ B cell precursor pool. These latter cells could be induced to respond only in carrier primed Igh allogeneic (Igh^a) mice (Froscher and Klinman 1985). Since in each of the other aforementioned responses sIg$^-$ precursors could respond in Igh syngeneic as well as Igh allogeneic environments, we presume the mechanism of their elimination is more likely to be tolerance than anti-idiotypic suppression which could be Igh restricted (Pierce and Klinman 1977). By this reasoning, the elimination of lambda bearing α(1–3)-dextran-specific B cells in Igh^b mice would be a likely candidate for anti-idiotypic modification of the expressed B cell repertoire. At the present time, the elimination of these B cells serves as the sole example of potential anti-idiotypic modification of the expressed repertoire. The presumption that the other specificities are eliminated by tolerance induction remains speculation since the responsible self antigen has not been definitively identified. In any case, the ease with which so many examples of clonotype elimination during B cell development have been identified would indicate that environmental down-regulation of repertoire expression may be quite extensive and could have a substantial impact on the functional primary B cell repertoire.

The relationship of sIg receptor affinity to responsiveness of the B cell repertoire

Can a repertoire of as many as 10^7–10^8 clonotypes be 'limited' with respect to the capacity to respond to given antigenic determinants? Since antibodies generally cross-react it should not be difficult to obtain at least low-affinity antibodies to any determinant. In this context, since antibody–antigen interactions are reversible and can be driven to the bound state by higher concentrations of reactants, why should it not be possible to stimulate at least some low-affinity B cell responses to a difficult antigen by simply raising the immunogen concentration?

Several years ago, in the course of analyzing monoclonal T cell-dependent B cell responses, an unusual relationship between immunogen concentration and antibody affinity was noted (Klinman 1972). At relatively low antigen concentrations (10^{-13}–10^{-7} M for hapten) there was a direct relationship between the number of B cells stimulated and antigen concentration. Consistently with the prediction that at high antigen concentrations low-affinity receptors would be adequate for stimulation, higher antigen concentrations were shown to stimulate more B cells, and B cells whose antibody product included those of relatively low affinity. However, whereas increasing antigen concentrations above a hapten determinant concentration of 10^{-7} M increased the number of cells whose sIg receptors bound antigen, no increase could be observed in the frequency of antigen responding cells nor was there any decrease in the average affinity of B cells that were stimulated (Klinman 1972; Klinman *et al.* 1976). Thus, it appeared that driving the antigen–receptor interaction by increasing antigen concentration could not enable T-dependent stimulation of B cells whose receptor affinity was below a threshold needed for stimulation.

In recent years, a considerable amount has been learned concerning the role of the sIg receptor in antigenic stimulation of B cells. It is now clear that the interaction of the sIg receptor with antigen can participate in the activation of B cells by several routes, all of which may operate simultaneously and in concert and all of which could be highly affinity-dependent (Klinman 1972; Klinman *et al.* 1976; Coutinho and Moller 1975; Pereira *et al.* 1986; Rock *et al.* 1984; Pierce *et al.* 1980; Kakiuchi *et al.* 1983; Lanzavecchia 1985; Casten *et al.* 1985; Mitchison 1967). For example, if the recognized antigen is itself a B cell mitogen, as would be true for many pathogens, then the antigen receptor may serve primarily as a focusing device to concentrate selectively the antigen on the surface of the B cell which would then be triggered by interaction with the appropriate mitogen receptor (Coutinho and Moller 1975). More recently it has been realized that, for the more general case of T cell dependent B cell stimulation, the function of the sIg receptor as an antigen focusing devise may be equally important (Kakiuchi *et al.* 1983; Lanzavecchia 1985; Casten *et al.* 1985). Numerous investigators have shown that B cells serve as a primary cell for antigen presentation to helper T cells (Pierce *et al.* 1980; Kakiuchi *et al.* 1983; Lanzavecchia 1985; Casten *et al.* 1985). Studies are also available that demonstrate that B cells with receptors for a given antigen can selectively take up that antigen, thus providing the opportunity for intracellular processing and presentation of that antigen on the cell surface in association with the B cell's class II MHC alloantigens (Kakiuchi *et al.* 1983; Lanzavecchia 1985). Since T cell/B cell interactions apparently require such presentation and since concentrations of natural antigens are likely to be exceedingly low, the role of the sIg receptor of B cells as a concentration device cannot be overestimated.

While the aforementioned antigen focusing functions of the sIg receptor appear to be both necessary and sufficient for T cell independent B cell stimulation on the one hand and T cell dependent stimulation on the other, antigen focusing is clearly not the only function subserved by the sIg receptor. For example, when appropriately engaged with antigen or anti-immunoglobulin the sIg receptor *per se* serves as a triggering receptor (Nossal 1987; Rock *et al.* 1984; Ashman 1984; Coggeshall and Cambier 1985; Teale and Klinman 1980, 1984; Moller 1976; Harris *et al.* 1982). This triggering function of the sIg receptor has been demonstrated at several levels. First, it appears that triggering via mitogen receptors is enhanced if sIg receptors are simultaneously engaged (Pereira *et al.* 1986). Second, it appears that triggering in a T-dependent fashion may be facilitated when sIg receptors are engaged (Casten *et al.* 1985). Third, the interlinkage of sIg receptors on mature or immature cells can initiate a cascade of intracellular processes typical of cell triggering events (Coggeshall and Cambier 1985). Fourth, interlinking the sIg receptor of mature B cells leads to enhanced expression of recognized MHC class II molecules on the B cell surface (Rock *et al.* 1984). And, fifth, tolerance induction of immature B cells appears solely dependent on the interlinkage of sIg receptors via high-affinity interactions with appropriate antigen (Teale and Klinman 1980, 1984). That the tolerance trigger is highly specific has been demonstrated directly by experiments wherein 2,4-dinitrophenyl (DNP)-specific immature neonatal B cells were shown to be highly susceptible to tolerance induction even with very low concentrations of DNP-carrier conjugates, but were not at all susceptible to tolerance induction by 2,4,6-trinitrophenyl (TNP)–carrier conjugates (Teale and Klinman 1980). Importantly, the antibodies produced by these DNP-specific antibodies were capable of binding TNP. Additionally, TNP–carrier conjugates when added to neonatal DNP specific B cells were able to bind the receptors of these cells so as to prohibit tolerance induction by DNP–carrier conjugates, yet TNP–carrier conjugates could not tolerize these B cells.

Given so highly specific and affinity-dependent a tolerance triggering mechanism, how is it possible to account for the presence of B cells responsive to self antigens within the mature B cell repertoire (Moller 1976; Harris *et al.* 1982; Jemmerson *et al.* 1985)? There are several plausible explanations for this phenomenon, some of which may provide useful insights into the challenges that must be met by effective vaccine programs. First, it is likely that certain self antigens (sequestered antigens) would not be accessible in the milieu of developing B cells in sufficient concentrations to render B cells unresponsive. As has been pointed out by many investigators, the danger of untoward reactions by surviving self-reactive B cells is lessened by the fact that T cell presentation for these antigens would likely be minimal.

A second explanation for the persistence of anti-self B cells is related to the affinity dependence of B cell tolerance induction. Since the affinity threshold for tolerance induction is relatively high, B cells with low affinity for self antigens would pass through the tolerance gauntlet. In general, these B cells could have sufficiently low-affinity receptors that they would not be triggered by self antigens. However, they may be triggered by foreign antigens and, under such circumstances, their capacity to bind to self antigens may be harmful.

Recently, two types of reactivity which would fit into this latter general category have gained considerably more interest. It has been found for several antigen systems including self antigens (Jemmerson *et al.* 1985), that immunization with peptides fashioned from sequences of native proteins can induce the production of anti-peptide antibodies which react, albeit at lower affinity, with the native antigen (Jemmersen *et al.* 1985; Hirayama *et al.* 1985;

Tainer *et al.* 1985). This type of reactivity could lead to the impression that repertoire potential for certain antigens is far greater than that which can be tapped by immunization with the antigen *per se*. Since the tolerance mechanism is permissive of low-affinity reactivities, the availability of a vast array of low-affinity reactivities that can be conjured up under appropriate circumstances is not contradictory to the concept of a limited specificity repertoire that is accessed by a highly specific and selective triggering mechanism. This is not to argue, however, that conjuring up low-affinity responses may not be helpful in certain vaccination programs.

A second example of this type of potential 'self' reactivity is that found with certain antibodies that, like T cell receptors, bind antigen only in the context of the MHC alloantigen of the presenting cell (Wylie *et al.* 1982; Froscher and Klinman 1986). In recent studies, using B cell recognition of SV40 transformed cells, it was found that some antibodies, while exhibiting a high affinity for SV40 antigens in conjunction with the class I MHC alloantigen of the immunizing cell, had a discernible but much lower affinity for the self-MHC alloantigen in the absence of SV40 transformation (Froscher and Klinman 1986). It now appears that such recognition might constitute an important component of B cell responses and could be of obvious interest in understanding T cell responses as well. As has been suggested for low-affinity reaction of anti-peptide antibodies with the homologous protein antigen (Hirayama *et al.* 1985), the low-affinity binding of these antibodies to self MHC may reflect the fact that these antibodies might induce a conformation of the MHC molecule similar to one induced by interaction of the MHC molecule with a foreign cell surface antigen.

Recent experiments in this laboratory have revealed yet another explanation for the persistence of B cells with low affinity for self antigens. In studies of the response of immature versus mature B cells to NP and its analog (4-hydroxy-5-iodo-3-nitrophenyl)acetyl (NIP), it was found that the population of lambda bearing B cells which dominate the response to NP were essentially the same B cells that responded to NIP and had a higher affinity for the NIP than NP (Riley and Klinman 1986). Importantly, while it was possible to both stimulate and tolerize immature B cells of this specificity with NIP–carrier conjugates, most of these cells could neither be stimulated nor tolerized as immature cells with NP–carrier conjugates. We have interpreted these findings as indicating that the affinity requisites for triggering or tolerizing immature B cells may be higher than is required for stimulating the same B cells expressing the same receptors once they are mature. If this is generally the case, then it is possible that many B cells that could respond to self antigens as mature cells would have too low an affinity to be tolerized during their tolerance-susceptible developmental stage. Given the availability of a tolerance mechanism, why would such a mechanism be so inefficient as to permit the persistence of cells which would ultimately have the capacity to respond to self antigens? It has been proposed by several investigators that, if a valid tolerance mechanism did in fact exist, because of the existence of a vast array of self-antigenic determinants and the high degree of antibody cross-reactivity, such a tolerance mechanism would likely eliminate the entire repertoire several times over. It is possible that by setting the tolerance threshold high, the immune system successfully eliminates only high-affinity self-reactive B cells while maintaining repertoire diversity. If broadly applicable, this could imply that many B cells that survive the tolerance gauntlet could have low affinity for self antigens, and may be potentially reactive to self antigens as mature B cells.

The consequences of secondary responses and somatic mutation

A severe test of the concept that tolerance to self antigens plays an important role in the elimination of potentially harmful self-reactive B cells comes from the finding that somatic mutations rapidly accumulate after immunization and during the generation of secondary B cells (Griffiths *et al.* 1984; McKean *et al.* 1984; Gearhart *et al.* 1981). Since these mutations change the specificities of the antibodies involved, it would seem essential that B cells pass through a second tolerance-susceptible phase to eliminate any new self reactivities that may be generated. Most importantly, for vaccination protocols, the accumulation of appropriate somatic mutations may enable the expression and increased affinity of responses that would otherwise be rare or of low affinity. Recent findings in this laboratory indicate that newly generated secondary precursors also pass through a tolerance-susceptible phase (Linton and Klinman 1986). Preliminary evidence indicates that this tolerance-susceptible phase of secondary cells may have a substantially lower affinity threshold than that required during the tolerance-susceptible phase of primary B cells. If this is true, then the immune system could eliminate not only potentially harmful newly generated secondary specificities but also potentially harmful primary specificities as these specificities are incorporated into the secondary B cell repertoire. As with the tolerance-susceptible phase of primary B cells (Metcalf and Klinman 1976), it is likely that the tolerance of secondary B cells may also be bypassed by antigenic stimulation in the presence of adequate T cell help. Thus, while many secondary precursor cells may be eliminated by their inherent capabilities of reacting with self antigens, those with sufficient affinity to capture antigen and T cell help could have a strong selective advantage. Given the potential of secondary responses to enhance markedly the number and affinity of specificities available for the immunizing antigen, it is likely that the most useful vaccination protocols would be those that successfully maximize the generation and selection of secondary B cells.

Acknowledgements

This work was supported by National Institutes of Health Grant Nos AI 15797 and T32 AG00080.

References

Ashman R 1984. Lymphocyte activation, in W Paul (ed) *Fundamental Immunology*. Raven Press, New York pp 267–300

Cancro M P, Gerhard W, Klinman N R 1978. Diversity of the primary influenza specific B cell repertoire in BALB/c mice, *Journal of Experimental Medicine* **147**: 776–87

Cancro M P, Wylie D E, Gerhard W, Klinman N R 1979. Patterned acquisition of the antibody repertoire: diversity of the hemagglutinin-specific B cell repertoire in neonatal BALB/c mice, *Proceedings of the National Academy of Sciences USA* **76**: 6577–81

Casten L A, Lakey E K, Jelachich M L, Margoliash E, Pierce S K 1985. Anti-immunoglobulin augments the B cell antigen-presentation function independently of internalization of receptor–antigen complex, *Proceedings of the National Academy of Sciences USA* **82**: 5890–4

Coggeshall K M, Cambier J C 1985. B cell activation. VI. Effects of exogenous diglyceride and modulators of phospholipid metabolism suggest a central role for diacylglycerol generation in transmembrane signaling by mIg, *Journal of Immunology* **134**: 101–7

Coutinho A, Moller G 1975. Thymus-independent B cell induction and paralysis, *Advances in Immunology* **21**: 113–236

Denis K A, Klinman N R 1983. Genetic and temporal control of neonatal antibody expression, *Journal of Experimental Medicine* **157**: 83

Early P, Huang H, Davis M, Calame K, Hood L 1980. An immunoglobulin heavy chain variable region gene is generated from three segments of DNA: V_H, D and J_H, *Cell* **19**: 981–92

Froscher B G, Klinman N R 1985. Strain-specific silencing of a predominant antidextran clonotype family, *Journal of Experimental Medicine* **162**: 1620–33

Froscher B G, Klinman N R 1986. Immunization with SV40 transformed syngeneic cells yields mainly MHC restricted monoclonal antibodies, *Journal of Experimental Medicine* **164**: 196–210

Fung S J, Kohler H 1980. Late clonal selection and expansion of the TEPC-15 germ-line specificity, *Journal of Experimental Medicine* **152**: 1262–73

Gearhart P J, Johnson H D, Douglas R, Hood L 1981. IgG antibodies to phosphorylcholine exhibit more diversity than their IgM counterparts, *Nature (London)* **291**: 29–34

Griffiths G M, Berek M C, Kaartinen M, Milstein C 1984. Somatic mutation and the maturation of immune response to 2-phenyl oxazolone, *Nature (London)* **312**: 271–5

Harris D E, Cairns L, Rosen F S, Borel Y 1982. A natural model of immunologic tolerance. Tolerance to murine C5 is mediated by T cells, and antigen is required to maintain unresponsiveness, *Journal of Experimental Medicine* **156**: 567–84

Hirayama A, Takagaki Y, Karush F 1985. Interaction of monoclonal anti-peptide antibodies with lysozyme, *Journal of Immunology* **134**: 3241–7

Jemmerson R R W, Morrow P R, Klinman N R, Paterson Y 1985. Analysis of an evolutionarily conserved antigenic site on mammalian cytochrome *c* using synthetic peptides, *Proceedings of the National Academy of Sciences USA* **82**: 1508–12

Juy D, Primi D, Sanches P, Casenave P-A 1983. The selection and maintenance of the V region determinant repertoire is germ-line encoded and T cell independent, *European Journal of Immunology* **13**: 326–31

Kakiuchi T, Chestnut R W, Grey H M 1983. B cells as antigen-presenting cells: the requirement for B cell activation, *Journal of Immunology* **131**: 109–14

Klinman N R 1972. The mechanism of antigenic stimulation of primary and secondary clonal precursor cells, *Journal of Experimental Medicine* **136**: 241–60

Klinman N R, Press J L 1975a. The characterization of the B cell repertoire specific for the DNP and TNP determinants in neonatal BALB/c mice, *Journal of Experimental Medicine* **141**: 1133–46

Klinman N R, Press J L 1975b. The B cell specificity repertoire: its relationship to definable subpopulations, *Transplantation Reviews* **24**: 41–83

Klinman N R, Stone M R 1983. Role of variable region gene expression and environmental selection in determining the antiphosphorylcholine B cell repertoire, *Journal of Experimental Medicine* **158**: 1948–61

Klinman N R, Pickard A R, Sigal N H, Gearhart P J, Metcalf E S, Pierce S K 1976. Assessing B cell diversification by antigen receptor and precursor cell analysis, *Annals of Immunology* **127**: 489–502

Kreth H W, Williamson A R 1973. The extent of diversity of anti-hapten antibodies in inbred mice: anti-NIP (4-hydroxy-5-iodo-3-nitrophenacetyl) antibodies in CBA/H mice, *European Journal of Immunology* **3**: 141–6

Lanzavecchia A 1985. Antigen-specific interactions between T and B cells, *Nature (London)* **314**: 537–9

Linton P J, Klinman N R 1986. The generation of secondary B cells *in vitro*, *Federation Proceedings* **45**: 378 (Abstract 1302)

Manser T, Wysocki L J, Gridley T, Near R I, Gefter M L 1985. The molecular evolution of the immune response, *Immunology Today* **6**: 3–5

Max E E, Seidman J G, Leder P 1979. Sequence of five potential recombination sites encoded close to an immunoglobulin κ constant region gene, *Proceedings of the National Academy of Sciences USA* **76**: 3450–4

McKean D, Huppi K, Bell M, Staudt L, Gerhard W, Weigert M 1984. Generation of antibody diversity in the immune response of BALB/c mice to influenza virus hemagglutinin, *Proceedings of the National Academy of Sciences USA* **81**: 3180–4

Metcalf E S, Klinman N R 1976. *In vitro* tolerance induction of neonatal murine B cells, *Journal of Experimental Medicine* **143**: 1327–40

Metcalf E S, Klinman N R 1977. *In vitro* tolerance induction of neonatal and adult bone marrow cells: a functional marker for B cell maturation, *Journal of Immunology* **118**: 2111–16

Mitchison N A 1967. Antigen recognition responsible for the induction *in vitro* of the secondary response, *Cold Spring Harbor Symposium on Quantitative Biology* **32**: 431–9

Moller G 1976. Mechanism of B cell activation and self–non-self discrimination, *Cold Spring Harbor Symposium on Quantitative Biology* **41**: 217–26

Morrow P R, Jemmerson R W, Klinman N R 1987. Disparities in the repertoire of B cells responsive to a native protein and those responsive to a synthetic peptide, in E E Sercarz, J Berzofsky (eds) *Immunogenicity of Protein Antigens: Repertoire and regulation.* Academic Press, Orlando (Florida) (in press)

Nishikawa S T, Takemori T, Rajewsky K 1983. The expression of a set of antibody variable regions in lipopolysaccharide-reactive B cells at various stages of ontogeny and its control by anti-idiotypic antibody, *European Journal of Immunology* **13**: 318–25

Nossal G J V 1987. Bone marrow pre B cells and the clonal anergy theory of immunologic tolerance, in H Kohler, C Bona (eds) *Pre-B Cells.* Gordon and Breach, New York (in press)

Osmond D G, Owens J J T 1984. Pre-B cells in bone marrow: size distribution profile, proliferative capacity and peanut agglutinin binding of cytoplasmic μ chain-bearing cell populations in normal and regenerating bone marrow, *Immunology* **51**: 333–42

Pereira P, Forsgren S, Portnoi D, Bandeira A, Martinez A C, Coutinho A 1986. The role of immunoglobulin receptors in 'cognate' T–B cell collaboration, *European Journal of Immunology* **16**: 355–61

Perlmutter R M, Kearney J F, Chang S P, Hood L 1985. Developmentally controlled expression of immunoglobulin V_H genes. *Science* **227**: 1597–601

Pierce S K, Klinman N R 1977. Antibody specific immunoregulation, *Journal of Experimental Medicine* **146**: 509–19

Pierce S K, Klinman N R, Maurer P H, Merryman C F 1980. Role of the MHC gene product in regulating the antibody response to DNP-GLφ9, *Journal of Experimental Medicine* **152**: 336–49

Riley R L, Klinman N R 1985. Differences in antibody repertoire for (4-hydroxy-3-nitrophenyl)acetyl (NP) in splenic vs immature bone marrow precursor cells, *Journal of Immunology* **135**: 3050–5

Riley R L, Klinman N R 1986. The affinity threshold for antigenic triggering differs for tolerance susceptible immature precursors vs mature primary B cells, *Journal of Immunology* **136**: 3147–54

Riley R L, Wylie D E, Klinman N R 1983. B cell repertoire diversification precedes immuno-globulin receptor expression, *Journal of Experimental Medicine* **158**: 1733–8

Riley S R, Connors S J, Klinman N R, Ogata R T 1986. Preferential expression of V_H gene segments by predominant DNP specific BALB/c neonatal antibody clonotypes, *Proceedings of the National Academy of Sciences USA* **83**: 2589–93

Rock K L, Benacerraf B, Abbas A K 1984. Antigen presentation by hapten-specific B lympho-cytes. I. Role of surface immunoglobulin receptors, *Journal of Experimental Medicine* **160**: 1102–13

Seidman J G, Leder A, Nau M, Norman B, Leder P 1978. Antibody diversity. The structure of cloned immunoglobulin genes suggests a mechanism for generating new sequences, *Science* **202**: 11–17

Sigal N H, Klinman N R 1978. B cell clonotype repertoire, *Advances in Immunology* **26**: 255–337

Sigal N H, Gearhart P J, Press J L, Klinman N R 1976. The late acquisition of a 'germ line' antibody specificity, *Nature (London)* **251**: 51

Sigal N H, Cancro M P, Klinman N R 1977. The significance of minor clonotypes in the dis-section of B cell diversification, in E E Sercarz, L A Herzenberg, C F Fox (eds) *ICN–UCLA Symposia on Molecular and Cellular Biology* vol VI *Immune system; genetics and regulation*. Academic Press, New York p 217

Tainer J A, Getzoff E D, Paterson Y, Olson A J, Lerner R A 1985. The atomic mobility component of protein antigenicity, *Annual Reviews of Immunology* **3**: 501–35

Teale J M, Klinman N R 1980. Tolerance as an active process, *Nature (London)* **288**: 385–7 Teale J M, Klinman N R 1984. Membrane and metabolic requirements for tolerance of neonatal B cells, *Journal of Immunology* **133**: 1811–17

Wylie D, Sherman L A, Klinman N R 1982. Participation of the major histocompatibility complex in antibody recognition of viral antigens expressed on infected cells, *Journal of Experimental Medicine* **155**: 403–14

Yancopoulos G D, Desiderio S V, Paskind M, Kearney J F, Baltimore D, Alt F W 1984. Pre-ferential utilization of the most J_H-proximal V_H gene segments in pre-B cell lines, *Nature (London)* **311**: 727–33

Zharhary D, Klinman N R 1986. A selective increase in the generation of phosphorylcholine specific B cells associated with aging, *Journal of Immunology* **136**: 368–70

Mucosal immune response to viral vaccines

Pearay L Ogra;* Tara R Dharakul; Joachim Freihorst†

* Departments of Pediatrics and Microbiology, State University of New York at Buffalo, and Division of Infectious Diseases, Children's Hospital, Buffalo, New York 14222, USA
† Medizinische Hochschule Hannover, Kinderklinik, D-3000 Hannover, West Germany

It is well known that most viral infections are acquired naturally via the mucosal portals of entry, especially through the mucosal surfaces of respiratory and intestinal tracts and, less frequently through genital mucosa (Ogra *et al.* 1980). Although the modern art of vaccine-induced protection against infectious diseases has been in practice for several decades, recent proliferation of knowledge in molecular biology of viruses, mechanisms of immunity and immunoregulation at mucosal and systemic sites, and introduction of several but unique biotechnologic approaches have opened new avenues of exploration in the field of vaccine development.

This report will briefly review the mucosal immune response to the conventional viral vaccines. An attempt will be made to examine the implication of mucosal immunity in newer aspects of viral vaccine development.

Conventional vaccines

The conventional vaccines currently in use include live attenuated, live cross-reactive, and inactivated (killed) organisms. No viral vaccines were available for human use prior to the 1960s for immunization via the mucosal routes. Since then, over 16 live or inactivated viral vaccines for veterinary use and three vaccines for human use have become available (Table 1).

Comparative evaluation of immunological efficiency of natural infection, or induced immunity with live or inactivated viral vaccines administered parenterally or mucosally, has provided a wealth of information concerning the development and possible functions of mucosal immunity. This information has been reviewed in several recent publications (Ogra *et al.* 1980, 1984; Ennis 1983). The factors which have been found to be of major importance in the development of mucosal immunologic reactivity are listed in Table 2.

Table 1 Available viral vaccines which can be administered via the mucosal route

Human		Non-human	
	Polio		NDV
	Rubella		Infectious bronchiolitis
	Adenovirus		Fowl pox
	Rotavirus*		Infectious laryngotracheitis
	Influenza*		Encephalomyelitis
	Measles*		Marek's disease
			IBD
			Parainfluenza
			Adenovirus
			Rotavirus
			Distemper
			TGE
			Duck hepatitis
			Rabies (fox, dog, bat)

* Candidate vaccines.

Table 2 Determinants of (mucosal) secretory immune response in the mammalian species

Pathogen determinant	Host determinant
Live	
virulent	Route and site of immunization
attenuated	
cold adapted	Genetic restrictions
Killed	
(altered) Ag	Age
Antigen dose	Level of prior systemic or mucosal immunity
Prior experience with host (homologous	
or cross-reactive)	

Live viruses

Studies carried out with a candidate live attenuated varicella zoster virus (VZV) vaccine and naturally acquired VZV infection have shown that replication of virus *per se* is not an adequate determinant of the mucosal immune response (Baba *et al.* 1982; Bogger-Goren *et al.* 1982, 1984). Naturally acquired infection, presumably via the respiratory route, was consistently followed by the development of secretory IgA response in nasopharyngeal secretions, VZV specific cell mediated immune response in tonsillar lymphocytes and antibody and cell mediated immune response to VZV in the peripheral blood. On the other hand, parenteral or inhalation induced immunization with the live vaccine failed to induce any secretory IgA response to VZV in the nasopharynx. It should, however, be pointed out that these

Table 3 Development of VZV specific immunity after natural or vaccine induced infection

Study group	Virus dose (PFU)	VZV specific antibody titer* after 4 months	
		Serum IgG	Secretory IgA
Natural infection	—	1552 ± 900	60 ± 21
VZV Vaccine†			
(a) S/C	500	44 ± 28	0
(b) I/H	2500	56 ± 15	0
(c) I/H	800	1.3 ± 0.5	0

* Expressed as geometric mean ± SD.
† S/C, subcutaneous; I/H, administered via inhalation; PFU, plaque-forming units of the virus.

vaccinees regularly developed antibody and cell mediated immunity (Bogger-Goren *et al.* 1984) in the peripheral blood (Table 3).

Immunization with other live viruses, such as different types of live attenuated rubella vaccines, e.g. RA27/3, has been shown to induce secretory antibody response in respiratory tract after intranasal immunization as well as after subcutaneous immunization. However, subcutaneous immunization with Cendehill or HPV-77 strains of live attenuated rubella vaccine result in minimal or no secretory antibody response in the nasopharynx when administered via either route of immunization (Fishaut *et al.* 1981; Ogra *et al.* 1983). Recently, it has been observed that despite the lack of significant nasopharyngeal antibody response following parenteral immunization with HPV or Cendehill strains, such immunization consistently results in the appearance of rubella specific IgA activity in milk after immunization in seronegative lactating females (Table 4). It is suggested that parenteral immunization with rubella vaccine probably permits some transport of viral antigens to the mucosal immunocompetent precursors in the respiratory tract, resulting in antigen-induced IgA–B cell activation and their possible migration to the mammary glands. As a result of vaccine-induced viremia, the availability of

Table 4 Development of rubella-specific antibody response in different body fluids

Rubella virus type and route†	Magnitude of Antibody Response* in:		
	NPS sIgA	Serum IgG	Milk sIgA
Natural infection	++	++	++
RA27/3 S/C	+	+	++
RA27/3 I/N	++	++	++
HPV-77 S/C	—	++	++

* — Essentially negative; + minimal; ++ strong.
† NPS, nasopharynx; S/C, subcutaneous; I/N, intranasal; sIgA, secretory IgA.

Table 5 Features of immune response to conventional viral vaccines*

Features of response	Immunization systemic		Immunization mucosal (enteric or respiratory)	
	Live vaccine	Killed vaccine	Live vaccine	Killed vaccine
Similar to natural infection	±	−	+	−
Systemic reponse observed	+	+	+	−
Persistence of systemic response	+	−	+	−
Viral antigen in mucosal surfaces	±	−	+	±
Secretory response observed	±	−	+	+
Persistence of secretory response	±	−	+	±
Immunity in other mucosal sites and milk	−	−	+	±
Protection against mucosal reinfection	±	±	+	+
Protection against systemic disease at reinfection	+	+	+	±
Herd immunity spread of vaccine virus to contacts	±	−	+	−
More serious disease on natural reinfection	−	±	−	?

* + Always; ± occasional or inconsistent; − absent; ? not known.

viral antigens from the blood stream to the breast may induce further proliferation of mucosally derived immunocompetent cells localized in the breast, resulting in development of significant immunologic reactivity in the milk in the absence of such reactivity in the nasopharyngeal secretions (Ogra *et al.* 1983). Based on the observations summarized above, immunization with live vaccine administered mucosally offers several unique advantages when compared to immunization via the systemic route (Table 5).

Inactivated vaccines

The patterns of immune response observed with a nonreplicating viral vaccine administered at mucosal or systemic sites exhibit many differences compared to the response observed with a live vaccine. This information is briefly summarized in Table 5. Killed viral vaccines are highly efficient in inducing serum antibody response and in prevention of viremia during reinfection challenge. Mucosal immunization, and in some studies systemic immunization with inactivated poliovaccine (IPV) has been shown to induce significant secretory IgA antibody response in the nasopharynx and intestine (Mellander 1985). It has also been proposed that prior parenteral priming with IPV results in significant enhancement of mucosal poliovirus IgA antibody response to subsequent oral immunization with live attenuated orally administered poliovaccine (OPV) (International Symposium on Poliomyelitis Control 1984).

There are at least two instances in which parenteral immunization with inactivated viral vaccines (measles and respiratory syncytial virus) have been associated with the appearance of more severe disease and development of pulmonary immunopathology following acquisition of natural infection with homologous wild virus. The observed enhancement of mucosal immune response and the development of increased mucosal immunopathology following parenteral priming or immunization respectively with inactivated virus vaccines has been recently shown to be related to induction of several distinct immunoregulatory abnormalities at the level of T cells, virus-specific IgE production and appearance of antibodies exhibiting cross-reactivity between the virus and the host tissues or tissue culture components in which the virus replication takes place (Ennis 1983; Wong *et al.* 1985; Welliver *et al.* 1980, 1981).

Notwithstanding the observed immunological differences between live or inactivated viral vaccines administered mucosally or via the blood stream, conventional vaccines employed to date have been amazingly successful in total or partial control of many devastating viral diseases. Most of these vaccines were developed with relatively minimal manipulation of the native virulent viruses rendering them either attenuated but still replicating, or inactivated (killed) but still immunogenic. Their success is especially impressive because their use preceded the acquisition of precise scientific information regarding mechanism of induced immunity.

Virtually all conventional vaccines contain varying amounts of nonviral but immunologically active contaminants such as tissue culture components, other viral induced neo-antigens and host proteins. In addition, inactivation procedures may result in loss or alteration of some viral glycoproteins or antigens important in the mechanism of protection. Thus, even with highly successful conventional viral vaccines, serious side effects and other risks may be potentially more harmful and socially unacceptable today than the actual risks associated with the natural infection itself. Furthermore, many conventional vaccines cannot be effectively delivered to subjects in many parts of the world because of cost and other socio-economic considerations.

Newer vaccines

The problems with conventional vaccines have identified a need for development of a new generation of viral vaccines, which would be highly efficient and cost-effective and at the same time do not exhibit limitations observed with conventional vaccines.

A number of approaches have been proposed in the recent years (Brown 1984; UytdeHaag *et al.* 1986; Boss and Wood 1985). These include: (a) subunit vaccines prepared in attenuated heterologous carriers or by recombinant DNA techniques; (b) idiotypic vaccines; (c) synthetic polypeptides or defined antigens; and (d) receptor-specific vaccines employing host cell receptors for virus binding or specific targets.

Unlike conventional vaccines, the successful use of newer candidate vaccines employing the approaches listed above will largely depend on identification and induction of mechanisms of specific immunity and a clear definition of viral epitopes or antigenic determinants necessary for such protective immune responses. Induction of such response in mucosal surfaces will be crucial especially for those infections which are limited to mucous membranes (RSV, parainfluenza, rotavirus, influenza viruses).

As pointed out earlier, replicating viral vaccines appear to be more efficient in inducing mucosal responses than nonreplicating inactivated vaccines. It is believed that the superior immunogenicity of live vaccines may be due in part to high efficiency in presentation of antigens in conjunction with the histocompatibility antigens of the host. This effect is possibly due to intracellular replication and formation of viral antigen–histocompatibility antigen complexes. This may explain the failure to induce development of viral specific cytotoxic T cell responses after immunization with nonreplicating viral vaccines. Although conventional replicating viral vaccines have been observed to induce cytotoxic T cell response in both systemic and mucosal sites, no information is available concerning the newer vaccines. It remains to be seen whether subunit or synthetic polypeptide or replicating recombinant vaccines will induce nonspecific, specific antibody, regulatory T cell, effector T cell (cytotoxic T cell), or other effector (intraepithelial lymphocytes, natural killer, delayed hypersensitivity) cellular responses in the mucosal surface, in a manner similar to natural disease, and thus provide superior protection for mucosally introduced viral pathogens.

Acknowledgements

This work was supported by National Institutes of Health Grant No AI 15939–7.

References

Baba K, Yabuuchi H, Takahashi M, Ogra P L 1982. Immunologic and epidemiologic aspects of varicella infection acquired during infancy and early childhood, *Journal of Pediatrics* **100**: 881

Bogger-Goren S, Baba K, Hurley P, Yabuuchi H, Takahashi M, Ogra P L 1982. Antibody response to varicella-zoster virus after natural or vaccine induced infection, *Journal of Infectious Diseases* **146**: 260–5

Bogger-Goren S, Bernstein J M, Gershon A A, Ogra P L 1984. Mucosal cell mediated immunity to varicella zoster virus: role in protection against disease, *Journal of Pediatrics* **105**: 195–9

Boss M A, Wood C R 1985. Genetically engineered antibodies, *Immunology Today* **6**: 12–13

Brown F 1984. Synthetic viral vaccines, *Annual Review of Microbiology* **3**: 221–35

Ennis F A 1983. *Human Immunity to Viruses*. Academic Press, New York

Fishaut M, Murphy D, Neifert M, McIntosh K, Ogra P L 1981. Bronchomammary axis in the immune response to respiratory syncytial virus, *Journal of Pediatrics* **99**: 186–91

International Symposium on Poliomyelitis Control 1984. *Reviews of Infectious Diseases* **6**: Supplement 2

Mellander L 1985. The development of mucosal immunity in relation to natural exposure and vaccination. Ph.D Thesis, University of Göteborg, Sweden

Ogra P L, Fishaut M, Welliver R C 1980. Mucosal immunity and immune response to respiratory viruses, in L Weinstein and B N Fields (eds) *Seminars in Infectious Disease*. Thieme-Stratton Inc, New York, vol III, pp 225–71

Ogra P L, Losonsky G A, Fishaut M 1983. Colostrum-derived immunity and maternal–neonatal interaction, in J R McGhee and J Mestecky (eds) *The secretory immune system, Annals of the New York Academy of Sciences* **409**: 81–95

Ogra P L, Cumella J C, Welliver R C 1984. Immune response to viruses, in J Bienenstock (ed) *Immunology of the Lung and Upper Respiratory Tract*, McGraw-Hill, New York, pp 242–63

UytdeHaag F G C M, Bunschoten H, Weijer K, Osterhaus A D M E 1986. From Jenner to Jerne: towards isotype vaccines, *Immunologic Reviews* **90**: 93–113

Welliver R C, Kaul T N, Ogra P L 1980. The appearance of cell-bound IgE in respiratory-tract epithelium after respiratory syncytial virus infection, *New England Journal of Medicine* **303**: 1198–202

Welliver R C, Wong D T, Sun M, Middleton E Jr, Vaughan R S, Ogra P L 1981. The development of respiratory syncytial virus-specific IgE and the release of histamine in nasopharyngeal secretions after infection, *New England Journal of Medicine* **305**: 841–6

Wong D T, Rosenband M, Hovey K, Ogra P L 1985. Respiratory syncytial virus infection in immunosuppressed animals: implications in human infection, *Journal of Medical Virology* **17**: 359–70

Multivalent synthetic peptide vaccines against group A streptococcal infections

Edwin H Beachey; James B Dale

Veterans Administration Medical Center and the University of Tennessee, Memphis, Tennessee 38104, USA

Introduction

It has been known for a long time that pharyngeal infections due to certain strains of group A streptococci can trigger acute rheumatic fever and rheumatic heart disease in a significant percentage of the infected population. Efforts to develop safe and effective vaccines against these streptococcal infections, however, have been hampered by toxic reactions to almost any streptococcal product injected into the human host (Stollerman 1967). Moreover, many streptococcal vaccine preparations have evoked autoimmune responses against host tissues, especially cardiac muscle (Kaplan and Meyeserian 1962). Such autoimmune responses have been particularly hampering because of the fear that the vaccine may actually provoke rather than prevent rheumatic heart disease.

After it was discovered that the surface M protein antigen is the major virulence determinant of group A streptococci, it seemed a relatively simple task to isolate and purify M protein and to use the purified material to formulate a protective vaccine free of toxic or tissue cross-reactive properties. Unfortunately, some of the purified M proteins appeared to be inseparably associated with tissue cross-reactive epitopes (Kaplan 1967). Limited peptic digestion appeared to overcome some of these problems by cleaving a polypeptide fragment from the M protein molecule that retained protective immunogenicity but lacked toxic moieties or autoimmune epitopes (Beachey *et al.* 1977a; 1977b). Such cleavage, however, was successful only with certain M proteins; such a peptic fragment of type 5 M protein retained tissue cross-reactive epitopes. Indeed, it was shown that this M protein fragment contained tissue cross-reactive epitopes within its covalent structure (Dale and Beachey 1982, 1985a, 1985b). These findings have necessitated detailed studies of the covalent structures of various rheumatogenic serotypes of streptococcal M proteins to define protective and tissue cross-reactive epitopes in a very precise way. The identification of these covalent structures should enable not only the development of a safe and effective streptococcal

143

vaccine(s) but also the elucidation of the mechanisms of the pathogenesis of acute rheumatic cardiac disease.

Biological properties of streptococcal M proteins

The M protein emanates as fibrils from the surface of virulent group A streptococci. In addition to its role as the protective antigen, M protein is the major virulence factor, conferring the ability of group A streptococci to resist ingestion by phagocytic cells of blood and tissues. Lancefield (1943) first showed that M protein was exposed on the surface of virulent hemolytic streptococci by demonstrating its release from viable organisms by proteolytic enzymes. Later on, electron microscopy of ultra-thin sections of group A streptococci revealed a fuzzy layer (Fig. 1) that reacted with ferritin-labeled M protein antibodies and that was removed with trypsin (Swanson *et al.* 1969). It is now known that the fibrillar surface layer is actually a complex matrix consisting not only of M protein, but also other surface proteins (T and R) as well as lipoteichoic acid (LTA) which is the ligand that mediates attachment of the organism to epithelial cells (Beachey 1981). Ofek and Beachey have recently provided evidence to support the concept that some of these surface proteins, particularly M protein, act as molecular anchors for LTA, and together they form the network of the surface fibrils (Ofek *et al.* 1982).

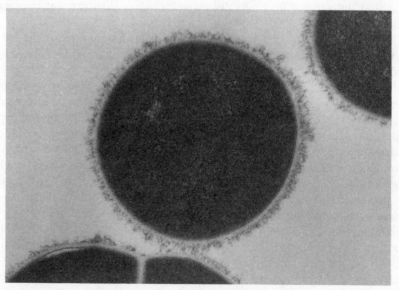

Figure 1. Electron micrograph of virulent group A streptococci illustrating the surface fimbriae.

Although the location of M protein on the surface of the organism has been known for a long time, the mechanisms of its 'antiphagocytic' effect have only recently been elucidated. Streptococci that lack M protein are readily opsonized by the alternate complement pathway (Bisno 1979; Peterson *et al.* 1979). Organisms rich in M protein also activate complement via the alternate pathway, but the activated C3 is bound less efficiently to the surface of the organisms (Jacks-Weiss *et al.* 1982). Whitnack and Beachey (1982, 1985) have recently shown that the antiopsonic effect of M protein is optimal only when the surface M proteins of the organisms bind fibrinogen or its D fragments generated by degradation of fibrinogen with plasmin; the fibrin(ogen) bound to the M protein completely blocks the binding of opsonic C3 to the surface of the bacteria.

Although organisms rich in M protein resist phagocytosis in the nonimmune host, antibodies against M protein epitopes not masked by fibrinogen are capable of opsonizing the organism by activating complement via the classical pathway (Whitnack and Beachey 1982, 1985). Epidemiologic studies have provided important data regarding immunity to M protein following streptococcal pharyngitis in humans, the only natural host for these bacteria. Most studies that have used human serum in bactericidal assays against group A streptococci suggest that pharyngeal infections with a given M protein serotype of streptococci provide lifelong, type-specific immunity (Lancefield 1962). Protective opsonic antibodies against M protein have been detected as long as 30 years following documented infections, and recurrent infections with the same M serotype of group A streptococci are rarely encountered (Lancefield 1959).

The finding that isolated M proteins were immunogenic in laboratory animals and that immunity to M protein following natural infection in humans was long-lasting prompted several investigators to undertake limited clinical trials with various M protein preparations in human volunteers. Early vaccines were simply cell wall preparations that contained variable amounts of M antigen (Stollerman 1967). Such crude preparations, which were undoubtedly contaminated with several toxic substances, were not well tolerated and produced local and systemic reactions (Stollerman 1967). One of the major problems was to isolate M protein in a form pure enough so that immunogenic amounts could be injected without adverse effects.

Hot hydrochloric acid extracts prepared by the method of Lancefield contained significant amounts of M protein polypeptides, but also were contaminated with toxic and so-called nontype-specific moieties, to which almost all humans were sensitized (Beachey *et al.* 1973). Other similar harsh treatments yielded M proteins that were also not well tolerated by human subjects. Although most of these crude vaccines evoked some degree of immunity in humans, the percentage of individuals that responded was generally low, and deciding whether the immune responses were primary or secondary was often difficult.

Some of the problems associated with toxicity of purified M proteins were

145

overcome by extraction of the M protein from the surface of virulent organisms by mild proteolysis with dilute solutions of pepsin (Beachey *et al.* 1974, 1977a, 1977b). The pepsin extract of type 24 streptococci contained a polypeptide fragment that could be purified to homogeneity free of toxic properties. The purified polypeptide retained protective immunogenicity in laboratory animals and when injected as an alum precipitate into humans it evoked opsonic antibodies in eight to ten individuals after three 200 µg injections (Beachey *et al.* 1979). There were no significant local or systemic toxic reactions to this vaccine material. Although these results were promising, other problems remained.

Immunological cross-reactivity between M proteins and host tissues

All cases of acute rheumatic fever are preceded by group A streptococcal pharyngitis; however, only a small percentage of individuals with streptococcal sore throat subsequently develop rheumatic fever. The disease has multiple 'autoimmune' features (Unny and Middlebrooks 1983), and the group A streptococcus is known to contain several antigens that are immunologically identical to host tissues (Kaplan and Meyserian 1962; Kaplan 1967; Lyampert *et al.* 1966; van de Rijn *et al.* 1977). The mechanisms involved in the pathogenesis of this often devastating disease remain an enigma. The most serious problem in the development of an M protein vaccine has been the fear that vaccine preparations might contain one or more of the tissue cross-reactive antigens that may actually evoke rather than prevent rheumatic heart disease.

Until recently, there was only circumstantial evidence to support the idea that M protein molecules themselves contained host tissue cross-reactive epitopes. Investigators believed that with improved methods of purification, homogeneous M protein preparations would be free of contaminating cell wall and membrane components which are known to contain tissue cross-reactive antigens. However, we have recently reported the most definitive evidence that types 5, 6 and 19 M proteins contain antigenic determinants within their covalent structures that are immunologically identical to sarcolemmal membrane proteins of human myocardium and to muscle myosin (Dale and Beachey 1982, 1985a, 1985b). The cross-reactive antibodies affinity-purified by adsorption to and elution from heart tissue opsonized types 5, 6 and 19 streptococci, indicating that they were directed against protective epitopes on the M protein molecules. These findings, which are of considerable concern, emphasize the need to understand fully the structure–function relationships of the M protein molecules that are to be used in vaccine preparations.

Biochemistry and structure of streptococcal M proteins

Considerable progress has recently been made in elucidating the primary structures of several M protein molecules (Beachey *et al.* 1977a; 1977b, 1978, 1980a, 1980b, 1983; Seyer *et al.* 1980; Manjula and Fischetti 1980a, 1980b; Manjula *et al.* 1983, 1984; Phillips *et al.* 1981; Scott *et al.* 1985; Hollingshead *et al.* 1986). First the covalent structure of a polypeptide fragment of type 24 M protein extracted from streptococci by limited pepsin digestion (pep M24) was described. The polypeptide fragment of molecular weight 33,000 was cleaved by cyanogen bromide into seven peptides, each of which contained type-specific epitopes (Beachey *et al.* 1978). Two of the cyanogen bromide peptides, CB1 and CB2, contained approximately 90 amino acid residues, and their amino-terminal sequences were identical to each other and to the parent pep M24 molecule. Five smaller peptides, CB3–7, contained 35–37 residues each and were identical to each other except for a few amino acid substitutions, but were different from CB1 and CB2. Each of the peptides was capable of evoking protective immune responses in rabbits (Beachey *et al.* 1978, 1980a, 1983). Thus, pep M24 is composed of long repeating covalent structures, each of which contains protective epitopes.

Similar structural analysis have been reported for types 5 and 6 M proteins. We found that, for the most part, the primary structures of these M proteins were entirely different from each other, although certain amino acid residues were conserved (Seyer *et al.* 1980; Beachey *et al.* 1980b). Manjula and Fischetti have recently reported the complete covalent structure of pep M5 and found no long internal repeating structures such as those in pep M24 (Manjula *et al.* 1984). These investigators compared the structures of types 5, 6 and 24 M proteins and found one common feature; each of the M proteins possesses a seven-residue periodicity with respect to the placement of charged and noncharged residues along the length of the molecule (Manjula and Fischetti 1980b). Based on the structural similarities between streptococcal M proteins and α-tropomyosin, Phillips *et al.* (1981) provided evidence that type 6 M protein exists as an α-helical coiled-coil. This conformation theoretically allows the paired molecules sufficient rigidity to project from the surface of the organism to form the fibrous coat. Thus, it appears that in order to maintain the functional characteristics of M protein, the seven-residue periodicity is retained from one serotype to another, while antigenicity is altered to enhance the survivability of the organism in the host.

Protective immunogenicity of native and synthetic peptide fragments of M protein

The notion that one might evoke protective immune responses by immunization with peptide fragments of M protein is based on several lines of evidence. First, the intact M protein molecule is considerably larger than the polypeptide fragments extracted by most methods from whole streptococci or cell walls. Second, several laboratories have presented evidence that individual M protein molecules contain many antigenic determinants, most of which are type-specific, but some of which are cross-reactive with other M serotypes (Fox 1974; Fischetti 1977; Dale *et al.* 1980; Dale and Beachey 1984). Third, purified subpeptides derived by cyanogen bromide cleavage of type 24 M protein each evoked protective antibodies against the homologous serotype of streptococci (Beachey *et al.* 1980a, 1983).

Having established the protective immunogenicity of small peptide fragments of cleaved M protein molecules, we proceeded chemically to synthesize selected regions of types 5, 6 and 24 M protein molecules. Synthetic copies of the three M proteins were based on the covalent structures determined by automated Edman degradation of the amino-termini of each of the proteins as well as of cyanogen bromide cleaved peptides of type 24 M protein (Beachey *et al.* 1981, 1983, 1984; Dale *et al.* 1983; Beachey and Seyer 1986). A summary of the immune responses in rabbits injected with each of the synthetic peptides is recorded in Tables 1 and 2. Most, but not all, of the synthetic peptides stimulated the production of antibodies that recognized the natural M protein fragments as measured by ELISA, or the intact M protein on the surface of the organisms as measured by opsonophagocytosis tests (Tables 1 and 2). Although we observed a few weak cross-reactions with heterologous sero-

Table 1 Immune responses in rabbits immunized with synthetic peptides of types 5, 6 and 24 streptococcal M proteins as measured by ELISA against the native M protein polypeptides

Synthetic peptide copies of:	ELISA titers against:		
	pep M5	pep M6	pep M24
Type 5 M protein			
S-M5(1–35)	12 800	200	<200
(1–20)	102 800	<200	<200
(20–40)	800	<200	<200
(26–35)	12 800	<200	<200
(14–26)	25 600	ND	ND
Type 6 M protein			
S-M6(1–20)	200	51 200	800
(10–20)	200	6400	200
(12–31)	200	6400	200
(22–31)	<200	<200	200
Type 24 M protein			
S-CB7(1–35)	<200	<200	102 400
(13–35)	<200	<200	102 400
(18–35)C	<200	<200	12 400
(18–35)C	<200	<200	12 800
(23–35)C	<200	<200	51 200
(23–32)KAMC	<200	<200	1600

ND – not determined.

Table 2 Opsonic antibody responses against types 5, 6 and 24 streptococci in rabbits immunized with synthetic peptide copies of the respective serotypes of M protein

Synthetic peptide copies of:	Opsonic antibodies; phagocytosis (%) of:		
	Type 5 strep	**Type 6 strep**	**Type 24 strep**
Type 5 M protein			
S-M5(1–35)	86	4	2
(1–20)	92	2	2
(20–40)	4	4	2
(26–35)	0	0	0
(14–26)	76	8	4
Type 6 M protein			
S-M6(1–20)	6	92	2
(10–20)	4	78	4
(12–31)	2	80	2
(22–31)	4	4	2
Type 24 M protein			
S-CB7(1–35)	4	2	88
(13–35)	0	4	86
(18–35)C	6	2	78
(23–35)C	4	4	84
(23–32)KAMC	2	2	2

types of M protein as measured by ELISA, the immune responses were entirely type-specific in the opsonophagocytosis tests. None of the immune sera cross-reacted with human cardiac sarcolemma or muscle myosin as determined by immunofluorescence tests or ELISA, respectively (Beachey *et al.* 1981, 1983; Beachey and Seyer 1986; Dale and Beachey 1986).

Interestingly, three peptides S-M5(26–35), S-M5(20–40), and S-M6(22–31) failed to evoke antibodies that reacted with the M proteins on the intact surfaces of the respective streptococcal cells even though they stimulated antibodies to the peptides themselves, and in the case of S-M5(26–35) to the isolated pep M5. These results indicated that the NH_2-terminal regions of these M proteins contain both protective and nonprotective epitopes. It should be noted that the nonprotective peptides of both M proteins were copied from a region that had previously been shown to have high α-helical potential (Manjula and Fischetti 1980a) and coiled-coil structure (Phillips *et al.* 1981). The greater rigidity conferred by this structure may render this part of the molecule less mobile and therefore less adaptable to the many different conformations recognized by the repertoire of antibodies raised against the more flexible synthetic peptides (Tainer *et al.* 1984).

The finding of multiple protective epitopes in the overlapping peptides is consistent with the previous findings that monoclonal antibodies against type 24 (Hasty *et al.* 1982) and type 5 (Dale and Beachey 1984) M proteins recognized multiple distinct epitopes. Moreover, some of the protective epitopes are shared with heterologous serotypes (Dale and Beachey 1984).

Synthetic hybrid peptide vaccines

Having established the protective immunogenicity of these small peptide fragments, we decided to prepare hybrid peptides in which immunogenic peptides of different M serotypes are synthesized in tandem (Beachey *et al.* 1986). Such hybrid peptides not only should produce a multivalent immune response but should have the added advantage that the synthetic peptides can be tailored in a predictable way to render the multivalent protective epitopes

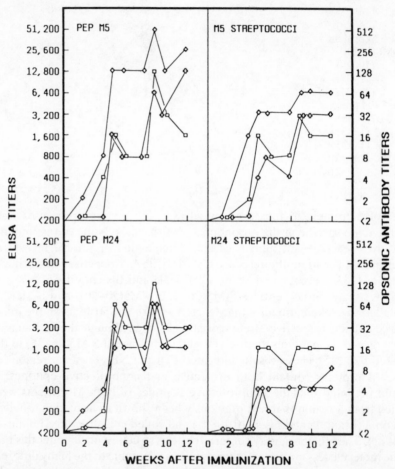

Figure 2. Immune responses of three rabbits (□, *, ◇) against synthetic M5–M24 hybrid peptide S-M5(1–20)–S-CB7(23–35)C emulsified in CFA as measured by ELISA against pep M5 or pep M24 (left) or by opsonic antibody assays against type 5 or type 24 streptococci (right). The rabbits were immunized with 50 nmol of the free peptide hybrid in CFA followed by booster injections subcutaneously of the same dose in saline at four and eight weeks. In control experiments none of the immune sera opsonized types 6 or 19 streptococci. Reproduced with the permission of Rockefeller University Press (Beachey *et al.* 1986).

optimally immunoaccessible. To test the feasibility of this aproach, we synthesized a hybrid of types 5 and 24 M proteins, S-M5(1–20)–S-CB7(23–35)C. Amino acid analysis and automated Edman degradation confirmed the amino acid sequence of the synthetic hybrid as corresponding to the respective regions of the related proteins.

Each of three rabbits injected with 50 nmol of S-M5(1–20)–S-CB7(23–35)C followed by booster injections with the same dose in saline at four, eight and ten weeks developed high titers of serum antibodies against both type 5 and 24 M protein as measured by ELISA, and against both serotypes of group A streptococci as measured by opsonophagocytic tests (Fig. 2). The immune sera were able to promote not only phagocytosis but also killing of both types 5 and 24 streptococci, indicating that the antibodies evoked by the synthetic hybrid peptide recognized protective antigenic determinants of both M serotypes exposed on the surfaces of the respective serotypes of streptococcal cells. None of the immune sera reacted with sarcolemmal membranes or muscle myosin (Beachey *et al.* 1986).

The specificities of the opsonic antibodies against the bivalent and trivalent hybrid peptides were determined by immunoabsorption and inhibition tests. In each case absorption of the opsonic antisera with the respective serotypes of whole streptococci was entirely type-specific (Beachey *et al.* 1986). Similarly, the peptide S-M5(1–20) inhibited opsonization only of type 5 streptococci, and S-CB7(23–35)C only of type 24 streptococci. The hybrid peptide used to immunize the rabbits inhibited opsonization of both M serotypes of streptococci represented in the tandem peptide hybrid (Beachey *et al.* 1986).

Summary and conclusions

The surface M protein of group A streptococci is the major virulence factor and protective antigen of the organisms; only antibodies against M protein are opsonic. The development of a safe and effective streptococcal vaccine composed of highly purified pepsin-extracted M proteins has been hampered by recent findings that such polypeptide fragments of several 'rheumatogenic' M protein serotypes contain epitopes that are shared with human tissues. To avoid these potentially harmful autoimmune reactions, we have undertaken studies to determine the protective immunogenicity of natural and synthetic subpeptides of several serotypes of M protein. Our studies clearly show that limited regions of the M protein molecule have the capacity to evoke protective immune responses against the related serotypes of group A streptococci. Chemically synthesized peptide fragments of carefully selected regions of various M protein molecules should provide vaccines that can be safely administered to humans without the fear that they might evoke tissue-cross-reactive antibodies. To our knowledge our studies are the first to show the opsonic protective immunogenicity of hybrid peptides containing virulence determinants of more than one strain of bacteria chemically synthesized in tandem. Of particular interest is the finding that the hybrid peptide of types 5 and 24 M proteins was immunogenic in the absence of a carrier. In fact, conjugation of the hybrid to tetanus toxoid suppressed the immune response to type 24 streptococci (Beachey *et al.* 1986). These findings have direct bearing on the development of safe and effective multivalent vaccines against group A streptococci, especially against the strains that trigger acute rheumatic fever and rheumatic heart disease.

Acknowledgements

The research of the authors is supported by research funds from the US Veterans Administration and by Research Grants AI-10085 and AI-13550 from the US Public Health Service. J B Dale is the recipient of a Clinical Investigatorship Award from the US Veterans Administration. The authors thank Mrs Johnnie Smith for expert secretarial assistance.

References

Beachey E H 1981. Bacterial adherence: Adhesin–receptor interactions mediating the attachment of bacteria to mucosal surfaces, *Journal of Infectious Diseases* **143**: 25–45

Beachey E H, Seyer J M 1986. Protective and nonprotective epitopes of chemically synthesized peptides of the NH_2-terminal region of type 6 streptococcal M protein, *Journal of Immunology* **136**: 2287–92

Beachey E H, Ofek I, Bisno A L 1973. Studies of antibodies to non-type specific antigens associated with streptococcal M protein in the sera of patients with rheumatic fever, *Journal of Immunology* **111**: 1361–6

Beachey E H, Campbell G L, Ofek I 1974. Peptic digestion of streptococcal M protein. II. Extraction of M antigen from group A streptococci with pepsin, *Infection and Immunity* **9**: 891–6

Beachey E H, Chiang E Y, Seyer J M, Kang A H, Chiang T M, Stollerman G H 1977a. Separation of the type-specific M protein from toxic cross-reactive antigen of group A streptococci, *Transactions of the Association of American Physicians* **90**: 390–400

Beachey E H, Stollerman G H, Chiang E Y, Chiang T M, Seyer J M, Kang A H 1977b. Purification and properties of M protein extracted from group A streptococci with pepsin. Covalent structure of the amino terminal region of type 24 M antigen, *Journal of Experimental Medicine* **145**: 1469–83

Beachey E H, Seyer J M, Kang A H 1978. Repeating covalent structure of streptococcal M protein, *Proceedings of the National Academy of Sciences USA* **75**: 3163–7

Beachey E H, Stollerman G H, Johnson R H, Ofek I, Bisno A L 1979. Human immune response to immunization with a structurally defined polypeptide fragment of streptococcal M protein, *Journal of Experimental Medicine* **150**: 862–77

Beachey E H, Seyer J M, Kang A H 1980a. Primary structure of protective antigens of type 24 streptococcal M protein, *Journal of Biological Chemistry* **255**: 6284–9

Beachey E H, Seyer J M, Kang A H 1980b. Studies of the primary structure of streptococcal M protein antigens, in J B Zabriskie, S E Read (eds) *Streptococcal Diseases and the Immune Response*. Academic Press, New York, pp 149–60

Beachey E H, Seyer J M, Dale J B, Simpson W A, Kang A H 1981. Type-specific protective immunity evoked by synthetic peptide of *Streptococcus pyogenes* M protein, *Nature (London)* **292**: 457–9

Beachey E H, Seyer J M, Dale J B, Hasty D L 1983. Repeating covalent structure and protective immunogenicity of native and synthetic polypeptide fragments of type 24 streptococcal M protein: mapping of protective and nonprotective epitopes with monoclonal antibodies, *Journal of Biological Chemistry* **258**: 13250–7

Beachey E H, Tartar A, Seyer J M, Chedid L 1984. Epitope-specific protective immunogenicity of chemically synthesized 13-, 18-, and 23-residue peptide fragments of streptococcal M protein, *Proceedings of the National Academy of Sciences USA* **81**: 2203–7

Beachey E H, Seyer J M, Gras-Masse H, Tarter A, Jolivet M, Chedid L, Audibert F 1986. Opsonic antibodies evoked by hybrid peptide copies of types 5 and 24 streptococcal M proteins synthesized in tandem, *Journal of Experimental Medicine* **163**: 1451–8

Bisno A L 1979. Alternate complement pathway activation by group A streptococci: role of M protein, *Infection and Immunity* **26**: 1172–6

Dale J B, Beachey E H 1982. Protective antigenic determinant of streptococcal M protein shared with sarcolemmal membrane protein of human heart, *Journal of Experimental Medicine* **156**: 1165–76

Dale J B, Beachey E H 1984. Unique and common protective epitopes among different serotypes of group A streptococcal M proteins defined with hybridoma antibodies, *Infection and Immunity* **46**: 267–9

Dale J B, Beachey E H 1985a. Multiple heart cross-reactive epitopes of streptococcal M proteins, *Journal of Experimental Medicine* **161**: 113–22

Dale J B, Beachey E H 1985b. Epitopes of streptococcal M proteins shared with cardiac myosin, *Journal of Experimental Medicine* **162**: 583–91

Dale J B, Beachey E H 1986. Localization of protective epitopes of the amino terminus of type 5 streptococcal M protein, *Journal of Experimental Medicine* **163**: 1191–1201

Dale J B, Ofek I, Beachey E H 1980. Heterogeneity of type-specific and cross-reactive antigenic determinants within a single M protein of group A streptococci, *Journal of Experimental Medicine* **151**: 1026–38

Dale J B, Seyer J M, Beachey E H 1983. Type-specific immunogenicity of a chemically synthesized peptide fragment of type 5 streptococcal M protein, *Journal of Experimental Medicine* **158**: 1727–32

Fischetti V A 1977. Streptococcal M protein extracted by nonionic detergent. II. Analysis of the antibody response to the multiple antigenic determinants of the M protein molecule, *Journal of Experimental Medicine* **146**: 1108–18

Fox E N 1974. M proteins of group A streptococci, *Bacteriological Reviews* **38**: 57–80

Hasty D L, Beachey E H, Simpson W A, Dale J B 1982. Hybridoma antibodies against protective and nonprotective antigenic determinants of a structurally defined polypeptide fragment of streptococcal M protein, *Journal of Experimental Medicine* **155**: 1010–18

Hollingshead S K, Fischetti V A, Scott J R 1986. Complete nucleotide sequence of type 6 M protein of the group A streptococcus, *Journal of Biological Chemistry* **261**: 1677–86

Jacks-Weis J, Kim Y, Cleary P P 1982. Restricted deposition of C3 on M+ group A streptococci: correlation with resistance to phagocytosis, *Journal of Immunology* **128**: 1897–2004

Kaplan M H 1967. Immunologic relation of streptococcal and tissue antigens. I. Properties of an antigen in certain strains of group A streptococci exhibiting an immunologic cross-reaction with human heart tissue, *Journal of Immunology* **90**: 595–603

Kaplan M H, Meyeserian H 1962. An immunologic cross-reaction between group A streptococcal cells and human heart, *Lancet* **i**: 706–8

Lancefield R C 1943. Studies on the antigenic compositions of group A hemolytic streptococci. I. Effect of proteolytic enzymes on streptococcal cells, *Journal of Experimental Medicine* **78**: 465–76

Lancefield R C 1959. Persistance of type-specific antibodies in man following infection with group A streptococci, *Journal of Experimental Medicine* **110**: 271–92

Lancefield R C 1962. Current knowledge of type-specific M antigens of group A streptococci, *Journal of Immunology* **89**: 307–13

Lyampert I M, Vvedenskaya O L, Danilova T A 1966. Study on streptococcus group A antigens common with heart tissue elements, *Immunology* **11**: 313–20

Manjula B N, Fischetti V A 1980a. Studies on group A streptococcal M proteins: purification of type 5 M protein and comparison of its amino terminal sequence with two immunologically unrelated M protein molecules, *Journal of Immunology* **124**: 261–7

Manjula B N, Fischetti V A 1980b. Tropomyosin-like seven residue periodicity in three immunologically distinct streptococcal M proteins and its implications for the antiphagocytic property of the molecule, *Journal of Experimental Medicine* **151**: 695–708

Manjula B N, Mische S M, Fischetti V A 1983. Primary structures of streptococcal pep M5 protein: absence of extensive sequence repeats, *Proceedings of the National Academy of Sciences USA* **80**: 5475–9

Manjula B N, Acharya A S, Mische S M, Fairwell T, Fischetti V A 1984. The complete amino acid sequence of a biologically active 197-residue fragment of M protein isolated from type 5 group A streptococci, *Journal of Biological Chemistry* **259**: 3686–93

Ofek I, Simpson W A, Beachey E H 1982. Formation of molecular complexes between a structurally defined M protein and acylated or deacylated lipoteichoic acid of *Streptococcus pyogenes*, *Journal of Bacteriology* **149**: 426–33

Peterson P K, Schmelling D, Cleary P P, Wilkinson B J, Kim Y, Quie P G 1979. Inhibition of alternative complement pathway opsonization by group A streptococcal M protein; *Journal of Infectious Diseases* **139**: 575–85

Phillips G N, Flicker P F, Cohen C, Manjula B N, Fischetti V A 1981. Streptococcal M protein: α-helical coiled-coil structure and arrangement on the cell surface, *Proceedings of the National Academy of Sciences USA* **78**: 4689–93

Scott J R, Pulliam W M, Hollingshead S K, Fischetti V A 1985. Relationship of M protein genes in group A streptococci, *Proceedings of the National Academy of Sciences USA* **82**: 1822–6

Seyer J M, Kang A H, Beachey E H 1980. Primary structural similarities between types 5 and 24 M proteins of *Streptococcus pyogenes*, *Biochemistry and Biophysical Research Communications* **92**: 546–53

Stollerman G H 1967. Prospects for a vaccine against group A streptococci: the problem of the immunology of M protein, *Arthritis and Rheumatism* **10**: 245–55

Swanson J, Hsu K C, Gotschlich E C 1969. Electron microscopic studies on streptococci. I. M antigen, *Journal of Experimental Medicine* **130**: 1063–91

Tainer J A, Gelzoff E D, Alexander H, Houghten R A, Olson A J, Lerner R A, Hendrickson W A 1984. The reactivity of anti-peptide antibodies is a function of the atomic mobility of sites in a protein, *Nature (London)* **213**: 127–34

Unny S K, Middlebrooks B L 1983. Streptococcal rheumatic carditis, *Microbiological Reviews* **47**: 97–120

van de Rijn I, Zabriskie J B, McCarty M 1977. Group A streptococcal antigens cross-reactive with myocardium. Purification of heart-reactive antibody and isolation and characterization of the streptococcal antigen, *Journal of Experimental Medicine* **146**: 579–99

Whitnack E, Beachey E H 1982. Antiopsonic activity of fibrinogen bound to M protein on the surface of group A streptococci, *Journal of Clinical Investigation* **69**: 1042–5

Whitnack E, Beachey E H 1985. Inhibition of complement-mediated opsonization and phagocytosis of *Streptococcus pyogenes* by D fragments and fibrin bound to cell-surface M protein, *Journal of Experimental Medicine* **162**: 1983–97

A mutans streptococcal enzyme-based vaccine for dental infection

Martin A. Taubman; Daniel J. Smith

Department of Immunology, Forsyth Dental Center, Boston, Massachusetts 02115, USA

Introduction

Dental caries and the mucosal immune system

Dental caries cannot develop in the absence of bacteria (Keyes 1960; Orland *et al.* 1955). Experiments of Fitzgerald and Keyes (1960) established the 'mutans' group of streptococci as primary pathogens in the etiology of dental caries. During the period when the infectious nature of dental caries was being established, Tomasi *et al.* (1965) identified an immune system specific to surfaces bathed by mucosal secretions. The presence of this mucosal immune system suggested that it might be possible to interfere with caries by stimulation of the salivary system. Such interference was observed in early experiments after salivary antibody was induced by local injection of mutans streptococci (Taubman 1973; Taubman and Smith 1974; McGhee *et al.* 1975). Similarly, protective effects were observed after oral immunization experiments in which salivary antibodies were demonstrated in the absence of serum antibody (Michalek *et al.* 1976; Smith *et al.* 1979, 1980).

Molecular pathogenesis of dental caries

Bare tooth enamel does not exist in the oral cavity but is covered with a membranous 'acquired pellicle' formed by selective adsorption of salivary components. The formation of *S. mutans* plaques appears to involve two mechanisms. The initial interaction between mutans streptococci and the tooth surface appears to be mediated by this pellicle (Clark and Gibbons 1977). The *S. mutans* receptors responsible for initial attachment seem to be protein since attachment can be inhibited by pretreatment with pepsin (Staat *et al.* 1980). Binding may involve α-galactoside moieties on the pellicle since adsorption of *S. mutans* to saliva-coated hydroxyapatite can be inhibited by α-galactosides (Gibbons and Qureshi 1979). Following this attachment,

S. mutans can accumulate on teeth by an independent mechanism that seems to be intimately related to the synthesis of extracellular glucose polymers. Water-soluble polyglucans (WSP) and water-insoluble polyglucans (WIP) are produced, although the WIP seem more important in accumulation of mutans streptococci. *Streptococcus mutans* strains that produce low amounts of WIP do not accumulate on hard surfaces (de Stoppelaar *et al.* 1971; Johnson *et al.* 1974; Tanzer *et al.* 1974; Tanzer and Freedman 1978) and are unable to produce experimental dental caries (Michalek *et al.* 1975; Tanzer *et al.* 1974). In contrast, mutants synthesizing increased amounts of WIP demonstrate greater cariogenicity than wild-type organisms (Michalek *et al.* 1975).

Glucosyltransferase

Glucosyltransferase (GTF) is an enzyme constitutively produced by the 'mutans' group of streptococci (Guggenheim and Newbrun 1969). At least two different gene products (GTF_S and GTF_I) are responsible for the synthesis of WSP and WIP from sucrose (Kuramitsu and Aoki 1986). A receptor-like protein, distinct from GTF, that will specifically bind glucan has been isolated from *S. sobrinus* cells (McCabe *et al.* 1977; Curtiss *et al.* 1985; Russell *et al.* 1983). GTF will bind glucan and in this respect may also act as a receptor. *Streptococcus sobrinus* cells can specifically bind preformed glucan, giving rise to aggregates of mutans streptococci (Gibbons and Fitzgerald 1969). The ability to aggregate is a property distinct from the ability to form WIP (Freedman and Tanzer 1974). Combinations of glucan-mediated aggregation, glucan to receptor, enzyme–glucan complex to receptor binding on the cell surface and cell multiplication can promote interactions between these organisms and promote accumulation of mutans streptococci. Although the production of acid by mutans streptococci directly causes disease, the ability to accumulate on tooth surfaces is an equally significant parameter of virulence (van Houte and Russo 1986). Specific polyclonal antibody to GTF has been clearly shown to interfere with *S. sobrinus* accumulation both *in vitro* and *in vivo* (Taubman *et al.* 1982, 1983).

Glucosyltransferase as antigen

Glucosyltransferase has been an effective antigen in eliciting secretory antibody following local injection or oral immunization of rodents (Taubman and Smith 1977; Smith *et al.* 1978a, 1979, 1980; Scholler *et al.* 1979). Secretory antibody produced after either route of immunization with GTF resulted in protection from caries by homologous or heterologous serotypes (relative to the GTF used for immunization; Smith *et al.* 1982; Taubman *et al.* 1983). A common mucosal immune system, primarily arising from the gut-associated lymphoreticular tissues, has been suggested and has been utilized as a route for induction of sIgA antibody to mutans streptococci (Mestecky *et al.* 1978, 1986).

Nature of antigen

The particulate nature of the antigen appears to be a critical feature in elicitation of a secretory immune response by this route (Cox and Taubman 1984). Thus, adjuvants which particularize antigen, including GTF, appear to enhance secretory responses after oral administration (Ebersole *et al.* 1983, 1986). Oral ingestion of particulate bacterial antigens can result in the appearance of sIgA antibodies in human external secretions such as tears and saliva (Mestecky *et al.* 1978).

Vaccine studies in humans

The vaccine studies that have been performed in humans are summarized in Table 1. Most studies have utilized whole *S. mutans* or *S. sobrinus* cells as antigen for immunization. Some studies have produced a secretory immune

Table 1 Mutans streptococci as antigen in human studies

Group	Number of subjects	Vaccine	Frequency	Route	Result
Mestecky *et al.* (1978)	4	Cells(*d*)	14d	Oral	Increased antibody
Krasse *et al.* (1978)	3	Cells(*c*)	8d	Topical	No change in antibody
Bonta *et al.* (1979)	4	Cells(*d*)	14d	Oral	No change in antibody; fewer bacteria
Cole *et al.* (1984)	8	Cells(*g*)	3(7)d	Oral	No change in antibody; fewer bacteria; reductions in levels & duration
Gahnberg and Krasse (1983)	11	Cells(*d*)	14d	Oral	No change in antibody; fewer bacteria
Gregory *et al.* (1985)	12	Indigenous antibody to serotype *g* not *c*	None	Bacterial challenge	Eliminate serotype *g* challenge, not serotype *c*
Hughes *et al.* (1986)	2	Antigen A(*c*) with alhydrogel	3X	Subcutaneous	Increased antibody
Mestecky *et al.* (1986)	6	Cells(*c*)	7d	Oral	Antibody increase; fewer bacteria

response both after primary and secondary immunization regimens (Mestecky *et al.* 1978). Others have not shown such pronounced elevated antibody levels but have demonstrated effects on bacteria (Cole *et al.* 1984). In general, the effects on bacteria have been more readily demonstrable than have changes in antibody levels. Recently the presence of specific IgA antibody producing mononuclear cells in serum after oral administration of mutans streptococci has been demonstrated (Mestecky *et al.* 1986). In this study we have investigated the appearance of IgA antibodies in saliva after oral ingestion of GTF by human volunteers.

Materials and methods

Preparation of glucosyltransferase (GTF)

Vaccine was derived from *S. sobrinus* strain 6715 (serotype *g*) grown anaerobically in chemically defined medium (Socransky *et al.* 1973). The GTF was prepared by affinity chromatography and gel filtration techniques which have been previously described (Smith *et al.* 1978b, 1984). Briefly, after mixture of cell-free supernatant with Sephadex G-100 and elution with 6M-guanidine–HCl the eluate was filtered on a column of Sepharose 4B-CL in guanidine–HCl. The peak containing GTF activity was filter sterilized and stored at −20°C. This GTF vaccine had been approved by the Food and Drug Administration – Bureau of Biologics, for use in the present study.

Antibody analyses

Parotid gland salivas were tested for IgA antibody to GTF and sera were tested for IgA and IgG antibody using the modified ELISA technique described previously (Smith *et al.* 1978a, 1985). Antibody levels were expressed as ELISA units (EU). Negative controls consisted of salivas or sera which had been repeatedly adsorbed with washed, sucrose-grown *S. sobrinus* cells. As a relative expression of changes in IgA antibody activity each individual antibody level was expressed as a ratio of the mean EU value of the six parotid samples taken from that subject during the initial screening plus one standard deviation of the mean. Serum values were also related to the serum EU obtained during the screen.

Subjects

Twenty-five adult males (aged 18–36 years) were selected for the study based on a screening of salivary antibody for activity to the GTF preparation. Subjects were assigned to the 'vaccine (GTF)' or 'placebo' group based on their mean IgA antibody activity to *S. sobrinus* 6715 GTF from the six parotid saliva samples taken in the initial screening. Subjects in both groups were paired with respect to their parotid saliva antibody activity to this antigen.

Experimental protocol

The clinical study was divided into three parts: (A) the Screening Phase (three months); (B) the First Immunization Phase including follow-up (42 days); (C) the Second Immunization Phase including follow-up (37 days) which was initiated 47 days after the final sampling of the First Immunization Phase. During Part A parotid saliva samples were taken (modified Curby cup) from 52 subjects on five separate occasions. The sixth saliva sample was taken two days prior to vaccine administration when all subjects were given a dental prophylaxis. Parotid saliva was collected on the first day of vaccine (or placebo) administration (First Immunization Phase) and on seven occasions (days 5, 9, 16, 21, 28, 35 and 42) thereafter. Blood was taken on days -2, 16 and 42 and whole saliva streptococci were obtained on days 2, 12, 21, 28, 35 and 42. Parotid saliva was also taken before the Second Immunization Phase was initiated by administering a dental prophylaxis and then presentation of vaccine or placebo. After this administration (day 0), parotid saliva (six occasions), blood (day 37) and salivary streptococci (six times) were collected. Physical examinations and clinical laboratory tests were performed at the beginning and the end of the study. Daily temperature measurements and recording of reactions were performed during the immunization periods. No detectable alterations in body temperature and no consistent reactions or changes in blood or urine clinical parameters were recorded.

Thirteen vaccine (or placebo) administrations were given in the first 17 days of the primary phase; five doses were administered in five days during the Second Immunization Phase. For each day of administration one aliquot of the GTF preparation was mixed with a sterile aluminum phosphate. Each dose contained 0.5 mg of GTF in phosphate buffer (PB) and 6.7 mg of aluminum phosphate. The placebo preparation consisted of equal volumes of PB and aluminum phosphate (6.7 mg). Individual doses consisted of 0.8 ml of vaccine or placebo in gelatin capsules given to the subject to swallow with water. All immunizations and antibody measurements were performed with the same lot of GTF.

Since a range of levels of antibody to the strain 6715 GTF pre-existed in both groups, each subject was compared with his own antibody or bacterial levels and served as his own control for the experiment. Treatment of the data in this way normalized the values among the subjects such that the 'vaccine' and 'placebo' groups could be compared.

Bacterial recoveries

Whole saliva was sonicated, diluted in one-quarter strength Ringer's solution and plated for total streptococci on Mitis–Salivarius (MS) agar and for *S. mutans* on MS agar with bacitracin. Colonies were counted after two days of incubation in 10% CO_2 and 90% N_2 at 35 °C. The bacterial counts determined prior to vaccine administration in each phase were taken for comparison with all subsequent bacterial measurements.

Results

Salivary IgA antibody

The parotid salivas collected after the first immunization regime were tested for IgA antibody activity to the immunizing antigen. The ratios of primary phase salivary IgA antibody to the mean of the screen value for each subject are summarized in Table 2. The data for the highest ratio of IgA antibody activity for each subject during the primary immunization phase are shown. The group of ratios observed for the GTF-vaccine group was significantly

Table 2 Levels of salivary IgA anti-GTF antibody after administration of oral GTF

	Vaccine*		Placebo*	
Subject	**Peak IgA antibody MSE + SD†**	**Subject**	**Peak IgA antibody MSE + SD†**	
1	2.8	15	1.2	
2	2.9	16	0.3	
3	0.6	17	0.9	
4	1.1	18	2.7	
5	2.4	19	2.2	
6	3.6	20	0.3	
7	1.1	21	0.7	
8	0.8	22	0.6	
9	1.1	23	0.1	
10	0.1	24	0.7	
11	1.9	25	0.7	
12	0.9			
13	3.4			
14	4.7			
Mean ± SEM‡	2.0 ± 0.4	Mean ± SEM‡	1.0 ± 0.2	

* Vaccine group data are significantly higher than placebo group data ($p < 0.05$) using the Mann–Whitney U test.
† Mean screen EU (antibody activity) + 1 standard deviation.
‡ SEM standard error of the mean.

($p<0.05$ – Mann–Whitney U test) higher than those obtained for the placebo group. Furthermore, only 3 of 11 (27%) subjects in the placebo group had IgA antibody levels to GTF which exceeded their screen values at any time during the First Immunization Phase, whereas 10 of 14 (71%) of the GTF-vaccine group had IgA antibody levels which exceeded screen values. The GTF-vaccine group also had a significantly higher distribution of IgA antibody levels ($p<0.05$) when the three highest ratios of the saliva collections were identified and compared for each group. Thus, most subjects receiving vaccine showed an antibody response whereas the placebo group showed virtually no response.

The peak IgA antibody response ratios compared with the mean of the screen values + one standard deviation identified during the Second Immunization Phase were determined. Statistically significant elevations in the levels of these ratios were found when the vaccine group was compared after the first and second phases. Although placebo group levels were also elevated, these were not statistically significant.

Serum antibody

Blood was collected five times during the course of the clinical trial for antibody evaluation. The sera were tested for IgG and IgA antibody to the immunizing GTF antigen. No significant increases in IgA and IgG serum antibody levels to the GTF antigen were observed during the First or Second Immunization Phases. Also, no significant differences between the groups were noted on any occasion.

Bacterial studies

The percentage of *S. mutans* of the total streptococci enumerated in whole saliva was used to monitor the effect of antibody to GTF on these organisms. The percentages were expressed as a ratio of the *S. mutans*/total streptococci relative to the percentage measured prior to the dental prophylaxis (day -2). The individual ratios were less than unity in the placebo group on 16 of 58 occasions (28%). In contrast, on 47 of 84 occasions (57%) the individual ratios were less than 1 in the GTF-vaccine group. On day 21, 40% of the placebo subjects had ratios below the pre-prophylaxis values, while 71% of the GTF-vaccine group remained beneath the pre-prophylaxis values. However, by day 42 (Table 3), nearly all the placebo group (89%) had reached the pre-prophylaxis *S. mutans*/total streptococcal percentage while only 27% of the GTF group reached this level. This difference was highly significant ($p<0.01$).

The *S. mutans*/total streptococcal percentages against which post second immunization percentages were compared were those obtained immediately prior to the second dental prophylaxis. On 22 of 54 (41%) of the occasions the

Table 3 Reduction in levels of salivary *S. mutans* 42 days after dental prophylaxis and oral administration of GTF or placebo

Vaccine*		Placebo*	
Subject	Reduction after prophylaxis (%)	Subject	Reduction after prophylaxis (%)
A	0	O	0
B	67	P	0
C	83	Q	0
D	0	R	0
E	0	S	0
F	89	T	0
G	17	U	0
H	59	V	22
I	51	W	0
J	20	X	—†
K	27	Y	—†
L	—†		
M	—†		
N	—†		
Mean ± SEM	38 ± 10	Mean ± SEM	2 ± 2

* Differences between groups statistically significant ($p<0.01$, Fisher Exact Test).
† Subjects with *S. mutans* beneath level of detection in whole saliva throughout course of study.

placebo subjects' individual ratios fell below the pre-prophylaxis values. On 36 of 78 (46%) of the sampling occasions, the GTF-vaccine subjects' individual ratios fell below their pre-prophylaxis values. No statistically significant differences were observed between the groups although the GTF-vaccine group mean ratios were less on days 5, 8 and 19. Importantly, both groups manifested diminished mean ratios throughout the observation period. These findings and the antibody data support a possible immunizing effect of the second prophylaxis (on the placebo group) and subsequent microbiological effects.

Discussion

The results of these studies verify the indications in humans that oral ingestion of microbial antigens can give rise to sIgA antibodies in external secretions of glands at remote sites (Mestecky *et al.* 1978, 1986; Clancy *et al.* 1983; Waldman *et al.* 1983). A probable explanation for our findings of IgA antibody to GTF derives from the migration of IgA-bearing lymphocytes from gut-associated lymphoid tissue (GALT) into salivary glands (Jackson *et al.* 1981). Such specific migrating IgA precursors have been demonstrated in human peripheral blood mononuclear cells after oral antigen administration (Mestecky *et al.* 1986).

A unique feature of the current study was the use of a defined soluble antigen combined in suspension with aluminum phosphate. Previously we reported that administration of a particulate antigen by gastric intubation generally elicited a greater salivary IgA response than an equivalent dose of the soluble form of the same antigen (Cox and Taubman 1984). These findings may be partially attributed to the enhanced uptake of particulate material by M cells in Peyer's patches (Wolf *et al.* 1982). We have also shown that particulate forms of GTF appear to promote enhanced salivary responses after intragastric administration (Ebersole *et al.* 1983).

A second significant finding was the retardation of reaccumulation of mutans streptococci after a dental prophylaxis had resulted in diminished numbers of these organisms. Presumably this effect was related to salivary IgA antibodies to *S. sobrinus* GTF. We have shown that antibody to the water-insoluble glucan synthesizing GTF (GTF$_1$) can markedly inhibit glucan synthesis and the accumulation of *S. mutans in vitro* (Taubman *et al.* 1983). The presence of salivary antibody to *S. sobrinus* GTF has also been shown to interfere with the accumulation of *S. sobrinus* (Taubman and Smith 1977) and other mutans streptococci in rodents (Smith *et al.* 1978a). This effect may result from direct inhibition of GTF-mediated glucan synthesis giving rise to alterations in the nature of dental plaque and thus eliminating glucan binding sites for *S. mutans* accumulation (Taubman *et al.* 1983). It should also be noted that in experiments where *S. mutans* was used as antigen, alterations in colonization were noted after antigen instillation (Table 1). Thus, IgA antibody to GTF in our system appears to interfere with reaccumulation of *S. mutans* on dental surfaces.

Although young adults were immunized in this study, it is clear that this would not necessarily be the target population for a dental caries vaccine because by this time of life most individuals are heavily colonized with mutans streptococci. The question then arises as to when would be the most appropriate time for immunization. Our recent studies on the ontogeny of secretory antibody to *S. mutans* antigens may shed some light on this dilemma. Salivary IgA levels in whole saliva of children show a significant increase in concentration at 12 to 17 months of age (Gahnberg *et al.* 1985). While IgA antibody to *S. sanguis* GTF could be detected in children aged two to four years with about 30–40% frequency, antibody to *S. mutans* GTF was virtually absent in children of this age group (Gahnberg *et al.* 1985). However, *S. mutans* could be recovered from 40% or more of the children above two years of age (Gahnberg *et al.* 1985). These data suggest the following: (1) children are immunocompetent with respect to salivary IgA after 12 months of age; (2) on average, children are colonized with mutans streptococci after the second year of age; (3) salivary antibody to *S. mutans* GTF is not detectable in the vast majority of children at four years of age. Therefore, it is clear that antibody to GTF is not present when children are colonized with *S. mutans*. Theoretically, immunization with GTF at approximately 12 months of age would encounter a competent immune system. Salivary IgA antibody to GTF formed at this time would be present to interfere with subsequent colonization or accumulation of *S. mutans* in the children. Employment of this strategy promises to provide a more effective mucosal approach to immunoprophylaxis of dental infections.

Acknowledgements

The research reported in this manuscript was supported by American Cyanamid Co. and DE-04733 and DE-06153 from the National Institute of Dental Research. We thank William King, Mary Ritchie and Donna Freedman for assistance.

References

Bonta C Y, Linzer R, Emmings F, Evans R T, Genco R J 1979. Human oral infectivity and immunization studies with *Streptococcus mutans* strain B13, *Journal of Dental Research* 58: 143

Clancy R, Cripps A W, Husband A J, Gleeson M 1983 Restrictions on mucosal B-lymphocyte function in man. *Annals of the New York Academy of Sciences* 408: 745–9

Clark W B, Gibbons R J 1977. Influence of salivary components and extracellular polysaccharide synthesis from sucrose on the attachment of *Streptococcus mutans* 6715 to hydroxyapatite surfaces. *Infection and Immunity* 18: 514–23

Cole M F, Emilson C-G, Hsu S D, Li S-H, Bowen W H 1984. Effect of peroral immunization of humans with *Streptococcus mutans* on induction of salivary and serum antibodies and inhibition of experimental infection, *Infection and Immunity* 46: 703–9

Cox D S, Taubman M A 1984. Oral induction of the secretory antibody response by soluble and particulate antigens, *Archives of Allergy and Applied Immunology* 75: 126–31

Curtiss R III, Murchison H H, Nesbitt W E, Barrett J F, Michalek S M 1985. Use of mutants and gene cloning to identify and characterize colonization mechanisms of *Streptococcus mutans*, in S Mergenhagen, B Rosan (eds) *Molecular Basis for Oral Microbial Adhesion*. American Society for Microbiology, Washington, DC, pp 187–93

de Stoppelaar J D, Konig D G, Plasschaert A J M, van der Hoeven J A 1971. Decreased cariogenicity of a mutant of *Streptococcus mutans*, *Archives of Oral Biology* 16: 971–5

Ebersole J L, Taubman M A, Smith D J 1983. Adjuvants, glucosyltransferases and caries vaccine, in R J Doyle, J E Ciardi (eds) *Glucosyltransferases, Glucans, Sucrose and Dental Caries*. Special Supplement. Chemical Senses, Washington, DC, pp 241–8

Ebersole J L, Taubman M A, Smith D J, Frey D E 1986. Regulation of salivary SIgA antibody, in S Hamada, A M Michalek, H Kiyono, L Menaker, J R McGhee (eds) *Molecular Microbiology and Immunology of Streptococcus mutans*. Elsevier, Amsterdam, pp 329–36

Fitzgerald R J, Keyes P H 1960. Demonstration of the etiologic role of *Streptococci* in experimental caries in the hamster, *Journal of the American Dental Association* 61: 9–19

Freedman M L, Tanzer J M 1974. Dissociation of plaque formation from glucan-induced agglutination in mutants of *Streptococcus mutans*, *Infection and Immunity* 10: 189–96

Gahnberg L, Krasse B 1983. Salivary immunoglobulin A antibodies and recovery from challenge of *Streptococcus mutans* after oral administration of *Streptococcus mutans* vaccine in humans, *Infection and Immunity* 39: 514–19

Gahnberg L, Smith D J, Taubman M A, Ebersole J L 1985. Salivary IgA antibody to glucosyltransferase of oral streptococcal origin in children, *Archives of Oral Biology* 30: 551–6

Gibbons R J, Fitzgerald R J 1969. Dextran-induced agglutination of *Streptococcus mutans*, and its potential role in the formation of microbial dental plaques, *Journal of Bacteriology* **98**: 341–6

Gibbons R J, Qureshi J V 1979. Inhibition of adsorption of *Streptococcus mutans* strains to saliva-treated hydroxyapatite by galactose and certain amines, *Infection and Immunity* **26**: 1214–17

Gregory R L, Michalek S M, Filler S J, Mestecky J, McGhee J R 1985. Prevention of *Streptococcus mutans* colonization by salivary IgA antibodies, *Journal of Clinical Immunology* **2**: 55–61

Guggenheim B, Newbrun E 1969. Extracellular glucosyltransferase activity of an HS strain of *Streptococcus mutans*, *Helvetica Odontologisk Acta* **13**: 84–97

Hughes M, Machardy S, Sheppard A, Langford D, Shepherd W 1986. Experiences in development of a dental caries vaccine, in S Hamada, S M Michalek, H Kiyono, L Menaker, J R McGhee (eds) *Molecular Microbiology and Immunology of Streptococcus mutans*. Elsevier, Amsterdam, pp 349–57

Jackson D E, Lally E T, Nakamura M C, Montgomery P C 1981. Migration of IgA-bearing lymphocytes into salivary glands, *Cellular Immunology* **163**: 203–9

Johnson M C, Bozzola J J, Schechmeister I L 1974. Morphological study of *Streptococcus mutans* and two extracellular polysaccharide mutants, *Journal of Bacteriology* **118**: 304–11

Keyes P H 1960. The infectious and transmissible nature of experimental dental caries. Findings and implications. *Archives of Oral Biology* **1**: 304–20

Krasse B, Gahnberg L, Bratthall D 1978. Antibodies reacting with *Streptococcus mutans* in secretions from minor salivary glands in humans, *Advances in Experimental Medicine and Biology* **109**: 349–54

Kuramitsu H K, Aoki H 1986. Isolation and manipulation of *Streptococcus mutans* glucosyltransferase genes, in S Hamada, S M Michalek, H Kiyono, L Menaker, J McGhee (eds) *Molecular Microbiology and Immunobiology of Streptococcus mutans*. Elsevier, Amsterdam, pp 199–215

McCabe M M, Hamelik R M, Smith E E 1977. Purification of dextran-binding protein from cariogenic *Streptococcus mutans*, *Biochemical and Biophysical Research Communications* **78**: 273–8

McGhee J R, Michalek S M, Webb J, Navia J M, Rahman A F R, Legler D W 1975. Effective immunity to dental caries: protection of gnotobiotic rats by local immunization with *Streptococcus mutans*, Journal of Immunology **114**: 300–5

Mestecky J, McGhee J R, Arnold R R, Michalek S M, Prince S J, Babb J L 1978. Selective induction of an immune response in human external secretions by ingestion of bacterial antigen, *Journal of Clinical Investigations* **61**: 731–7

Mestecky, J, Czerkinsky C, Brown T A, Prince S J, Michalek S M, Russell M W, Jackson S, Scholler M, McGhee J R 1986. Human immune responses to *Streptococcus mutans*, in S Hamada, S M Michalek, H Kiyono, L Menaker, J R McGhee (eds) *Molecular Microbiology and Immunobiology of Streptococcus mutans*. Elsevier, Amsterdam, pp 207–306.

Michalek S M, Shiota T, Ikeda T, Navia J M, McGhee J R 1975. Virulence of *Streptococcus mutans*; biochemical and pathogenic characteristics of mutant isolates, *Proceedings of the Society of Experimental Biology and Medicine* **150**: 498–502

Michalek S M, McGhee J R, Mestecky J, Arnold R R, Bozzo L 1976. Ingestion of *Streptococcus mutans* induces secretory immunoglobulin A and caries immunity, *Science* **192**: 1238–40

Orland F J, Blayney J R, Harrison R W, Reyniers J A, Trexler P C, Ervin R F, Gordon H A, Wagner M 1955. Experimental caries in germfree rats inoculated with enterococci, *Journal of the American Dental Association* **50**: 259–72

Russell R R B, Donald A C, Douglas C W I 1983. Fructosyltransferase activity of a glucan-binding protein from *Streptococcus mutans*, *Journal of General Microbiology* **129**: 3242–50

Scholler M, Klein J P, Frank R M 1978. Dental caries in gnotobiotic rats immunized with purified glucosyltransferase from *Streptococcus sanguis*, *Archives of Oral Biology* **23**: 501–9

Smith D J, Taubman M A, Ebersole J L 1978a. Effects of local immunization with glucosyltransferase fractions from *Streptococcus mutans* on dental caries in hamsters caused by homologous and heterologous serotypes of *Streptococcus mutans*, *Infection and Immunity* **21**: 843–51

Smith D J, Taubman M A, Ebersole J L 1978b. Preparation of glucosyltransferase from *Streptococcus mutans* by elution from water-insoluble polysaccharide with a dissociating solvent, *Infection and Immunity* **23**: 446–52

Smith D J, Taubman M A, Ebersole J L 1979. Effect of oral administration of glucosyltransferase antigens on experiment dental caries, *Infection and Immunity* **26**: 82–9

Smith D J, Taubman M A, Ebersole J L 1980. Local and systemic antibody response to oral administration of glucosyltransferase antigen complex, *Infection and Immunity* **28**: 441–50

Smith D J, Taubman M A, Ebersole J L 1982. Effects of local immunization on colonization of hamsters by *Streptococcus mutans*, *Infection and Immunity* **37**: 656–61

Smith D J, King W, LaVangie D C, Gahnberg L, Taubman M A, Ebersole J L 1984. Preparation and characteristics of glucosyltransferase from *Streptococcus mutans*, *Journal of Dental Research* **63**: 675

Smith D J, Taubman M A, Ebersole J L 1985. Salivary IgA antibody to glucosyltransferase in man, *Clinical and Experimental Immunology* **61**: 416–24

Socransky S, Smith D, Manganello A J 1973. Defined media for the cultivation of oral Gram positive rods, *Journal of Dental Research* **52**: 88

Staat R H, Langley S D, Doyle R J 1980. *Streptococcus mutans* adherence: presumptive evidence for protein-mediated attachment followed by glucan-dependent cellular accumulation, *Infection and Immunity* **27**: 675–81

Tanzer J M, Freedman M L 1978. Genetic alterations of *Streptococcus mutans* virulence, *Advances in Experimental Medicine and Biology* **107**: 661–72

Tanzer J M, Freedman M L, Fitzgerald R J, Larson R H 1974. Diminished virulence of glucan synthesis-defective mutants of *Streptococcus mutans*, *Infection and Immunity* **10**: 197–203

Taubman M A 1973. Role of immunization in dental disease, in S Mergenhagen, H Scherp (eds) *Comparative Immunology of the Oral Cavity*. US Government Printing Office, Washington, DC, pp 138–58

Taubman M A, Smith D J 1974. Effects of local immunization with *Streptococcus mutans* on induction of salivary immunoglobulin A antibody and experimental dental caries in rats, *Infection and Immunity* **9**: 1079–91

Taubman M A, Smith D J 1977. Effects of local immunization with glucosyltransferase fractions from *Streptococcus mutans* on experimental dental caries in rats and hamsters, *Journal of Immunology* **118**: 710–20

Taubman M A, Smith D J, Ebersole J L, Hillman J D 1982. Immunological interference with accumulation of cariogenic microorganisms on tooth surfaces, in W Strober, L A Hanson, K W Sell (eds) *Recent Advances in Mucosal Immunity*. Raven Press, NY, pp 371–82

Taubman M A, Smith D J, Ebersole J L, Hillman J D 1983. Protective aspects of immune response to glucosyltransferase in relation to dental caries, in R J Doyle, J E Ciardi (eds) *Glucosyltransferase, Glucans Sucrose and Dental Caries*. Special Supplement. Chemical Senses, Washington, DC, pp 249–58

Tomasi T B Jr, Tan E M, Solomon A, Prendergast R A 1965. Characteristics of an immune system common to certain external secretions, *Journal of Experimental Medicine* **121**: 101–24

van Houte J, Russo J 1986. Factors influencing the cariogenicity of *Streptococcus mutans*, in S Hamada, S M Michalek, H Kiyono, L Menaker, J R McGhee (eds) *Molecular Micriobiology and Immunology of Streptococcus mutans*. Elsevier, Amsterdam, pp 157–69

Waldman R H, Stone J, Lazzel V, Bergmann K Ch, Khakoo R, Jacknowitz A, Howard S, Rose C 1983. Oral route as method for immunizing against mucosal pathogens, *Annals of New York Academy of Sciences* **409**: 510–16

Wolf J L, Rubin D H, Finberg R, Kaufman R S, Sharpe A H, Trier J S, Fields B N 1982. Intestinal M cells: a pathway of entry for reovirus into the host, *Science* **212**: 471–2

Regulation of complement activation on bacterial surfaces

J McLeod Griffiss*; Susan Schecter†; Michael M Eads†; Ryohei Yamasaki*;
Gary A Jarvis*

* The Centre for Immunochemistry and the Departments of Laboratory
Medicine and Medicine, University of California at San Francisco, San
Francisco, California 94143, USA
† The Channing Laboratory and Department of Medicine, Brigham and
Women's Hospital and Harvard Medical School, Boston, Massachusetts
02115, USA

Introduction

Bacteria that enter the circulation are cleared by complement-mediated
immune effector mechanisms. Activation and deposition of complement onto
the bacterial surface is a complex interaction between the chemical environment presented by the bacterium and initiator and regulatory components of the complement cascade. Circulating antibodies interact with the
bacterial surface and initiator and regulatory components to either promote
(up-regulate) *or* prevent (down-regulate) effective complement activation
(Griffiss 1983; Griffiss and Goroff 1983; Apicella *et al.* 1986). An individual
acquires antibodies over a lifetime by sequential encounters with organisms; a
mother may pass some of these antibodies to her fetus, thereby providing a
potential for protection during the first six to ten months of life.

The presence of circulating antibodies that focus deposition of complement
onto the bacterial surface and insure its effective activation can prevent
diseases for which bloodstream dissemination and survival are essential parts
of the pathogenesis. Vaccination seeks to provide the infant or child with
adult-levels of such antibodies prior to an encounter with the potentially
pathogenic strain. Development of vaccines to accomplish this goal has
focused on the capsular polysaccharides of *Streptococcus pneumoniae*,
Haemophilus influenzae and *Neisseria meningitidis*, as these polysaccharides
have long been known to be 'anticomplementary'.

In this review, we will summarize our current understanding of
complement-activation regulation by bacterial surfaces and by antibody
molecules that bind to them.

The chemical structure of bacterial capsules

The hydrophilic capsules that surround *S. pneumoniae, H. influenzae*, and *N. meningitidis* protect them from desiccation during passage from the mucosa of one individual to another (Griffiss 1982). They also render their surfaces 'anticomplementary' and 'antiphagocytic'.

Differences among the various capsules of these bacteria were originally found serologically, i.e. by differences in the antigenic structures, or epitopes, that they form, and that could be recognized by antibodies. They are thus separated and denominated by their *antigenic* specificities. The *chemical* structures of many of these polysaccharides are known with great certainty, but the *physical* structures of epitopes formed within them remain unknown. It is, however, clear that epitope structure is independent of chemical structure *per se*. That is, epitopes represent shapes that are provided by the spatial conformation of the chemical structures. As a given shape can be formed by chemically different molecules, epitopes may overlap, or be common to, several chemically different polysaccharides.

Because monosaccharides, unlike peptides, can be linked in multiple ways, the number of chemical structures represented by bacterial capsules is enormous. But they share certain attributes. Almost all are acidic, with the acidic function provided by ketulosonic, uronic or phosphoric acid constituents, or by organic acid substituents, such as pyruvic acid. Most contain amino sugars, and these are invariably acetylated.

Neisseria meningitidis is capable of elaborating 12 serogroup-specific capsules. They are chemically related and their synthesis from glucosamine phosphate is rather straightforward – at least for a bacterium (Griffiss 1981). They can be chemically divided into those that are hexosamine polymers with phosphoric, ketulosonic or uronic substituents (groups A, H, I, J, K, L, X, Z and 29E), and those that are sialic (neuraminic) acid polymers, with or without

Table 1 Chemical and structural relationships of *N. meningitidis* capsules that have been evaluated as vaccines in man

Serogroup	Chemical structure	Immunologic relationship
A	α1–6 Mannosamine phosphate	Unknown
X	α1–4 Glucosamine phosphate	
B	α2–8 Sialic acid	Shared minor epitopes
C	α2–9 Sialic acid	
Y	4-Sialic acid α2–6 glucose α1–	Heteroclitic
W	4-Sialic acid α2–6 galactose α1–	
Z	3-Galactosamine α1–1 glycerol phosphate 3–	Shared major epitope
29E	3-Galactosamine α1–7 deoxyoctulosonic acid α2–	Heteroclitic

interposed hexose components (groups B, C, Y and W) (Griffiss 1981). Four structurally and immunologically related pairs have been used as vaccines in man (Table 1). Shared immunogenicity reflects both shared epitopes (B/C and Z/29E) and the induction of an heteroclitic response (Y/W and Z/29E) (Griffiss *et al.* 1981, 1983).

Regulation of complement activation by the bacterial surface

Complement molecules interact with *physical and chemical* structures on the bacterial surface, not necessarily with their *antigenic* structures. The capsule, as the outermost organelle, is the most important surface receptor for complement molecules. The anticomplementarity, or down-regulating capacity, of capsules has *chemical specificity* that is distinct from the *antigenic specificity* by which we know and denominate them. Up-regulation of complement activation by antibodies, on the other hand, has *antigenic specificity* that may be independent of *chemical specificity*. In the absence of circulating antibody, complement molecules are ineffectively deposited onto bacterial surfaces and the organisms multiply intravascularly until concentrations are reached that are capable of producing circulatory collapse and/or secondary localization.

Down-regulation by the capsules of bacteria involves both the classical and alternative pathways of complement activation. We have studied the antigenic independence of down-regulation using immune lysis of *N. meningitidis* and opsonophagocytosis of group B, type III streptococci as indicators of effective complement activation (Griffiss *et al.* 1984). For the two pathways combined, group B meningococcal polysaccharide ($\alpha 2$–8 NeuNAc) is twice as effective, on a weight basis, as group A or C meningococcal, or B/III streptococcal capsules; the latter three are equimolar in their inhibitory capacities. The 2:1 molar ratio holds for both opsonophagocytosis of the streptococcus and immune lysis of the various meningococci – but only in the absence of capsular antibody. That is, group A meningococcal polysaccharide (ManNAc-*P*) inhibits opsonophagocytic killing of the streptococcus just as well as the streptococcal capsule; $\alpha 2$–8 NeuNAc inhibits killing of streptococci, and meningococci of other serogroups, twice as effectively as do their respective capsules.

The chemical basis of down-regulation of the classical pathway is unexplored; down-regulation of the alternative pathway is a function of amide-linked acetyl groups (Varki and Kornfeld 1980). This exquisite chemical specificity is seen in Fig. 1, where we used immune lysis of rabbit erythrocytes by MgEGTA-chelated serum as the indicator. The three meningococcal capsules (ManNAc-*P;* $\alpha 2$–8 NeuNAc; $\alpha 2$–9 NeuNAc) contain one *N*-acetyl group per monosaccharide; the streptococcal capsule (Glc-GlcNAc-(Gal)$_2$-NeuNAc) contains 0.4 moles of *N*-acetyl per mole of monosaccharide. The

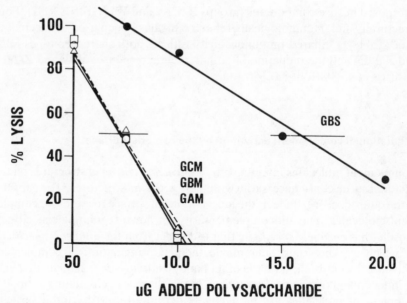

Figure 1. Fluid-phase inhibition of alternative complement pathway-mediated immune lysis of rabbit erythrocytes by the capsular polysaccharides of group A ($\triangle$——$\triangle$; GAM), group B (○———○; GBM), and group C (□———□; GCM) *N. meningitidis*, and group B, type III streptococcus (●———●; GBS). Human serum without measurable antibody to any of the four polysaccharides was chelated with MgEGTA and used to support lysis. The difference in weight of polysaccharide required to produce 50% inhibition reflects the molar ratios of *N*-acetyl groups to monosaccharides (1:1 for the meningococcal polysaccharides; 0.4:1 for the streptococcal polysaccharide).

inhibitory capacities of the meningococcal polysaccharides are equimolar and slightly more than twice that of the streptococcal capsule. Although these data reflect fluid-phase inhibition, there is no reason to believe that similar interactions do not take place on the cell surface (Griffiss *et al.* 1984).

Epitope expression within polar polysaccharides

We have only recently begun to explore how bacterial polysaccharides conform, or shape themselves, into epitopes. The α2–8 and α2–9 NeuNAc capsules of *N. meningitidis* provide an illustrative model system.

Sialic acid is a nine-carbon ketulosonic acid that is *N*-acetylated at C5. It is synthesized by the condensation of pyruvic acid to ManNAc. The three additional carbons (C7–C9) stick out like a tail from the pyranose ring formed by C2–C6. Linkage of adjacent residues to this 'tail' provides a molecule with the potential for considerably more molecular motion than it would have if the monosaccharides were linked to the rigid, box-like, pyranose rings (Fig.

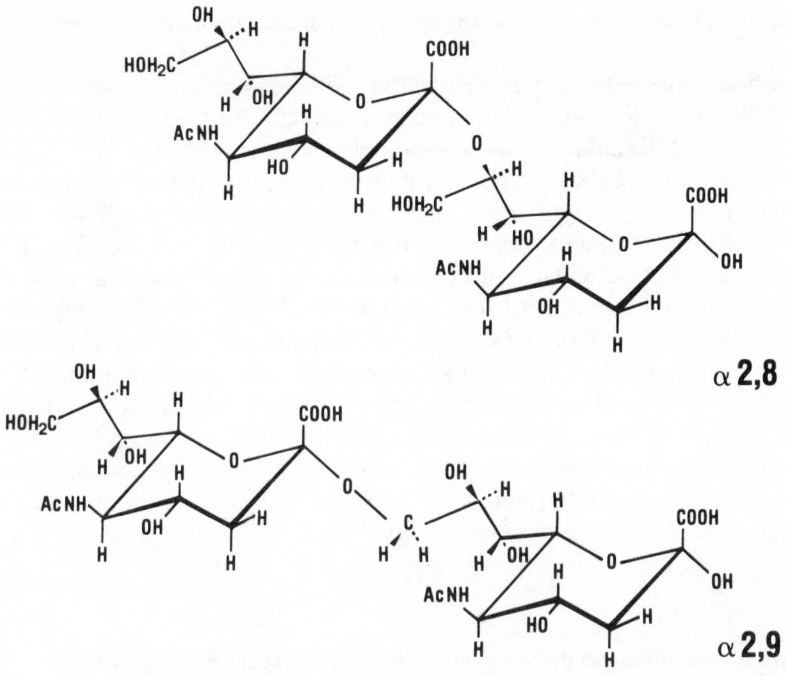

Figure 2. Sialic acid disaccharides linked α2–8 (upper; group B) and α2–9 (lower; group C) showing the potential molecular motion conferred by linkage of the adjacent monosaccharides to the C7–C9 'tail' that extends from the rigid pyranose ring structures. C7–C9 are the sites of variable *O*-acetylation.

2). The α2–8 NeuNAc residues produced by most strains of *N. meningitidis* are not substituted at the C7 position (Lifely *et al.* 1984; Lindon *et al.* 1984). When produced by *Escherichia coli* and a few strains of *N. meningitidis*, α2–8 NeuNAc residues are often *O*-acetylated at C7 (Jennings *et al.* 1985). As C7 is in the hinge region between adjacent pyranose rings, substitution of a polar acetyl group at this position would be expected to 'direct' intramolecular motion and alter conformation. α2–9 NeuNAc polymers have two potential sites for acetylation within the hinge regions of their constituents, C7, and C8, and are usually fully acetylated.

One epitope presented by the *O*-acetylated α2–8 NeuNAc polymer (group B) is identical to an epitope within the α2–9 NeuNAc polymer (group C). We currently believe that acetylation at C7 conforms the two sialic acid polymers into the same epitopic 'shape' despite their different linkages. The unacetylated α2–8 linkage, and α2–9 disaccharides that are acetylated at C8 or at both C7 and C8 would each form different epitopic shapes. By this reasoning, the two polysaccharides should contain at least four separate epitopes. Although much uncertainty remains, it is clear that epitope expression within polysaccharides is complex, independent of linkage, *per se*, and dependent upon chemical fine structure.

Immunoglobulin isotypes and the activation of complement

Antibodies of the three major circulating isotypes vary greatly in their ability to induce complement-mediated immune effector mechanisms (Griffiss and Goroff 1983). Immune lysis and opsonophagocytosis, initiated by 'bactericidal' antibodies, are the effector mechanisms that prevent dissemination of *N. meningitidis* and *H. influenzae* in the first instance, (Fothergill and Wright 1932; Griffiss 1982) and *Streptococcus* in the second (Brown *et al.* 1983). IgM is invariably bactericidal; the bactericidal capacity of IgG is, at best, only one-half that of IgM (Griffiss and Goroff 1983), and the complement-activating capacity of the IgG isotypes that bind these polysaccharides has not been determined. IgA *never* initiates complement-mediated immune effector mechanisms (Griffiss and Goroff 1983; Griffiss 1983). More importantly, circulating IgA *blocks* immune lysis induced by IgM and IgG (Griffiss 1975; Griffiss and Goroff 1983; Griffiss *et al.*1978). What makes an antibody, of whatever isotype, bactericidal and the molecular mechanism by which IgA blocks complement activation remain elusive.

Immunoglobulin isotype response to meningococcal polysaccharides

ManNAc-*P* (group A) and *O*-Ac-α2–9 NeuNAc (group C) polymers induce IgM, IgG and IgA in more than 90% of adults (Artenstein *et al.* 1971; Gotschlich *et al.* 1969; Käyhty *et al.* 1981). IgA is rapidly removed (? days) by hepatic clearance (Griffiss 1983); IgM wanes more slowly, over the ensuing 12–18 months; IgG is long-lived. Groups Y (NeuNAc α2–6 Glc) and W (NeuNAc α2–6 Gal) polysaccharides induce heteroclitic responses similar to that to group C (Griffiss *et al.* 1981, 1982, 1985a).

Pure α2–8 NeuNAc is not immunogenic in man when hydrophobically complexed with outer membrane proteins; it induces bactericidal IgM, but neither IgG nor IgA (Zollinger *et al.* 1979). The IgM response is very short-lived, and the avidity of the IgM is considerably lower than that of IgM induced by α2–9 NeuNAc (Mandrell and Zollinger 1982).

Functional response to meningococcal polysaccharides

Antibodies induced by these polysaccharides do not invariably activate complement in such a way that it mediates bactericidal activity. The lytic efficacy of IgG binding to ManNAc-*P* is dependent upon the lipooligosaccharide serotype of the group A strain used in the assay, but the relationship of this *in vitro* phenomenon to vaccine efficacy has not been explored.

There is a ceiling on production of complement-activating antibody, and the total and lytic antibody responses are de-coupled (Griffiss *et al.* 1981, 1983). Individuals reach the same titer of bactericidal activity regardless of pre-vaccination levels, but do not exceed the ceiling. The total antibody response is unlimited; the higher the pre-vaccination level, the greater is the incremental response. But much of this augmented antibody is not bactericidal.

Antibodies that bind both GalNAc-d0clA (group 29E) and GalNAc-glycerol-*P* (group Z) polysaccharides are induced by vaccination with 29E polysaccharide; however, in some individuals a portion of the induced antibody, presumably IgA, blocks the bactericidal activity of other pre-existing and induced antibodies, and total bactericidal activity is lost (Griffiss *et al.* 1983). The blocking antibody declines by four weeks, at which time lytic antibody responses are seen. The shift occurs without appreciable change in antibody levels. Antibodies induced by 29E polysaccharide that bind Z polysaccharide are not bactericidal (Griffiss and Brandt 1983).

How does complement kill a meningococcus?

Theories of the molecular basis of complement-mediated lysis of bacteria are inadequate to explain recent data, but two conclusions seem clear: first, whether lysis occurs is independent of the quantity of complement components deposited on the cell surface; and second, alternative complement pathway (ACP) activation must be involved for lysis to proceed efficiently.

Both IgA and IgG increase the deposition of C3 onto the bacterial surface as they block effective lysis, and antibody binding to $\alpha2-8$ NeuNAc reverses the latter's down-regulation of the ACP and permits ACP-mediated lysis without increasing the quantity of either C3 or factor B deposited onto the surface (Jarvis and Vedros, 1985). Up-regulation of ACP augmentation of CP-mediated killing is also not accompanied by quantitative increases in the deposition of C3 or factor B (Schneider *et al.* 1985). We conclude that lysis can occur only when complement components are assembled in a favorable chemical environment, and that antibody molecules differ in their ability to provide such an environment.

Neisserial surfaces variably bind properdin (P) (Griffiss *et al.* 1985b), and quantitative differences in P-binding account for differences in sensitivity to lysis by the CP. Studies of two families with X-linked P-deficiency and multiple episodes of fulminant meningococcal disease confirm that an intact ACP is necessary to prevent disseminated meningococcal disease in individuals who lack capsular antibody (Sjöholm *et al.* 1982).

Summary

We have presented a complex picture of the regulation of complement-activation by the bacterial surface. The effectiveness of complement molecules in initiating lysis of an organism is a function of the chemical environment in which they are activated, rather than the quantity of their deposition. Different antibody isotypes vary in their ability to provide an environment that supports the effective activation of complement, and the isotypes induced by polysaccharides may be restricted.

Augmentation of antibody-initiated, CP-mediated deposition of C3 by the ACP is critical to the effectiveness of antibody. ACP augmentation requires binding of properdin.

Acknowledgements

This is paper No. 5 from the Centre for Immunochemistry of the University of California at San Francisco. The manuscript was prepared by Ms May Fong.

References

Apicella, M A, Westerink J A J, Morse S A, Schneider H, Rice P A, Griffiss J McL 1986. Bactericidal antibody response of normal human serum to the lipooligosaccharide of *Neisseria gonorrhoeae*, *Journal of Infectious Diseases* 153: 520–6

Artenstein M S, Brandt B L, Tramont E C, Branche W C Jr, Fleet H D, Cohen R L 1971. Serologic studies of meningococcal infection and polysaccharide vaccination, *Journal of Infectious Diseases* 124: 277–88

Brown E J, Hosea W, Frank M M 1983. The role of antibody and complement in the reticuloendothelial clearance of pneumococci from the bloodstream, *Reviews of Infectious Diseases* 5: 5797–805

Fothergill L D, Wright J 1932 Influenzal meningitis. The relation of age incidence to the bactericidal power of blood against the causal organism, *Journal of Immunology* 24: 273–84

Gotschlich E C, Goldschneider I, Artenstein M S 1969. Human immunity to the meningococcus. IV. Immunogenicity of group A and group C meningococcal polysaccharides in human volunteers, *Journal of Experimental Medicine* 129: 1367–84

Griffiss J McL 1975. Bactericidal activity of meningococcal antisera: blocking by IgG of lytic antibody in human convalescent sera, *Journal of Immunology* 114: 1779–84

Griffiss J McL 1981. Immune response to meningococcus antigens, in G Torrigiani, R Bell (eds) *Immunological Recognition and Effector Mechanisms in Infectious Diseases*. Schwabe, Basel, pp 137–52

Griffiss J McL 1982. Epidemic meningococcal disease: synthesis of a hypothetical immunoepidemiologic model, *Reviews of Infectious Diseases* 4: 159–71

Griffiss J McL 1983. Biologic function of the serum IgA system: modulation of complement-mediated effector mechanisms and conservation of antigenic mass, *Annals of the New York Academy of Sciences* 409: 697–707

Griffiss J McL, Brandt B L 1983. Immunological relationship between the capsular polysaccharides of *Neisseria meningitidis* serogroups Z and 29E. *Journal of General Microbiology* **129**: 447–52

Griffiss J McL, Goroff D K 1983. IgA blocks IgM and IgG-initiated immune lysis by separate molecular mechanisms, *Journal of Immunology* **130**: 2882–5

Griffiss J McL, Bertram M A, Broud D D 1978. Separation and purification of immunoglobulins M, A and G from small volumes of human sera by a continuous, in-line chromatographic process (GV-2), *Journal of Chromatography* **156**: 121–30

Griffiss J McL, Brandt B L, Altieri P L, Pier G B, Berman S L 1981. Safety and immunogenicity of group Y and group W135 meningococcal capsular polysaccharide vaccines in adults, *Infection and Immunity* **34**: 725–32

Griffiss J McL, Brandt B L, Broud D D 1982. Human immune response to various doses of group Y and W135 meningococcal polysaccharide vaccines, *Infection and Immunity* **37**: 205–8

Griffiss J McL, Brandt B L, Altieri P L, Pier G B, Berman S L 1983. Safety and immunogenicity of a group 29E meningococcal capsular polysaccharide vaccine in adults, *Infection and Immunity* **39**: 247–52

Griffiss J McL, Brandt B L, Broud D D, Goroff D K, Baker C J 1984. Immune response of infants and children to disseminated *Neisseria meningitidis* infection, *Journal of Infectious Diseases* **150**: 71–9

Griffiss J McL, Brandt B L, Broud D D, Altieri P L, Berman S L 1985a. Relationship of dose to the reactogenicity and immunogenicity of meningococcal polysaccharide vaccines in adults, *Military Medicine* **150**: 529–33

Griffiss J McL, Schnieder H, O'Brien J P 1985b. Lysis of *Neisseria gonorrhoeae* initiated by binding of normal human IgM to an hexosamine-containing LOS epitope is augmented by strain permissive feedback through the alternative pathway of complement activation, in G K Schoolnik, G F Brooks, S Falkow, C E Frasch, J S Knapp, J A McCutchan, S A Morse (eds) *The Pathogenic Neisseriae*. Proceedings of the Fourth International Symposium. American Society for Microbiology, Washington, DC, pp 456–61

Jarvis G A, Vedros N A 1985. Antibody-dependent alternative complement pathway killing of group B meningococci, in G K Schoolnik, G F Brooks, S Falkow, C E Frasch, J S Knapp, J A McCutchan, S A Morse (eds) *The Pathogenic Neisseriae*. Proceedings of the Fourth International Symposium. American Society for Microbiology, Washington, DC, pp 592–6

Jennings H J, Roy R, Michon F 1985. Determinant specificities of the groups B and C polysaccharides of *Neisseria meningitidis*, *Journal of Immunology* **134**: 2651–7

Käyhty H, Jousimies-Somer H, Peltola H, Mäkelä P H 1981. Antibody response to capsular polysaccharides of groups A and C *Neisseria meningitidis* and *Haemophilus influenzae* type b during bacteremic disease, *Journal of Infectious Diseases* **143**: 32–41

Lifely M R, Gilbert A S, Moreno C 1984. Rate, mechanism, and immunochemical studies of lactonisation in serogroup B and C polysaccharides of *Neisseria meningitidis*, *Carbohydrate Research* **134**: 229–43

Lindon J C, Vinter J G, Lifely M R, Moreno C 1984. Conformational and dynamic differences between *N. meningitidis* serogroup B and C polysaccharides, using NMR spectroscopy and molecular mechanics calculations, *Carbohydrate Research* **133**: 59–74

Mandrell R E, Zollinger W D 1982. Measurement of antibodies to meningococcal group B polysaccharide: low avidity binding and equilibrium binding constants, *Journal of Immunology* **129**: 2172–8

Schneider H, Griffiss J McL, Mandrell R E, Jarvis G A 1985. Elaboration of a 3.6-kilodalton lipooligosaccharide, antibody against which is absent from human sera, is associated with serum resistance of *Neisseria gonorrhoeae*, *Infection and Immunity* **50**: 672–7

Sjöholm A G, Braconier J-H, Söderström C 1982. Properdin deficiency in a family with fulminant meningococcal infections, *Clinical and Experimental Immunology* **50**: 291–7

Varki A, Kornfeld S 1980. An autosomal dominant gene regulates the extent of 9-*O*-acetylation of murine erythrocyte sialic acids. A probable explanation for the variation in capacity to activate the human alternate complement pathway, *Journal of Experimental Medicine* **152**: 532–44

Zollinger W D, Mandrell R E, Griffiss J McL, Altieri P, Berman S 1979. Complex of meningococcal group B polysaccharide and type 2 outer membrane protein immunogenic in man, *Journal of Clinical Investigation* **63**: 836–48

Interactions of antibodies and complement on bacterial surfaces: lessons learned from the gonococcus

Peter A Rice*; Milan S Blake†; Keith A Joiner‡;

* *The Maxwell Finland Laboratory for Infectious Diseases, Boston City Hospital, Boston University School of Medicine, Boston, MA 02118, USA*
† *The Rockefeller University of New York, NY 10021, USA*
‡ *The National Institute of Allergy and Infectious Diseases, National Institutes of Health, Bethesda, Maryland 20205, USA*

Introduction

Direct complement-mediated killing, in the case of several Gram-negative bacteria, may both require and be prevented by antibodies of diverse specificity that are present in human serum (Neisser and Wechsberg 1901; Thomas and Dingle 1943; Waisbren and Brown 1966; Taylor 1972; Griffiss *et al.* 1975; Guttman and Waisbren 1975; Rice and Kasper 1977; McCutchan *et al.* 1978; Rice and Kasper 1982; Rice *et al.* 1986). This disparate effect is well characterized for serum killing of *Neisseria gonorrhoeae* (McCutchan *et al.* 1978; Rice and Kasper 1982; Joiner *et al.* 1985b; Rice *et al.* 1986). The mechanisms of serum killing and resistance to serum killing of *N. gonorrhoeae* are directly related to the efficiency of insertion of the membrane attack complex of complement (C5b–9) (Joiner *et al.* 1983). Activation and deposition of individual complement components onto the surface of organisms either directly or via antibody is not sufficient, however, to ensure complete insertion of the membrane attack complex (MAC) (Joiner *et al.* 1983). Natural antibodies of the IgG class may subvert adequate insertion of the MAC. These have been described in human sera, and are termed blocking antibodies (McCutchan *et al.* 1978; Rice and Kasper 1982; Joiner *et al.* 1985a; Rice *et al.* 1986). These antibodies interfere with the efficient insertion of the MAC by as-yet unknown mechanism(s); however, binding of these antibodies to particular antigenic targets on the surface of the gonococcus may divert the necessary localization of C away from bactericidal sites (Joiner *et al.* 1985a). Recent studies with monoclonal antibody have shown that antibody specific for gonococcal surface protein, Protein III, is able to block killing of gonococci by bactericidal antibody directed against a separate epitope (Joiner *et al.* 1985b). Protein III appears to be not only present in all strains of gonococci (Judd

1982a, 1982b), but is biochemically and immunochemically identical (Judd 1982b; Swanson *et al.* 1982).

The studies reported here investigate the unique antigenic specificity of human blocking antibody and demonstrate the blocking action of purified IgG antibodies directed against gonococcal outer membrane Protein III. Furthermore, blocking F(ab')$_2$ as well as blocking IgG inhibits binding of bactericidal antibody to *N. gonorrhoeae*. These studies also indicate that blocking IgG and F(ab')$_2$ enhance rather than inhibit complement deposition on *N. gonorrhoeae*, leading to relocation of complement binding at new sites on the outer membrane.

Results

Specificity of immunopurified IgG

A single serum-resistant strain of *N. gonorrhoeae* (IB-3 serovar [Knapp *et al.* 1984]) isolated from a patient with disseminated gonococcal infection (designated as DGI-1 [Rice *et al.* 1986] and elsewhere as *ser*^{r} [Rice and Kasper 1982] or WG [Joiner *et al.* 1985a]) was used in these studies. Isolated outer membranes and derived molecules were prepared from this strain. These included lipooligosaccharides (LOS) (Gnehm *et al.* 1985; Rice *et al.* 1986), Proteins III (Lytton and Blake 1986) and Protein I (Blake and Gotschlich 1982) antigens.

IgG was prepared by anion exchange methods from normal human serum and shown to contain blocking activity. IgG was further purified (immunopurified) against Proteins III and I antigens (Rice *et al.* 1986). Immunopurified IgG was assessed for specificity in Western blotting experiments that employed the whole outer membrane as target antigen (Fig. 1). While whole IgG was seen to bind to a number of proteins in addition to major gonococcal Proteins III and I (also Proteins II [Swanson 1980], lane 3), immunopurified antibody against Protein III bound only to the Protein III antigen (lane 4). Antibody purified against Protein I, tested subsequently in the blocking experiments as a negative control, was shown to bind principally at the location of Protein I (36,200 MW, lane 5).

Specific antibody activity against the two isolated proteins, in addition to LOS antigens, were determined by quantitative ELISA (Table 1) (Rice *et al.* 1986). The specific activity of Protein III antibody was enhanced 47-fold in the Protein III eluent compared to the whole IgG preparation. The specific activity of Protein I antibody was enhanced 25-fold in the Protein I eluent. LOS antibody was not detected in either preparation by ELISA.

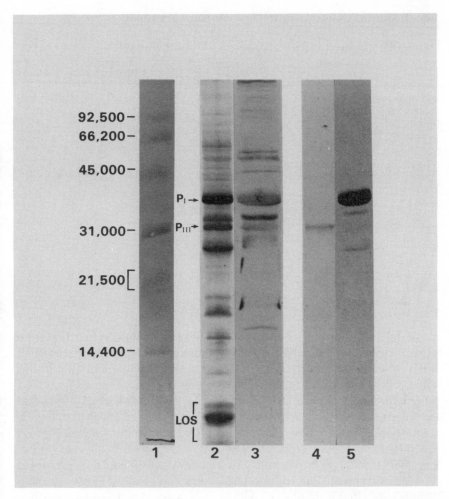

Figure 1. SDS–PAGE analysis of *N. gonorrhoeae* strain DGI-1 outer membranes and Western blots of whole IgG and purified IgG antibodies reacted with outer membrane antigens. Lane 1, standards; lane 2, SDS–PAGE of outer membranes of strain DGI-1; lane 3, human IgG reacted with outer membranes in Western blot; lane 4, human IgG immunopurified against Protein III (P_{III}) and reacted with outer membranes in Western blots; lane 5, human IgG immunopurified against Protein I (P_I) and reacted with outer membranes in Western blots. Reproduced with the permission of Rockefeller University Press (Rice *et al.* 1986).

Table 1 Specific Antibody Activity* in serum derived fractions

Preparation	Target Antigens†		
	Protein III	Protein I	LOS
IgG preparation	2.08 ± 0.06	3.01 ± 1.0	0.70 ± 0.04
Protein III eluent	98.0 ± 7.2	<0.06‡	<0.06‡
Protein I eluent	0.07 ± 0.01	75.1 ± 10.1	<0.06‡

* $\dfrac{\mu\text{g of measured antibody (IgG)}}{\mu\text{g IgG}} \times 10^{-4}$.

† Antigens used in ELISA were prepared from DGI-1.
‡ ODs (optical densities) were less than negative controls.

Blocking by specific IgG

Whole IgG and Protein III and Protein I antibodies immunopurified from IgG were tested for their ability to block complement-dependent bactericidal activity present in convalescent DGI serum. Bactericidal antibody in this serum is directed against LOS similarly to other serums obtained from DGI patients in convalescence (Rice and Kasper 1977; Hook *et al.* 1984) that sometimes express bactericidal activity against strains resistant to killing by normal human sera (Schoolnik *et al.* 1976; Rice and Kasper 1982; O'Brien *et al.* 1983). As previously reported (Rice and Kasper 1982; Joiner *et al.* 1985a; Rice *et al.* 1986), IgG blocks killing by human convalescent (DGI) serum of gonococci that resist killing by normal human serum (Fig. 2). Purified Protein III antibody effectively blocked killing in a dose-related fashion. Purified Protein I antibody displayed no blocking activity.

The requirement for Protein III antibody concentration necessary for blocking in whole IgG was compared to that needed in the purified Protein III antibody preparation. This comparison revealed that purified Protein III antibody maintained equivalent blocking activity at similar concentrations to Protein III antibody in whole IgG and indicates that blocking activity in whole IgG may be caused predominantly by the action of antibodies directed against Protein III (experiments not shown). Further evidence for this was shown by examining a second immune DGI serum (DGI-2) that had been chosen for study because it lacked killing activity at high concentration against the DGI-1 test strain. DGI-2 serum was depleted of Protein III antibody and tested in the bactericidal assay. Serum passed over the Protein III immunoabsorbent column was depleted of 96% of Protein III antibody while Protein I and LOS antibody concentrations were maintained. Bactericidal assays were

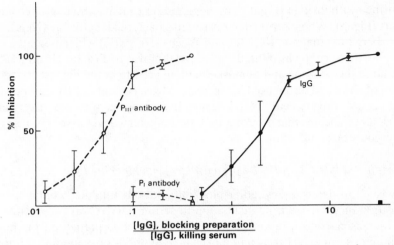

Figure 2. Inhibition of convalescent immune serum killing of *N. gonorrhoeae* strain DGI-1 by IgG isolated from normal human serum and by purified antibodies P_{III} and P_I. Percentage inhibition is expressed as a function of the ratio of IgG concentration in the blocker preparation to IgG concentration in the killing serum. □, P_{III} antibody heated to 65 °C; ■, IgG heated to 65 °C. For each point, $n = 2$ experiments; the bars indicate ± range. Reproduced with the permission of Rockefeller University Press (Rice *et al.* 1986).

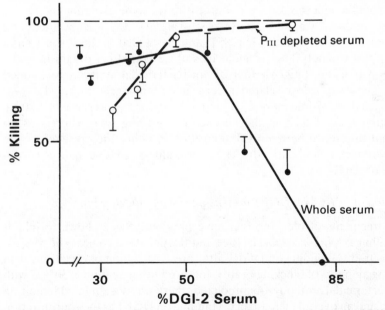

Figure 3. Killing action of DGI-2 serum and DGI-2 serum depleted of 96% of P_{III} antibody against *N. gonorrhoeae* strain DGI-1. Percentage killing is expressed as a function of percentage of serum in the bactericidal reaction mixture. For each point, $n = 2$ experiments; the bars indicate ± range. Reproduced with the permission of Rockefeller University Press (Rice *et al.* 1986).

performed with Protein III antibody-depleted sera and its whole serum counterpart (Fig. 3). Whole serum demonstrated a bactericidal prozone (Neisser–Wechsberg phenomenon (Neisser and Wechsberg 1901)) with emergence of killing as the serum was diluted. Selective removal of Protein III antibody eliminated the prozone and unmasked killing activity at the highest concentration of absorbed serum used in the assay. Measurement of PIII antibody in early versus convalescent DGI-2 serum had shown a five-fold rise. This experiment indicates that blocking PIII antibody may develop in response to active gonococcal infection.

Deposition of ^{125}I-C3 on DGI-1 presensitized with blocking IgG

We wished to determine whether blocking antibody inhibited complement deposition on DGI-1 during incubation in serum. DGI-1 was presensitized with increasing concentrations of purified blocking IgG prepared from normal human serum (NHS) by anion exchange methods or octonoic acid precipitation, then incubated in 30% complement (C) source in the presence or absence of convalescent DGI-1 serum that contained bactericidal antibody. A pool of normal human serum was used as a source of complement (C) activity. Before use, the serum was absorbed at $0\,°C$ with glutaraldehyde-fixed strain DGI-1 to remove specific antibody (absorbed pooled normal human serum (Abs PNHS, Joiner *et al.* 1983)). Serum from a patient with acquired hypogammaglobulinemia was used as a source of C for some experiments (IgG < $20\,mg/dl$; IgM < $5\,mg/dl$; and IgA < $4\,mg/dl$). C3 was purified and radiolabeled (Joiner *et al.* 1983, 1985a) and was added to the C source as a tracer. Approximately 1×10^5 molecules of C3 bound per organism in the absence of blocking IgG, whether or not bactericidal antibody was added (Fig. 4). There was a dose-related increase in C3 binding as blocking IgG was added, such that 2.5-fold more C3 bound to DGI-1 in the presence of $0.80\,mg$ of blocking IgG/ml than in the absence of blocking IgG. There was no significant difference between C3 deposition in either the presence or the absence of bactericidal antibody. Therefore, blocking IgG enhances C3 deposition on DGI-1 in C.

Deposition of ^{125}I-C3 on DGI-1 presensitized with blocking F(ab')$_2$

F(ab')$_2$ fragments of blocking IgG have previously been shown to inhibit serum killing of *N. gonorrhoeae* (Rice and Kasper 1982; Joiner *et al.* 1985a). We measured C3 binding on DGI-1 after presensitization of organisms with increasing amounts of blocking F(ab')$_2$ followed by incubation in 30% C with added bactericidal antibody. As predicted, there was dose-related inhibition of killing and an overall increase in C3 binding on DGI-1 as the concentration of blocking F(ab')$_2$ was increased to $0.96\,mg/ml$ (Fig. 5). Concentrations of blocking F(ab')$_2$ that were higher (>$0.12\,mg/ml$) than those of blocking IgG were required to increase C3 binding significantly in comparison to C3 binding on organisms not incubated with antibody. At low concentrations of

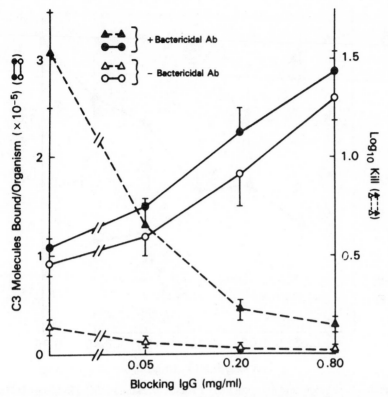

Figure 4. C3 binding and $\log_{10}$ kill of DGI-1 versus blocking IgG concentration. Binding of C3 and killing of DGI-1 were measured after presensitization with IgG blocking antibody, followed by incubation in Abs PNHS containing ^{125}I-C3. Results were compared in the presence and absence of added bactericidal antibody. Each point represents the mean ± SD for two experiments. C3 binding at blocking IgG inputs of 0.20 and 0.80 mg/ml was significantly greater than in the absence of added antibody. Reproduced with the permission of Rockefeller University Press (Joiner *et al.* 1985a).

blocking $F(ab')_2$ that were still capable of blocking (<0.12 mg/ml), no increase in C3 deposition was noted, suggesting that complement deposition mediated by blocking antibody may not be necessary for the observed inhibition of killing.

Binding of C9 to DGI-1 presensitized with blocking IgG

A dissociation between binding of C3 and binding of the bactericidal C5b–9 complex to the bacterial surface has been reported previously for serum-

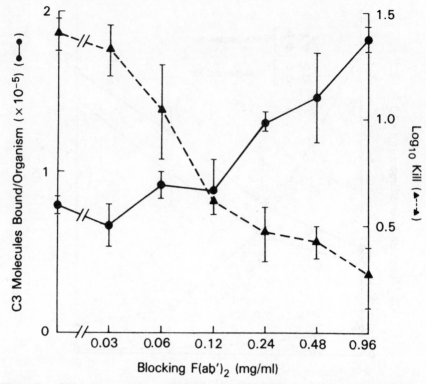

Figure 5. C3 binding and $\log_{10}$ kill DGI-1 versus blocking $F(ab')_2$. Binding of C3 and killing of DGI-1 were measured after presensitization with $F(ab')_2$ blocking antibody followed by incubation in Abs PNHS containing ^{125}I-C3 and added bactericidal antibody. Results shown are the mean ± SD for two experiments. C3 binding was significantly higher at blocking $F(ab')_2$ inputs of $0.24\,\mathrm{mg\,ml^{-1}}$ or greater when compared with organisms not presensitized with blocking $F(ab')_2$. Reproduced with the permission of Rockefeller University Press (Joiner *et al.* 1985a).

resistant strains of *Salmonella* and *E. coli* (Joiner *et al.* 1982). To address this issue for DGI-1 incubated in serum, we first measured deposition of radiolabeled C9 (Joiner *et al.* 1983, 1985b) onto DGI-1 during incubation in 30% C with added bactericidal antibody. C9 was purified and radiolabeled (Joiner *et al.* 1983, 1985a) and was added to the C source as a tracer. C9 binding on DGI-1 increased significantly after presensitization with 0.40 or 1.60 mg of blocking IgG, and killing was blocked substantially at both inputs of blocking IgG (Table 2). This experiment indicates that blocking IgG enhances deposition of the terminal complement complex C5b–9 on DGI-1 and shows that blocking IgG does not function by selective inhibition of either the C5 convertase or at a later step in C5b–9 formation; rather blocking IgG leads to deposition of C5b–9, which is in a nonbactericidal configuration.

Table 2 C9 binding and Log_{10} kill on DGI-1 presensitized with blocking IgG

Blocking IgG (mg/ml)	$10^{-4} \times$ Molecules C9/organism	Log_{10} kill
0.00	4.62 ± 1.15*	1.52 ± 27*
0.40	6.27 ± 0.96	0.19 ± 0.09
1.60	7.63 ± 0.74†	0.14 ± 0.01

Strain DGI-1 was presensitized with dilutions of purified blocking IgG or buffer for 15 min at room temperature, then incubated for 60 min in 30% complement (Abs PNHS) containing ^{125}I-C9 and bactericidal IgG.
* Mean ± sd for three experiments.
† $p<0.05$ in comparison to 0.00 mg/ml blocking IgG.

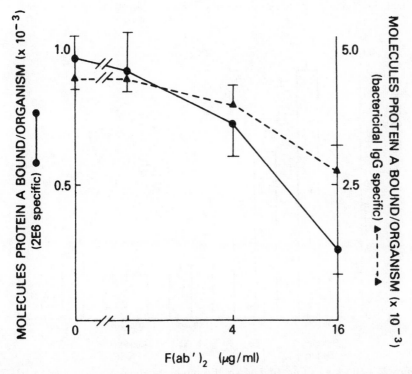

Figure 6. Blocking F(ab′)$_2$ inhibits binding of bactericidal IgG and MAb 2E6. DGI-1 was sensitized with increasing amounts of blocking F(ab′)$_2$, then incubated with bactericidal antibody or MAb 2E6. The organisms were washed, ^{125}I-protein A was added, and the molecules of protein A bound were determined. The assay was based on the fact that F(ab′)$_2$ fragments will not bind ^{125}I-protein A with high affinity, whereas bactericidal IgG and MAb 2E6 bind ^{125}I-protein A avidly. Results represent the mean ± sd for three experiments. Reproduced with the permission of Rockefeller University Press (Joiner *et al.* 1985a).

Competition binding studies with blocking and bactericidal antibody

We next investigated whether presensitization of DGI-1 with blocking antibody could interfere with subsequent binding of bactericidal antibody. Two approaches were used. First, uptake of radiolabeled protein A was determined on DGI-1 that was presensitized with increasing concentrations of purified $F(ab')_2$ blocking antibody, then with a fixed amount of convalescent DGI serum that contained bactericidal IgG. Protein A (Sigma Chemical Co., St Louis, MO) was radiolabeled with ^{125}I (Joiner *et al.* 1985a). $F(ab')_2$ fragments will not bind ^{125}I-protein A with high affinity, whereas intact IgG binds ^{125}I-protein A avidly. A dose-related inhibition of ^{125}I-protein A binding was observed as the concentration of $F(ab')_2$ blocking antibody was increased (Fig. 6), which suggests that $F(ab')_2$-inhibited binding of bactericidal IgG present in DGI-1 convalescent serum. The capacity of $F(ab')_2$ blocking antibody to inhibit the binding of the Protein III monoclonal antibody (MAb) 2E6 to DGI-1 was also tested. Nearly 75% inhibition of 2E6 binding, also

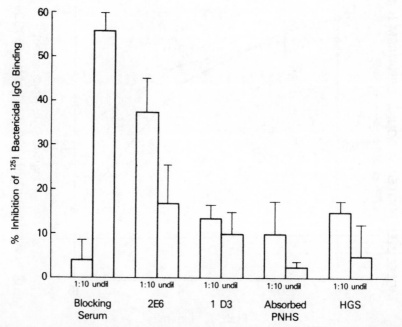

Figure 7. Blocking serum and MAb 2E6 inhibit binding of ^{125}I bactericidal IgG. strain DGI-1 was sensitized with either blocking serum, MAb 2E6, MAb 1D3 (which does not bind to DGI-1), or with each of two sources of antibody free serum, heated to 56 °C × 30 min (Δ56) to inactivate C (Δ56, Absorbed [Abs], PNHS and Δ56 hypogammaglobulinemic [HGS] serum). Binding of ^{125}I-bactericidal IgG was then measured. Results are expressed as the percentage inhibition of specific ^{125}I-labelled bactericidal IgG uptake compared to binding on DGI-1 sensitized in buffer alone. Results shown are the mean ± SD for three experiments. Reproduced with the permission of Rockefeller University Press (Joiner *et al.* 1985a).

shown in Fig. 6, occurred at a concentration of $F(ab')_2$ blocking antibody of only 16 μg/ml. This efficient inhibition suggests that $F(ab')_2$ blocking antibody, like whole IgG, is directed, at least in part, against Protein III.

Next, the capacity of blocking serum and other antibody sources to inhibit binding of ^{125}I-labeled bactericidal IgG to DGI-1 was measured (Fig. 7). Both blocking serum and Protein III specific MAb 2E6 significantly inhibited binding of ^{125}I-labeled bactericidal IgG to DGI-1, in comparison to C sources or MAb ID3 (Protein I-A specific), none of which contains specific antibodies for strain DGI-1. Therefore, by two separate techniques, we have shown that blocking antibody inhibited binding to DGI-1 of IgG present in DGI-1 convalescent serum.

Determination of C3 binding to biotinylated blocking IgG during serum incubation

We considered the possibility that the blocking IgG for *N. gonorrhoeae* did not serve as an acceptor for C3 deposition during complement activation. DGI-1 presensitized with biotinylated blocking IgG (Joiner *et al.* 1985a) was incubated in serum that contained ^{125}I-C3, and the percentage of C3 covalently attached to biotinyl IgG was determined by affinity purification of the SDS-solubilized organisms on avidin agarose (Table 3). Between 18.9 and 24.4% of the total available C3 that attached to DGI-1 was bound to biotinyl blocking IgG, in comparison to ~1% binding in controls. C3 binding to blocking IgG was not significantly altered by bactericidal antibody, although in separate experiments (not shown) we have found that bactericidal IgG for DGI-1 serves as an acceptor for C3 deposition. These results indicate that the blocking IgG on *N. gonorrhoeae* serves as an acceptor for C3 deposition and that antibody molecules that bind C3 during complement activation are not necessarily bactericidal.

Table 3 Binding of C3 to biotinylated blocking IgG on DGI-1

Antibody	Serum	Percent of ^{125}I-C3 on DGI-1 that bound to avidin agarose
Biotinyl blocking IgG	20%C (Abs PNHS) + bactericidal antibody	18.9 ± 3.6
Biotinyl blocking IgG	20%C (Abs PNHS)	24.4 ± 4.7
Biotinyl blocking IgG	20%Δ56C (Abs PNHS)	0.8 ± 0.4
None	20%C (Abs PNHS)	1.2 ± 0.3

DGI-1 was presensitized with biotinyl blocking IgG. Biotinyl blocking antibody was used at a final concentration of 0.72 mg/ml, and the final concentration for bactericidal antibody used in the first reaction mixture was 0.20 mg/ml. Opsonized DGI-1 was incubated in 20%C (Abs PNHS) containing ^{125}I-C3, solubilized in 1% SDS, and applied to avidin agarose; the percentage of ^{125}I-C3 bound was then determined. Results shown are the mean ± SD for two experiments.
C = complement.

Determination of C3 acceptor site on DGI-1

We examined the possibility that the site of C3 deposition (C3 acceptor) on DGI-1 differed, depending on whether blocking IgG was present or absent. Surface-iodinated DGI-1 (Joiner *et al.* 1983) were presensitized with blocking IgG or bactericidal antibody, incubated in serum, and the ^{125}I gonococcal constituents bearing C3 were affinity-purified on anti-C3 Sepharose (Joiner *et al.* 1985a) (Table 4). Significantly more ^{125}I-labeled gonococcal constituents

Table 4 Binding of ^{125}I-labelled *N. gonorrhoea* (DGI-1) constituents to anti-C3 Sepharose

Antibody	Serum	Percent of total ^{125}I-DGI-1 that bound to anti-C3 Sepharose
None	20%C# (Abs PNHS)	6.60 ± 1.41*
Bactericidal antibody	20%C (Abs PNHS)	5.27 ± 0.65†
Blocking IgG	20%Δ56C (Abs PNHS)	4.57 ± 1.00†
None	20%C (Abs PNHS)	2.02 ± 0.84

Surface-iodinated *N. gonorrhoeae* (DGI-1) was presensitized with the indicated antibody source, then incubated in Abs PNHS. ^{125}I-DGI-1 was solubilized in 1% SDS; the sample was diluted to achieve a final SDS concentration of 0.04% and then applied to anti-C3 Sepharose. The percentage of total available ^{125}I-DGI-1 that bound to anti-C3 Sepharose was determined. Results shown are means ± SD for two experiments.
complement.
* $p < 0.02$ compared with organisms incubated in 20% Δ56C (Abs PNHS).
† $p < 0.05$ compared with organisms incubated in 20% Δ56C (Abs PNHS).

bound to anti-C3 Sepharose for samples incubated in 20% Abs PNHS as a source of C than for the control sample incubated in 20% PNHS heated to 56°C × 30 min (Δ56) to inactivate C.

^{125}I-DGI-1 constituents linked to C3 by an ester bond were released with hydroxylamine (>87% release) and analyzed by 10% SDS–PAGE (Joiner *et al.* 1985a). The only major difference between experimental and control samples, as determined by densitometric scanning, was the presence of a prominent 40,000-MW band in the organisms presensitized with blocking IgG (experiments not shown). This band was six- to nine-fold more intense in this sample compared to controls and was barely discernible in native ^{125}I-DGI-1. These results indicate that blocking antibody changes the C3 acceptor on DGI-1.

Discussion

We have shown in these studies that blocking IgG with specificity for a common gonococcal surface protein, Protein III, contributes a major portion of blocking activity in normal and immune serums. Blocking IgG competes for binding sites on gonococcal surfaces with bactericidal antibody, and results in effective prevention of complement (C) dependent killing (Joiner *et al.* 1985a). This provides a partial explanation of why certain strains of *N. gonorrhoeae* are resistant to killing by normal human serum. Immune and normal bactericidal antibodies against both serum-resistant and serum-sensitive strains of *N. gonorrhoeae*, respectively, are directed mainly against LOS antigens (Glynn and Ward 1970; Rice and Kasper 1977). Normal and convalescent serum may contain antibodies that recognize Protein I; these antibodies may also be bactericidal (Hook *et al.* 1984), particularly when they are tested in the absence of blocking antibodies (unpublished observations). The intimate relationship of Proteins III and I (McDade and Johnston 1980; Swanson 1981; Swanson *et al.* 1982), which in turn appears to be tightly bound to LOS (Hitchcock 1984), indicates that binding sites for bactericidal and blocking antibodies are in close proximity. Based on estimates of the density distribution of LOS and Protein I molecules on the surface of gonococci and their relationship to Protein III, antibody binding to Protein III might be expected to obscure certain binding sites present on either LOS or Protein I.

We have also shown here that blocking IgG and $F(ab')_2$ enhance complement deposition on a strain of *N. gonorrhoeae* that resists killing by normal but not by convalescent DGI serum. This resulted in the inhibition of killing by convalescent serum. Complement deposition is increased through C9, as shown by binding of C9 to the bacterial surface. As demonstrated, blocking IgG and $F(ab')_2$ are at least in part directed against an antigenically conserved gonococcal outer membrane protein, Protein III (Swanson *et al.* 1982). These blocking antibodies or fragments compete with binding of bactericidal IgG to the strain. These results suggest that the mechanism of action of blocking antibody is to replace binding of bactericidal IgG with an antibody that leads to deposition of nonbactericidal C5b–9.

Extensive serologic testing for the presence of Protein III antibodies in normal human sera have not been performed; however, many sera that have been tested contain IgG antibodies against this antigenically conserved surface protein (Lammel *et al.* 1985; Rice P A, unpublished observations). In addition, the observation that the development of bactericidal activity in patients convalescing from disseminated gonococcal infection (DGI) is often nonexistent or meager (O'Brien *et al.* 1983), despite high-titered antibody rises measured by indirect immunofluorescence (Hess *et al.* 1965) or ELISA (Rice P A, unpublished data), suggests that blocking antibodies may result from specific antigenic challenge. We have shown in these studies that selective Protein III antibody depletion from DGI convalescent serum with unexpressed bactericidal activity, restores killing activity to the serum.

Evidence of the specificity of binding of blocking antibody is also provided by these and earlier studies that have demonstrated equivalent blocking activity by $F(ab')_2$ fragments pepared from normal IgG (Rice and Kasper 1982; Joiner *et al.* 1985a). We have also found that low concentrations of

$F(ab')_2$ blocking antibody effectively inhibited the binding of the Protein III specific monoclonal antibody 2E6 to DGI-1, the strain used in these studies (Joiner *et al.* 1985a). In a study that used a different serum-resistant strain, FA171, normal human serum (NHS) was also shown to inhibit binding of MAb 2E6 (Sarafian *et al.* 1983). In those studies, most of the inhibition of MAb 2E6 binding was removed by absorption of NHS with purified Protein I, which suggests that steric hindrance to nearby antibody combining sites also played a critical role in those competition binding studies. Using a third serum-resistant strain, R11 (Joiner *et al.* 1985b), it has also been demonstrated that MAb 2E6 can inhibit binding of a Protein I MAb to yet another gonococcal surface.

The capacity of serum-resistant strains of *N. gonorrhoeae* to activate the alternative pathway in the absence of serum killing has been shown previously (Densen *et al.* 1982). $F(ab')_2$ fragments cannot activate complement via the classical pathway, but are capable of initiating or facilitating alternative pathway activation in many systems (Ratnoff *et al.* 1983). It is possible, therefore, that blocking antibody mediated alternative pathway activation by serum-resistant gonococci (Densen *et al.* 1982) although in our experiments low concentrations of $F(ab')_2$ blocked killing, but did not fix C3 (Fig. 5).

The mechanisms of action of the blocking antibody for *N. gonorrhoeae* has not previously been known. In addition to displacing bactericidal antibody from gonococcal surfaces, it has been speculated that like blocking antibodies for *N. meningitidis* (Griffiss *et al.* 1975; Griffiss and Bertram 1977) and *B. abortus* (Hall *et al.* 1971), which are of the IgA isotype and therefore unable to activate complement effectively, blocking IgG for *N. gonorrhoeae* and for other Gram-negative organisms (Waisbren and Brown 1966; Taylor 1972; Guttman and Waisbren 1975) may be predominantly those isotypes of IgG that activate C poorly. Blocking IgG, used in our studies, contained exclusively C-fixing subclasses (IgG4 was excluded). We have also shown that organisms opsonized with blocking IgG increase consumption and deposition of the third (C3) and ninth (C9) components of complement. In earlier studies we have also demonstrated increased consumption of C3 and C9 by opsonized organisms (Joiner *et al.* 1985).

Blocking IgG alters the site of C3 deposition on *N. gonorrhoeae*, both by serving as an acceptor for C3 deposition and by redirecting C3 deposition to different bacterial constituents. The percentage of ^{125}I-*N. gonorrhoeae* constituents that were affinity-purified on anti-C3 Sepharose was lower in the presence than in the absence of blocking IgG (Table 4); this is due in part to the fact that a substantial fraction of C3 deposited by blocking IgG redirects C3 to nonlabeled constituents, such as lipooligosaccharide, or that multiple C3 molecules are deposited on individual gonococcal constituents. These experiments do not exclude the possibility that the redistribution of C3 initiated by blocking IgG may be a passive phenomenon dictated by a masking of certain C3 acceptor sites by the blocking IgG molecule. This possibility is supported by the observation that C3 deposition is directed to a 40,000-MW constituent on *N. gonorrhoeae* presensitized with blocking IgG; yet the blocking antibody itself recognizes predominantly Protein III and does not recognize the 40,000-MW molecule by immunoprecipitation (experiments not shown).

Although our studies have shown that human sera contain Protein III specific antibodies that are predominantly responsible for blocking activity, nonetheless it is possible that the nature of the antibody itself or the location of the epitope on the organism recognized by the antibody, in addition to the antigenic specificity, may dictate whether killing or blocking will supervene. Such an assumption is based on several observations: (a) different ratios of Protein III blocking antibody to bactericidal antibody are required in individual sera to achieve constant blocking (Rice P A, unpublished observations); (b) different MAbs, all directed at a single Protein I, can vary in bactericidal activity for *N. gonorrhoeae*, and, indeed, nonkilling MAbs against Protein I can effectively block killing antibodies that recognize different epitopes on this protein (Joiner *et al.* 1985b); (c) IgA blocking antibody, which is specific for LOS, can sometimes block IgG anti-LOS killing of serum-resistant gonococci (Apicella *et al.* 1986); (d) Protein III MAb 2E6 is bactericidal for some strains of *N. gonorrhoeae* at high concentrations (Joiner K A and Swanson J, unpublished observations; Rice P A, unpublished observations). In humans, however, Protein III antibody competes for binding with bactericidal antibody, leads to deposition of nonbactericidal C5b–9, and can prevent killing of gonococci by bactericidal antibody.

Acknowledgements

This research was supported in part by grants AI 15633, AI 10615 and AI 18637 from the National Institutes of Health. Dr Blake is the recipient of the Irma T. Hirschl Award.

References

Apicella M A, Westerink M A J, Morse S A, Schneider H, Rice P A, Griffiss J McL 1986. Bactericidal antibody response of normal human serum to the lipooligosaccharide of *Neisseria gonorrhoeae*, *Journal of Infectious Diseases* **153**: 520–6

Blake M S, Gotschlich E C 1982. Purification and partial characterization of the major outer membrane protein of *Neisseria gonorrhoeae*, *Infection and Immunity* **36**: 277–83

Densen P, MacKeen L A, Clark R A 1982. Dissemination of gonococcal infection is associated with delayed stimulation of complement-dependent neutrophil chemotaxis *in vitro*, *Infection and Immunity* **38**: 563–72

Glynn A A, Ward M E 1970. Nature and heterogeneity of the antigens of *N. gonorrhoeae* involved in the serum bactericidal reaction, *Infection and Immunity* **2**: 162–8

Gnehm H E, Pelton S I, Gulati S, Rice P A 1985. Characterization of antigens from nontypable

Haemophilus influenzae recognized by human bactericidal antibodies, *Journal of Clinical Investigations* **75**: 1645–58

Griffiss J McL, Bertram M A 1977. Immunoepidemiology of meningococcal disease in military recruits. II. Blocking of serum bactericidal activity by circulating IgA early in the course of invasive disease, *Journal of Infectious Diseases* **36**: 733–9

Griffiss J McL, Broud D D, Bertram M A 1975. Bactericidal activity of meningococcal antisera blocking by IgA of lytic antibody in human convalescent sera, *Journal of Immunology* **14**: 1779–84

Guttman R M, Waisbren B A 1975. Bacterial blocking activity of specific IgG in chronic *Pseudomonas aeruginosa* infection, *Clinical and Experimental Immunology* **19**: 121–30

Hall W H, Manion R E, Zinneman H H 1971. Blocking of serum lysis of *Brucella abortus* by hyperimmune rabbit immunoglobulin A, *Journal of Immunology* **107**: 41–6

Hess E V, Hunter D K, Ziff M 1965. Gonococcal antibodies in acute arthritis, *Journal of the American Medical Association* **191**: 531–4

Hitchcock P J 1984. Analyses of gonococcal lipopolysaccharide in whole-cell lysates by sodium dodecylsulfate–polyacrylamide gel electrophoresis: stable association of lipopolysaccharide with the major outer membrane protein (Protein I) of *Neisseria gonorrhoeae*, *Infection and Immunity* **46**: 202–12

Hook E W III, Olsen D A, Buchanan T M 1984. Analysis of the antigen specificity of the human serum immunoglobulin G immune response to complicated gonococcal infection, *Infection and Immunity* **43**: 706–9

Joiner K A, Hammer C H, Brown E J, Cole R J, Frank M M 1982. Studies on the mechanism of bacterial resistance to complement-mediated killing. I. Terminal complement components are deposited and released from *Salmonella minnesota* S218 without causing bacterial death, *Journal of Experimental Medicine* **55**: 797–808

Joiner K A, Warren K A, Brown E J, Swanson J, Frank M M 1983. Studies on the mechanism of bacterial resistance to complement-mediated killing IV. C5b–9 forms high molecular weight complexes with bacterial outer membrane constituents on serum-resistant but not on serum-sensitive *Neisseria gonorrhoeae*, *Journal of Immunology* **131**: 1443–51

Joiner K A, Warren K A, Tam M, Frank M M 1985b. Monoclonal antibodies directed against protein I vary in bactericidal activity, *Journal of Immunology* **134**: 3411–19

Joiner K A, Scales R, Warren K A, Frank M M, Rice P A 1985a. Mechanism of action of blocking immunoglobulin G for *Neisseria gonorrhoeae*, *Journal of Clinical Investigations* **76**: 1765–72

Judd R C 1982a. ^{125}I-Peptide mapping of protein III isolated from four strains of *Neisseria gonorrhoeae*, *Infection and Immunity* **37**: 622–31

Judd R C 1982b. Surface peptide mapping of protein I and protein III of four strains of *Neisseria gonorrhoeae*, *Infection and Immunity* **37**: 632–41

Knapp J S, Tam M R, Nowinsky R C, Holmes K K, Sandstrom E G 1984. Serologic classification of *Neisseria gonorrhoeae* with use of monoclonal antibodies to gonococcal outer membrane protein I, *Journal of Infectious Diseases* **150**: 44–8

Lammel C J, Sweet R L, Rice P A, Knapp J S, Schoolnik G K, Heilbrun D C 1985. Antibody–antigen specificity in the immune response to infection with *Neisseria gonorrhoeae*, *Journal of Infectious Diseases* **152**: 990–1001

Lytton E J, Blake M S 1986. Isolation and partial characterization of the reduction-modifiable proteins of *Neisseria gonorrhoeae*, *Journal of Experimental Medicine* **164**: 1749–59

McCutchan J A, Katzenstein D, Norquist D, Chikami G, Wunderlich A, Braude A I 1978. Role of blocking antibody in disseminated gonococcal infection, *Journal of Immunology* **121**: 1884–8

McDade R I, Johnston K H 1980. Characterization of serologically dominant outer membrane proteins of *Neisseria gonorrhoeae*, *Journal of Bacteriology* **141**: 1183–91

Neisser M, Wechsberg F 1901. Ueber die wirkungsart bactericider sera, *Munchener Medicinische Wochenschrift* **18**: 697–700

O'Brien J P, Goldenberg D L, Rice P A 1983. Disseminated gonococcal infection: a prospective analysis of 49 patients and a review of pathophysiology and immune mechanisms, *Medicine* **62**: 395–406

Ratnoff W P, Fearon D T, Austen K F 1983. The role of antibody in the activation of the alternative complement pathway, *Springer Seminars in Immunopathology* **6**: 361–72

Rice P A, Kasper D L 1977. Characterization of gonococcal antigens responsible for induction of bactericidal antibody in disseminated infection: the role of gonococcal endotoxins, *Journal of Clinical Investigations* **60**: 1149–58

Rice P A, Kasper D L 1982. Characterization of serum resistance of *Neisseria gonorrhoeae* that disseminate, *Journal of Clinical Investigations* **70**: 157–67

Rice P A, Vayo H E, Tam M R, Blake M S 1986. Immunoglobulin G antibodies directed against PIII block killing of serum-resistant *Neisseria gonorrhoeae* by immune serum, *Journal of Experimental Medicine* **164**: 1735–48

Sarafian S K, Tam M R, Morse S A 1983. Gonococcal protein I-specific opsonic IgG in normal human serum, *Journal of Infectious Diseases* **148**: 1025–32

Schoolnik G K, Buchanan T M, Holmes K K 1976. Gonococci causing disseminated gonococcal infections are resistant to the bactericidal action of normal human sera, *Journal of Clinical Investigations* **58**: 1163–73

Swanson J 1980. ^{125}I-labeled peptide mapping of some heat-modifiable proteins of the gonococcal outer membrane, *Infection and Immunity* **28**: 54–64

Swanson J 1981. Surface-exposed protein antigens of the gonococcal outer membrane, *Infection and Immunity* **34**: 804–16

Swanson J, Mayer L W, Tam M R 1982. Antigenicity of *Neisseria gonorrhoeae* outer membrane proteins III detected by immunoprecipitation and Western blot transfer with a monoclonal antibody, *Infection and Immunity* **38**: 668–72

Taylor P W 1972. An antibactericidal factor in the serum of two patients with infection of the upper respiratory tract, *Clinical Science (London)* **43**: 23–7

Thomas L, Dingle J H 1943. Investigations of meningococcal infection. III. The bactericidal action of normal and immune sera for the meningococcus, *Journal of Clinical Investigations* **22**: 375–85

Waisbren B A, Brown I 1966. A factor in the serum of patients with persisting infection that inhibits the bactericidal activity of normal serum against the organism that is causing the infection, *Journal of Immunology* **97**: 431–7

A survey of vaccine strategies and T cell response to vaccination

N A Mitchison

Imperial Cancer Research Fund, Tumour Immunology Unit, Department of Zoology, University College London, Gower Street, London WC1E 6BT, United Kingdom

How close are we to major advances in vaccine development? The three great challenges to our age are tropical disease, viral cancer and birth control, and each is likely to be met only by the development of second-generation vaccines. Our decade has seen a resurgence of interest in vaccine development, based on the possibilities created by advances in biotechnology, and supported by a growing commitment from the First to the Third World evident in such new enterprises as the Special Programmes of the World Health Organization (WHO) in Tropical Disease Research (TDR) and in Human Reproduction (HRP), the effort of the United Kingdom Cancer Research Campaign to develop an Epstein–Barr Virus (EBV) vaccine, and similar initiatives launched by other agencies. I have been associated with each of these three enterprises, and for further reading particularly recommend the annual reports of the two WHO Special Programmes (World Health Organization, 1985a, 1985b).

Tropical disease

The Special Programme identifies six major diseases, in order of importance: malaria, schistosomiasis, filariasis, trypanosomiasis, leprosy and leishmaniasis. Vaccines for all of these diseases are under development, each offering particular opportunities and problems.

In leprosy the breakthrough came when Tore Godal determined that the disease organism *Mycobacterium leprae* grown in armadillos should be used to provide a first-generation (i.e. whole-organism-based) vaccine. This vaccine, in the form of killed whole organisms extracted from the animal's organs, has passed its Phase I trial in Norway, and is about to enter field trials in Malawi and South India. These trials aim to answer the important question of whether protection against leprosy can be obtained by vaccination. This will be a long and difficult task, mainly because most people recover from infection naturally without developing overt symptoms. The longer-term objective of disease control by vaccination is further off, and can hardly be achieved by an armadillo-based vaccine. For this reason great efforts are being made worldwide to develop a second-generation vaccine, based on antigens manu-factured by biotechnology. The cloning into an expression vector, bacter-iophage lambda gt11, of DNA from *M. leprae* by Richard Young and Barrie Bloom (Young *et al.* 1985) represented an important step forward. We and others, as outlined below, are now trying to develop this library into a usable vaccine.

Next in stage of development come the malaria vaccines. Independent vaccines are being developed against the sporozoite, merozoite and gameto-cyte stages of *Plasmodium falciparium*, the principle killer form of malaria. (One might argue that high priority should also be given to *P. vivax*, which, if it kills less, probably troubles more.) Here the breakthrough was the discov-ery by Ruth and Victor Nussenzweig (Cochrane *et al.* 1982) that the malarial sporozoite has a surprisingly simple coat, made of a single circumsporozoite protein. Later it was found that this and many other parasite proteins have an unusually simple structure, consisting of repeating oligopeptides. Alas, as discussed below, what seems at first sight to offer an opportunity to build an astonishingly simple vaccine may turn out to be a trap laid by the parasite for the immune system of the host.

The United States army is preparing extensive field trials of a sporozoite vaccine based on a recombinant circumsporozoite fusion protein. A vaccine of this sort may well prove useful for military personnel or tourists entering an endemic area for a brief period. But for local inhabitants, apart perhaps from nomads or migrants passing in and out, it could well be dangerous to grow up devoid of the usual partial immunity to the main blood forms of the parasite. These are structurally more complex, and the best antigens for vaccine development have yet to be selected. In spite of considerable effort, we still have a great deal to learn about immunity to merozoites: do antibodies block transmission between erythrocytes *in vivo*, or do macrophages kill the para-sites in passing erythrocytes? Less effort has been devoted to gametocytes, and yet this interesting and altruistic form of vaccination may have much to offer in the long run.

Vaccines against leishmaniasis are of special interest from a theoretical standpoint because mouse experiments indicate that immunization can per-turb the delicate balance between T lymphocyte subsets in unexpected ways (Liew *et al.* 1985; Milton *et al.* 1986). Caution is needed therefore in human trials, and it is agreed that vaccination against visceral leishmaniasis (far the most dangerous form of the disease) remains a distant goal. But in the Old-World cutaneous form of the disease, caused by *Leishmania major*, an unusual opportunity is presented by certain high-risk populations which currently undergo 'leishmanization', that is to say, protective inoculation with live parasites. Here it would be possible, and I believe acceptable, to exam-ine the effect of a first-generation, killed-organism-based vaccine on the subsequent reaction to leishmanization. One thing clear about this work is that it provides a perfect example of how it takes a parasite to bring out the full flavour of the immune system.

Anti-cancer virus vaccines

As an example of the important group of anti-cancer virus vaccines which includes hepatitis and papiloma viruses, let us take Epstein–Barr Virus. In the United Kingdom the Cancer Research Campaign has supported strong efforts to develop a vaccine made by the groups of Epstein in Bristol (Epstein 1984) and by Arrand and Mackett in Manchester (Arrand and Mackett 1984). A virion 340 kD glycoprotein able to generate a protective antibody response has been identified as a candidate vaccine molecule, and recombinant vaccine constructs prepared and tested in animals. But many questions remain. Some of these are common to most viral vaccines: will an antibody approach be sufficient, or must LYDMA (lymphocyte defined membrane antigens) epitopes also be included? If a T cell response proves necessary, what is the magic in live-virus immunization, and can it be duplicated with biotechnology-produced antigens? Others are unique to cancer viruses: is it acceptable to immunize people, knowing that only poorly understood variations in the immune response determine whether the outcome of viral infection is oncogenic or not?

One thing is clear to me. It may take a long time to control, say, nasopharyngeal cancer, but the sooner very small trials can be started in fully informed volunteers, the sooner we shall know whether it is possible to vaccinate against the virus in man. Note, in passing, that exactly the same consideration applies to vaccination against human immunosuppressive (AIDS) virus: the regulations which delay the onset of such trials have much to answer for.

Birth-control vaccines

In February 1986 in South Australia, WHO–HRP started the first trial of a synthetic birth-control vaccine. This vaccine was conceived and largely developed by Vernon Stevens in Ohio (reviewed in World Health Organization 1985b; Mitchison 1984), and is an anti-hormone vaccine composed of C-terminal peptides(CTP) of the β chain of chorionic gonadotrophin coupled to a protein carrier. Any birth-control vaccine has vast potential benefits in terms of long duration, ease of administration, lack of side-effects and low cost; and a peptide vaccine has the merit of minimizing the danger of generating an anamnastic response and thereby producing irreversible sterility. Other somewhat similar anti-hormone vaccines are also entering trials this year (1986), particularly those developed by the Population Council and by the Institute of Immunology at Delhi. So within a year or two we should know whether this approach is likely to work. What will take longer is finding out whether these vaccines live up to the high hopes entertained of them.

Because the CTP vaccine is only marginally effective, and this kind of weak isoimmunization evidently needs all the help that it can get, it may be necessary to include other supplementary peptides. Choosing peptides rationally should be easier now that S Cooper and T Blundell (Birbeck College London, personal communication) have formulated a three-dimensional structure for Beta chorionic gonadotrophin (βCG). In particular they have been able to list six candidate loop peptides in order of decreasing homology to the β chains of the structurally related pituitary hormones. Meanwhile a homologous immunization model within a suitable primate is badly needed, but at the moment baboon studies have run into trouble.

If the anti-hormone vaccines look at all encouraging, they should provide a strong incentive for developing other birth-control vaccines. Sperm, zona and trophoblast are all reasonable candidates (Ada *et al.* 1986). Developing a sperm vaccine ought to involve antibodies, recombinant DNA technology and the developmental biology of a highly specialized cell used together in a coordinated effort.

Screening an expression library for T epitopes

In the wake of successes achieved by scanning recombinant DNA libraries with antibodies, attempts are being made to do likewise with T cells. Where cytotoxic T cells constitute a conspicuous feature of the immune response, as is the case for tumor antigens, transplantation antigens such as H-Y, and many viruses, the usual approach seems to be via transfection of genomic DNA. One problem with this is that expression is variable and selection for high levels is not easy. It is tempting to use cloned T cells, but this involves a strong element of selection. With these problems in mind Dr P Salgame and I, in collaboration with Dr J Colston of the Medical Research Council Leprosy Research Unit, chose to scan the Young–Bloom DNA lambda gt11 library from *M. leprae* for antigens able to elicit a proliferative T cell response.

In this system the *M. leprae* antigens are expressed as fusion proteins in bacterial lysates. We partially purified them by extractions with the weak detergents deoxycholate and Triton-X, solubilized in SDS, dialyzed, and assayed at an optional concentration of 100 ng protein/ml. Alternatively, the SDS-solubilized antigen can be absorbed on to nitrocellulose disks and put directly into the assay. From these preparations signals adequate for screening purposes have been obtained from T cells isolated from lymph nodes of mice primed with whole killed *M. leprae*, and we are making progress in fractionating the library by this means.

The use of biotechnology to circumvent molecular evasion

Every textbook of parasitology has a list of the tactics employed by parasites to evade the immune response of the host: antigenic variation, cleavage of antibodies by parasite enzymes, coating with host glycolipids and so on. What is only beginning to emerge is that potential antigens can also select molecular structures that tend to minimize or render ineffective the immune response towards them. Figures 1, 2 and 3 illustrate some of the tactics that a parasite might use to protect a receptor which is vital for its survival – for instance the erythrocyte receptor on the surface of a malarial merozoite. In one the receptor is protected by distractor antigens which successfully compete for the attention of the host's immune system, possibly by competing for desotope sites on major histocompatibility complex (MHC) molecules (Fig. 1). In another the receptor is surrounded by a stockade of suppressor epitopes (Fig. 2). In the third the receptor protein cleaves preferentially at a site which splits an otherwise vulnerable epitope away from the agretope to which the host's MHC molecule binds (Fig. 3). We do not know to what extent these mechanisms are in fact used by parasites. All of them are documented in the literature of cellular immunology, and by and large parasites have been found to exploit any conceivable opportunity offered by chinks in the host's armour (for discussion of the first two tactics, see Mitchison 1984; and of the third see Manca *et al.* 1984). The repeating oligopeptides of the circumsporozoite protein may well have something to do either with Ts epitopes or competition

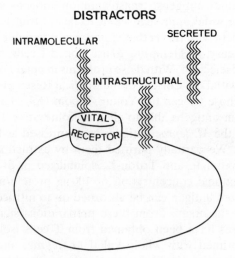

DISTRACTORS

Figure 1. A survival strategy.

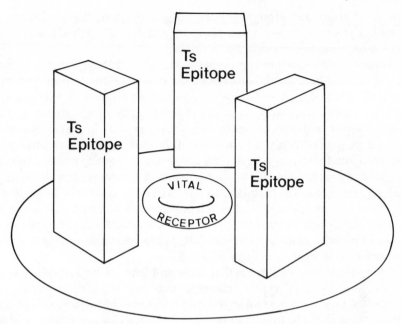

Figure 2. Another survival strategy.

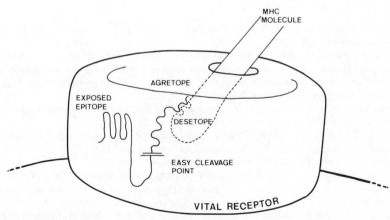

Figure 3. Yet another survival strategy.

from distractors; and strong, secreted antigens such as the S antigens of plasmodia (McGregor 1972) and those of hydatids (Lingelbach and Hinz 1984) must come under suspicion as distractors.

First-generation vaccines can perhaps skirt around these parasite tactics, but only second-generation ones can tackle them directly. In principle, one should be able to design and construct molecules with their Ts epitopes and distractors amputated, with agretopes placed in judicious proximity to key target epitopes, and with helper epitopes appropriately available. But how close are we to achieving this in practice? It is one thing to sort through easy model proteins for the appropriate bits and pieces, but quite another to do the same for the poorly defined, often insoluble, and sometimes heavily glycosylated macromolecules of parasites. In fact, we hardly know how to begin the task. Also the grave theoretical problem confronts us that many of the Ts epitopes, agretopes, etc, that have been identified thus far have turned out to behave quite differently in different MHC haplotypes; and indeed there are good reasons for expecting them to do so.

Perhaps the important thing is that these problems are beginning to attract the attention of very clever scientists who are pursuing a variety of approaches. Some concentrate on the empirical screening of large numbers of proteins, such as can be found in a parasite expression library. Others analyze in detail the epitopes of one or two proteins, or simply scan the presently available information about T-cell epitopes for common structural features. And yet others attempt to circumvent epitopes analysis by constructing mimetopes. In the long run all these streams should run into the same pool. Biotechnology may feed on optimism, but here at least some optimism is justified.

References

Ada G L, Basten A, Jones W R 1986. Prospects for developing vaccines to control fertility, *Nature (London)* **317**: 288–9

Arrand J R, Macket M 1984. In *Annual Report of the Paterson Laboratories*, Manchester, UK

Cochrane A H, Samboro F, Nussenzweig V, Gwadz R W, Nussenzweig R S 1982. Monoclonal antibodies identify the protective antigens of sporozoites of *Plasmodium knowlesi, Proceedings of the National Academy of Sciences USA* **79**: 5651–5

Epstein M A 1984. A prototype vaccine to prevent Epstein–Barr virus-associated tumours, *Proceedings of the Royal Society of London B* **221**: 1–20

Liew F Y, Howard J G 1985. Role of T cells in the unusual cutaneous responses to leishmania in Balb/c mice, *Current Topics in Microbiology and Immunology* **122**: 122–7

Lingelbach K, Hinz E 1984. *Echinococcus multiocularis* identification of proteins inducing antibody formation in metacestode infections, *Journal of Helminthology* **58**: 1–6

Manca F, Clarke J A, Miller A, Sercarz E, Shasti N 1984. A limited region within hen egg-white lysozyme serves as the focus for a diversity of T cell clones, *Journal of Immunology* **133**: 2075–8

McGregor I A 1972. Immunology of malaria infection and its possible consequences, *British Medical Bulletin* **28**: 22–7

Milon G, Titus R G, Cerottini J-C, Marchal G, Louis J A 1986. Higher frequency of Leishmania major-specific L3T4$^+$ T cells in susceptible Balb/c as compared with resistant CBA mice, *Journal of Immunology* **136**: 1467–71

Mitchison 1984. Strategies for optimal T-cell activation, in *New Approaches to Vaccine Development*, R Bell, G Torrigiani (eds) Proceedings of World Health Organization Meeting October 1983. Schwabe, Basel, pp 93–112

World Health Organization 1985a. *Tropical Disease Research (TDR)*. Seventh Programme Report 1 January 1983–31 December 1984. WHO, Geneva.

World Health Organization 1985b. *Special Programme of Research, Development and Research Training in Human Reproduction*. Fourteenth Annual Report. WHO, Geneva.

Young R A, Mehra V, Sweetser D, Buchanan T, Clark-Curtiss J, Davis R W, Bloom B R 1985. Genes for the major protein antigens of the leprosy parasite *Mycobacterium leprae*, *Nature (London)* **316**: 450–1

Recognition of cloned influenza virus gene products by cytotoxic T lymphocytes

Jonathan W Yewdell*; Jack R Bennink*; Geoffrey L Smith†; Bernard Moss‡

* *Wistar Institute, Philadelphia, Pennsylvania, USA*
† *University of Cambridge, Addenbrooke's Hospital, Cambridge, United Kingdom*
‡ *Laboratory for Viral Diseases, National Institute of Allergy and Infectious Diseases, National Institutes of Health, Bethesda, Maryland, USA*

Cytotoxic T lymphocytes (CTL) arise during the immune response to many viruses (Zinkernagel and Doherty 1979). *In vitro*, CTL recognize viral antigens on cells bearing self major histocompatibility complex (MHC) class I antigens and respond by lysing the infected cell and releasing gamma inteferon (Ennis 1982). Although the anti-viral function of CTL *in vivo* has been studied in only a few instances, it appears that they can play a critical role in limiting virus dissemination and eradicating established infections (Yap *et al.* 1978; Lin and Askonas 1981; Lukacher *et al.* 1984; Bennink *et al.* 1984a; Oldstone *et al.* 1986). Under certain circumstances, they can also cause severe immunopathology (Doherty and Zinkernagel 1975).

Understanding of the CTL response has been hindered by difficulties in determining the specificity of CTL for viral antigens. A number of strategies have been employed to determine which viral antigens serve as CTL target structures. The most straightforward (and recent) approach is to produce target cells expressing individual antigens in complete isolation from other viral components. This has been achieved mainly by genetic means (Braciale *et al.* 1984; Townsend *et al.* 1984; Yamada *et al.* 1985), although recently it has been demonstrated that chemically synthesized oligopeptides may play an important role in elucidating CTL recognition structures (Townsend *et al.* 1986). To study CTL recognition of viral antigens, we have used recombinant vaccinia (Vac) viruses containing cloned copies of viral genes derived from influenza A virus (an orthomyxovirus) or vesicular stomatitis virus (VSV) (a rhabdovirus).

CTL recognition of individual influenza A virus antigens

Influenza A viruses acquire their envelope by budding through the host cell plasma membrane. The virion contains eight segmented genes which are known to code for ten proteins (Lamb 1983). Two integral membrane gly-coproteins (the hemagglutinin (HA) and neuraminidase (NA)) are expressed in relatively large quantities on infected cell surfaces and form a dense layer of spikes on the virion surface. The matrix protein (M1) forms a sub-envelope shell encasing the ribonucleoprotein complex which is comprised of the RNA segments, nucleoprotein (NP), and small amounts of three viral polymerases (PA, PB2, PB1). During the infectious cycle three proteins are synthesized which appear to be completely excluded from virions. Non-structural 1 (NS1) and NS2 are located in the cytoplasm and nucleus of infected cells and are produced via alternative splicing from the same gene segment. M2 is an integral membrane protein produced via alternative splicing from the gene segment which encodes M1.

Initial studies found that anti-influenza CTL could be divided into two major categories, those specific for the immunizing strain and closely related strains ('strain-specific'), and those able to lyse cells infected with any human influenza A virus subtype ('cross-reactive') (Effros *et al.* 1977; Yap and Ada 1977; Zweerink *et al.* 1977a). (Human type A influenza viruses are grouped into three subtypes, designated H1N1, H2N2 and H3N2. H1, H2, and H3 and N1 and N2 each designate non-cross-reactive serotypes of the HA and NA molecules, respectively.) While it was clear from this early work that at least some of the strain-specific CTL recognized the HA (Ennis *et al.* 1977; Zweerink *et al.* 1977b; Braciale 1979), the viral antigens recognized by cross-reactive CTL remained uncertain. The existence of cross-reactive CTL was surprising since at that time it was thought that only the serologically non-cross-reactive glycoproteins were expressed on infected cell surfaces. It was proposed that either CTL recognized the glycoproteins in a manner different from antibodies, or that one or a number of the highly conserved internal proteins were expressed on infected cell surfaces. This problem proved to be of general interest since similar types of cross-reactivity were observed in CTL responses to a number of other viruses (Zinkernagel and Doherty 1979).

To examine anti-influenza CTL recognition of individual viral components, we constructed recombinant vaccinia viruses containing cloned copies of influenza virus genes (Table 1) (Smith *et al.* 1983; Mackett *et al.* 1984). These recombinants had the following properties:

1. Following infection of simian cells, each of the Vac recombinants produced influenza virus proteins of the proper mobility when ^{35}S-methionine-labeled cell extracts were immunoprecipitated with anti-influenza antisera and analyzed in SDS–PAGE.
2. Where monoclonal antibodies were available for antigenic analysis (HA, NP, M1, NS1, PB2), influenza virus proteins produced during infection of murine cells with Vac recombinants were found to be antigenically indis-tinguishable from authentic viral proteins.
3. Immunization of mice with a number of these recombinants was found to prime mice for secondary *in vitro* anti-influenza CTL responses.

Table 1 Vac recombinants used to study CTL recognition

Recombinant	Influenza virus gene
H2-Vac	JAP HA
H1-Vac	PR8 HA
NP-Vac	PR8 NP
PA-Vac	PR8 PA
PB1-Vac	PR8 PB1
PB2-Vac	PR8 PB2
M1-Vac	PR8-M1
NS1-Vac	PR8 NS1
M2-Vac	UDORN M2

The JAP (A/JAPAN/305/57 (H2N2) HA gene was provided by M-J Gething (University of Texas Health Science Center, Dallas, Texas, USA). All PR8 (A/PR/8/34 (H1N1) genes were provided by P Palese (Mount Sinai School of Medicine, New York, USA). The Udorn (A/Udorn/72 (H3N2) M2 gene was provided by R Lamb (Northwestern University, Evanston, Illinois, USA).

Additionally, some of the viruses could stimulate secondary anti-influenza CTL responses using splenocytes derived from influenza virus primed mice.

Results obtained using the recombinants to examine the specificity of anti-influenza CTL derived from BALB/c (H-2^d) mice are described below by gene product (references are given where these results have been described in published accounts). CTL activity was measured in ^{51}Cr release assays using influenza or recombinant Vac infected P815 cells (DBA/2 (H-2^d) mastocytoma cell line). To produce CTL populations, splenocytes from mice immunized with live influenza virus or Vac recombinants were co-incubated for six days with autologous splenocytes infected with influenza A virus.

HA (Bennink et al *1984b*; Bennink et al. *1986*)

Recognition of H1-Vac and H2-Vac infected cells by anti-influenza CTL populations was predominantly strain-specific. CTL populations induced by priming and/or *in vitro* stimulation with H1-Vac or H2-Vac also demonstrated predominantly strain-specific recognition. A moderate amount of cross-reactive recognition was detected between H1 and H2 HAs, but did not extend to the H3 HA. This pattern of recognition is consistent with the amino acid homologies of the HAs (H1 and H2 are among the most closely related of the 13 known HA serotypes, while H1 and H3, and H2 and H3 are among the most distantly related HAs). Unlabeled target inhibition studies confirmed that the HA is, at most, only a minor target antigen for cross-reactive CTL.

NP *(Yewdell* et al *1985)*

NP was found to be a major target antigen for cross-reactive CTL. NP-Vac infected cells were consistently lysed by all cross-reactive CTL populations tested. Unlabeled target inhibition experiments and limiting dilution analysis of CTL precursor frequency confirmed that a substantial portion of second-arily *in vitro* stimulated BALB/c CTL recognize NP. Inoculation of mice with NP-Vac primed splenocytes for vigorous secondary CTL responses following *in vitro* stimulation with influenza viruses from all three human subtypes. NP-Vac also primed mice for an accelerated pulmonary CTL re-sponse following aerosol infection with PR8.

NS1

NS1-Vac infected cells were consistently lysed by cross-reactive CTL, but generally at lower levels than NP-Vac infected cells. The comparative fre-quencies of BALB/c NP- and NS1-specific CTL precursors, as determined by limiting dilution analysis, were consistent with this finding. Curiously, although inoculation of mice with NS1-Vac primed their splenocytes for a vigorous secondary *in vitro* anti-Vac CTL response, priming for anti-influenza responses was not observed.

Polymerases

PB2-Vac infected cells were consistently lysed by cross-reactive BALB/c CTL, and inoculation with PB2-Vac primed mice for secondary *in vitro* cross-reactive responses. Levels of lysis were generally similar to those observed on NS1-Vac infected cells; again this was consistent with precursor frequencies. PA-Vac infected cells were usually lysed by cross-reactive CTL populations. Levels of lysis were always lower than those observed for PB2-Vac infected cells. PB1-Vac infected cells were only occasionally lysed by cross-reactive (or strain-specific) CTL populations, and then only at low levels.

M1

In a large number of experiments M1-Vac infected cells were not specifically recognized by any anti-influenza CTL population tested. This was not due to low levels of expression of M1, since M1-Vac infected cells expressed anti-genically active M1 at levels comparable to influenza A virus infected cells. Nor is this attributable to the resistance of these cells to lysis by CTL, since they were lysed by anti-Vac CTL with identical efficiency to cells infected with other Vac recombinants. M1-Vac also failed to prime for secondary *in vitro* responses.

M2

M2-Vac infected cells were not recognized by most CTL populations tested. Occasionally, using high effector-to-target ratios, lysis at levels marginally above control values were observed. Whether this represents specific recognition by a very minor CTL population can probably only be determined using CTL clones. The failure to observe greater levels of CTL recognition is not due to the lack of surface expression of this integral membrane protein, since in the presence of complement, M2-Vac infected cells were efficiently lysed by an antiserum which demonstrates the same cross-reactive recognition of influenza A virus infected cells as CTL. This antiserum was produced by immunization of goats with purified M1, and its cross-reactive recognition of influenza A virus infected cells provided evidence for the expression of M1 on infected cell surfaces (Biddison *et al.* 1977). These findings could not be confirmed using monoclonal antibodies specific for M1 (Hackett *et al.* 1980; Yewdell *et al.* 1981). This cell surface reactivity, and probably the reactivity of other anti-M1 antisera used in other studies (Ada and Yap 1977; Braciale 1977; Reiss and Schulman 1980), is apparently entirely due to its cross-reaction with M2, since we found that it does not lyse cells infected with M1-Vac or with any of the other Vac recombinants. The basis for this cross-reaction is easily explained, since M1 and M2 have the same nine amino-terminal residues, and M2 has been shown to be oriented in the plasma membrane so that at least 18 of its amino terminal residues are exposed at the cell surface (Lamb *et al.* 1985).

CTL recognition of individual VSV antigens

Our study of anti-influenza CTL resulted in two major findings. First, integral membrane proteins as well as internal viral proteins can serve as CTL recognition structures. Second, the cross-reactive CTL response is almost exclusively directed against internal viral components. To determine whether these findings extend to CTL recognition of other viruses, we performed similar experiments using Vac recombinants containing genes derived from VSV.

To examine anti-VSV CTL recognition we used recombinant Vac viruses containing G genes derived from Indiana and New Jersey serotypes, and the nucleocapsid (N) gene derived from Indiana (all VSV genes were provided by Dr J Rose, Salk Institute, San Diego, California, USA). G and N are functionally analogous to the influenza virus HA and NP respectively. The recombinant Vac viruses were used to both elicit anti-VSV CTL and to sensitize target cells for lysis by CTL induced by VSV.

The results of these experiments were completely consistent with the influenza virus studies. As with anti-influenza CTL, anti-VSV CTL can be divided into cross-reactive and serotype-specific categories (Rosenthal and

Zinkernagel 1980). CTL recognition of G was found to be largely serotype-specific, while recognition of N was highly cross-reactive (Yewdell *et al.* 1986). Although it will be important to examine CTL recognition of proteins derived from other viruses, these findings suggest that recognition of internal viral proteins comprises a critical portion of the CTL response.

CTL recognition of individual viral antigens occurs in conjunction with only a limited number of the available class I restriction elements

As described above, BALB/c CTL demonstrated marked differences in responsiveness to individual influenza virus proteins. To examine the possible role of the MHC in this phenomenon, cross-reactive CTL derived from C57BL/6 (H-2^b) and CBA (H-2^k) mice were tested for their ability to lyse Vac-recombinant infected MC57G (H-2^b) and L (H-2^k) cells respectively (Bennink *et al.* 1986). In contrast to BALB/c CTL, C57BL/6 CTL only consistently recognized NP and NS1 (Table 2). CBA CTL yielded still another pattern of recognition, in only recognizing NP, NS1 and PB1 (Table 2). We failed to detect recognition of either M1 or M2 in any of these experiments.

The differential responsiveness to PB1 and PB2 by BALB/c and CBA/J CTL was further examined using cross-reactive CTL populations derived from BALB/c and BALB/K (H-2^k), and B10.D2 (H-2^d) and B10.BR (H-2^k) congenic strains. Responsiveness to PB1 was found to co-segregate with

Table 2 Recognition of *Influenza A* virus proteins by cross-reactive CTL derived from different mouse strains

	BALB/c	CBA	C57B1/6
NP	+++++	+++++	++
PA	++	0	++
PB1	+/−	+++++	0
PB2	+++	0	+/−
NS1	+++	+++	+/−
M1	0	0	0
M2	0	0	0

This table summarizes the results of a large number of assays performed using BALB/c and CBA anti-influenza CTL and recombinant Vac infected P815 and L cells respectively. Recognition of each recombinant is graded from 0 to +++++ based on the levels of lysis generally obtained, as well as the consistency of responses observed between different CTL populations. Similar criteria were used to summarize the recognition of recombinant Vac infected MC57G cells by CTL derived from C57B1/6 mice. This was assessed in a much smaller number of experiments however (three), and was hindered by low levels of anti-influenza CTL activity.

$H-2^k$, while PB2 responsiveness co-segregated with $H-2^d$. By using target cells derived from C3H × DBA/2 ($H-2^{kxd}$) F1 mice we eliminated the possibility that these results were due to differential expression of PB1 and PB2 in L cells versus P815 cells since an identical pattern of recognition of PB1 and PB2 was observed.

The effect of the MHC on CTL recognition of individual antigens was further studied by testing the ability of cross-reactive CTL derived from A/J (K^kD^d) and C3H.OH (K^dD^k) to lyse Vac recombinant infected P815 and L cells. With a single exception (recognition of PB1 by $H-2^k$ CTL), recognition of individual viral antigens could be mapped to the K or D end of the MHC. These data suggest that CTL recognition of many viral antigens occurs only in association with a limited number of the available MHC class I restriction elements.

Implications for vaccine design

Our findings have two major implications for the design of vaccines meant to elicit maximal CTL immunity. First, these vaccines should include internal viral antigens. From the present work it is clear that many of these proteins can be recognized by CTL, and that their generally high degree of conservation between virus serotypes will insure the broadest induction of immunity. Second, to avoid potential difficulties of MHC-linked non-responsiveness to individual viral components, vaccines should be composed of a number of viral proteins.

It must be stressed that the utility of such anti-viral 'CTL vaccines' remains to be determined. Although CTL appear to play an important role in eradicating established influenza, vaccinia and LCM virus infections (Yap *et al.* 1978; Lin and Askonas 1981; Bennink *et al.* 1984a; Lukacher *et al.* 1984; Oldstone *et al.* 1986), the anti-viral activity of CTL in other viral infections must be determined for each individual virus. Furthermore, as suggested by Zinkernagel *et al.* (1985), vaccination for CTL memory may be a pointless exercise since CTL memory could be short-lived, and in any event, primary and secondary *in vivo* CTL responses differ little in their kinetics and magnitude. However, while such vaccines may not prove to be useful in cases where vigorous CTL responses arise during the immune response, they may be important in circumstances where CTL responses are low or absent, such as chronic virus infections and tumors.

Acknowledgements

This work was supported by grants AI 22114, AI 14162 and AI 20338 from the National Institutes of Health, Bethesda, Maryland, USA.

References

Ada G L, Yap K L 1977. Matrix protein expressed at the surface of cells infected with influenza viruses, *Immunochemistry* **14**: 643–51

Bennink J R, Yewdell J W, Feldman A, Gerhard W, Doherty P C 1984a. The role of virus-specific CTL *in vivo*, in H von Boehmer, W Haas (eds) *T Cell Clones*. Elsevier, New York

Bennink J R, Yewdell J W, Smith G L, Moller C, Moss B 1984b. Recombinant vaccinia virus primes and stimulates influenza haemagglutinin-specific cytotoxic T cells, *Nature (London)* **311**: 578–9

Bennink J R, Yewdell J W, Smith G L, Moss B 1986. Recognition of cloned influenza virus hemagglutinin gene products by cytotoxic T lymphocytes, *Journal of Virology* **57**: 786–91

Biddison W E, Doherty P C, Webster R G 1977. Antibody to influenza virus matrix protein detects a common antigen on the surface of cells infected with type A influenza virus, *Journal of Experimental Medicine* **146**: 690–7

Braciale T J 1977. Immunologic recognition of influenza virus-infected cells. II. Expression of influenza A matrix protein on the infected cell surface and its role in recognition by cross-reactive cytotoxic T cells, *Journal of Experimental Medicine* **146**: 673–89

Braciale T J 1979. Specificity of cytotoxic T cells directed to influenza virus hemagglutinin, *Journal of Experimental Medicine* **149**: 856–69

Braciale T J, Braciale V L, Henkel T J, Sambrook J, Gething M-J 1984. Cytotoxic T lymphocyte recognition of the influenza hemagglutinin gene product expressed by DNA-mediated gene transfer, *Journal of Experimental Medicine* **159**: 341–54

Doherty P C, Zinkernagel R M 1975. Capacity of sensitized thymus derived lymphocytes to induce fatal lymphocytic choriomeningitis is restricted by the H-2 gene complex, *Journal of Immunology* **114**: 30–3

Effros R B, Doherty P C, Gerhard W, Bennink J 1977. Generation of both cross-reactive and virus-specific T-cell populations after immunization with serologically distinct influenza A viruses, *Journal of Experimental Medicine* **145**: 557–68

Ennis F A 1982. Some newly recognized aspects of resistance against and recovery from influenza, *Archives of Virology* **73**: 207–17

Ennis F A, Martin W J, Verbonitz M W, Butchko G M 1977. Specificity studies on cytotoxic thymus-derived lymphocytes reactive with influenza virus infected cells: evidence for dual recognition of H-2 and viral hemagglutinin antigens, *Proceedings of the National Academy of Sciences USA* **74**: 3006–10

Hackett C J, Askonas B A, Webster R J, van Wyke K 1980. Quantitation of influenza virus antigens on infected target cells and their recognition by cross-reactive cytotoxic T cells, *Journal of Experimental Medicine* **151**: 1014–25

Lamb R A 1983. The influenza virus RNA segments and their encoded proteins, in P A Palese, D W Kingsbury (eds) *Genetics of Influenza Viruses*. Springer Verlag, New York

Lamb R A, Zebedee S L, Richardson C D 1985. Influenza virus M2 protein is an integral membrane protein expressed on the infected-cell surface, *Cell* **40**: 627–33

Lin Y L, Askonas B A 1981. Biological properties of an influenza A virus specific killer T cell clone, *Journal of Experimental Medicine* **154**: 225–34

Lukacher A E, Braciale V L, Braciale T J 1984. *In vivo* effector function of influenza virus specific cytotoxic T lymphocyte clones is highly specific, *Journal of Experimental Medicine* **160**: 814–26

Mackett M, Smith G L, Moss B 1984. General method for production and selection of infectious vaccinia virus recombinants expessing foreign genes, *Journal of Virology* **49**: 857–64

Oldstone M B A, Blount P, Southern P J, Lampert P W 1986. Cytoimmunotherapy for persistent virus infection reveals a unique clearance pattern from the central nervous system, *Nature (London)* **321**: 239–3

Reiss C S, Schulman J L 1980. Influenza type A M protein: expression on infected cells is responsible for cross-reactive recognition by cytotoxic thymus derived lymphocytes, *Infection and Immunity* **29**: 719–23

Rosenthal K L, Zinkernagel R M 1980. Cross-reactive cytotoxic T cells to serologically distinct vesicular stomatitis viruses, *Journal of Immunology* **124**: 2301–8

Smith G L, Mackett M, Moss B 1983. Infectious vaccinia virus recombinants that express hepatitis B virus surface antigens, *Nature (London)* **302**: 490–5

Townsend A R M, McMichael A J, Carter N P, Huddleston J A, Brownlee G G 1984. Cytotoxic T cell recognition of the influenza nucleoprotein and hemagglutinin expressed in transfected mouse L cells, *Cell* **39**: 13–25

Townsend A R M, Rothbard J, Gotch F M, Bahdur G, Wraith D, McMichael A J 1986. The epitope of influenza nucleoprotein recognized by cytotoxic T lymphocytes can be defined with short synthetic peptides, *Cell* **44**: 959–68

Yamada A, Young, J F, Ennis F A 1985. Influenza virus subtype-specific cytotoxic T lymphocytes lyse target cells coated with a protein produced in *E. coli*, *Journal of Experimental Medicine* **162**: 1720–5

Yap K L, Ada G L 1977. Cytotoxic T cells specific for influenza virus-infected target cells, *Immunology* **32**: 151–60

Yap K L, Ada G L, McKenzie I F C 1978. Transfer of specific cytotoxic T lymphocytes protects mice inoculated with influenza virus, *Nature (London)* **273**: 236–7

Yewdell J W, Frank E, Gerhard W 1981. Expression of influenza A virus internal antigens on the surface of infected P815 cells, *Journal of Immunology* **126**: 1814–19

Yewdell J W, Bennink J R, Smith G L, Moss B 1985. Influenza A virus nucleoprotein is a major target antigen for cross-reactive anti-influenza A virus cytotoxic T lymphocytes, *Proceedings of the National Academy of Sciences USA* **82**: 1785–89

Yewdell J W, Bennink J R, Mackett M, LeFrancois L, Lyles D S, Moss B 1986. Recognition of cloned vesicular stomatitis virus internal and external gene products by cytotoxic T lymphocytes, *Journal of Experimental Medicine* **163**: 1529–38

Zinkernagel R M, Doherty P C 1979. MHC-restricted cytotoxic T cells, *Advances in Immunology* **27**: 51–177

Zinkernagel R M, Hengartner H, Stitz L 1985. On the role of viruses in the evolution of immune responses, *British Medical Bulletin* **41**: 92–7

Zweerink H J, Courtneidge S A, Skehel J J, Crumpton M J, Askonas B A 1977a. Cytotoxic T cells kill influenza virus infected cells but do not distinguish between serologically distinct type A viruses, *Nature (London)* **267**: 354–6

Zweerink H J, Askonas B A, Millican D, Courtneidge S A, Skehel J J 1977b. Cytotoxic T cells to type A influenza virus; viral hemagglutinin induces A-strain specificity while infected cells confer cross-reactive cytotoxicity, *European Journal of Immunology* **7**: 630–5

Immunochemical studies of T and B cell responses to a protein epitope

Eli Benjamini; Charles D Estin; Frank L Norton; Matthew L Andria; Anne M Wan; Beatrice C Langton; C Y Leung

Department of Medical Microbiology and Immunology, School of Medicine, University of California, Davis, California 95616, USA.

Introduction

Recent advances in immunology, molecular biology and peptide synthesis have intensified research towards their application for vaccine development, particularly vaccines where the immune response is directed towards proteins. It is now clear that the immune response to antigenic stimuli is complex and is highly regulated. Only recently is it becoming possible to answer such important questions as what are the attributes of B and/or T cell recognizable determinants and how does the immunized individual regulate the B and T cell responses?

Using the tobacco mosaic virus protein (TMVP) as a model antigen, recent work in our laboratory has been performed in an attempt to elucidate some of the attributes of a single epitope of a protein antigen and to elucidate some of the mechanisms which operate in the B and T cell responses to this epitope. It is realized that the investigations pertain to a single epitope and that a protein antigen consists of many epitopes. However, it is felt that consideration of the response to a single epitope is of utmost importance since the response to a single given epitope may be crucial in the ability of the host to survive the invasion of a certain pathogen or the action of its toxin.

The B cell response

Immunization of many animal species with TMVP leads to the induction of antibodies directed against several areas of the protein. One such area consists of residues 93–112; this is tryptic peptide number 8, having the amino acid sequence Ile-Ile-Glu-Val-Glu-Asn-Gln-Ala-Asn-Pro-Thr-Thr-Ala-Glu-Thr-Leu-Asp-Ala-Thr-Arg.Further investigations revealed that antibodies produced in rabbits, guinea pigs and many (but not all) strains of mice are directed to the *C*-terminal decapeptide portion of tryptic peptide 8 (referred to as 'decapeptide') (summarized in Benjamini 1980) and that the responsiveness of various strains of mice to this decapeptide is linked to the immunoglobulin allotype (Morrow *et al.* 1984). Moreover, depending on the strain, even within 'responder' strains consisting of genetically identical (or very closely related) syngeneic individuals, the antibody responses to the decapeptide are not uniform, either with respect to the total antibody response or with respect to the fine specificity of antibodies as determined by the capacity of the anti-decapeptide antibodies to bind with a series of synthetic analogues related to the decapeptide. Characterization of the anti-decapeptide antibody responses of individual mice following immunization with the whole TMVP revealed that while the antibody response to TMVP was, as expected, i.e. heterogeneous, the response to the decapeptide appeared to be of a rather restricted heterogeneity (Morrow *et al.* 1984). Moreover, the responsiveness (or nonresponsiveness) and fine specificity of the anti-decapeptide antibodies of a given individual appear to be 'locked in' for the life of the individual, unchanged upon repeated reimmunization with TMVP.

In an attempt to elucidate the reason for the failure of approximately half of syngeneic C3H.SW animals to respond to the decapeptide, an experiment was performed in which a pool of spleen cells from 48 naive syngeneic mice was transferred into 400 R irradiated syngeneic recipients. One-half of the spleen cells were treated with anti-theta serum and complement; the other half were not. After a few days all the recipients were immunized with TMVP. It was anticipated that the donors' spleen cells representing a B cell pool containing decapeptide-specific B cells would confer upon every recipient the

Table 1 The frequency of mice producing antibodies capable of binding with TMVP or with the *C*-terminal decapeptide of tryptic peptide 8 following transfer of pooled naive spleen cells*

Treatment of recipients							
Recipients received naive spleen cells				Recipients received naive spleen cells treated with anti-theta serum and complement			
Test antigen†				Test antigen†			
TMVP		Decapeptide		TMVP		Decapeptide	
positive/total	(%)	positive/total	(%)	positive/total	(%)	positive/total	(%)
21/21	100	10/21	48	22/22	100	11/22	50

* Each C3H.SW recipient received 400 R and transplanted with 1×10^8 naive syngeneic cells; each recipient was subsequently immunized with 100 μg TMVP in Freund's Complete Adjuvant followed 20 days later by an aqueous boost with 100 μg TMVP. Sera were obtained 10 days after the boost.
† Assayed by solid-phase radioimmunoassay.

ability to make anti-decapeptide antibodies. Data presented in Table 1 indicate that this is not the case. While all the recipients made anti-TMVP antibodies, again approximately only half produced antibodies binding with the decapeptide. Moreover, the frequency of animals responding to the decapeptide was approximately the same regardless of whether or not the donors' spleen cells were treated with anti-theta serum and complement. Further investigations were performed to assess the fine specificity of anti-decapeptide antibodies produced in 400 R irradiated recipients which had received a pool of naive syngeneic spleen cells and had subsequently been immunized with TMVP. The fine specificity was assessed by the ability of the anti-decapeptide antibodies to bind with synthetic analogs of the decapeptide which were previously shown to define best the fine specificity of this strain of mice (Morrow *et al.* 1984; Norton *et al.* 1985). Here again it was anticipated that every recipient would respond with anti-decapeptide antibodies exhibiting the sum of all the fine specificities of this strain of mice. Instead, less than half of the recipients responded with antibodies to the decapeptide and the frequency of the fine specificity of these anti-decapeptide antibodies was approximately the same as that exhibited by naive individuals of this strain

Table 2 The frequency of donor and recipient C3H.SW mice making antibodies exhibiting binding with the *C*-terminal decapeptide or tryptic peptide 8 of TMVP and its synthetic analogues*

| | Donors | | | Recipients | | | | |
| | | | | Before transfer | | After transfer | | |
Analog†	positive total	(%)		positive total	(%)		positive total	(%)
Decapeptide	22/22	100		19/27	70		25/27	93
(Ala)$_5$	6/22	27		10/19	53		18/19	95
Cys$_{112}$	13/22	59		11/19	58		18/19	95
Tyr$_{106}$	10/22	45		13/19	68		18/19	95

* Donors were immunized with 100μg TMVP in Freund's Complete Adjuvant followed by an aqueous boost with 100μg TMVP. Each recipient was irradiated with 600 R, received 1×10^8 cells consisting of a pool of donors immune spleen cells and subsequently boostered with 100 g TMVP. Approximately 60% of the animals in the donor group made anti-decapeptide antibodies. Only mice making anti-decapeptide antibodies were selected as donors.

† Position	103	104	105	106	107	108	109	110	111	112
Decapeptide	Thr–	Thr–	Ala–	Glu–	Thr–	Leu–	Asp–	Ala–	Thr–	Arg
(Ala)$_5$ analog	Ala–	Ala–	Ala–	Ala–	Ala					
Cys$_{112}$ analog										Cys
Tyr$_{106}$ analog				Tyr						

(which did not receive a pool of B cells) immunized with TVMP (data not shown).

In another transfer experiment, mice were first immunized with TMVP and their anti-decapeptide responses and the fine specificity of the anti-decapeptide antibodies was determined. The animals were then rested until their anti-decapeptide titers decreased to insignificant amounts (approximately eight months). They were then irradiated with 600 R and transplanted with a pool of primed spleen cells from animals which had been immunized with TMVP and whose response to TMVP, to the decapeptide and to several of its synthetic analogs had been determined. Results in Table 2 clearly demonstrate that while prior to transfer the donors and the recipients had the restricted pattern of the response characteristic to this strain of mice (C3H.SW) (Morrow *et al.* 1984), virtually all of the recipients produced antibodies reactive with the decapeptide. Moreover, the fine specificity of the anti-decapeptide antibodies of virtually every recipient individual consisted of the total fine specificity exhibited by all the donors.

The results of the transfer experiments indicate that the antibody responsiveness to the decapeptide and the fine specificity of these antibodies are governed by mechanism(s) other than just the availability of a suitable B cell repertoire. If the availability of the appropriate B cell repertoire was the only factor, it would be expected that following immunization with TMVP every recipient would respond to all of the synthetic analogs. This was not the case. Moreover, it appears that the pattern of responsiveness was not governed by T cells (either helper or suppressor) since the responsiveness was the same whether the pooled spleen cells were treated with anti-theta serum and complement or not.

The above pertains to primary responses and virgin B cells. However, whatever the mechanism which restricts the primary response in spite of the availability of an extended repertoire of virgin B cells, it does not appear to operate on the activation of memory B cells where the responsiveness of mice which had received a pool of memory B cell appears unrestricted. Work is currently in progress to elucidate the mechanism(s) which restrict the primary response.

The above findings pertain to one single epitope of a protein antigen. They are however significant if this epitope gives rise to antibodies with fine specificities which are essential for the neutralization of the antigen's biological activity and the survival of the individual.

The antibody response to an epitope following immunization with related but different immunogens

We have previously shown that tryptic peptide 8 of TMVP is immunogenic in mice, leading to the induction of antibodies to the decapeptide which also exhibit binding with TMVP (Wan *et al.* 1985). We have also shown that while the decapeptide is not immunogenic it is immunogenic when conjugated to keyhole limpet hemocyanin (KLH); the conjugate induces antibodies capable of binding with the decapeptide as well as with the whole protein TMVP (Wan *et al.* 1985). Additionally, we have established that all three immunogens (TMVP, peptide 8, and decapeptide–KLH conjugate) are T cell dependent and induce anti-decapeptide antibodies of similar isotypes (Wan *et al.* 1985; Benjamini *et al.* 1985). In view of these findings it was of interest to compare the fine specificity of the anti-decapeptide antibodies induced by TMVP, by peptide 8 and by the decapeptide–KLH conjugate. This was performed by assessing the binding between anti-decapeptide antibodies induced by these immunogens in C3H.SW mice and several selected synthetic analogs of the decapeptide which have been found useful in assessing the fine specificity of anti-decapeptide antibodies in this mouse strain (Morrow *et al.* 1984; Norton *et al.* 1985). Results of these experiments showed that most (75–100%) anti-decapeptide antibodies induced by immunization with TMVP, with decapeptide–KLH conjugate, or with peptide 8 exhibited binding with the Met_{107} analog (in which Thr at position 107 was substituted with methionine). Also 50–85% of anti-decapeptide antibodies induced TMVP or by decapeptide–KLH conjugate exhibited binding with the $(Ala)_4$ analog [in which the four *N*-terminal residues consisted of alanine]. However, no binding with the $(Ala)_4$ analog was exhibited by any of the anti-decapeptide antibodies induced by immunization with peptide 8 (Benjamini *et al.* 1985).

The lack of binding with the $(Ala)_4$ analog suggests that the central area of peptide 8, where the alanine substitutions are made, is crucial for the interaction with antibodies or B cells of a certain specificity. Studies conducted recently in our laboratory indicate that some T cell populations of this strain recognize this central area on peptide 8 (Wan *et al.* 1986 and *vide infra*) and thus overlap with certain B cells which recognize the same area. This may preclude effective antigen participation in the interaction between T cells and certain B cell clonotypes. The interaction and activation of such B cell clonotypes with T cells directed to more distant areas on the immunogen would however take place, as in the case of immunization with TMVP or with decapeptide–KLH conjugate.

Comparison of the anti-decapeptide antibodies induced by TMVP, peptide 8 and decapeptide–KLH conjugate indicate that, by and large, their isotype composition and fine specificities are similar (Wan *et al.* 1985; Benjamini *et al.* 1985). However, immunization with immunogens consisting of relatively short peptides such as peptide 8 may impose constraints on cellular interactions during immunogenesis so that one or more B cell clonotypes of certain antibody specificities will not become activated.

The induction of immunological memory

An important attribute of an effective immunogen is its ability to induce long-lived immunological memory such that even when the antibody titer to the antigen is low, encounter of the memory cells with the antigen results in a rapid memory response consisting of cellular proliferation, differentiation and antibody synthesis. Since it has been previously established in our laboratory that TMVP-immunized mice exhibited a memory response when reinjected with TMVP (Rennick *et al.* 1983), experiments were performed to assess whether immunization with peptide 8 or with the decapeptide–KLH conjugate would also induce a state of immunologic memory such that an enhanced anamnestic booster response would occur upon subsequent reimmunization with the native protein TMVP. Results of these experiments demonstrated that immunization with peptide 8 induced this state of immunological memory. In contrast, immunization with decapeptide–KLH conjugate did not induce the necessary memory cells capable of responding to subsequent challenge with TMVP: encounter with TMVP did not result in increased anti-TMVP titers (Benjamini *et al.* 1985).

The above results are not unexpected. The decapeptide by itself is not immunogenic and can thus be considered a hapten. For the induction of anti-hapten antibodies it is imperative that the hapten, recognizable by B cells, be conjugated to a carrier recognizable by T cells. Thus, the decapeptide in the context of TMVP or peptide 8, or conjugated to KLH, is immunogenic, with B cells directed towards the decapeptide and T cells directed to other areas on TMVP, to various areas on KLH, or to the *N*-terminal portion of peptide 8 (see below). For a memory response to take place it is imperative that the immunogen consist of the same hapten on the same carrier (Mitchison 1971). Thus, when the primary immunogen is TMVP or peptide 8 and the secondary immunogen is TMVP, the secondary immune response will be developed through the same hapten (i.e. the decapeptide) on the same carrier (i.e. the *N*-terminal portion of peptide 8, in the context of the whole protein TMVP). In contrast, when the primary immunogen is decapeptide–KLH conjugate and the secondary immunogen is TMVP, a secondary response will not develop since the carriers of the decapeptide hapten were different for the primary immunization (KLH) and the secondary immunization (TMVP). These observations are important in the design of synthetic vaccines which must be able to induce a state of immunological memory such that a future encounter with the pathogen will lead to an anamnestic response with a rapid production of high titers of antibodies against the pathogen. Such vaccines must share both B cell recognizable epitopes and T cell recognizable epitopes with the challenging antigen against which vaccination is attempted.

T cell responses

Structural antigenic features required for T cell activation

Immunization of mice with peptide 8 induces T cells capable of proliferating, *in vitro*, in response to stimulation with peptide 8 (Wan *et al.* 1986). In an attempt to define the structural features of peptide 8 required for this activation of peptide-8-specific T cells, various portions of peptide 8 were synthesized. These included residues 101–112 (*C*-decapeptide), 97–112 (*C*-hexadecapeptide), 98–107 (central peptide) and 93–103 (*N*-undecapeptide). The peptides were tested for their capacity to stimulate lymph node cells from A/J, C57BL/10 and B10.BR mice immunized with peptide 8. Results of these experiments indicate that none of the peptides was stimulatory except in the case of C57BL/10 mice where the *C*-terminal hexadecapeptide was stimulatory (Wan *et al.* 1986).

Since peptide 8 in its entirety was stimulatory while most synthetic portions of peptide 8 were not, it is conceivable that the latter lacked part or all of a T cell recognizable epitope. It is also possible that since T cell activation requires not only a T cell recognizable epitope but also an area of the antigen capable of interacting with Ia of the major histocompatibility complex (MHC) of antigen presenting cells (APC) (Babbit *et al.* 1985) to which the term agretope was coined (Heber-Katz *et al.* 1983), part or all of a region capable of interacting with the Ia was missing from the synthetic portions of peptide 8. To ascertain these possibilities, the *N*-terminal undecapeptide representing residues 93–103 and the *C*-terminal decapeptide representing residues 103–112 were conjugated to several protein carriers or to their succinylated derivatives. Tests for the capacity of these conjugates to stimulate peptide-8-primed cells of A/J, C57BL/10 and B10.BR mice revealed that none of the conjugates of the *C*-decapeptide was stimulatory. In contrast, several conjugates of the *N*-undecapeptide were stimulatory. These results indicate that the *N*-undecapeptide contains an area recognized by T cells of the three strains. Moreover, this area seems to be recognized either in the context of the entire peptide 8 or when this area is conjugated to proteins. It is postulated that the *C*-terminal decapeptide portion of peptide 8 or some portions of the 'carrier' proteins either stabilized a conformation of the *N*-undecapeptide or provided areas (agretopes) for interaction with the Ia of APC. The finding that *N*-undecapeptide conjugated to succinylated BSA but not to the unsuccinylated protein was stimulatory indicates that the interaction with Ia, leading to T cell activation, involves some degree of specificity. However, since the *N*-undecapeptide was stimulatory when 'attached' to the *C*-terminal nonapeptide of peptide 8, to transferrin, to succinylated bovine serum albumin (BSA) or to succinylated transferrin, it appears that the specificity of interaction with Ia leading to T cell activation is limited (Wan *et al.* 1986).

The exact nature of the interaction between the epitope, the putative agretope, the Ia and the T cell receptor remains to be elucidated.

Genetic control of T cell activation

During the course of our investigations it became apparent that immunization of some strains of mice with either TMVP or with peptide 8 induced T cells capable of responding, *in vitro*, either to TMVP or to peptide 8. Such strains (e.g. C57/BL/10) are referred to as cross-reactive (CR). Other strains do not exhibit such cross-reactivity. Thus, immunization with TMVP induces T cells capable of responding, *in vitro*, to TMVP but not to peptide 8 and vice versa. Such strains (e.g. A/J) are referred to as non-cross-reactive (NCR). This non-cross-reaction, on the T cell level, is expressed in spite of the cross-reaction on the B cell level seen in CR as well as NCR strains (Wan *et al.* 1985).

Using congenic and recombinant strains of mice, we have shown that $H-2^k$ are NCR, and that the non-cross-reactivity is mapped to the I-A, with $I-A^k$ being NCR. Furthermore, we have shown that the cross-reactivity may be attributed to antigen presentation by macrophages, and the non-cross-reactivity attributed to the inability of macrophages with $I-A^k$ to present effectively peptide 8 to the TMVP-immune T cells (Benjamini *et al.* 1987).

In an attempt to elucidate the molecular basis for this phenomenon we tried to delineate the fine specificity of the T cells induced in CR as well as in NCR mice in response to immunization with peptide 8. Results of these experiments indicated that peptide-8-immune lymph node cells from CR but not from NCR mice could be stimulated by the *C*-terminal hexadecapeptide of peptide 8 (residues 97–112 of TMVP). Moreover, while none of the cells could be stimulated by the *C*-terminal decapeptide or its conjugates, lymph node cells from CR mice immunized with peptide 8 responded to the *N*–undecapeptide conjugated to BSA, transferrin or to their succinylated derivatives. In contrast, cells from peptide-8-immunized NCR animals responded to the *N*-undecapeptide conjugated to succinylated BSA or succinylated transferrin but generally not to the conjugates with the non-succinylated forms of the protein carrier. The findings that peptide-8-immune cells from CR as well as from NCR mice can be stimulated with the *N*-undecapeptide conjugated through the *N*-terminus to the succinylated proteins, indicate that T cells of both strains overlap in their specificity. Whether the CR strain which responds *in vitro* to the *C*-hexadecapeptide has additional T cell populations remains to be investigated. The findings that peptide-8-immune T cells of the CR or the NCR strain did not respond to the conjugates of the *C*-terminal decapeptide suggest that there are no T cell populations which recognize this *C*-terminal half of peptide 8 (Benjamini *et al.* 1986).

It appears that a major difference between the CR and NCR strains is not so much in the area of peptide which their corresponding peptide-8-immune T cells recognize, but rather in how this area is presented to the T cell: both the CR and NCR peptide-8-immune strains contain T cells which recognize the *N*-undecapeptide. However, it appears that the CR cells recognize the peptide when it is conjugated through the *N*- or *C*-terminus while the NCR cells recognize it only when conjugated through the *N*-terminus. It is tempting to speculate that the difference between the CR and NCR strains which maps to the I-A of the APC is attributed to the orientation in which a T cell recognizable area is presented. It is further tempting to speculate that when a native protein does not induce T cells to a certain accessible area of the protein it may be because of shortcomings in presentation. Denaturing the protein, excising the portion of the protein containing this area, or conjugating the area to heterologous proteins may result in immunogens which will be correctly presented and will lead to the induction of T cells to that area. This may be of practical importance in vaccine production where it may be desirable to induce T cells to a certain area of a protein to which no T cells are induced by immunization with the native protein.

Acknowledgements

The work described herein was supported in part by grants PCM 8103264 and PCM 8411235 from the National Science Foundation and by grants IM291 and IM401 from the American Cancer Society.

References

Babbitt B, Allen P M, Matsueda H, Haber E, Unanue E R 1985. Binding of immunogenic peptides to Ia histocompatibility molecules, *Nature (London)* **317**: 359–61

Benjamini E 1980. Immunochemistry of the tobacco mosaic virus protein, in M Z Atassi (ed) *Immunochemistry of Proteins*. Plenum Press, New York, vol. 2, pp 265–310

Benjamini E, Wan A M, Langton C B, Andria M L 1985. Induction of immunity by a model synthetic vaccine from the tobacco mosaic virus protein, in G R Dreesman, J G Bronson, R C Kennedy (eds) *High Technology Route to Virus Vaccines*. American Society for Microbiology, Washington, DC, pp 30–42.

Benjamini E, Langton B C, Wan A M, Andria M L, Leung C Y 1986. Cellular and molecular aspects of the genetic control of the T cell response to a defined protein epitope, in R Bell and G Torrigiani (eds) *Progress Towards Better Vaccines* Oxford University Press

Heber-Katz E, Hansburg D, Schwartz R H 1983. The Ia molecule of the antigen presenting cell plays a critical role in immune response gene regulation of T cell activation, *Journal of Molecular and Cellular Immunology* **1**: 3–14

Mitchison N A 1971. The carrier effect in the secondary response to hapten protein conjugates. II: Cell cooperation, *European Journal of Immunology* **1**: 18–27

Morrow P R, Renninck D M, Benjamini E 1984. The antibody response to a single antigenic determinant of the tobacco mosaic virus protein (TMVP): effect of allotype-linked genes and restricted heterogeneity of the response, *Journal of Immunology* **131**: 2875–81

Norton F L, Morrow P R, Leung C Y, Benjamini E 1985. The idiotypic characterization of the immune response to a defined epitope of a protein antigen and the specific *in vivo* suppression of the immune response to this epitope by anti-idiotypic antibodies, *Journal of Immunology* **134**: 3226–32

Rennick D M, Morrow P R, Benjamini E 1983. Functional heterogeneity of memory B lymphocytes: *in vivo* analysis of TD-primed B cells responsive to secondary stimulation with TD and TI antigens, *Journal of Immunology* **131**: 561–6

Wan A M, Estin C D, Langton B C, Andria M L, Benjamini E 1985. Immune induction by a protein antigen and by a peptide segment of the protein, in M Z Atassi, H L Bachrach (eds) *Immunobiology of Proteins and Peptides* Plenum Press, New York, vol 3, pp 175–91

Wan A M, Langton B C, Andria M L, Benjamini E 1986. Antigenic requirements for T cell activation: reconstitution of a functional antigen from an inactive peptide portion of an antigen conjugated to protein carriers, *Molecular Immunology* **23**: 467–74

Production and utilization of chimeric immunoglobulin molecules

Sherie L Morrison*; Letitia A Wims*; Vernon T Oi†

* Department of Microbiology and the Cancer Center/Institute for Cancer Research, Columbia University College of Physicians and Surgeons, 701 West 168th Street, New York, New York 10032, USA
† Becton–Dickinson Monoclonal Center, Mountain View, California 94043, USA

Introduction

Antibodies have long been recognized for the role they play in protection against disease. Therefore, antibody molecules and the genes that control their expression have been the objects of investigation for several decades. Early studies showed that the gamma globulins, the proteins with the least electrophoretic mobility, were specifically removed upon reaction with antigen (Tiselius and Kabat, 1939). However, studies of these proteins were hindered by their structural heterogeneity.

With the realization that myeloma proteins represent monoclonal antibodies, great progress was made in the understanding of immunoglobulin (Ig) structure. However, in most cases, myeloma proteins could not be demonstrated to react with a specific antigen.

A major breakthrough was made when Kohler and Milstein demonstrated that it was possible to immortalize individual antibody-producing cells by fusing them to mouse myeloma cells. The ability to generate hybridoma cell lines producing antibodies with desired binding specificities has provided the means to identify, purify, characterize and quantitate biologically important molecules in every scientific discipline. The antigenic determinants recognized by hybridoma antibodies include, among other things, cell surface and tumor antigens, small molecules such as drugs, and soluble proteins. The limitless availability of these antibodies has enabled investigators to standardize their reagents.

However, even with the development of hybridomas, limitations persisted. Although hybridoma proteins that bind a defined antigen can be identified, the affinity of that binding cannot be determined by the researcher. Furthermore, the isotype of the antibody is determined by the constant-region gene used by the normal cell at the time of fusion. Therefore it is not always possible to generate antibodies with the precise specificity desired or with the appropriate combination of specificity and effector function. An additional problem with hybridomas is their species limitations. While it is relatively easy to produce mouse or rat monoclonals, it has been difficult to produce human monoclonals which would be desirable for certain applications.

One approach to resolving these limitations has been the isolation of somatic mutants of hybridoma cells. Cell lines with both decreased and increased affinity for antigens can be isolated (Cook and Scharff 1977; Cook *et al.* 1982). In addition it is possible to isolate isotype switch variants and variants with structural changes in their Fc region (Preud'homme *et al.* 1975; Liesegang *et al.* 1978; Yelton and Scharff 1982; Muller and Rejewsky 1983).

An alternative approach to overcoming these limitations is provided by the development of transfectomas in which a combination of recombinant DNA techniques and gene transfection can be used to create novel immunoglobulin molecules.

Approaches to gene transfection in lymphoid cells

To produce large quantities of a novel protein, stable transfectants which provide a continuous source of that protein need to be isolated. Because only a small percentage (10^{-3}–10^{-4}) of the lymphoid cells exposed to foreign DNA become stably transformed, selective techniques which permit the isolation of these rare transformed cells are required. Dominant selectable markers are preferred since they can produce a selectable change in the phenotype of a normal, non-drugmarked cell.

The most commonly used vectors have been the pSV2 vectors (Mulligan and Berg 1980, 1981) in which bacterial genes have been placed in mammalian transcription units under the control of the SV40 early promoter. Two selectable bacterial genes have been used: (1) the xanthine–guanine phosphoribosyl transferase gene (*gpt*) (Mulligan and Berg 1981); and (2) the phosphotransferase gene from Tn5 (*neo*) (Southern and Berg 1982). The enzyme encoded by the *gpt* gene can use xanthine as a substrate for purine nucleotide synthesis, whereas the analogous endogenous enzyme cannot. Thus normal cells, in which the conversion of inosine monophosphate to xanthine monophosphate is blocked by mycophenolic acid, will die if xanthine is provided as a substrate, while cells expressing *gpt* will survive. The product of the *neo* gene inactivates the antibiotic G418 (Franklin and Cook 1969; Davies and Jiminez 1980) which blocks protein synthesis in eukaryotic cells. It is important to note that these two selection procedures depend on two entirely different mechanisms.

To create a transfectoma cell line both the heavy and light chain of an immunoglobulin must be transfected into the same myeloma cells. In initial experiments two approaches were used: (1) heavy and light chains were placed on vectors with different selectable markers (*neo* and *gpt*); first a cell line expressing heavy chain was isolated and this was transfected with light chains to produce a transfectoma synthesizing both heavy and light chains (Morrison *et al.* 1984); (2) heavy and light chains were both cloned into the same transfection vector (Boulianne *et al.* 1984). The first approach requires multiple steps and is very time-consuming while the second approach makes genetic manipulations of heavy and light chains difficult.

To overcome both of these problems we have developed new transfection vectors (Oi and Morrison 1986) that can compatibly replicate and amplify in *Escherichia coli* (Fig. 1). This means the plasmids can be genetically manipulated separately but can be placed and maintained together in the same bacterium and, therefore, can be simultaneously delivered to a myeloma cell by protoplast fusion (see below).

The light chain vector (pSV184ΔH*neo*) is derived from the pACYC184 plasmid and contains the pACYC origin of replication, a chloramphenicol resistance gene for selection in *E. coli* and the *neo* gene for selection of eukaryotic cells. The immunoglobulin heavy chain transfection vector (pSV2ΔH*gpt*) is derived from pSV2*gpt* and contains the pBR322 origin of

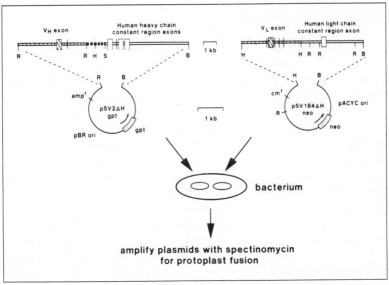

Figure 1. Simultaneous gene transfer using replication compatible plasmid vectors. The vectors contain origins of replication from either pBR or pACYC and hence are compatible. The existence of a chloramphenicol resistance gene on one (*cm*^r) and of an ampicillin resistance gene on the other (*amp*^r) permits their simultaneous selection in *E. coli*. The *neo* and *gpt* genes provide independent dominant selectable markers in eukaryotic cells. Cloned heavy chain variable regions can be inserted into the *Eco*R1 site of the heavy chain vectors. The heavy chain constant regions are on a unique Sal-Bam fragment; therefore, any constant region can easily be inserted 3' of the variable region. The light chain variable region can be inserted as a *Hind*III fragment. (From Oi and Morrison 1986.)

replication, an ampicillin resistance gene for selection in *E. coli* and the *gpt* gene for selection in eukaryotic cells. The pBR and pACYC origins of replication are compatible so selection with chloramphenicol and ampicillin permits isolation of bacteria with normal copy numbers of both plasmids. Since, as described above, *neo* and *gpt* are also independent selectable markers, eukaryotic cells expressing both transfected genes can be isolated in one step. These vectors are illustrated in Fig. 1.

Several methods exist for introducing DNA into eukaryotic cells; however, protoplast fusion has been shown to be an efficient method for introducing DNA into lymphoid cells (Sandri-Goldin *et al.* 1981; Oi *et al.* 1983). In this method, lysozyme is used to remove the bacterial cell walls from *E. coli* bearing the plasmids of interest and the resulting spheroplasts are fused with myeloma cells by means of polyethylene glycol using the same procedures used to produce hybridomas (Oi and Morrison 1986). Stable transfectants can be isolated at frequencies ranging from 10^{-3} to 10^{-7} depending on the recipient cell line and the transfection vectors which are used.

Production of novel Ig molecules

Both the heavy and light chains of Ig are encoded by multiple DNA segments. A functional Ig gene is generated only after somatic rearrangement of distinct DNA segments. However, in the functional Ig gene, intervening sequences separate the hydrophobic leader sequence from the variable region and also the variable-region gene segment from the constant region; in addition, intervening sequences separate the different domains of the constant region so that each functional region of the heavy chain constant region is on a separate exon (Fig. 2).

This exon organization of the antibody molecule greatly facilitates its genetic manipulation. Since the intervening sequences (IVS) are removed by splicing and are not present in the mature mRNA, joining of different DNA segments within the intervening sequences does not have to pay attention to reading frame. In addition, large segments of the IVS are not necessary for Ig gene function so these regions can be removed or duplicated and functional Ig genes are still produced.

Since the variable-region domains which determine the antigen-binding specificity of the antibody molecule are encoded in distinct exons, antibody molecules of different specificities can be produced by changing these exons. Variable regions can be expressed associated with different constant regions. Thus the isotype and hence the effector function of an antibody molecule can be changed. This can be done within a species to produce intraspecies isotype switch molecules. In addition antibody-combining sites from one species can be expressed associated with constant regions from a different species, resulting in interspecies isotype switching. An example of this type of molecule in

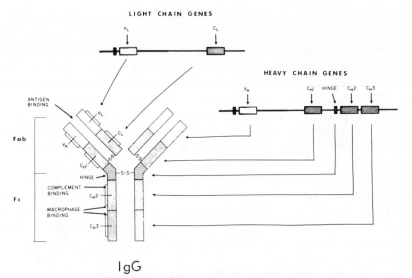

LIGHT CHAIN GENES

HEAVY CHAIN GENES

IgG

Figure 2. Structure of an IgG molecule and the genes that encode it. The regions of the molecule that participate in antigen binding (Fab) or different effector functions (Fc) are indicated. Arrows indicate the correspondence between the DNA segments and the different domains of the Ig polypeptide chain they encode. The existence of intervening sequences between the domains of the Ig greatly facilitates its genetic manipulation. The hydrophobic leader sequence of both heavy and light chains is removed immediately after synthesis and so is absent in the mature Ig molecule. (From Morrison 1985.)

which the variable region from a mouse myeloma protein is expressed associated with human constant regions will be discussed below. In addition hybrid antibodies can be produced by exchanging exons from different heavy chain isotypes and joining them in novel combinations.

The expression vectors which we have developed have been designed as cassette vectors to facilitate the genetic engineering of antibody molecules. Novel restriction sites have been introduced into the intervening sequences separating the variable regions from the constant regions. Thus it is easy to insert any variable region 5' of either the heavy or light chain constant regions.

Among the interesting Ig molecules which can be created by gene transfection are those in which the variable regions from the heavy and light chains of a mouse myeloma are joined to human constant regions. These molecules should have the antigen-binding specificity of the mouse hybridoma but they should exhibit the effector functions of the human constant regions and should be less antigenic in humans than are totally mouse antibodies.

Initially the variable region from the heavy chain of the anti-phosphocholine myeloma was joined to either human γ_1 or γ_2 heavy chain, and the variable region of the light chain was joined to human C_κ. Transfectants synthesizing both chimeric heavy and light chains were isolated (Morrison *et al.* 1984). The chimeric heavy and light chains were of the expected molecular weight and assembled into H_2L_2 molecules which were secreted. The chimeric H_2L_2 molecules bound the antigen phosphocholine and were recognized by both the monoclonal antibodies specific for human κ chain and by monoclonal antibodies specific for the idiotype of the S107 myeloma (Fig. 3). The cells from the transfectoma produced an ascites after being injected into a mouse and the chimeric proteins were present in the ascitic fluid.

Chimeric human–mouse molecules have also been produced in which the variable regions of heavy and light chains were linked to human μ and κ genes respectively (Boulianne *et al.* 1984). In addition a chimeric molecule was produced in which the variable region from a mouse antibody to 4-hydroxy-3-nitrophenacetyl (NP) was joined to human ε heavy chain and expressed associated with a mouse λ light chain of the appropriate sequence (Neuberger *et al.* 1985). In both cases the chimeric molecule had the predicted properties; however, the chimeric anti-TNP antibody showed a displaced binding curve in hapten inhibition assays.

More recently chimeric antibodies have been produced which recognize cell surface antigens. These include chimeric antibodies which recognize the Leu 3 antigen characteristic of a subset of human T lymphocytes (Oi *et al.* in preparation) and antibodies which recognize tumor-associated antigens (Sahagan *et al.* 1986; Sun *et al.* 1986). These engineered antibodies are exactly what would be expected based on their genetic blueprint. Thus this approach is generally applicable to the production of functional antibody molecules.

Heavy chain proteins can exist as either membrane or secreted immunoglobulins. In B lymphocytes heavy chains are primarily of the membrane form; as differentiation to plasma cells takes place, there is an increase in the level of heavy chain synthesis and a switch from being primarily of the membrane form to being primarily of the secreted form. The processing of transfected heavy chain genes mirrors the processing seen in the recipient cell type (Kobrin *et al.* 1986). That is, when the recipient cell type is a lymphoma, processing is largely to the membrane form. When the recipient cell is of the plasma cell lineage, the heavy chain gene transcripts are processed primarily to the secreted form.

Alterations in the sequences 3' of Ig genes can lead to alterations in the processing of the transcripts to either the membrane or the secreted form. When a deletion of 830 bases beginning 22 base pairs beyond the AATAA polyA additional signal was made in the intervening sequence between CH_3 and the first membrane exon in the γ_{2b} heavy chain gene, the processing pattern of this gene following transfection was found to be changed so that when this gene was transfected into a myeloma recipient it was processed primarily to the membrane form. A second deletion beginning 53 bases 3' of the first deletion was found to give rise to transcripts which were processed in the same pattern as transcripts from the unaltered gene. These experiments suggest that within the 53 bases absent in the first deletion but present in the second, are signals important for heavy chain processing (Kobrin *et al.* 1986).

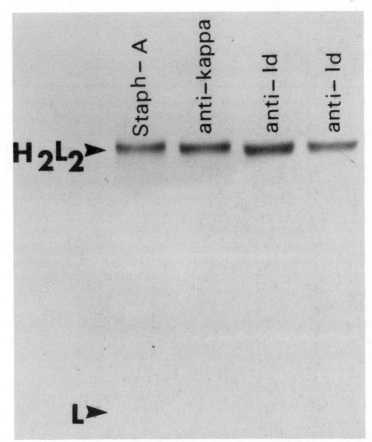

Figure 3. Chimeric Igs produced by a transfectoma. A transfectoma synthesizing a chimeric Ig with V_H and V_L from the anti-phosphocholine myeloma S107 and human γ_2 and κ constant regions was grown in medium containing ^{14}C-valine, threonine and leucine. Secreted Igs were passed through a phosphocholine column and specifically bound protein eluted with phosphocholine. The eluted proteins were precipitated using either *Staph* protein A, a monoclonal anti-human κ, or two different monoclonal anti-idiotype recognizing the idiotype present on the S107 myeloma (gift of A. Giusti and M D Scharff). The precipitated proteins were fractionated on 5% SDS–polyacrylamide gels and the position of the radioactive proteins determined by auto-radiography. (Figure from Morrison *et al.* 1984.)

In addition to using gene transfection to study the signals necessary for mRNA processing, it is also possible to use transfection to produce cell lines producing predominately membrane Ig. The new cell lines can then be used to study the mechanisms of signaling using membrane Ig. In initial studies, it has been shown that cross-linking of Ig expressed from transfected gene induces a calcium flux, in much the same way as does crosslinking of the normal membrane Ig (Mizuguchi *et al.* 1986). The ability to produce such cell lines provides a potential means to identify and characterize the protein sequences important for intracellular signaling.

Application to additional antibody molecules

A functional Ig gene is produced only after DNA rearrangement. Therefore the antibodies produced by myeloma and hybridoma cells are encoded by the V_H and V_L genes that have been rearranged next to the expressed heavy and light chain genes. The strategy to identify the expressed variable-region genes from among the many non-expressed variable regions relies on identifying which variable regions have been rearranged. In each case functional re-arrangement requires joining a variable region to a J region segment. There-fore, a DNA probe hybridizing to sequences immediately 3' of the J regions can be used to identify rearranged V region genes. Unrearranged germ-line DNA can be distinguished from expressed rearranged V region by Southern blot analysis of genomic DNA from antibody-producing cells cleaved with the appropriate restriction endonuclease. A complete genomic library or an enriched DNA restriction fragment library is then screened to clone the appropriate V genes. The use of probes hybridizing to sequences 3' of the rearranged V region permits one to use the same probes to isolate any variable region. Therefore expressed variable regions can be cloned without any specific knowledge of their sequence.

The fact that myeloma and hybridoma cell lines frequently contain more than one rearranged V_H and V_L gene complicates this analysis and often requires the cloning of more than one V region. Since these additional rearranged V regions are frequently found as aberrant transcripts in the cytoplasm, the use of cDNAs in screening the genomic library does not necessarily solve this problem. If only one Ig light chain mRNA and one heavy chain mRNA is present, confirmation that the correct V region gene has been cloned is done by Northern blot analysis using the cloned V gene as a probe. When more than one Ig light chain or heavy chain mRNA is present in an antibody-producing cell line, the correct V gene can be identified by expressing the cloned V genes and determining which gene encodes the desired immunoglobulin polypeptide chain.

Production of other novel molecules

The ability to manipulate genetically and express Ig genes by gene transfec-tion provides the virtually unlimited potential to produce novel antibody molecules.

Antibody combining regions can be placed on sequences with which they are not normally associated. V_H from an anti-azophenylarsonate myeloma was joined to C_κ. When introduced into a light-chain-producing variant of the same myeloma from which the gene was isolated, the V_H–C_κ protein was synthesized and assembled with the endogenous light chain to yield a secreted light chain heterodimer which bound antigen (Sharon *et al.* 1984). A chimeric molecule was also produced in which V_H from human was joined to mouse C_κ (Tan *et al.* 1985). This chimeric protein was synthesized but not secreted. Light chain heterodimers represent an antibody-combining site with no associated effector functions, as light chain constant regions have no known effector function.

Chimeric molecules can also be produced in which Ig and non-Ig sequences are joined (Neuberger *et al.* 1984), The gene for *Staphylococcus aureus* nuclease was inserted into the CH_2 exon of a mouse γ_2 heavy chain specific for NP. When this construction was transfected into J558L, it was synthesized and assembled with the λ light chain to form an NP-binding protein. Molecules of the appropriate size to be H_2L_2 were isolated from the secretions: these molecules bound the antigen NP and had a nuclease activity similar to that of the *S. aureus* nuclease. In the same study the CH_2 and CH_3 domains of the heavy chain were replaced with the third exon of *c-myc*. The chimeric proteins produced following transfection bound antigen and were recognized by a monoclonal antibody to *c-myc*.

Future directions and applications

All experiments to date have demonstrated the feasibility of producing novel Ig molecules by gene transfection. Myeloma cells appear to be the best recipient for Ig genes because the transfected Ig genes are faithfully transcribed, translated and glycosylated in them. Protoplast fusion is an efficient method of introducing genes into most lymphoid cells.

Chimeric Ig molecules provide a new family of reagents with wide potential application. Changing the Fc portion of the Ig can alter its ability to bind staphylococcal protein A, to be multivalent, or to fix complement and therefore affect the usefulness of the Ig for many *in vitro* assays. Molecules with increased or decreased binding affinity can be useful in creating detection assays with differing levels of sensitivity and stringency.

In addition to creating large changes in Ig molecules by moving exons, small changes can be made using *in vitro* mutagenesis. It should be possible to generate molecules lacking only one specific effector function, to eliminate or generate glycosylation sites or, through small changes in the variable region, to increase or decrease affinity for antigen.

The new technology provides tools which expand the utility of rodent hybridoma antibodies and complements the developing human hybridoma technology. Chimeric human–mouse antibodies should be less immunogenic when used in man than totally mouse antibodies. In addition, chimeric Igs have the advantage that they can be optimized for a specific, desired effector function. Thus even if more human monoclonals become available, chimeric molecules might be preferred because of the feasibility of 'tailormaking' their effector functions.

Acknowledgements

This study was supported by Public Health Service grants AI 19042, CA 16858, CA 22376 and CA 13696 (to the Cancer Center) from the National Institutes of Health and by grant IMS-360 from the American Cancer Society.

References

Boulianne G L, Hozumi N, Shulman M J 1984. Production of functional chimaeric mouse/human antibody, *Nature (London)* **312**: 643–6

Cook W D, Scharff M D 1977. Antigen-binding mutants of mouse myeloma cells, *Proceedings of the National Academy of Sciences USA* **74**: 5687–91

Cook W D, Rudikoff S, Giusti A M, Scharff M D 1982. Somatic mutation in a cultured mouse myeloma cell affects antigen binding, *Proceedings of the National Academy of Sciences USA* **79**: 1240–4

Davies J, Jiminez A 1980. A new selective agent for eukaryotic cloning vectors, *American Journal of Tropical Medicine and Hygiene* **29**(5) (Supplement): 1089–92

Franklin T J, Cook J M 1969. The inhibition of nucleic acid synthesis by mycophenolic acid, *Biochemical Journal* **113**: 515–24

Kobrin B J, Milcarek C, Morrison S L 1986. Sequences near the 3' secretion-specific polyadenylation site influence levels of secretion-specific and membrane-specific IgG$_{2b}$ mRNA in myeloma cells, *Molecular and Cellular Biology* **6**: 1687–97

Kohler G, Milstein C 1974. Continuous cultures of fused cells secreting antibodies of predefined specificity, *Nature (London)* **256**: 495–7

Liesegang B, Radbruch A, Rajewsky K 1978. Isolation of myeloma variants with predefined variant surface immunoglobulin by cell sorting, *Proceedings of the National Academy of Sciences USA* **75**: 3901–5

Mizuguchi J, Tsang W, Monion S L, Bevan M A, Paul W E 1986. Membrane IgM, IgD and IgG act as signal transmission molecules in a series of B lymphomas. *Journal of Immunology* **137**: 2162–7

Morrison S L 1985. Transfectomas provide novel chimeric antibodies *Science* **229**: 1202–7

Morrison S L, Johnson M J, Herzenberg L A, Oi V T 1984. Chimeric human antibody molecules: mouse antigen-binding domains with human constant region domains, *Proceedings of the National Academy of Sciences USA* **81**: 6851–5

Muller C E, Rajewsky K 1983. Isolation of immunoglobulin class switch variants from hybridoma lines secreting anti-idiotope antibodies by sequential sublining, *Journal of Immunology* **131**: 877–81

Mulligan R C, Berg P 1980. Expression of a bacterial gene in mammalian cells, *Science* **209**: 1422–7

Mulligan R C, Berg P 1981. Selection for animal cells that express the *Escherichia coli* gene coding for xanthine–guanine phosphoribosyltransferase. *Proceedings of the National Academy of Sciences USA* **78**: 2072–6

Neuberger M S, Williams G T, Fox R O 1984. Recombinant antibodies possessing novel effector functions, *Nature (London)* **312**: 604–8

Neuberger M S, Williams G T, Mitchell E B, Jonhal S S, Flanagan J G, Rabbitts T H 1985. A hapten-specific chimaeric IgE antibody with human physiological effector function, *Nature (London)* **314**: 268–70

Oi V T, Morrison S L 1986. Chimeric antibodies, *BioTechniques* **4**: 214–21

Oi V T, Morrison S L, Herzenberg L A, Berg P 1983. Immunoglobulin gene expression in transformed lymphoid cells, *Proceedings of the National Academy of Sciences USA* **80**: 825–9

230

Oi V T, Federspiel N, Hinton P, McNally M, Roark L, Waters V 1987. (In preparation)

Preud'homme J-L, Birshtein B K, Scharff M D 1975. Variants of a mouse myeloma cell line that synthesize immunoglobulin heavy chains having an altered serotype, *Proceedings of the National Academy of Sciences USA* **72**: 1427–30

Sahagan B K, Dorai H, Saltzgaber-Muller J, Toneguzzo F, Gundon C A, Lilly S P, McDonald K W, Morrissey D V, Stone B A, Davis G L, McIntosh P K, Moore G P 1986. A genetically-engineered murine/human chimeric antibody retains specificity for human tumor-associated antigen, *Journal of Immunology* **137**: 1066–74

Sandri-Goldin R M, Goldin A L, Levine M, Glorioso J C 1981. High frequency transfer of cloned herpes simplex virus type 1 sequences to mammalian cells by protoplast fusion, *Molecular and Cellular Biology* **1**: 743–52

Sharon J, Gefter M L, Manser T, Morrison S L, Oi V T, Ptashne M 1984. Expression of a $V_H C_\kappa$ chimeric protein in mouse myeloma cells. *Nature (London)* **309**: 364–7

Southern P J, Berg P 1982. Transformation of mammalian cells to antibiotic resistance with a bacterial gene under control of the SV40 early region promoter, *Journal of Molecular and Applied Genetics* **1**: 327–41

Sun L K, Curtis P, Rakowicz-Szulczynska E, Ghrayeb J, Morrison S L, Chang N, Koprowski H 1986. Chimeric antibodies with 17-1A-derived variable and human constant regions, *Hybridoma* **5** (Supplement 1): S17–S20

Tan L K, Oi V T, Morrison S L 1985. A human–mouse chimeric immunoglobulin gene with a human variable region is expressed in mouse myeloma cells, *Journal of Immunology* **135**: 3564–7

Tiselius A, Kabat E A 1939. An electrophoretic study of immune sera and purified antibody preparation, *Journal of Experimental Medicine* **69**: 119–31

Yelton D E, Scharff M D 1982. Mutant monoclonal antibodies with alterations in biological functions, *Journal of Experimental Medicine* **156**: 1131–48

Humoral and cellular responses in man to hepatitis B vaccination: analysis with synthetic peptides

Michael W Steward; Barbara M Sisley; Carolynne M Stanley; Sheila E Brown; Colin R Howard

Department of Medical Microbiology, London School of Hygiene and Tropical Medicine, Keppel Street, London WC1E 7HT, United Kingdom

Introduction

There are more than 280 million persistent carriers of hepatitis B virus (HBV) throughout the world, representing a major risk of transmission via contaminated blood, via blood products and via maternal or close personal contact (Tiollais *et al.* 1985). Furthermore, there is a clear association of the development of primary liver cancer with HBV infection (Zuckerman 1982). This situation has led to intense effort in the development of an HBV vaccine. A vaccine derived by extensive purification of the surface antigen (HBsAg) from plasma is available (Hilleman *et al.* 1983) but its restricted availability and expense make it of limited value for use in regions of high endemicity. There is thus an urgent need for the development of a cheap and efficacious hepatitis B vaccine for mass vaccination. New vaccines comprised of synthetic polypeptides which mimic naturally occurring antigenic structures present on infectious agents would offer many advantages over current vaccines, particularly in terms of uniformity, safety and cost (Steward and Howard 1987). In this context, the recent rapid advances in protein chemistry and molecular biology have provided the impetus for the identification of immunogenic determinants of infectious agents, their chemical synthesis and subsequent testing as components of potential vaccines.

HBsAg particles contain a major 25,000 MW protein consisting of 226 amino acids which also exists in a glycosylated form of MW 30,000. Both these forms bear the antigenic determinants responsible for the induction of protective antibody (Szmuness *et al.* 1980). These determinants, termed group 'a' determinants, are expressed by all virus isolates and have been shown to lie within the region spanned by amino acid residues 110–155 (Bhatnager *et al.* 1982). Within this sequence, residues 139–147 represent the major hydrophilic area of the predominantly hydrophobic molecule and it is this region which we and others have proposed as an important component of any potential synthetic hepatitis B vaccine (Brown *et al.* 1984a, 1984b;

Bhatnager *et al.* 1982). Additional sequences expressed by the pre-S region of the genome are also to be found as major components of HBV virions. Pre-S determinants expressed by initiation of translation upstream to the gene coding for the HBsAg p25 polypeptide are thought important for the binding of virus to hepatocytes and therefore their presence is desirable in future hepatitis B vaccines (reviewed by Howard 1986).

Work from other laboratories has shown that synthetic peptides mimicking selected regions of HBsAg, and coupled to carrier molecules, induce antibodies in experimental animals which cross-react with the native molecule (Lerner *et al.* 1981; Bhatnager *et al.* 1982). We have used sera from infected individuals and recipients of the licensed hepatitis B vaccine and a number of polyclonal and monoclonal antibodies to assess the extent to which synthetic peptide antigens (derived from the sequence 124–147 of HBsAg) mimic antigens which are expressed by the virus and are recognized by the immune system. Our strategy has included the measurement of the affinity of the antibodies induced by the native antigen for the synthetic peptides (Steward and Steensgaard 1983). Since the affinity of antibody binding to a peptide reflects the closeness or 'fit' or complementarity of the antibody combining site to the conformation of the peptide, then the higher the affinity constant for the reaction, the closer the similarity of the peptide to the determinant expressed in the native molecule. The affinity of antibodies to HBsAg in human sera for a linear synthetic peptide representing residues 139–147 was significantly higher than for a linear peptide representing residues 124–137 (a second hydrophilic region) in HBsAg. Furthermore, the cyclization of these peptides resulted in a significant increase in the observed affinity values. The cyclized 139–147 (C139) peptide was bound with a higher affinity than was the cyclical 124–137 peptide (C124) by antibodies from vaccine recipients, patients who had recovered from acute hepatitis B and by pooled anti-HBs antibodies (Brown *et al.* 1984a, 1984b; and Table 1).

At the cellular level of response to HBsAg, there have been several reports on the absence of HBsAg-induced lymphocyte proliferation in acute hepatitis and chronic HBsAg carriers (e.g. Hanson *et al.* 1984) although such stimulation has been demonstrated using purified peripheral T cells and monocytes

Table 1 The affinities ($\times 10^6 \, \text{M}^{-1} \pm$ SD) of anti-HBs antibodies for linear and cyclical synthetic peptides representing residues 124–147 of HBsAg

Peptide	Anti-HBs sera	
	From recovered acute hepatitis B patients	From vaccine recipients (after 3 doses)
Linear 139–147	3.6 ± 3.2	4.8 ± 2.7
Cyclical 138–147	21.0 ± 22.0	50.0 ± 44.0
Linear 124–137	0.5 ± 0.3	0.4 ± 0.2
Cyclical 124–137	2.5 ± 1.4	1.8 ± 1.6

from asymptomatic carriers (Sylvan *et al.* 1985). Lymphocyte stimulation in vaccine recipients has been studied, but only limited information is available on responses to synthetic HBsAg peptides (Milich *et al.* 1985). In this paper, we describe sequential studies of antibody and lymphocyte responses to HBsAg and synthetic HBsAg peptides in recipients of a plasma-derived vaccine during the course of immunization.

Materials and methods

Sera and lymphocytes

Serum samples and peripheral blood lymphocyte preparations were obtained at various times during immunization of six healthy laboratory personnel with a plasma-derived HBV vaccine (Hep-B vax; Merck Sharp and Dohme).

Antigens

HBsAg was purified from a pool of serum from asymptomatic carriers of hepatitis B (Skelly *et al.* 1979). Native HBsAg was dissociated by overnight incubation at 37 °C in 2% Triton X-100. The soluble complex of the HBsAg polypeptide (p25) and its glycosylated form (gp30) was isolated by binding to a concanavalin A–Sepharose column and subsequent elution with 0.01 M-Tris/HCl buffer, pH 7.3, containing 0.2% Triton X-100 and 5% methyl-D-mannoside (Young *et al.* 1982). Synthetic peptides representing regions within amino acid residues 124–147 of the HBsAg and residues 126–140 of the pre-S2 region were produced by solid-phase synthesis. Peptides representing residues 124–137 and 139–147 were synthesized in both linear and cyclical forms.

Antibody assays

Levels of serum anti-HBs antibodies were assessed by commercial solid-phase radioimmunoassay (AUSAB; Abbott Laboratories, Chicago). The affinities of anti-HBs antibodies for the radiolabeled gp30p25 polypeptide complex and synthetic peptides were determined as previously described (Steward 1978; Brown *et al.* 1984a).

Lymphocyte stimulation assays

Peripheral blood lymphocytes (2×10^5) were isolated from heparinized blood samples drawn at various times during immunization with the HBV vaccine by centrifugation on Ficoll-hypaque and were incubated for four days with either HBsAg or synthetic peptides, pulsed with $1\,\mu\text{Ci}$ [³H]thymidine (Amersham) and harvested 18 hours later. Stimulation indices (SI) were calculated as the ratio of the mean [³H] counts per minute of quadruplicate samples of cells incubated with antigen or peptides to the mean [³H] counts per minute of quadruplicate samples cultured in the absence of antigen and peptide. A stimulation index of greater than 2.0 was considered positive.

Results

Immune responses following two doses of vaccine

Antibody and lymphocyte responses in the six vaccine recipients were analysed with HBsAg, the gp30p25 polypeptide complex and the synthetic C139 peptide.

Antibody responses

As demonstrated in previous studies (Brown *et al.* 1984b), serum antibody levels assessed by the AUSAB assay and by radioimmunoassay for binding to gp30p25 polypeptide complex and the cyclical 139–147 peptide (C139) increased with time after the second vaccine dose in four of the six recipients. One recipient had no demonstrable antibody to either HBsAg or the peptides and a second received passive immunoglobulin at the time of the first vaccine dose. Antibodies binding to HBsAg in the AUSAB assay and to gp30p25 in

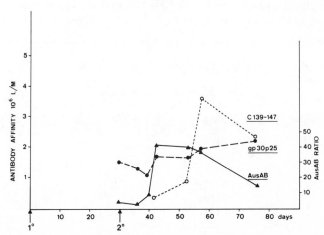

Figure 1. Sequential serum antibody responses in one recipient following two doses of the vaccine. ▲——▲, AUSAB titre; ●——● affinity for gp30p25; ○——○, affinity for the C139 peptide.

the radioimmunoassay were demonstrable before those capable of binding to the C139 peptide. Furthermore, there was a progessive increase in affinity of antibodies for both the gp30p25 and C139 following the second dose of vaccine. Data on the antibody responses of one of the six recipients studied after two vaccine doses are shown in Fig. 1.

Lymphocyte stimulation

In contrast to data published by others, we have demonstrated positive lymphocyte stimulation to HBsAg in six out of six recipients of the HB vaccine. In addition, of these six individuals, five showed a positive lymphocyte stimulation by the C139 but not to the linear form of the same peptide. Positive lymphocyte stimulation by HBsAg (between 7 and 20 days following second vaccine dose) precedes that for the peptide (between 15 and 60 days following second vaccine dose) and corresponded to the time when antibody to the surface antigen could be detected in the serum. In one individual, lymphocyte stimulation by both HBsAg and the C139 was observed in the absence of detectable serum antibody. Maximum stimulation by HBsAg was greater than for that by C139 and occurred earlier following the second dose of vaccine (Table 2).

The ability of C139 to stimulate lymphocytes was demonstrated after the detection of serum antibodies to the peptide. Figure 2 represents the sequential lymphocyte responses of one recipient after two vaccine doses.

Immune responses following three doses of vaccine

The responses of four of the six original vaccine recipients after the third dose of vaccine were analyzed with HBsAg, gp30p25 and a panel of synthetic HBsAg peptides: cyclical and linear 139–147; cyclical and linear 124–137 and a pre-S2 peptide, representing residues 126–140 of the pre-S2 region.

Table 2 Lymphocyte stimulation following two doses of vaccine

Vaccine recipient	Maximum stimulation index*	
	HBsAg	C139
BS	3.5 (30)	2.8 (60)
MS	3.5 (45)	4.0 (45)
KM	9.6 (60)	2.5 (30)
CS	3.0 (15)	2.2 (15)
FI	2.0 (10)	2.1 (10)
KB	2.2 (2)	1.9 (65)
Average	4.0 (27)	2.6 (38)

* Numbers in parentheses represent day of maximum response post-second vaccine dose.

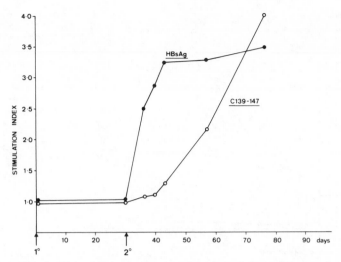

Figure 2. Sequential lymphocyte responses in one recipient after two doses of the vaccine. Stimulation indices following incubation with ●——●, HBsAg and ○——○, C139 peptide.

Antibody responses

Following the third dose of vaccine, levels and affinities of antibodies for HBsAg and related peptides showed a progressive increase. Maximum affinity values for the gp30p25 polypeptide complex and the C139 peptide were of the order of five- and ten-fold higher respectively than the corresponding maximum values after two doses of vaccine. Furthermore, in all four recipients, the affinities of antibodies for the C139 peptide were considerably higher (up to 50-fold) than for the cyclical 124–137 (C124) peptide. Figure 3 represents antibody responses, analyzed by AUSAB, synthetic peptides and the gp30p25 polypeptide complex, in one vaccine recipient following the third dose of vaccine.

Lymphocyte stimulation

At intervals following the third dose of vaccine, lymphocytes from the four recipients were cultured in the presence of each of the panel of antigens and their stimulation indices determined (Table 3). In all recipients, stimulation indices with HBsAg were significantly higher than with the peptides and maximum stimulation by HBsAg preceded that for the peptides. Of the peptides studied, only C139 induced lymphocyte stimulation in all vaccine recipients. There were individual variations in both the time and level of maximum stimulation by the peptides and in addition, differences were observed in lymphocyte stimulation induced by the cyclical and linear forms of the peptides. Thus in two individuals, C139 showed a greater ability to stimulate primed lymphocytes than did the linear form, whereas in others the

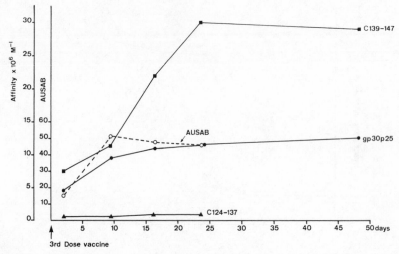

Figure 3. Sequential serum antibody responses in one recipient following the third dose of vaccine. ○---○, AUSAB titre; ●——●, affinity for gp30p25; ▲——▲, affinity for C124 and ■——■, affinity for C139 peptide.

Table 3 Lymphocyte stimulation following three doses of vaccine

Vaccine recipient	Maximum stimulation index					
	HBsAg	C139	L139	C124	L124	PreS
BS	7.0	2.1	4.0	2.3	2.4	4.9
MS	15.0	2.8	1.4	1.9	1.8	1.7
CS	31.6	2.3	3.3	3.0	1.6	1.2
KM	26.6	2.3	2.2	3.1	2.6	2.0
Average	20.0	2.4	2.7	2.6	2.1	2.5

converse was observed. The C124 peptide appeared to be more effective than the corresponding linear form.

Lymphocytes from two recipients showed repeated positive stimulation by the pre-S2 peptide following the third dose of vaccine. Neither of these individuals had demonstrable serum antibody to the pre-S2 peptide or a hepatitis B core peptide, nor did these lymphocytes proliferate in the presence of the HB core peptide.

Discussion

We have demonstrated that synthetic peptides can be used to probe both the humoral and cellular immune responses to hepatitis B vaccine in man. Antibody responses following immunization were analyzed by the assessment of the affinity of the antibodies for synthetic peptides representing the region spanning amino acids 124–147, a region of the HBsAg molecule in which the 'a' group determinants are located. The affinities of antibodies for these antigens increased during the immunization protocol. However, cyclical forms of the peptides were bound with higher affinity than were the linear forms. Furthermore, C139 was bound with a significantly higher affinity compared to the C124 peptide. Thus, in view of the superiority of high-affinity antibody over lower-affinity antibody in a number of biological functions (Steward and Steensgaard 1983) we consider that a synthetic peptide based on the region 139–147 is likely to be a more effective component of a synthetic peptide vaccine than a peptide representing residues 122–137 (Dreesman *et al.* 1982).

Peripheral blood lymphocytes isolated from individuals during the course of vaccination showed *in vitro* stimulation following culture in the presence of HBsAg and a panel of synthetic peptides. All vaccine recipients showed lymphocyte stimulation to HBsAg and to the C139 peptide. There were variations in responsiveness to the other peptides. The observed stimulation of lymphocytes by the pre-S2 peptide was of particular interest since the plasma-derived vaccine is not thought to express a pre-S component as assessed by its absence of reactivity with anti-pre-S antibodies. The data presented here suggest that the vaccine may have pre-S determinants capable of priming T cells but not B cells or, alternatively, pre-S sequences may be closely associated with S sequences. The possibility exists that the pre-S2 peptide could assume a conformation in solution which mimicked an S sequence and thus stimulate T cells.

It is thought that B cells recognize tertiary structures on native protein antigens and that T cells recognize short sequences of amino acids or antigenic fragments. The question of whether T and B cells can recognize the same determinants has been extensively investigated. There are reports that the two cell types recognize the same or overlapping determinants (Bixler and Atassi 1984; Berzofsky *et al.* 1979) whereas others suggest that T and B cells recognize different sites (Berkower *et al.* 1982; Maizels *et al.* 1980) and that T helper cells and T suppressor cells recognize non-overlapping determinants (Wicker *et al.* 1984). Our data suggest that C139 can be recognized by both T and B cells and thus may well be a valuable component of a synthetic hepatitis B vaccine. Further support for the view that this peptide represents an important HBsAg epitope(s) comes from work with monoclonal internal image anti-HBs idiotypes (Thanavala *et al.* 1985). In inhibition radioimmunoassays, the internal image anti-idiotypes can inhibit the binding of both monoclonal and polyclonal anti-HBs antibodies to the C139 peptide (Thanavala *et al.* 1986).

On the basis of the high-affinity binding of anti-HBs antibodies to the C139 peptide, the ability of the peptide to stimulate primed T cells and its similarity to monoclonal internal image anti-HBs idiotypes, we consider this peptide to be the basis of a synthetic hepatitis B vaccine.

Summary

Immune responses in human recipients of a hepatitis B virus vaccine were analyzed with synthetic peptides representing various residues 124–147 of the surface antigen of the virus (HBsAg) and residues 126–140 of the pre-S2 region. Antibody levels and affinities were assessed in radioimmunoassays with synthetic linear and cyclical forms of peptides 124–137 and 139–147, and with the gp30p25 polypeptide complex of HBsAg. Anti-HBs levels were measured by AUSAB assays. Cellular responses were assessed by *in vitro* stimulation of peripheral blood lymphocytes by HBsAg and by the synthetic peptides.

Levels and affinities of antibodies to the antigens increased with time during immunization. However, antibodies binding the cyclical peptide representing amino acids 139–147 (C139) were present at higher levels and had higher affinities than antibodies binding the other peptides, indicating that C139 more closely approximates a domain on the native antigen than do the other peptides.

All vaccine recipients had demonstrable lymphocyte responsiveness to HBsAg after both second and third doses of the vaccine. Of the peptides, only the C139 induced lymphocyte stimulation in all recipients. However, there were individual variations both in the time of initial responsiveness to peptides and in the level and time of maximal stimulation. Stimulation by native HBsAg particles, which corresponded to the appearance of anti-HBs antibody, preceded that observed using synthetic peptides. In all recipients, maximum stimulation indices with HBsAg were significantly higher than those observed with the peptides.

The lymphocytes from three recipients showed positive stimulation in response to the pre-S2 peptide and of these, two showed repeated positivity after the third vaccine dose. None of these individuals had antibodies to pre-S or HB core peptides, nor did their lymphocytes respond to synthetic peptides representing HB core determinants.

These results show that: (1) synthetic peptides can be used effectively to analyze humoral and cellular immune responses; (2) peptides which are bound by serum anti-HBs antibodies are also able to stimulate T cells; and (3) these peptides form the basis of a vaccine for hepatitis B.

Acknowledgement

This work was supported by grants from the Wellcome Trust and the Medical Research Council (U.K.).

References

Berkower I, Buckenmeyer G K, Gurd F R N, Berzofsky J A 1982. A possible immunodominant epitope recognized by murine T lymphocytes immune to different myoglobulins, *Proceedings of the National Academy of Sciences USA* **79**: 4723–7

Berzofsky J A, Richman L K, Killion D J 1979. Distinct H-2 linked Ir genes control both antibody and T-cell responses to different determinants on the same antigen, myoglobin, *Proceedings of the National Academy of Sciences USA* **76**: 4046–50

Bhatnager P K, Papas E, Blum H E, Millich D R, Nitecki D, Karels M J, Vyas G N 1982. Immune response to synthetic peptide analogues of hepatitis B surface antigen specific for the a determinant, *Proceedings of the National Academy of Sciences USA* **79**: 4400–4

Bixler G S, Atassi M Z 1984. T-cell recognition of lysozyme. III. Recognition of the surface simulation synthetic antigen sites, *Journal of Immunogenetics* **11**: 245–50

Brown S E, Howard C R, Zuckerman A J, Steward M W 1984a. Determination of the affinity of antibodies to hepatitis B surface antigen in human sera, *Journal of Immunological Methods* **72**: 41–8

Brown S E, Howard C R, Zuckerman A J, Steward M W 1984b. Affinity of antibody responses in man to hepatitis B vaccine determined with synthetic peptides, *Lancet*, **ii**: 184–7

Dreesman G R, Sanchez Y, Ionescu-Matiu I, Sparro J–T, Six H R, Peterson D L, Hollinger F B, Melnick J L 1982. Antibody to hepatitis B surface antigen after a single inoculation of uncoupled synthetic HBsAg peptides, *Nature (London)* **295**: 158–60

Hanson R G, Hoofnagle J H, Minuk G Y, Purcell R H, Gerin J L 1984. Cell mediated immunity to HBsAg in man, *Clinical and Experimental Immunology* **57**: 257–64

Hilleman M R, McAleer W J, Buynak E B, McLean A A 1983. Quality and safety of human hepatitis B vaccine, *Developments in Biological Standardisation* **54**: 3–12

Howard C R 1986. The biology of hepadnaviruses, *Journal of General Virology* **67**: 1215–35

Lerner R A, Green N, Alexander H, Liu F T 1981. Chemically synthesized peptides predicted from the nucleotide sequence in common with a fragment of a virus protein, the hepatitis B surface antigen, *Proceedings of the National Academy of Sciences USA* **78**: 3403–7

Maizels R M, Clarke J A, Harvey M A, Miller A, Sercarz E E 1980. Epitope specificity of the T-cell proliferative response to lysozyme: proliferative T cells react predominantly to different determinants from those recognised by B cells, *European Journal of Immunology* **10**: 509–15

Milich D R, Peterson d L, Leroux-Roels G G, Lerner R A, Chisari F V 1985. Genetic regulation of the immune response to hepatitis B surface antigen (HBsAg). VI. T-cell fine specificity, *Journal of Immunology* **134**: 4203–11

Skelly J, Howard C R, Zuckerman A J 1979. Analysis of hepatitis B surface antigen components solubilised with Triton X-100, *Journal of General Virology* **44**: 679–89

Steward M W 1978. Introduction to methods used to study antibody–antigen reactions, in D M Weir (ed) *Handbook of Experimental Immunology*, 3rd edn. Blackwell, Oxford

Steward M W, Howard C R 1987. Synthetic peptides: the next generation of vaccines? *Immunology Today* **8**: 51–8

Steward M W, Steensgaard J 1983. *Antibody Affinity: thermodynamic aspects and biological significance*. CRC Press, Boca Raton, Florida

Sylvan S P E, Hellstrom U B, Lundbergh P R 1985. Detection of cellular and humoral immunity to hepatitis B surface antigen in asymptomatic HBsAg carriers, *Clinical and Experimental Immunology* **62**: 288–95

Szmuness W, Stevens C E, Marley E J, Zang E A, Oleszko W R, Williams D C, Sedovsky R, Morrison J M, Kellner A 1980. Hepatitis B vaccine: demonstration of efficacy in a controlled clinical trial in a high-risk population in the United States, *New England Journal of Medicine* **303**: 833–41

Thanavala Y, Bond A, Tedder R, Hay F C, Roitt I M 1985. Monoclonal internal image anti-idiotypic antibodies of hepatitis B surface antigen, *Immunology* **55**: 197–204

Thanavala Y, Brown S E, Howard C R, Roitt I M, Steward M W 1986. A surrogate hepatitis B virus antigenic epitope represented by a synthetic peptide and an internal image anti-idiotype antibody, *Journal of Experimental Medicine* **164**: 227–6

Tiollais P, Pourcell C, Dejean A 1985. The hepatitis B virus, *Nature (London)* **317**: 489–95

Wicker L S, Katz M, Sercarz E E, Miller A 1984. Immunodominant protein epitopes. I. Induction of suppression to hen egg-white lysozyme is obliterated by removal of the first three *N*-terminal amino acids, *European Journal of Immunology* **14**: 442–7

Young P R, Vaudin M, Dixon J, Howard C R and Zuckerman A J 1982. preparation of hepatitis B polypeptide micelles from human carrier plasma, *Journal of Virological Methods* **4**: 177

Zuckerman A J 1982. Primary hepatocellular carcinoma and hepatitis B virus, *Transactions of the Royal Society of Tropical Medicine and Hygiene* **76**: 711–18

5 Production of vaccines by recombinant DNA techniques

Mycobacterial antigens, genes and vaccines

Richard A Young

Whitehead Institute for Biomedical Research, Nine Cambridge Center, Cambridge, Massachusetts 02142, USA
Department of Biology, Massachusetts Institute of Technology, Cambridge, Massachusetts 02139, USA

Several laboratories have pooled their expertise in recombinant DNA expression technology and immunology to describe the immune response to infection by *Mycobacterium leprae* and *M. tuberculosis*. This manuscript briefly summarizes the isolation of genes that encode the major protein antigens of the etiologic agents of leprosy and tuberculosis and the indication that these particular antigens are among those important for the cell-mediated immune response. Laboratories whose work I will summarize include those headed by Dr Barry Bloom (Albert Einstein), Dr Tore Godal (Norwegian Radium Hospital) and my own.

Leprosy is a chronic infectious disease afflicting between 10 and 15 million people and is caused by the obligate intracellular parasite *Mycobacterium leprae* (Bloom and Godal 1983). Although *M. leprae* was the first identified bacterial pathogen of man (Hansen 1874), basic biochemical, immunologic, diagnostic and therapeutic investigations have been severely limited because it remains one of the few human pathogens that has not been cultivated *in vitro*.

Tuberculosis, recognized as the major cause of infectious mortality in Europe and the United States in the 19th and early 20th centuries (Dubos and Dubos 1952), remains a significant global health problem. In the United States there are over 20,000 new cases of tuberculosis annually and the steadily declining incidence of tuberculosis in the preceding several decades appears to have changed course, reaching a plateau in 1985 and showing an actual increase in the first half of 1986. Worldwide, tuberculosis remains widespread and constitutes a health problem of major proportions, particularly in developing countries. The World Health Organization (WHO) recently estimated that there are ten million new cases of active tuberculosis per year with an annual mortality of approximately three million (Joint International Union Against Tuberculosis and World Health Organization Study Group 1982). Tuberculosis is caused by *M. tuberculosis* or *M. bovis*, the 'tubercle bacilli' of the family Mycobacteriaceae.

In 1984 and 1985 WHO sponsored two workshops to characterize murine monoclonal antibodies against mycobacteria (Engers *et al.* 1985, 1986). Fifty-six monoclonal antibodies developed by several independent investigators were analyzed in multiple laboratories and the reactivity of the monoclonal antibodies with several species of mycobacteria was determined. Fourteen of the anti-*M. leprae* protein monoclonal antibodies recognized antigens of sizes 12 kD, 18 kD, 28 kD, 36 kD and 65 kD. Nineteen of the anti-*M. tuberculosis* antibodies bound to seven protein antigens of sizes 12 kD, 14 kD, 19 kD, 23 kD, 38 kD, 65 kD and 71 kD. These antibodies were used as tools to probe recombinant DNA expression libraries to isolate the genes that encode these antigens.

Mycobacterium leprae and *M. tuberculosis* genes encoding immunologically relevant proteins were isolated by systematically screening λgt11 recombinant DNA expression libraries with the collection of murine monoclonal antibodies directed against protein antigens of these pathogens that were characterized by WHO Workshops. DNA sequences encoding five major protein antigens of *M. leprae* were isolated and studied (Young *et al.* 1985). These genes encode the 12 kD, 18 kD, 28 kD, 36 kD and 65 kD antigens. Similarly, *M. tuberculosis* genes encoding 12 kD, 14 kD, 19 kD, 65 kD and 71 kD protein antigens were isolated and characterized (Husson and Young 1987).

The insert DNAs of the recombinant DNA clones were mapped with restriction endonucleases. Figure 1 shows the genomic DNA restriction maps deduced for the genes encoding each of the five *M. leprae* and each of the five *M. tuberculosis* antigens and illustrates how each of the cloned DNAs aligns with that map. All clones isolated with monoclonal antibodies directed against any single antigen align with a single genomic DNA segment. This result indicates that all clones were isolated because they express the protein of interest rather than an unrelated polypeptide containing a similar or identical epitope. In addition this result suggests that each antigen is the product of a single gene.

The recombinant DNA strategy used here to express the coding capacity of the *M. leprae* and *M. tuberculosis* genomes in *Escherichia coli* and detect specific antigenic determinants with monoclonal antibodies appears to be an effective one. Each of the genes of interest were isolated by screening no more than 10% of the recombinant DNA library. These results suggest that a similar approach is feasible with genomic DNA from parasites with more complex genomes, such as schistosomes, filaria, leishmania and plasmodia, parasites that cause disease in hundreds of millions of people.

Because cell-mediated immunity plays a major role in resistance to mycobacterial infection, it was important to determine whether the antigens whose genes we isolated were relevant to T cell responses. To assess the T cell response, T cells were cloned from infected mice, vaccinated humans and patients with leprosy or tuberculosis. Recombinant antigens were produced in *E. coli* and the crude lysate was presented to the T cell clones with the appropriate feeder cells (Mustafa *et al.* 1986). The results were very encourag-

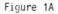

Figure 1A

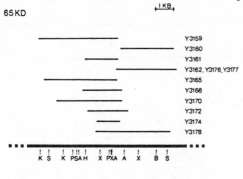

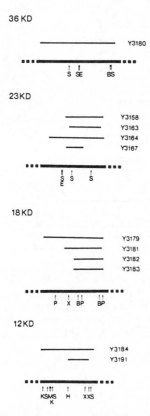

Figure 1A. Restriction maps of *M. leprae* DNA. Recombinant DNA clones isolated by using antibodies directed against the 65 kD, 36 kD, 28 kD, 18 kD and 12 kD antigens were subjected to restriction endonuclease mapping. A, *Sac*I; B, *Bgl*II; E, *Eco*RI; H, *Hind*III; K, *Kpn*I; M, *Bam*HI; P, *Pvu*I; S, *Sal*I; X, *Xho*I.

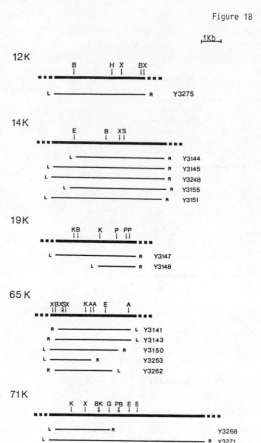

Figure 1B. Restriction maps of *M. tuberculosis* DNA. Recombinant DNA clones isolated with monoclonal antibodies directed against the 12 kD, 14 kD, 19 kD, 65 kD and 71 kD protein antigens were mapped with restriction endonucleases. The insert DNA endpoints are designated left (L) or right (R) in relation to *lac* Z transcripts which traverse the insert from right to left. Restriction enzymes: A, *Sal*I; B, *Bam*HI, E, *Eco*RI; G, *Bgl*II; K, *Kpn*I, P, *Pvu*I; S, *Sac*I; X, *Xho*I.

ing: reactive T helper cells were observed for many of the recombinant antigens. A brief and incomplete summary of these results and further results obtained with antibodies follows.

Among the major antigens of the leprosy bacillus, the 65 kD antigen elicits strong antibody and T cell responses. Both serum antibodies (Britton *et al.* 1985) and T cells (Mustafa *et al.* 1986) directed against the 65 kD *M. leprae* antigen have been observed in patients with leprosy. In addition, T cell clones from leprosy patients have been found to respond to recombinant 65 kD protein of *M. bovis* (Shankar *et al.* 1986; Emmrich *et al.* 1986).

The 18 kD antigen of *M. leprae* is the major antigen recognized by T cells isolated from individuals immunized with killed *M. leprae*.

Considerable evidence indicates that *M. tuberculosis* 65 kD antigen plays an important role in the human immune response to tuberculosis. Antibodies directed against this protein can be detected in the serum of patients with tuberculosis (Thole *et al.* 1985). The 65 kD antigen is present in purified protein derivatives (PPDs) of *M. tuberculosis*, *M. bovis*, and other mycobacteria (Thole *et al.* 1985). Finally, helper T cell clones reactive with recombinant 65 kD antigen have been isolated from patients with tuberculosis (Oftung *et al.* 1987), indicating that this antigen is involved in the cell-mediated, as well as the humoral, immune response to tuberculosis.

In addition to the 65 kD antigen, there is evidence that the 19 kD and 71 kD antigens of *M. tuberculosis* may be particularly important in the immune response to this bacillus. Helper T cell clones from tuberculosis patients have been isolated which respond to the recombinant 19 kD protein (Oftung *et al.* 1987). The 71 kD antigen is recognized by the humoral immune system of both mice and rabbits, and we have shown that antibody to this antigen is a prominent component of hyperimmune anti-*M. tuberculosis* rabbit sera (Husson and Young 1987).

The isolation of genes for major protein antigens of *M. leprae* and *M. tuberculosis* should permit the development of improved reagents for diagnosis and immunoprophylaxis of these diseases. For example, proteins encoded by some of these DNA sequences may be a source of specific serodiagnostic and skin test antigens, reagents which would be valuable for monitoring disease transmission and the effectiveness of vaccination or therapy. Finally, it is now possible to introduce into viruses, and possibly into cultivable mycobacteria, genes that specify polypeptides which may provide immunological protection, in order to produce more specific and effective vaccines.

Acknowledgements

I am very grateful to my colleagues Barry Bloom, Bob Husson, Vijay Mehra, Tore Godal, Douglas Young, Jurai Ivanyi, Thomas Shinnick, Doug Sweetser and Bobby Cherayil for advice and discussion. Supported by grants from the NIH (AI23545), and the WHO/World Bank/ UNDP Special Program for Research and Training in Tropical Diseases.

Mycobacterial antigens, genes and vaccines

References

Bloom B R, Godal T 1983. Selective primary health care: strategies for control of disease in the developing world. V. Leprosy, *Reviews of Infectious Diseases* **5**: 765–80

Britton W J, Hellqvist L, Basten A, Raison R L 1985. *Mycobacterium leprae* antigens involved in human immune responses. I. Identification of four antigens by monoclonal antibodies, *Journal of Immunology* **135**: 4171–7

Dubos R, Dubos J 1952. In *The White Plague: Tuberculosis Man and Society*. Little Brown & Co., Boston, Massachusetts

Emmrich F, Thole J, van Emden J, Kaufmann S H E 1986. A recombinant 64 kilodalton protein of *Mycobacterium bovis* Bacillus Calmette–Guerin specifically stimulates human T4 clones reactive to mycobacterial antigens, *Journal of Experimental Medicine* **163**: 1024–9

Engers H D *et al.* 1985. Results of a World Health Organization-sponsored Workshop on Monoclonal Antibodies to *Mycobacterium leprae*, *Infection and Immunity* **48**: 603–5

Engers H D *et al.* 1986. Results of a World Health Organization-sponsored Workshop to Characterize Antigens Recognized by Mycobacterium-Specific Monoclonal Antibodies, *Infection and Immunity* **51**: 718–20

Hansen G A 1874. *Norsk Magasin for Laegezitenskapen* **4**: 1–88 I–L III

Husson R, Young R A 1987. Genes for the major protein antigens of *M. tuberculosis*: the etiologic agents of tuberculosis and leprosy share a major protein antigen. *Proceedings of the National Academy of Sciences USA* **84**: 1679–83

Joint International Union Against Tuberculosis and World Health Organization Study Group 1982. Tuberculosis control, *Tubercle* **63**: 157–69

Mustafa A S, Gill H K, Nerland A, Britton W J, Mehra V, Bloom B R, Young R A, Godal T 1986. Human T-cell clones recognize a major *M. leprae* protein antigen expressed in *E. coli*, *Nature (London)* **319**: 63–6

Oftung F, Mustafa A S, Husson R N, Young R A, Godal T 1987. Human T-cell clones recognize two abundant *M. tuberculosis* protein antigens expressed in *E. coli*, *Journal of Immunology* **138**: 927–31

Shankar P, Agis F, Wallach D, Flageul B, Cottenot F, Augier J, Bach M 1986. *M. leprae* and PPD-triggered T cell lines in tuberculoid and lepromatous leprosy, *Journal of Immunology* **136**: 4255–63

Thole J E R, Dauwerse H G, Das P K, Groothuis D G, Schouls L M, van Emden J D A 1985. Cloning of *Mycobacterium bovis* BCG DNA and expression of antigens in *Escherichia coli*, *Infection and Immunity* **50**: 800–6

Young R A, Mehra V, Sweetser D, Buchanan T, Clark-Curtiss J, Davis R W, Bloom B R 1985. Genes for the major protein antigens of the leprosy parasite *Mycobacterium leprae*, *Nature (London)* **316**: 450–2

Expression of *Plasmodium falciparum* antigens in *Escherichia coli* for the development of a human malaria vaccine

James F Young*; Mitchell S Gross*; W. Ripley Ballou†; Wayne T Hockmeyer†

* *Smith Kline and French Laboratories, Department of Molecular Genetics, 709 Swedeland Avenue, Swedeland, Pennsylvania 19479, USA*
† *Walter Reed Army Institute of Research, Department of the Army, Walter Reed Army Medical Center, Washington, DC 20307, USA*

Introduction

Malaria is a great medical problem that threatens nearly two billion people worldwide. The World Health Organization estimates that nearly three million people die from this disease annually. Attempts to reduce the prevalence and geographic spread of the disease by chemotherapy and spraying with insecticides to eliminate the mosquito vector have been hindered by the emergence of resistant strains of both the parasite and the vector. Recent advances in the identification and characterization of parasite antigens using the techniques of immunochemistry and molecular cloning now offer opportunities for vaccination as a strategy for disease control. The most encouraging effort to date is aimed at the sporozoite, the stage of the parasite transmitted by Anopheline mosquitoes, which initiates the infection in man. An effective vaccine against this stage of the parasite would thus prevent infection. However, since immunity to the sporozoite has no effect on the development of the clinically important blood stages, a single sporozoite escaping the primed immune system could cause disease. Thus, the ideal vaccine should also contain immunogens which provoke a response against the asexual erythrocytic stages. The effort to develop such molecules is complex due to the plethora of antigens displayed on the surface of these stages, many of which are strain variant and are thus not ideal vaccine candidates.

The ability to immunize against the sporozoite stage has been demonstrated. Irradiated sporozoites have been used successfully to immunize and protect rodents, nonhuman primates and a small number of human volunteers from challenge with live sporozoites (Nussenweig *et al.* 1969; Clyde *et al.* 1975; Rieckmann *et al.* 1979). This protection is at least in part mediated by antibodies directed against the major protein found on the surface of sporozoites termed the circumsporozoite (CS) protein (Vanderberg *et al.* 1969; Cochrane *et al.* 1980; Potocnjak *et al.* 1980; Yoshida *et al.* 1980; Nardin *et al.* 1982). Nevertheless, vaccination with sporozoites or a CS subunit vaccine has not been feasible due to an inability to culture this stage of the parasite *in vitro*.

Recently, the genes coding for the CS proteins of *Plasmodium knowlesi* (Godson *et al.* 1983), *P. falciparum* (Dame *et al.* 1984; Enea *et al.* 1984a), *P. cynomolgi* (Enea *et al.* 1984b) and *P. vivax* (Arnot *et al.* 1985; McCutchan *et al.* 1985) have been cloned and sequenced. These studies revealed a class of proteins which are structurally analogous, yet differ significantly in their primary amino acid sequence. In fact, only two small regions of approximately 15 amino acids each, termed region I and region II, are conserved between *P. knowlesi* and *P. falciparum* (Dame *et al.* 1984) and were viewed as potential targets for a cross-reactive vaccine. These two regions have also now been shown to be conserved in *P. vivax* (Arnot *et al.* 1985; McCutchan *et al.* 1985), strengthening this hypothesis. The most striking feature of these proteins is a large central repeat domain. In the case of the *P. falciparum*, this region is composed of 37 Asn-Ala-Asn-Pro tetrapeptide repeats interspersed with four Asn-Val-Asp-Pro tetrapeptide repeats. Since neutralizing monoclonal antibodies and serum from protected individuals react with this immunodominant repeat domain, it was seen as an important vaccine target in addition to the two conserved regions.

Peptide studies

Since there appeared to be at least three regions of the CS protein which might form the basis for a malaria sporozoite vaccine, we decided to undertake studies to determine which of these would be most efficacious (Ballou *et al.* 1985). In particular, if a protective response could be raised to region I or region II, this would serve as the basis for a cross-reactive vaccine. Therefore, peptides were synthesized corresponding to the repeat region and the two conserved regions with the sequences shown in Table 1. The peptides were

Table 1 Sequence of synthetic *P. falciparum* CS protein peptides

Peptide	Sequence
Repeat 8-mer	NPNANPNAC–
Repeat 16-mer	NPNANPNANPNANPNAC–
Region I	–CKHKKLKQPGDG
Region II	–TEWSPCSVTCGNGIQ

Synthetic peptides corresponded to eight (two tetrapeptide repeats) and 16 (four tetrapeptide repeats) residues of the repeat domain as well as the conserved regions I and II as described (Dame *et al.* 1984).

conjugated to thyroglobulin or keyhole limpet hemocyanin, emulsified in Complete Freund's Adjuvant (CFA), and used to immunize C57/BL/6 mice or rabbits. High-titered antibody responses to all peptides was observed by an enzyme-linked immunosorbent assay (ELISA). These sera were then tested in an indirect immunofluorescent antibody assay against sporozoites (Ballou *et al.* 1985). Antisera to the repeat peptides and the region I peptide reacted with the sporozoites whereas the antisera to the region II peptide did not (data not shown).

The next question was whether these antisera possessed any biological activity indicative of protection. It has been observed that sera from animals and humans immune to sporozoites produce a circumsporozoite precipitin (CSP) reaction on live sporozoites and inhibit sporozoite invasion (ISI assay) of human hepatoma cells *in vitro*. These assays are therefore accepted as good correlates of protection *in vivo* (Yoshida *et al.* 1980; Nardin *et al.* 1982; Hollingdale *et al.* 1984). The sera raised against the peptides were tested in these assays for activity and the results are shown in Table 2. Only antisera raised against the repeat peptides produced strong CSP reactions and inhibited the invasion of hepatoma cells, whereas antisera to regions I and II showed no activity (Ballou *et al.* 1985).

These data were important since they clearly showed that the repeat region of the CS protein, and not the conserved sequences, was a more likely vaccine target. More encouraging was that biologically active antibodies could be raised to a synthetic derivative of the native CS molecule. Although these experiments demonstrated the feasibility of a synthetic peptide vaccine approach, we felt that such a vaccine might have a number of potential limitations: (1) in order to be immunogenic the peptide must be linked to a carrier protein which may be difficult to standardize; (2) the amount of

Table 2 Circumsporozoite precipitin (CSP) reactivity and percentage inhibition of sporozoite invasion (ISI) of HepG2-A16 hepatoma cells by antisera to repeat, region I and region II peptides *in vitro*

Immunogen	CSP*	Inhibition (%)
8 residues	23/25 (4+)	100
16 residues	21/25 (4+)	100
Region I	0/25 (0)	0
Region II	0/25	0

* The CSP reactions were performed as described (Vanderberg *et al.* 1969). Twenty-five random sporozoites were examined for each serum sample and the number of CSP-positive organisms is indicated. The degree of CSP reactive is shown in parentheses (0, no CSP reactivity detectable; 2+, a granular precipitate on the surface of the sporozoites; 4+, a long thread-like filament at one end of the sporozoites). Inhibition of sporozoite invasion was performed as described (Hollingdale *et al.* 1984) and indicates the percentage inhibition as compared to a normal serum control. CS reactive monoclonal antibody 2F1.6 (Dame *et al.* 1984) gave 100% inhibition at a dilution of 1:20.

peptide that can be conjugated to the carrier may limit the ability to induce a strong anti-peptide response; (3) CFA was required to elicit a strong response in mice and rabbits (data not shown) and is not approved for use in humans; (4) the peptide-carrier conjugate may increase reactogenicity and sensitization of the host, leading to an enhanced clearance of the vaccine; (5) epitope-specific suppression may occur (Chedid *et al.* 1982) as has been observed with peptides from streptococcal M protein and diphtheria peptides conjugated to tetanus toxoid (Schutze *et al.* 1985). We therefore decided to produce larger molecules based on the repeat domain using recombinant DNA techniques with the hope of circumventing these problems.

Production of CS protein derivatives in *E. coli*

The data derived from studies using antisera generated to synthetic peptides indicated that the repeat region of the CS protein was capable of eliciting protective antibodies. We therefore concentrated on producing recombinant derivatives based on this repeat domain (Young *et al.* 1985). A recombinant plasmid containing the *P. falciparum* CS gene was the source of DNA for these studies (Dame *et al.* 1984). Figure 1a shows a schematic of the CS gene insert contained in this plasmid. Restriction endonuclease *Xho*II was used to excise a 192 base pair fragment from the gene (Fig. 1a) coding for 16 tetrapeptide repeats. This fragment was isolated and ligated into the *Bam*HI of λP_L *E. coli* expression plasmid pAS1 (Fig. 1b) (Rosenberg *et al.* 1983; Shatzman *et al.* 1983). Three clones were isolated: pR16tet$_{86}$, pR32tet$_{86}$, and pR48tet$_{86}$, which had inserts of one, two or three *Xho*II fragments, respectively, in-frame with the ATG initiation codon adjacent to the *Bam*HI site. The proteins produced from these plasmids, R16tet$_{86}$, R32tet$_{86}$ and R48tet$_{86}$, would contain 15, 30 or 45 Asn-Ala-Asn-Pro tetrapeptide repeats and one, two or three Asn-Val-Asp-Pro tetrapeptide repeats, respectively. In all three constructs, the repeat portion was fused to a downstream open reading frame coding for 86 amino acids in the tetracycline resistance (*tet*[r]) region of the plasmid (out-of-frame with the *tet*[r] protein). The proteins expressed by these clones was examined by immunoblot analysis. A heterogeneous set of products was observed (Young *et al.* 1985). The size of the smallest species in the three clones was proportional to the number of repeats present. Therefore, it appeared that the degradation observed was due to cleavages within the tet$_{86}$ tail. In an attempt to produce a more homogeneous product, a 14 base pair *Ban*II fragment was deleted from the *tet*[r] region in each clone (Fig. 1b). This manipulation resulted in the introduction of a stop codon after only 32 codons of the *tet*[r] region. The resulting truncated products, R16tet$_{32}$, R32tet$_{32}$ and R48tet$_{32}$, should now contain only 32 amino acids derived from the plasmid sequence (Fig. 2). The expression of these constructs resulted in the production of a single immunoreactive species in each case which could be easily purified (Young *et al.* 1985).

a)

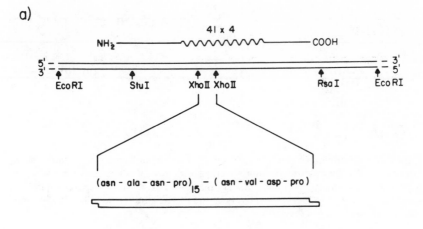

b)

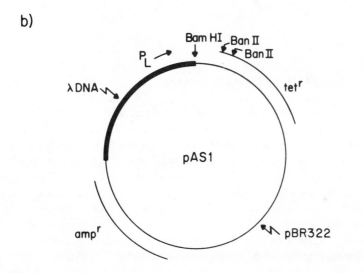

Figure 1. (a) Schematic of the *Eco*RI insert from the λmPF1 (Dame *et al.* 1984) encompassing the CS gene and a diagram of the protein encoded by this gene showing the central repeat domain as a wavy line. The 192 base pair *Xho*II fragment encodes 15 Asn-Ala-Asn-Pro tetrapeptide repeats and one Asn-Val-Asp-Pro repeat, as indicated. (b) Diagram of the *E. coli* expression plasmid pAS1 (Rosenberg *et al.* 1983; Shatzman *et al.* 1983). The segments of DNA from λ phage and pBR322 are indicated. The complete ampicillin resistance region (*amp*[r]) and part of the *tet*[r] derive from pBR322. Expression of genes inserted into the *Bam*HI site is under control of the λ P_L promoter, whose transcription is controlled by a cI repressor protein. Vector constructs are therefore transformed and maintained in a cI[+] lysogenic host (MM294cI[+]) to prevent expression of protein that may be toxic to the host strain. To obtain expression of the inserted DNA, the plasmid is transformed into a lysogenic host carrying a temperature-sensitive cI857 repressor (Sussman and Jacob 1962). Bacteria can then be grown at 32 °C in the absence of expression (repressor active), and then shifted to 42 °C to inactivate the repressor and turn on transcription from the P_L promoter (Young *et al.* 1983).

255

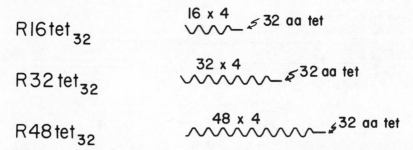

Figure 2. Schematic of three CS protein derivatives produced in *E. coli*. The wavy lines represent the immunodominant tetrapeptide repeat segment and the number of repeats in each construct is indicated over this line. The R16tet$_{32}$, R32tet$_{32}$ nd R48tet$_{32}$ contain 16, 32 or 48 repeats respectively, fused to a 32 amino acid tail coded by an open reading frame in the *tet^r* region.

Immunogenicity of the recombinant CS proteins

The R16tet$_{32}$, R32tet$_{32}$ and R48tet$_{32}$ proteins (50 µg) were used to immunize C57BL/6 mice either alone, emulsified with CFA, or adsorbed to aluminum hydroxide (alum), with a booster dose four weeks later. Animals were bled one week after the boost; sera from five animals in each group were pooled and tested for CS antibody by an ELISA. As shown in Fig. 3, R32tet$_{32}$ and R48tet$_{32}$ produced high-titer antibody, even without adjuvants, whereas the smaller R16tet$_{32}$ was less immunogenic. As expected, alum and CFA both enhanced the antibody response to all three proteins. These sera were then tested for activity against sporozoites by their ability to produce CSP reactions and inhibit sporozoite invasion of hepatoma cells *in vitro*. As shown in Tables 3 and 4, these sera produced strong CSP reactions and blocked the invasion of hepatoma cells by sporozoites in a manner that paralleled the ELISA titers. As indicated above, the CSP and ISI are considered predictive of *in vivo* protection. These sera were also screened in a primary human hepatocyte assay where complete development of the sporozoite into merozoites occurs. In this system, these antibodies not only inhibited invasion by sporozoites, but also hindered the development of those parasites which did enter the cell (Mazier *et al.* 1986). More recently we have examined the antibody titers in these animals eight months after their last immunization with protein. Animals vaccinated with alum-adjuvanted R32tet$_{32}$ still exhibited high-titered antibody levels which gave strong CSP and ISI reactivities (Wirtz *et al.* 1987). Taken together, these data suggest that the R32tet$_{32}$ molecule is a promising vaccine candidate against *P. falciparum* human malaria.

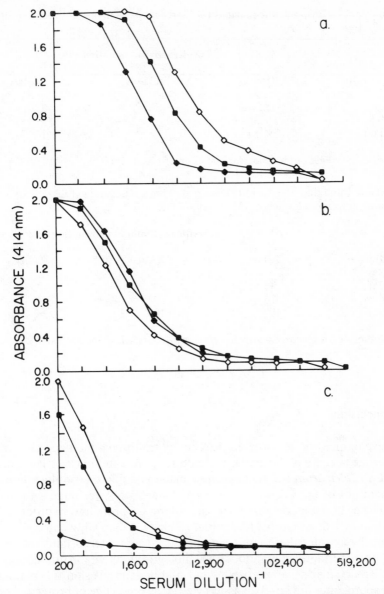

Figure 3. Antibody responses of mice to recombinant *P. falciparum* CS proteins R16tet$_{32}$, R32tet$_{32}$, or R48tet$_{32}$ were determined by ELISA using as antigen a 16 amino acid synthetic peptide consisting of four repeats of the *P. falciparum* CS protein (Asn-Ala-Asn-Pro) (Dame *et al.* 1984; Ballou *et al.* 1985). Assays were run in triplicate and the means and SEMs were calculated. In all instances the SEM was less than 0.09. Symbols for the antisera are: ◆, R16tet$_{32}$; ◇, R32tet$_{32}$; ■, R48tet$_{32}$. Animals were immunized with (a) proteins in CFA; (b) proteins with aluminum hydroxide; or (c) proteins in PBS without adjuvant.

Table 3 Circumsporozoite precipitin (CSP reactivity of mouse antisera to R16tet$_{32}$, R32tet$_{32}$ and R48tet$_{32}$

	Reactivity* of antisera to:		
Adjuvant	R16tet$_{32}$	R32tet$_{32}$	R48tet$_{32}$
None	0/25 (0)	17/25 (2+)	21/25 (4+)
CFA	23/25 (4+)	21/25 (4+)	21/25 (4+)
Alum	25/25 (4+)	25/25 (4+)	16/27 (2+,4+)

* The CSP reactions were performed as described in Table 2.

Table 4 Inhibition of sporozoite invasion* of human hepatoma cells *in vitro* by mouse antisera to R16tet$_{32}$, R32tet$_{32}$ and R48tet$_{32}$

	Percentage of inhibition by antisera to:		
Adjuvant	R16tet$_{32}$	R32tet$_{32}$	R48tet$_{32}$
None	46	95	92
CFA	76	92	94
Alum	100	100	96

* Inhibition of sporozoite invasion was performed as described in Table 2.

Conclusions

Development of a sporozoite vaccine by traditional methods has not been feasible because of the inability to culture sporozoites *in vitro*. The cloning of the *P. falciparum* CS gene has now made possible the production of large quantities of the CS protein by recombinant DNA techniques for use in a vaccine. In this study, three derivates of the CS protein were produced in *E. coli*, purified, and tested for immunogenicity. When adjuvanted with aluminum hydroxide, these constructs produced high-titered antibody in mice. More importantly, this antibody was biologically active and produced positive CSP reactions on live sporozoites and inhibited the invasion of hepatoma cells by sporozoites *in vitro*, two assays viewed as predictive of protection *in vivo*. We have also determined, by Southern blot analysis of the CS gene, that the repeat domain of the protein is conserved in a wide distribution of geographical isolates (Weber and Hockmeyer 1985). Since the molecules produced in this study are based on the repeat region, we would expect them to induce antibodies which are protective against all strains of *P. falciparum*.

Of those molecules so far examined, alum-adjuvanted R32tet$_{32}$ appears to be the primary candidate for the first sporozoite vaccine against *P. falciparum* induced malaria in man. This material has been produced on a large scale and has been approved by the US Food and Drug Administration for human use. Clinical trials have begun at Walter Reed Army Institute for Research and results are expected later this year.

References

Arnot D E, Barnwell J W, Tam J P, Nussenzweig V, Nussenzweig R S, Enea V. 1985. Circumsporozoite protein of *Plasmodium vivax*: gene cloning and characterization of the immunodominant epitope, *Science* **230**: 815–18

Ballou W R, Rothbard J, Wirtz R A, Gordon D M, Williams J S, Gore R, Schneider I, Hollingdale M R, Beaudoin R L, Maloy W L, Miller L H, Hockmeyer W T 1985. Immunogenicity of synthetic peptides from circumsporozoite protein of *Plasmodium falciparum*, *Science* **228**: 996–9

Chedid L A, Parant M A, Audibert F M, Riveau G J, Parant F J, Lederer E, Choay J P, Lefrancier P L 1982. Biological activity of a new synthetic muramyl peptide adjuvant devoid of pyrogenicity, *Infection and Immunity* **35**: 417–24

Clyde D F, McCarthy V C, Miller R M, Woodward W E 1975. Immunization of man against *falciparum* and *vivax* malaria by use of attenuated sporozoites, *American Journal of Tropical Medicine and Hygiene* **24**: 397–401

Cochrane A H, Nussenzweig R S, Nardin E H 1980. In J P Kreier (ed) *Malaria in Man and Experimental Animals.* Academic Press, New York, pp 163–202

Dame J B, Williams J L, McCutchan T F, Weber J L, Wirtz R A, Hockmeyer W T, Maloy W L, Haynes J D, Schneider I, Roberts D, Sanders G S, Reddy E P, Diggs C L, Miller L H 1984. Structure of the gene encoding the immunodominant surface antigen on the sporozoite of the human malaria parasite *Plasmodium falciparum*, *Science* **225**: 593–9

Enea V, Arnot D, Schmidt E C, Cochrane A, Gwadz R, Nussenzweig R S 1984a. cDNA cloning and expression of the repetitive circumsporozoite epitope, *Proceedings of the National Academy of Sciences USA* **81**: 7520–4

Enea V, Ellis J, Zavala F, Arnot D E, Asavanich A, Masuda A, Quakyi I, Nussenzweig R S 1984b. DNA cloning of *Plasmodium falciparum* circumsporozoite gene: amino acid sequence of repetitive epitope, *Science* **225**: 628–30

Godson G N, Ellis J, Svec P, Schlesinger D H, Nussenzweig V 1983. Identification and chemical synthesis of a tandemly repeated immunogenic region of *Plasmodium knowlesi* circumsporozoite protein, *Nature (London)* **305**: 29–33

Hollingdale M R, Nardin E H, Tharavanij S, Schwartz A L, Nussenzweig R S 1984. Inhibition of entry of *Plasmodium falciparum* and *P. vivax* sporozoite into cultured cells; and *in vitro* assay of protective antibodies, *Journal of Immunology* **132**: 909–13

Mazier D, Mellouk S, Beaudoin R L, Texier B, Druilhe P, Hockmeyer W, Trosper J, Paul C, Charoenvit Y, Young J, Miltgen F, Chedid L, Chigot J P, Galley B, Brandicourt O, Gentilini M 1986. Effect of antibodies to recombinant and synthetic peptides on *P. falciparum* sporozoites *in vitro*, *Science* **231**: 156–9

McCutchan T F, Lal A A, de la Cruz V F, Miller L H, Maloy W L, Charoenvit Y, Beaudoin R L, Guerry P, Wistar R Jr, Hoffman S L, Hockmeyer W T, Collins W E, Wirth D 1985. Sequence of the immunodominant epitope for the surface protein on sporozoites of *Plasmodium vivax*, *Science* **230**: 1381–3

Nardin E H, Nussenzweig V, Nussenzweig R S, Collins W E, Harinasuta K T, Tapchaisri P, Chomcharn Y 1982. Circumsporozoite proteins of human malaria parasites *Plasmodium falciparum* and *Plasmodium vivax*, *Journal of Experimental Medicine* **156**: 20–30

Nussenzweig R, Vanderberg J, Most H 1969. Protective immunity produced by the injection of X-irradiated sporozoites of *Plasmodium berghei*, *Military Medicine* **134**: 1176–82

Potocnjak P, Yoshida N, Nussenzweig R, Nussenzweig V 1980. Monovalent fragments (Fab) of monoclonal antibodies to a sporozoite surface antigen (Pb44) protect mice against malaria infection, *Journal of Experimental Medicine* **151**: 1504–13

Rieckmann K H, Beaudoin R L, Cassells J S, Sell K W 1979. Use of attenuated sporozoites in the immunization of human volunteers against falciparum malaria, *Transactions of the Royal Society of Tropical Medicine and Hygiene,* Supplement 1: 261–5

Rosenberg M, Ho Y S, Shatzman A R 1983. The use of pKC30 and its derivatives for controlled expression of genes, in R Wu (ed) *Methods in Enzymology.* Academic Press, London, vol 101, pp 123–38

Schutze M P, Leclerc C, Jolivet M, Audibert F, Chedid L 1985. Carrier-induced epitopic suppression, a major issue for future synthetic vaccines, *Journal of Immunology* **135**: 2319–22

Shatzman A, Ho Y S, Rosenberg M 1983. Using phage λ regulatory signals to obtain efficient expression of genes in *E. coli,* in M Inouye (ed) *Experimental Manipulation of Gene Expression.* Academic Press, New York, pp 1–14

Sussman R, Jacob F. 1962. Sur un systeme de repression thermosensible chez le bacteriophage d'*Escherichia coli, Comptes Rendus de l'Academie des Sciences* **254**: 1517–19

Vanderberg J, Nussenzweig R, Most H 1969. Protective immunity produced by the injection of X-irradiated sporozoites of *Plasmodium berghei.* V. *In vitro* effects of immune serum on sporozoites, *Military Medicine* **134**: 1183–90

Weber J L, Hockmeyer W T 1985. Structure of the circumsporozoite protein gene in 18 strains of *Plasmodium falciparum, Molecular and Biochemical Parasitology* **15**: 305–16

Wirtz R A, Ballou W R, Schneider I, Chedid L, Gross M S, Young J F, Hollingdale M, Diggs C L, Hockmeyer W T 1987. *Plasmodium falciparum*: immunogenicity of circumsporozoite protein constructs produced in *E. coli, Experimental Parasitology* **63** (in press)

Yoshida N, Nussenzweig R S, Potochjak P, Nussenzweig V, Aikawa M 1980. Hybridoma produces protective antibodies directed against the sporozoite stage of malaria parasite, *Science* **207**: 71–3

Young J F, Desselberger U, Palese P, Ferguson B, Shatzman A R, Rosenberg M 1983. Efficient expression of influenza virus NS1 nonstructural proteins in *Escherichia coli, Proceedings of the National Academy of Sciences USA* **80**: 6105–9

Young J F, Hockmeyer W T, Gross M S, Ballou W R, Wirtz R A, Trosper J H, Beaudoin R L, Hollingdale M R, Miller L H, Diggs C L, Rosenberg M 1985. Expression of *Plasmodium falciparum* circumsporozoite proteins in *Escherichia coli* for potential use in a human malaria vaccine, *Science* **228**: 958–62

Recombinant avirulent *Salmonella* for oral immunization to induce mucosal immunity to bacterial pathogens

Roy Curtiss III*; Raul Goldschmidt*; Sandra Kelly*; Mary Lyons*;Suzanne M Michalek†; Russell Pastian*; Sidney Stein*

* *Department of Biology, Washington University, St Louis, Missouri 63130, USA*
† *Department of Microbiology, University of Alabama in Birmingham, Birmingham, Alabama 35294, USA*

Introduction

Several observations have led us (Curtiss *et al.* 1983a, 1986; Curtiss 1986) to devise a strategy to develop live oral vaccine strains to immunize against *Streptococcus mutans*-induced dental caries.

First, antigen delivery to the gut-associated lymphoid tissue (GALT or Peyer's patches) leads to a generalized secretory immune response (Cebra *et al.* 1976; Bienenstock *et al.* 1978; Weisz-Carrington *et al.* 1979). Second, as originally noted by Carter and Collins (1974), orally fed *Salmonella typhimurium* initially attach to and invade the GALT in mice before colonizing in the liver and spleen. Third, enteric bacteria can be attenuated by mutation to prevent disease without preventing initial tissue tropism (Bacon *et al.* 1951; Jackson and Burrows 1956; Germanier and Furer 1975; Hoiseth and Stocker 1981). Fourth, oral administration of formalin-killed *S. mutans* cells induces secretory IgA in saliva and other secretions and confers protective immunity against *S. mutans*-induced dental caries (Michalek *et al.* 1976; Mestecky *et al.* 1978). Fifth, by using gene cloning, mutant isolation and virulence testing, we and others have identified several *S. mutans* gene products essential for *S. mutans* colonization on teeth and these constitute prime candidates for use to induce protective immunity (Curtiss 1985, 1986; Curtiss *et al.* 1986).

Streptococcus mutans-induced dental caries and virulence attributes

A group of microorganisms often collectively called *Streptococcus mutans* constitutes the principal etiologic agents of dental caries. Since *S. mutans* infects some 95% of the human population, it is one of the most ubiquitous bacterial infectious diseases. There are at least five genospecies (*S. mutans*, *S. sobrinus*, *S. cricetus*, *S. ferrus*, *S. rattus*), each with different DNA G + C contents (range of 36% to 46%) and with different group-specific carbohydrate surface antigens (Curtiss 1985).

Colonization on the tooth surface occurs soon after tooth eruption and initially involves a sucrose-independent phase requiring that surface protein antigen A and, presumably, lipoteichoic acids on the bacterial surface interact with salivary glycoprotein(s) forming a pellicle on the tooth surface. In the second phase, which is dependent upon the presence of sucrose, glucosyl-transferases synthesize water-insoluble glucans that cause cells to attach tenaciously to the tooth surface and also to aggregate to each other to result in the formation of dental plaque. In the last and continuous stage, various enzymes metabolize mono-, di-, and tri-saccharides to produce lactic acid which demineralizes tooth enamel and leads to the onset of tooth decay. When free sugars are plentiful, *S. mutans* enzymatically synthesizes intra- and extra-cellular carbohydrate storage reserves that are metabolized to generate energy and lactic acid when free sugars are unavailable.

Gene cloning and immunological screening by Holt *et al.* (1982) led to the identification of recombinant clones of *Escherichia coli* expressing the *S. sobrinus* surface protein antigen A (SpaA). The SpaA protein is released into the periplasmic space of *E. coli* by cold osmotic shock. It is readily purified from either *S. mutans* or *E. coli*. Antibodies to the SpaA protein from the serotype *g S. sobrinus* strain 6715 react with the proteins present in all of the serotypes known to cause carious lesions in humans. In spite of a substantial conservation of antigenic similarity, there is little or no DNA sequence homology in that the gene specifying the SpaA protein for serotype *g* is unable to hybridize with DNA sequences from any of the other serotypes except from the closely related serotype *d* strains. Antibodies against the SpaA protein have been used to isolate mutants that lack SpaA protein. These mutants are unable to cause dental caries in germ-free rats (Curtiss *et al.* 1986).

In summary, the SpaA protein is a 210,000 molecular weight protein that accounts for some 35% of the cell surface protein on *S. mutans*. The protein is involved in sucrose-independent adherence to the saliva-coated tooth surface (Douglas and Russell 1984; Russell 1986) and also is involved in sucrose-induced aggregation (Curtiss *et al.* 1983b). An identical or cross-reactive protein is present in *S. mutans* serotypes *a*, *c* (also known as antigen I/II, B, and P1), *d*, *e*, *f*, *g* and *h*. Antibodies against the SpaA protein made by *E. coli* react with dextranase and glucan-binding protein (Barrett *et al.* 1986). Most important, the protein seems to be essential for *S. mutans* virulence in germ-free animals. A number of different glycosyltransferase genes have been cloned in *E. coli* (Robeson *et al.* 1983; Gilpin *et al.* 1985; Jacobs *et al.* 1986) and work to clone and characterize others is proceeding in several labs. Obviously, these enzymes play a key role in maintaining *S. mutans* on the tooth surface.

Both the SpaA protein (Russell *et al.* 1980) and glucosyltransferases (Taubman *et al.* 1986) have been evaluated as potential antigens. Both have been found to be highly immunogenic and able to confer protective immunity against *S. mutans*-induced dental caries when used for immunization of rats or rhesus monkeys.

Ability of *Salmonella typhimurium* to colonize the GALT

As originally noted by Carter and Collins (1974), *S. typhimurium*, upon oral ingestion by the mouse, invades the deep tissues by first passing through the GALT or Peyer's patches. Table 1 displays data of the titers of *S. mutans*, *E. coli* and *S. typhimurium* in various regions of the gastrointestinal tract as a function of time after oral ingestion of differentially marked antibiotic-resistant isolates. *Streptococcus mutans* seems to pass right through the intestinal tract with little or no detectable attachment of cells either within Peyer's patches or to the epithelial lining of the small intestine. *Escherichia coli*, however, is able to be taken up by Peyer's patches, but the cells fail to survive

Table 1 Bacterial titers in mice after oral feeding of 2×10^8 *S. mutans* (UAB66), 2×10^8 *E. coli* K-12 (χ2900) and 1×10^8 *S. typhimurium* SR-11 (χ3338)*

Time	Peyer's patches	Small intestinal wall (−PP)	Small intestinal contents	Colon contents	Spleen
S. mutans					
1 hr	<10	<10	1×10^3	$>5 \times 10^4$	
5 hr	<10	<10	<10	2×10^5	
26 hr	<10	<10	<10	<10	
4 d	<10	<10	<10	<10	<10
E. coli					
1 hr	8×10^1	3×10^3	2×10^5	$>1 \times 10^5$	
5 hr	<10	<10	2×10^3	5×10^7	
26 hr	<10	<10	<10	1×10^4	
4 d	<10	<10	<10	<10	<10
S. typhimurium					
1 hr	7×10^1	4×10^2	2×10^5	$>1 \times 10^5$	
5 hr	6×10^1	3×10^1	5×10^2	9×10^7	
26 hr	6×10^2	<10	1×10^1	2×10^4	
4 d	5×10^4	5×10^3	1×10^5	2×10^4	6×10^5

* Mice were mixedly infected with *E. coli* (resistant to streptomycin and nalidixic acid), *S. typhimurium* (resistant to tetracycline and nalidixic acid), and *S. mutans* (resistant to streptomycin and spectinomycin). These antibiotics were used to monitor the recovery of each strain from mouse tissue using as basal medium Difco Penassay Base Agar (*E. coli* and *S. typhimurium*) and Difco Brain Heart Infusion Agar (*S. mutans*).
−PP: without Peyer's Patches.

even for a five-hour period. They, too, seem to pass right through the GI tract. *Salmonella typhimurium*, on the other hand, attaches to and invades the GALT and is able to proliferate there. It is also evident that *S. typhimurium* cells attach to the walls of the small intestine and proliferate there as they do within the contents of the small and large bowel. It remains to be determined whether *S. typhimurium* has a specific surface attribute or other mechanism for attachment to and invasion of the GALT or whether the ability of the organism to proliferate in the intestinal contents provides a sufficient inoculum over a period of time to result in nonspecific uptake by the activities of the M cells overlying each Peyer's patch.

Strain construction and immunization results

We have employed transposon mutagenesis of *S. typhimurium* to generate avirulent strains still capable of attaching to and invading Peyer's patch cells (Curtiss *et al.* 1986). The transposon Tn*10* (Kleckner *et al.* 1977) confers resistance to tetracycline and sensitivity to fusaric acid and can insert into or adjacent to genes. Selection of fusaric acid-resistant isolates (Bochner *et al.* 1980; Maloy and Nunn 1981) selects for loss of Tn*10* which is often caused by deletion of Tn*10* and DNA sequences adjacent to the site of Tn*10* insertion. Deletion mutations so generated are very stable and cannot revert. We have generated or made use of Δ*asd* mutations which impose the requirement for diaminopimelic acid (DAP) and these strains lyse and liberate their antigenic contents when taken up by mammalian cells that are devoid of DAP. The Δ*thyA* mutation imposes a requirement for thymine or thymidine, the absence of which leads to thymine-less death. The Δ*aroA* mutation isolated by Hoiseth and Stocker (1981) imposes a requirement for *p*-aminobenzoic acid, a compound which is not present in mammalian tissues, and which is needed for the synthesis of folate. Δ*purA* mutations impose a requirement for adenine and have been known to confer avirulence to *Salmonella* and *Yersinia* strains for over thirty years (Bacon *et al.* 1951; Jackson and Burrows 1956). The *galE* mutation originally employed by Germanier and Furer (1975) blocks synthesis of UDP-Gal, which is needed for synthesis of a normal LPS core and O-antigen side chain in *S. typhimurium*. In the absence of galactose, strains become rough and are now susceptible to nonspecific host defenses. Strains with Δ*thyA* mutations and with Δ*purA* mutations alone have a moderately reduced virulence but are still able to kill mice. Strains with a Δ*asd* mutation with or without a Δ*thyA* mutation never kill mice even when 10^9 organisms are fed orally or given by gastric intubation or when 10^8 organisms are injected intraperitoneally. Strains with Δ*aroA* mutation sometimes kill mice but the addition of the Δ*purA* mutation prevents this.

All of the vaccine strains constructed were derived from the mouse virulent *S. typhimurium* strains SR-11 or SL1344. All have the *gyrA1816* mutation conferring resistance to nalidixic acid thus facilitating their recovery from mouse tissues. χ3266 is derived from SR-11, has the Δ*asdA3* mutation and possesses plasmids pYA601 producing glucosyltransferase A and pYA727 producing SpaA protein. χ3267 is an SR-11 derivative with Δ*asdA3* and Δ*thyA42* mutations with the pYA727 plasmid specifying the SpaA protein. χ3270 is a derivative of SL1344 with Δ*aroA544* and *his G46* mutations and has both pYA601 and pYA727. Immunization of mice by the oral route with high concentrations of χ3266 and χ3267 does not result in a high level of immunity

Table 2 Mortality of BALB/c mice immunized by oral administration of live *S. typhimurium* SR-11 χ3266 Δ*asdA3* (pYA601, pYA727) SR-11, χ3267 Δ*asdA3* Δ*thyA42* (pYA727) SR-11 and χ3270 Δ*aroA554 his G46* (pYA601, pYA727) SL1344 and challenged by oral administration of live, virulent *S. typhimurium* SR-11 or SL1344*

Immunization schedule		χ3266		χ3267		χ3270	
No. of doses	Time between doses (days)						
		Dead (%)	MDD‡	Dead (%)	MDD‡	Dead (%)	MDD‡
1	—	100	8	100	8	0	—
3	1	100	9	100	9	0	—
3	4	100	10	100	10	20	7

* Mice were challenged with 1×10^8 CFU χ3339 SL1344 and 2×10^9 χ3306 SR-11 at approximately 25 days post-immunization. All unimmunized control mice died within ten days after challenge.
† Mice were immunized with approximately 5×10^8 CFU/dose.
‡ Mean day of death for mice which died after challenge.

Table 3 Mortality of BALB/c mice immunized by oral administration of live *S. typhimurium* SR-11 χ3266 Δ*asdA3* (pYA601, pYA727) and χ3267 Δ*asdA3* Δ*thyA42* (pYA727) and challenged by i.p. administration of various doses of live, virulent *S. typhimurium* SR-11 χ3306 at 30 days post-immunization.

I.p. challenge dose (CFU χ3306)	χ3266		χ3267		None	
	Dead (%)	MDD†	Dead (%)	MDD†	Dead (%)	MDD†
1.4×10^3	100	8	100	7	—	—
2.7×10^2	100	14	100	10	100	8
1.3×10^2	100	21	100	13	100	10
6.4×10^1	33	13	100	9	100	5

* Mice were immunized with approximately 1×10^9 CFU/day for three consecutive days.
† Mean day of death for mice which died after challenge.

Table 4 Mortality of BALB/c mice immunized by oral administration of live *S. typhimurium* SR-11 χ3266 Δ*asdA3* (pYA601, pYA727) and χ3267 Δ*asdA3* Δ*thyA42* (pYA727) and challenged by oral administration of various doses of live, virulent *S. typhimurium* SR-11 χ3306 at 30 days post-immunization.

Oral challenge dose (CFU χ3306)	Immunization treatment*					
	χ3266		χ3267		None	
	Dead (%)	MDD†	Dead (%)	MDD†	Dead (%)	MDD†
1.2×10^8	33	13	83	18	—	—
1.5×10^7	50	18	83	34	100	20
1.5×10^6	83	19	66	18	100	12
2.0×10^5	50	25	50	17	83	17

* Mice were immunized with approximately 1×10^9 CFU/day for three consecutive days.
† Mean day of death for mice which died after challenge.

to oral challenge with virulent wild-type *S. typhimurium* whereas oral immunization with the Δ*aroA* strain χ3270 does induce a high level of protective immunity (Table 2). These results were confirmed in experiments in which mice orally immunized with either χ3266 or χ3267 were challenged either by the i.p. (Table 3) or oral (Table 4) routes with differing lower doses of the virulent wild-type SR-11 strain. As noted by the date (Table 3), oral immunization, with either χ3266 or χ3267, does not alter in any significant way the response to challenge with *S. typhimurium* by the i.p. route. On the other hand, when the wild-type virulent *Salmonella* is orally administered to mice orally immunized with χ3266 or χ3267, it is evident that some protection is afforded (Table 4). Thus, oral immunization with Δ*asd* (+/− Δ*thyA*) strains does not confer significant immunity against i.p. challenge with a wild-type virulent *S. typhimurium* strain but does confer some protection against oral challenge.

Serum and salivary antibody titers have been determined, using ELISA, following oral immunization of BALB/c mice immunized with various avirulent *S. typhimurium* strains expressing *S. mutans* serotype *g* SpaA protein or the serotype *c* GtfA protein. These data are presented in Table 5. The results demonstrate that the secretory IgA (sIgA) response in saliva is delayed in appearance compared to the detection of serum antibody. Note that the titers of antibody reacting with antigens present on *S. mutans* serotype *g* or *c* are at values not much lower in relation to serum and salivary IgA antibody titers against *S. typhimurium*. It should be evident that the secretory IgA antibody against *S. typhimurium* in saliva is indicative of this antibody in all secretions and is undoubtedly responsible for the slight protection observed in orally immunized mice to oral challenge with *S. typhimurium* noted in Table 4. The results with χ3267, which only expresses the serotype *g* SpaA protein, are

Table 5 Serum and salivary antibody titers (ELISA) in BALB/c mice immunized with avirulent *S. typhimurium* expressing *S. mutans* serotype *g* SpaA and/or serotype *c* GtfA proteins*

Immunizing strain	Day assayed	Serum Ig (1/100) against:			Salivary IgA (1/10) against:		
		S. typhimurium	*S. mutans* serotype: *g*	*c*	*S. typhimurium*	*S. mutans* serotype: *g*	*c*
χ3266 SR-11 Δ*asd* SpaA⁺ GtfA⁺	1	<0.1	<0.1	0.10	—	0.21	0.16
	16	0.51	0.11	0.57	0.13	<0.1	<0.1
	23	0.58	0.14	0.98	0.50	<0.1	<0.1
	30	0.90	0.38	1.15	0.49	0.32	0.51
χ3267 SR-11 Δ*asd* Δ*thyA* SpaA⁺	4	0.21	<0.1	0.15	<0.1	<0.1	<0.1
	16	0.32	0.16	0.25	0.13	<0.1	<0.1
	23	0.33	0.17	0.40	0.13	<0.1	<0.1
	30	1.81	0.18	0.68	0.71	0.25	0.65
χ3270 SL-1344 Δ*aroA* SpaA⁺ GtfA⁺	1	<0.1	<0.1	<0.1	—	0.10	<0.1
	16	1.53	0.18	0.68	0.18	0.13	<0.1
	23	1.18	0.17	1.00	0.18	0.14	0.30
	30	1.77	0.18	1.11	1.01	0.38	0.90

* Mice immunized with 1×10^9 CFU on each of three successive days. Individual mice were sacrificed for collection of serum and saliva. Microtiter wells were coated with extracts of *S. typhimurium* LT2, *S. mutans* serotype *g* (6715) or with (MT8148).

Table 6 Caries scores in mice immunized orally with avirulent *S. typhimurium* strains expressing *S. mutans* antigens and then challenged with virulent *S. mutans**

Treatment	Mean caries score
Control, no infection	15 ± 13
Control, infected with UAB765	44 ± 36
Immunized with χ3266, infected with UAB765	43 ± 11
Immunized with χ3267, infected with UAB765	60 ± 30
Immunized with χ3270, infected with UAB765	40 ± 20

* Mice were immunized at 4–5 weeks of age with 1×10^9 CFU χ3266, χ3267 or χ3270 and challenged with 2×10^7 CFU UAB765 30 days later. Caries scored 45 days after challenge.

interesting since it is evident that antibodies are produced which react with the serotype *c S. mutans*. This demonstrates that the immunological cross-reaction is induced in this immunization procedure as it is in rabbits immunized with purified SpaA protein.

These results were encouraging and we next embarked on animal protection studies. Rather than switch to germ-free rats, which would require development of assays for serum and salivary antibodies, we developed a mouse caries model for this purpose. Three- to five-week-old BALB/c mice, fed a soft diet containing sucrose (Tanzer 1979), were challenged with 2×10^7 CFU of a spectinomycin-resistant serotype *c S. mutans* strain (UAB765). As shown in Table 6 control mice not infected with *S. mutans* develop a low level of caries on this soft diet. The level of caries was only one-third that of animals infected with UAB765. In this particular experiment, results with mice immunized three times on successive days with approximately 10^9 χ3266, χ3267 or χ3270 and challenged with UAB765 four weeks later were most disappointing. In this experiment serum and salivary titers against *S. mutans* antigens were very low and in most instances were not significantly higher than controls when measured either four weeks after immunization or ten weeks after immunization in those mice not challenged with UAB765. However, in those mice challenged with UAB765 we observed that the titers of antibody in serum and saliva against *S. mutans* antigens increased by ten weeks after the initial immunization as though oral challenge with *S. mutans* acted as a secondary immunization. In any event, the low sIgA titers against *S. mutans* at the time of challenge with UAB765 were insufficient to prevent colonization and thus there was no reduction in caries incidence (Table 6). Evaluation of the *S. typhimurium* strains used to immunize these mice by Western blot analysis with anti-SpaA sera indicated that they produced either little or no SpaA protein or, in some instances, produced SpaA protein derivatives with an altered molecular weight.

Subsequently, we have modified the recombinant clones producing SpaA protein to produce high amounts of SpaA antigen in either *E. coli* or *S. typhimurium*. The recombinant plasmid pYA770 causes *E. coli* to produce about ten times more SpaA protein than does the pYA727 plasmid. *S. typhimurium* strains with pYA770 produce about 50 times more SpaA protein than strains with pYA727. Experiments to evaluate immunogenicity of and protection by avirulent *S. typhimurium* strains with this recombinant clone pYA770 are in progress.

Conclusions

Avirulent derivatives of *S. typhimurium* harboring plasmids expressing *S. mutans* colonization protein antigens are often effective in stimulating a secretory immune response against both *S. typhimurium* and *S. mutans*. The genetic stability of strains can sometimes be a problem. This requires that further work be conducted to stabilize the genetic properties of the strains and even to construct those that express the *S. mutans* antigens on the *S. typhimurium* cell surface. Based on studies in humans, rats and monkeys, the titers of secretory IgA achieved in saliva of mice immunized with these bivalent vaccines should be protective and prevent colonization of teeth by *S. mutans*. A similar immunization strategy should be effective in contending with bacterial, viral and mycotic pathogens that colonize on or invade through a mucosal surface.

Acknowledgements

Research was supported by US Public Health Service Grant DE06669 from the National Institute of Dental Research. We thank Margaret Buoncristiani and Christine Pearce for editorial assistance with the manuscript.

References

Bacon G A, Burrows T W, Yates M 1951. The effects of biochemical mutation on the virulence of *Bacterium typhosum*: the loss of virulence of certain mutants, *British Journal of Experimental Pathology* **32**: 85–96

Barrett J F, Barrett T A, Curtiss R III 1986. Biochemistry and genetics of dextranase from *Streptococcus mutans* 6715, in S Hamada, S M Michalek, H Kiyono, L Menaker, J R McGhee, (eds) *Molecular Microbiology and Immunobiology of Streptococcus mutans*. Elsevier Publishers BV, Amsterdam, pp 205–15

Bienenstock J, McDermott M, Befus D, O'Neill M 1978. A common mucosal immunologic system involving the bronchus, breast and bowel, *Advanced Experimental Medical Biology* **107**: 53–9

Bochner B R, Huang H, Schieven G L, Ames B N 1980. Positive selection for loss of tetracycline resistance, *Journal of Bacteriology* **143**: 926–33

Carter P B, Collins F M 1974. The route of enteric infection in normal mice, *Journal of Experimental Medicine* **139**: 1189–203

Cebra J J, Gearhart P J, Kamat R, Robertson S M, Tseng J 1976. Origin and differentiation of lymphocytes involved in the secretory IgA response, *Cold Spring Harbor Symposia of Quantitative Biology* **41**: 201–15

Curtiss R III 1985. Genetic analysis of *Streptococcus mutans* virulence, in W Goebel (ed) *Current Topics in Microbiology and Immunology: genetic approaches to microbial pathogenicity.* Springer-Verlag, Berlin, vol 118, pp 253–77

Curtiss R III 1986. Genetic analysis of *S. mutans* virulence and prospects for an anticaries vaccine, *Journal of Dental Research* **65**: 1034–45

Curtiss R III, Holt R G, Barletta R, Robeson J P, Saito S 1983a. *Escherichia coli* strains producing *Streptococcus mutans* proteins responsible for colonization and virulence, in J R McGhee, J Mestecky (eds) *The secretory immune system. Annals of the New York Academy of Sciences* **409**: 688–96

Curtiss R III, Larrimore S A, Holt R G, Barrett J F, Barletta R, Murchison H H, Michalek S M, Saito S 1983b. Analysis of *Streptococcus mutans* virulence attributes using recombinant DNA and immunological techniques, in R J Doyle, J E Ciardi (eds) *Glucosyltransferases, Glucans, Sucrose and Dental Caries*, Special Supplement of Chemical Senses, IRL, pp 95–104

Curtiss R III, Goldschmidt R, Pastian R, Lyons M, Michalek S M, Mestecky J 1986. Cloning virulence determinants from *Streptococcus mutans* and the use of recombinant clones to construct bivalent oral vaccine strains to confer protective immunity against *S. mutans*-induced dental caries, in S Hamada, S M Michalek, H Kiyono, L Menaker, J R McGhee (eds) *Molecular Microbiology and Immunobiology of Streptococcus mutans.* Elsevier Publishers BV, Amsterdam, pp 173–80

Douglas C W I, Russell R R B 1984. Effect of specific antisera upon *Streptococcus mutans* adherence to saliva-coated hydroxylapatite, *FEMS Microbiology Letters* **25**: 211–14

Germanier R, Furer E 1975. Isolation and characterization of *galE* mutant Ty21a of *Salmonella typhi*: a candidate strain for a live oral typhoid vaccine, *Journal of Infectious Diseases* **131**: 553–8

Gilpin M L, Russell R R B, Morrissey P 1985. Cloning and expression of two *Streptococcus mutans* glucosyltransferases in *Escherichia coli* K-12, *Infection and Immunity* **49**: 414–16

Hoiseth S K, Stocker B A D 1981. Aromatic-dependent *Salmonella typhimurium* are non-virulent and effective as vaccines, *Nature (London)* **291**: 238–9

Holt R G, Abiko Y, Saito S, Smorawinska M, Hansen J B, Curtiss R III 1982. *Streptococcus mutans* genes that code for extracellular proteins in *Escherichia coli* K-12, *Infection and Immunity* **38**: 147–56

Jackson S, Burrows T W 1956. The pigmentation of *Pasteurella pestis* on a defined medium containing haemin, *British Journal of Experimental Pathology* **37**: 570–6

Jacobs W R, Barrett J F, Clark-Curtiss J E, Curtiss R III 1986. *In vivo* repackaging of recombinant cosmid molecules for analyses of *Salmonella typhimurium*, *Streptococcus mutans* and mycobacterial genomic libraries, *Infection and Immunity* **52**: 101–9

Kleckner N, Roth J R, Botstein D 1977. Genetic engineering *in vivo* using translocatable drug-resistance elements, *Journal of Molecular Biology* **116**: 125–59

Maloy S R, Nunn W D 1981. Selection for loss of tetracycline resistance by *E. coli*, *Journal of Bacteriology* **145**: 1110–12

Mestecky J, McGhee J R, Arnold R R, Michalek S M, Prince S J, Babb J L 1978. Selective induction of an immune response in human external secretions by ingestion of bacterial antigen, *Journal of Clinical Investigation* **61**: 731–7

Michalek S M, McGhee J R, Mestecky J, Arnold R R, Bozzo L 1976. Ingestion of *Streptococcus mutans* induces secretory IgA and caries immunity, *Science* **192**: 1238–40

Robeson J P, Barletta R, Curtiss R III 1983. Expression of *Streptococcus mutans* glucosyltransferase gene in *Escherichia coli*, *Journal of Bacteriology* **153**: 211–21

Russell M W 1986. Protein antigens of *Streptococcus mutans*, in S Hamada, S M Michalek, H Kiyono, L Menaker, J R McGhee (eds) *Molecular Microbiology and Immunobiology of Streptococcus mutans.* Elsevier Publishers BV, Amsterdam, pp 51–60

Russell M W, Challacombe S J, Lehner T 1980. Specificity of antibodies induced by *Streptococcus mutans* during immunization against dental caries, *Immunology* **40**: 97–106

Tanzer J M 1979. Essential dependence of smooth surface caries on, and augmentation of fissure caries by, sucrose and *S. mutans* infection, *Infection and Immunity* **25**: 526–31

Taubman M A, Smith D J, Ebersole J L, Stack W E, Tsukuda T, Trocme M C 1986. Caries immunity and immune responses to *Streptococcus mutans* glucosyltransferase, in S Hamada, S M Michalek, H Kiyono, L Menaker, J R McGhee (eds) *Molecular Microbiology and Immunobiology of Streptococcus mutans*. Elsevier Publishers BV, Amsterdam, pp 279–86

Weisz-Carrington P, Roux M, McWilliams M, Phillips-Quagliata J M, Lamm M E 1979. Organ and isotype distribution of plasma cells producing specific antibody after oral immunization: evidence for a generalized secretory immune system, *Journal of Immunology* **123**: 1705–8

Immunization against the AIDS retrovirus: facts and prospects

L Montagnier*; J P Lecocq†; M P Kieny†; and M Girard‡

* Institut Pasteur, Unité d'Oncologie Virale, 25–28 rue du Dr Roux, 75724 Paris Cédex 15, France
† Transgène SA, 11 rue de Molsheim, 67082 Strasbourg Cédex, France
‡ Pasteur Vaccins SA, 1 Bld R. Poincaré, 92340 Marnes-la-Coquette, France

The rapid spread of Human Immunodeficiency Virus (HIV) is alarming, and an important increase of the number of HIV-infected individuals as well as of AIDS cases is expected in the coming years throughout North and South America, Africa and Western Europe. In the past, control of important virus-induced diseases was achieved by preventive immunization, i.e. vaccination, and we clearly need to apply the same approach to the AIDS epidemic. What are the present prospects for an AIDS vaccine?

The AIDS virus is a retrovirus, and more precisely a retro-lentivirus. Its characteristics raise some particular problems for the design of an efficient vaccine. First, let us recall the relevant characteristics of HIV.

HIV is a lentivirus

HIV, a retrovirus, has the capacity to integrate its genetic material (RNA, reverse-transcribed into DNA) into the host genome. In consequence, the viral proviral DNA can persist in a latent state in some infected cells without detectable gene expression. In such a situation the virus is invisible from the immune system of the host and virus-infected cells cannot be eradicated. The virus intrinsically has the potential to establish a lifelong chronic infection.

HIV is a retro-lentivirus and considerable similarities between HIV and the more general group of Ungulate lentiviruses have been demonstrated (Montagnier *et al.* 1984; Gonda *et al.* 1985; Wain-Hobson *et al.* 1985a; Sonigo *et al.* 1985). From its ultrastructure and morphogenesis, as well as nucleic acid homology within its most conserved genes, HIV resembles the lentiviruses such as Visna Virus, Equine Infectious Anemia Virus (EIAV), and the Caprine-Encephalitis Arthritis Virus (CAEV). The structure of the Visna and CEAV genomes (Sonigo *et al.* 1985; Wain-Hobson, personal communication 1985) are similar to that of HIV, all presenting a central region containing the Q, R and s/TAT genes. In addition, there is some immunologic cross-reactivity between the major core protein of HIV and that of EIAV.

In vivo, lentiviruses are characteristically cyolytic when expressed in infected cells. *In vivo*, they are all associated with chronic, severe diseases, with a long incubation period. None is directly associated with the production of tumors.

Their main *in vivo* targets are white blood cells. Although all lentiviruses have been shown to replicate in macrophages or in cells derived from monocytes, HIV has acquired a novel tropism for T4 lymphocytes (Klatzmann *et al*. 1984a; Clavel *et al*. 1986). The virus receptor present on $T4^+$ lymphocytes appears to be the T4 (CD4) molecule itself (Klatzmann *et al*. 1984b; Dalgleish *et al*. 1984; Wain-Hobson *et al*. 1985b).

This new tropism is shared by retro-lentiviruses isolated from primates such as macaques and African green monkeys. Other cells which are susceptible to virus infection include B lymphoblastoid cells, macrophages, and follicular dendritic cells of the germinative centers of lymph nodes which also seem to express the T4 gene to some extent. The situation is less clear for infected brain cells, which involve not only $T4^+$ macrophages (Koenig *et al*. 1986) but also $T4^-$ microglial cells (Vaseux *et al*. 1987). In the latter case it is possible that a related gene may be expressed or that a different processing of the T4 messenger RNA might occur.

HIV induces an atypical immune response in the host

Antibodies

It was not difficult from the onset of the discovery of HIV to detect antibodies raised against viral proteins (Barré-Sinoussi *et al*. 1983). The presence of antibodies remains the best sign of HIV infection. All viral proteins are antigenic, including nonstructural proteins such as the polymerase polypeptides and proteins coded by genes only expressed in infected cells, such as F, Q and TAT (Kan *et al*. 1986; Allan *et al*. 1985; Aldovini *et al*. 1986). However, there are variations both from one individual to another and also between different stages of the disease.

Asymptomatic carriers and Lymphadenopathy Syndrome (LAS) patients have, in general, the richest and broadest antibody response, directed towards core proteins p25 and p18 as well as to the envelope glycoproteins. In patients with advanced AIDS the antibody titers tend to decrease, particularly that of antibodies directed against core proteins, and in roughly one-half of cases only antibodies against gp41, gp110 (envelope glycoproteins) can still be detected. A striking feature which has to be taken into consideration for the design of vaccines is the fact that these antibodies poorly neutralize virus infectivity in classical *in vitro* neutralization tests (Weiss *et al*. 1985; Robert-Guroff *et al*. 1985; Clavel *et al*. 1985).

Reasons for this discrepancy are not clear. The higher degree of glycosylation of the outer membrane protein (32 potential glycosylation sites) may lead to protection by polysaccharides of the most critical regions of the protein. Another feature of this glycoprotein is its lack of stability at the viral envelope. The gp110 can be easily lost from the virus during purification. Such shedding of free protein into the circulation may also play a role *in vivo* in saturating plasma antibodies before they reach viral particles or infected cells.

Another likely explanation is that the critical sites of the viral glycoprotein, including the site which binds to the T4 molecule, may not be highly immunogenic due to similarities to host proteins involved in the interaction with T4, such as the DR HLA molecules.

Analysis of the more immunogenic regions of the envelope proteins has revealed that they correspond to very limited sites on the viral glycoproteins. For instance, a peptide of 25 amino acids (p39), located at the *N*-terminus of gp41, is the major antigen recognized by host antibodies in nearly 100% of the cases (Clavel *et al.* 1985; Goldstein, personal communication 1986). A site situated towards the *C*-terminus of the gp110 is also recognized, but not as frequently. These sites probably correspond to highly exposed regions of the molecules but unfortunately are not involved in the virus binding.

Cellular immune response

The detection of specific Cytotoxic Lymphocytes (CTL) in patients has been made difficult due to the fact that it is difficult to distinguish the *in vitro* CTL-induced lysis of target cells (T4 lymphocytes) from virus-induced lysis.

The appearance of a strong specific cellular immunity may explain the observed resistance to virus infection of some regular sexual partners of HIV-infected individuals, in the absence of detectable antibodies.

High genetic variability of HIV

The genetic variability of HIV has been abundantly documented by restriction map analysis of cloned isolates and by comparison of nucleic acid sequences of various isolates (Shaw *et al.* 1984; Willey *et al.* 1986; Starcich *et al.* 1986; Sanchez-Pescador *et al.* 1985).

In particular we have compared the nucleic acid sequences of two African (Zairian) isolates to that of the prototype LAV1 BRU (Alizon *et al.* 1986). Most of the variation occurs in the genes of envelope proteins, particularly those of the outer membrane proteins (up to 25% amino acid changes). Interestingly, the same extent of variation exists between the two African isolates, suggesting more protracted (or faster) molecular evolution of HIV in Central Africa.

Some regions of the envelope gene are highly variable, whereas some regions remain conserved. This stability is particularly the case in the p39 region mentioned above, explaining why by using one single strain (LAV/ HTLV-IIIB) it has been possible to detect infection of individuals by many other strains of the virus.

The mechanism of this genetic variation is likely to be caused by errors made during reverse transcription which include point mutations, frame shift mutations, deletions and repetitions. Its occurrence is probably highly signifi- cant for the pathogenic role of the virus. For both HIV and the animal lentiviruses variation may provide a means for escaping the host immune response or, possibly, permit a better match with the genotype of the infected cells (if for instance HLA genes play an accessory role in virus binding or penetration). It is interesting to note that some genetic variation has also been observed within one host according to time of virus isolation, although to a lesser extent than observed between isolates from different individuals (Hahn *et al.* 1986).

The discovery of HIV type 2

We have mentioned that most of the virus strains share common epitopes at the level of their glycoproteins. However, we find a few exceptions. Some AIDS patients present antibodies against their own virus but not against the envelope of the prototype LAVI/HTLV-IIIB. Most of these patients origin- ate in West Africa, particularly Guinea-Bissau. Furthermore, RNA of such isolates did not hybridize under high-stringency conditions with DNA probes of LAVI. In fact, only limited regions of the *gag-pol* regions and of the LTR hybridize under low-stringency conditions with the corresponding probes of LAVI. Only limited immunologic cross-reactivity between *gag* proteins was observed.

In contrast, there is a close relationship between this new type of virus (named LAV-II or HIV-2) with Simian Immunodeficiency Virus (SIV), a primate lentivirus causing AIDS in colonies of macaques (Desrosiers *et al.* 1986). In particular, the glycoproteins of HIV-2 and SIV show some immuno- logic cross-reactivity. However, their transmembrane and core proteins have different sizes, and molecular hybridization data suggest important sequence differences. HIV-2 is as pathogenic as HIV-1, and patients infected with this virus show typical clinical signs of AIDS, with opportunistic infections and a strong depression of the T4 subset.

Table 1 compares the major characteristics of this new type of HIV with those of HIV-1 and SIV. Since the virus displays the same tropism for T4 lymphocytes and probably binds to the same site on T4 molecules, examina- tion of its genetic sequence may well allow regions of the outer membrane glycoprotein involved in this binding to be defined. These regions should be expected to be highly conserved.

275

Table 1 Comparison of properties of HIV-1, HIV-2, SIVmac

Same ultrastructure

Similar *in vitro* biological properties (T4 tropism, cytopathic effect)

Similar pathogenic power

Weak sequence homology between HIV-1 and HIV-2 DNAs, mostly in *gag* and *pol* genes

No detectable cross-reacting epitopes in envelope glycoproteins of HIV-1 and HIV-2, some found between HIV-2 and SIV

Size of core and envelope proteins slightly different for HIV-1, HIV-2 and SIV.

Animal models

Many viruses possess immunosuppressive capacity and this may confer considerable selective advantage. Retroviruses, for instance the oncoviruses AKV of mice and feline Leukemia Virus, are no exception. In these cases the immunosuppressive activity has been linked to a particular region of the transmembrane segment of the envelope protein, p15. This region is not found in HIV, and immune suppression caused by this virus probably has a more complex origin, possibly involving an autoimmune reaction in the infected host (see for discussion of this hypothesis Klatzmann and Montagnier 1986).

Soon after the isolation of the AIDS retrovirus, preparations of live virus were inoculated into various species of primates. Only chimpanzees were found to be reproductively infected by some strains of the virus, as demonstrated by a rise in antibodies against viral proteins and virus isolation from peripheral blood lymphocytes. However, inoculated animals have remained asymptomatic for more than three years and it is unlikely that clinical symptoms of AIDS will appear. The use of chimpanzees will therefore be limited to the testing of the efficacy of subunit vaccines to prevent asymptomatic infection: the protecting power of a vaccine using the envelope protein as immunogen may be assessed by the lack of appearance of antibodies against core proteins and the lack of virus isolation from blood lymphocytes upon challenge by complete live virus.

Another possibility for the testing of retro-lentivirus vaccines will be to use macaques infected with SIV virus as an animal model, assuming that the lessons learned from this system could be applied to the human AIDS virus.

A further approach is suggested by the isolation of HIV type 2. The envelope glycoprotein of this virus is related to that of SIV and the virus may proliferate in one of the lesser primates such as the macaque. Indeed, recent results obtained independently by Patricia Fultz at CDC and Donald

Desrosiers at the New England Primate Center seem to confirm this hypothesis. Both groups could, at least transiently, raise antibodies against HIV-2 in inoculated macaques, and Desrosiers could show transient replication of the virus in baboons. Further adaptation of the virus to these monkeys will be required in order to use the latter for testing vaccines elaborated using this virus type.

Present and future strategies for vaccines

Although Essex has recently proposed the use of HTLV-IV virus isolated from healthy carriers in Senegal it is, in our opinion, not advisable to use 'attenuated' strains of HIV as vaccines. The extreme genetic instability of this group of viruses, as well as the risk of recombination with virulent wild strains, would make unrealistic the use of such viruses. Neither does the use of killed complete virus (inactivated for instance with formaldehyde or with psoralen derivatives) seem to be very promising, for recent experiments upon macaques by Desrosiers with formol-inactivated SIV indicate no protection against challenge virus.

The use of subunit vaccines appears more attractive. Recombinant DNA techniques can now be used to produce large quantities of viral antigen, and the *env* protein of HIV and other structural proteins have been expressed in *Escherichia coli*, yeast and in cultured mammalian cells (Dowbenko *et al.* 1985; Cabradilla *et al.* 1986; Hu *et al.* 1986; Chakrabart *et al.* 1986; Kieny *et al.* 1986; Franchini *et al.* 1986; Aldovini *et al.* 1986; Tanese *et al.* 1986).

Evaluation of the immunogenicity of such material is now on the way. Lasky *et al.* (1986) have recently succeeded in producing the extracellular NH_2-terminal segment (gp120) of the HIV I *env* glycoprotein in mammalian cells. Nevertheless, antibodies obtained in mice had only low neutralizing activity.

A further approach involves the construction of recombinant vaccinia virus expressing HIV proteins. This system was shown to be very efficient for other diseases (Mackett and Smith 1986) and is particularly well documented for rabies (Kieny *et al.* 1984; Wiktor *et al.* 1984; Blancou *et al.* 1986). In a first set of experiments we have integrated the HIV *env* gene into the vaccinia virus genome. Tissue-culture cells infected with the recombinant virus produce an authentic *env* protein which is recognized by sera from AIDS patients; the gp160 precursor is further processed to generate gp120 (the extracellular NH_2-terminal segment) and gp41 (the transmembrane COOH terminus).

Mice and rabbits inoculated with such recombinants however present only low titers of circulating antibodies capable of recognizing the *env* protein. Further, we have demonstrated that the low immunogenicity of the *env* protein may be due to the shedding of gp120 from the cell surface. Shedding may also occur in the human host and soluble *env* glycoprotein may disrupt the normal immune response by binding to $T4^+$ lymphocytes.

Similar vaccinia recombinant viruses have also been constructed by other laboratories and induction of a cellular immune response in macaques has been reported (Zarling *et al.* 1986). It remains to be seen whether such recombinant vaccinia virus expressing the *env* protein can induce an anti-viral response in chimpanzees.

Substantial engineering of the HIV surface antigen is likely to be necessary in order to improve its immunogenicity, and co-expression with other viral proteins may merit consideration.

Although there have been objections that complete protection may not be achieved with any of these approaches, for the reason that infection can spread from cell to cell with the production of little or no free virus, in our opinion this contention is unsubstantiated. Initial primary infection with HIV is likely to require a certain dose of virus and very probably involves amplification by means of infected cells producing free viral particles. Further, although many other viruses (e.g. the paramyxoviruses) induce cell fusion and proliferate by direct cell-to-cell transmission, vaccination against such viruses (for instance against measles virus) has been highly effective.

A more serious objection is that if we succeed in identifying highly immunogenic peptide sequences, we may also run the risk of eliciting auto-antibodies in view of the homology between certain viral polypeptides and cellular proteins. This objection was also raised in the past for hepatitis B vaccines and proved to be not confirmed by experimental results. The only way to evaluate such objections is to proceed to test of HIV vaccines designed in the laboratory, first in nonhuman primates, then in human volunteers.

Acknowledgements

The authors are grateful to Rick Lathe for critical reading of the manuscript. They also thank all their collaborators who participated in some experiments described in this paper.

References

Aldovini A, Debouck C, Feinberg M B, Rosenberg M, Arya S K, Wong-Staal F 1986. Synthesis of the complete trans-activation gene product of human T-lymphotropic virus type III in *Escherichia coli*: demonstration of immunogenicity *in vivo* and expression *in vitro*, *Proceedings of the National Academy of Sciences USA* **83**: 6672–7

Alizon M, Wain-Hobson S, Montagnier L, Sonigo P 1986. Genetic variability of the AIDS virus: nucleotide sequence analysis of two isolates from African patients, *Cell* **46**: 63–74

Allan J S, Coligan J E, Lee T H, McLane M F, Kanki P J, Groopman J E, Essex M 1985. A new HTLV-III/LAV antigen detected by antibodies from AIDS patients, *Science* **230**: 810–3

Barré-Sinoussi F, Chermann J C, Rey F, Nugeyre M T, Chamaret S, Gruest J, Dauguet C,

Axler-Blin C, Vézinet-Brun F, Rouzioux C, Rozenbaum W, Montagnier L 1983. Isolation of a T-lymphotropic retrovirus from a patient at risk for acquired immune deficiency syndrome (AIDS), *Science* **220**: 868–71

Blancou J, Klieny M P, Lathe R, Lecocq J P, Pastoret P P, Soulebot J P, Desmettre P 1986. Oral vaccination of the fox against rabies using a live recombinant vaccinia virus, *Nature (London)* **322**: 373

Cabradilla C D, Groopman J E, Lanigan J, Renz M, Lasky L A, Capon D J 1986. Serodiagnosis of antibodies to the human AIDS retrovirus with a bacterially synthesized *env* polypeptide, *Biotechnology* **4**: 128

Chakrabart S, Robert-Guroff M, Wong-Staal F, Gallo R C, Moss B 1986. Expression of the HTLV-III envelope gene by a recombinant vaccinia virus, *Nature (London)* **320**: 535

Clavel F, Klatzmann D, Montagnier L 1985. Deficient LAV, neutralizing capacity of sera from patients with AIDS or related syndromes, *The Lancet* **i**: 879–80

Clavel F, Guétard D, Brun-Vézinet F, Chamaret S, Rey M A, Santos-Ferreira M O, Laurent A G, Dauguet C, Katlama C, Rouzioux C, Klatzmann D, Champalimaud J L, Montagnier L 1986. Isolation of a new human retrovirus from West African patients with AIDS, *Science* **233**: 343–6

Dalgleish A G, Beverley P C L, Clapham P R, Crawford D H, Greaves M F, Weiss R A 1984. The CD4 (T4) antigen is an essential component of the receptor for the AIDS retrovirus, *Nature (London)* **312**: 763–7

Desrosiers R C, Daniel M D, Hunt R D, King N W, Arthur L O, Letvin N L 1986. An HTLV-III/LAV related virus from macaques. *International Conference on AIDS*, Paris, June 1986.

Dowbenko D J, Bell J R, Benton C V, Groopman J E, Nguyen H, Vetterlein D, Capon D J, Lasky L A 1985. Bacterial expression of the acquired immunodeficiency syndrome retrovirus p24 *gag* protein and its use as a diagnostic reagent, *Proceedings of the National Academy of Sciences USA* **82**: 7748

Franchini G, Robert-Guroff M, Wong-Staal F, Ghrayeb J, Kato I, Chang T W, Chang N T 1986. Expression of the protein encoded by the 3′ open reading frame of human T-cell lymphotropic virus type III in bacteria: demonstration of its immunoreactivity with human sera. *Proceedings of the National Academy of Sciences USA* **83**: 5282–7

Goldstein L 1986 (personal communication)

Gonda M A, Wong-Staal F, Gallo R C, Clements J E, Narayan O, Gilden R V 1985. Sequence homology and morphologic similarity of HTLV-III and Visna virus, a pathogenic lentivirus, *Science* **227**: 173

Hahn B H, Shaw G M, Taylor M E, Redfield R R, Markham P D, Salhuddin S Z, Wong-Staal F, Gallo R C, Parks E S, Parks W P 1986. Genetic variation in HTLV-III/LAV over time in patients with AIDS or at risk of AIDS, *Science* **232**: 1458–553

Hu S L, Kosowski S G, Dalrymple J M 1986. Expression of AIDS virus envelope gene in recombinant vaccinia viruses, *Nature (London)* **320**: 537

Kan N C, Franchini G, Wong-Staal F, Dubois G C, Robey W G, Lautenberger J A, Papas T S 1986. Identification of HTLV-III/LAV sor gene product and detection of antibodies in human sera, *Science* **231**: 1553–5

Kieny M P, Lathe R, Drillien R, Spehner D, Skory S, Schmitt D, Wiktor T, Koprowski H, Lococq J P 1984. Expression of rabies virus glycoprotein from a recombinant vaccinia virus, *Nature (London)* **312**: 163

Kieny M P, Rautmann G, Schmitt D, Dott K, Wain-Hobson S, Alizon M, Girard M, Chamaret S, Laurent A, Montagnier L, Lecocq J P 1986. AIDS virus *env* protein expressed from a recombinant vaccinia virus, *Biotechnology* **4**: 90

Klatzmann D, Montagnier L 1986. Approaches to AIDS therapy, *Nature (London)* **319**: 10–11

Klatzmann D, Barré-Sinoussi F, Nugeyre M T, Dauguet C, Vilmer E, Griscelli C, Brun-Vézinet F, Rouzioux C, Gluckman J C, Chermann J C, Montagnier L 1984a. Selective tropism of Lymphadenopathy Associated Virus (LAV) for helper-inducer T lymphocytes, *Science* **225**: 59–63

Klatzmann D, Champagne E, Chamaret S, Gruest J, Guétard D, Hercend T, Gluckman J C,

Montagnier L 1984b. T-lymphocyte T4 molecule behaves as the receptor for human retrovirus LAV, *Nature (London)* **312**: 767–8

Koenig S, Gendelman H E, Orenstein J M, Dal Canto M C, Pezeshkpour G H, Yungbluth P, Janotta F, Aksamit A, Martin M, Fauci A S 1986. Detection of AIDS virus in macrophages in brain tissue from AIDS patients with encephalopathy, *Science* **233**: 215–9

Lasky L A, Groopman J E, Fennie C W, Benz P M, Capon D J, Dowbenko D J, Nakamura G R, Nunes W M, Renz M E, Berman P W 1986. Neutralization of the AIDS retrovirus by anti-bodies to a recombinant envelope glycoprotein, *Science* **233**: 209

Mackett M, Smith G L 1986. Vaccinia virus expression vectors, *Journal of General Virology* **67**: 2067

Montagnier L, Dauguet C, Axler C, Chamaret S, Gruest J, Nugeyre M T, Rey F, Barré-Sinoussi F, Chermann J C 1984. A new type of retrovirus isolated from patients presenting with lymphadenopathy and acquired immune deficiency syndromes: structural and antigenic re-latedness with Equine Infectious Anemia Virus, *Annales de Virologie (Institut d'Pasteur)* **135E**: 119–34

Robert-Guroff M, Brown M, Gallo R C 1985. HTLV-III-neutralizing antibodies in patients with AIDS and AIDS-related complex, *Nature (London)* **316**: 72

Sanchez-Pescador R, Power M D, Barr P J, Steimer K S, Stempien M M, Brown-Shimer S L, Gee W W, Renard A, Randolph A, Levy J A, Dina D, Luciw P A 1985. Nucleotide sequence and expression of an AIDS-associated retrovirus (ARV-2), *Science* **227**: 484

Shaw G M, Hahn B H, Arya S K, Groopman J E, Gallo R C, Wong-Staal F 1984. Molecular characterization of human T-cell leukemia (lymphotropic) virus type III in the acquired immune deficiency syndrome, *Science* **226**: 1165

Sonigo P, Alizon M, Staskus K, Klatzmann D, Cole S, Danos O, Retzel E, Tiollais P, Haase A T, Wain-Hobson S 1985. Nucleotide sequence of the visna lentivirus: relationship to the AIDS virus, *Cell* **42**: 369–82

Starcich B R, Hahn B H, Shaw G M, McNeely P D, Modrow S, Wolf H, Parks E S, Parks W P, Josephs S F, Gallo R C, Wong-Staal F 1986. Identification and characterization of conserved and variable regions in the envelope gene of HTLV-III/LAV, the retrovirus of AIDS, *Cell* **45**: 637–48

Tanese N, Sodroski J, Haseltine W A, Goff S P 1986. Expression of reverse transcriptase activity of human T-lymphotropic virus type III (HTLV-III/LAV) in *Escherichia coli*, *Journal of Virology* **59**: 743

Vazeux R, Brousse N, Jarry A, Henin D, Marche C, Vedrenne C, Michon C, Rozenbaum W, Bureau J F, Montagnier L, Brahic M 1987. AIDS subacute encephalitis: identification of HIV infected cells, *American Journal of Pathology* (in press)

Wain-Hobson S 1985. (personal communication)

Wain-Hobson S, Alizon M, Montagnier L 1985a. Relationship of AIDS to other retroviruses, *Nature (London)* **313**: 743

Wain-Hobson S, Sonigo P, Danos O, Cole S, Alizon M 1985b. Nucleotide sequence of the AIDS virus, LAV, *Cell* **40**: 9–17

Weiss R A, Clapham P R, Cheingsong-Popov R, Dalgleish A G, Carne C A, Weller I V D, Tedder R S 1985. Neutralization of human T-lymphotropic virus type III by sera of AIDS and AIDS-risk patients, *Nature (London)* **316**: 69

Wiktor T J, Macfarlan R I, Reagan K J, Dietzschold B, Curtis P J, Wunner W H, Kieny M P, Lathe R, Lecocq J P, Mackett M, Moss B, Koprowski H 1984. Protection from rabies by a vaccinia virus recombinant containing the rabies virus glycoprotein gene, *Proceedings of the National Academy of Sciences USA* **81**: 7194

Willey R L, Rutledge R A, Dias S, Folks T, Theodore T, Buckler C E, Martin M A 1986. Identification of conserved and divergent domains within the envelope gene of the AIDS retrovirus, *Proceedings of the National Academy of Sciences USA* **83**: 5038–42

Zarling J M, Morton W, Moran P A, McClure J, Kosowski S G, Hu S L 1986. T-cell responses to human AIDS virus in macaques immunized with recombinant vaccinia viruses, *Nature (London)* **323**: 344

Molecular approaches to foot-and-mouth disease vaccines

Howard L Bachrach

Plum Island Animal Disease Center, Agricultural Research Service, US Department of Agriculture, Greenport, New York 11944, USA

Introduction

Foot-and-mouth disease (FMD) affects all domesticated and wild cloven-footed animals; but cattle, swine, sheep and goats – in that order – are the most important to animal agriculture. The disease is so infectious that it spreads to most, if not all, animals in unvaccinated herds of cattle and swine. There are seven viral immunotypes – A, O, C; SAT 1, 2, 3; and Asia 1 – which are further divided into 70 or more subtypes. The duration of immunity in recovered cattle is about two years and in swine only a few months. A post-recovery carrier state of virus in the esophageal and pharyngeal tissues of cattle, sheep and goats can act to propagate the disease further. The diagnosis of FMD from clinical signs alone is often uncertain, because several other animal diseases produce, initially, similar vesicular lesions. Direct losses in meat, milk and fiber production can amount to 25% or more, and mortality from myocarditis in young cattle sometimes exceeds 50%. Indirect losses are usually far larger than direct losses, because of embargos placed on exportations until the disease is officially eradicated. There have been nine outbreaks of FMD in the United States, the first in 1870 and the last in 1929; however, outbreaks occurred in Mexico from 1946 to 1954 and in Canada in 1952. Import restrictions of the Smoot–Hawley Tariff Act of 1930 have helped to keep the USA free of FMD since its last eradication in 1929.

Foot-and-mouth disease was the first animal disease shown to be caused by a filterable agent (Loeffler and Forsch 1897). More than 50 years then passed, however, before the agent was shown to be a 22 nm viral nucleoprotein (31% RNA/69% protein) with a sedimentation rate of approximately 140 S Svedberg units (Bachrach 1977). The virus contains 60 copies each of four capsid proteins VP_{1-4} which encapsidate a single strand of infectious-messenger sense 5' VP_g-linked RNA, approximately 8500 nucleotides long. (Actually, two or three copies of VP_2 and VP_4 are present as uncleaved VP_0 precursor molecules). The genome order is: 5' VP_g——poly C-L-VP_4-VP_2-VP_3-VP_1-?-$VP_{g1,2,3}$-Pro-Pol-poly A 3'. Noncapsid proteins L (Strebel and Beck 1986) and

Pro are proteases, and Pol is the viral-coded RNA polymerase. The three variant VP_gs link covalently in equimolar proportions to the 5' terminus (Forss and Schaller 1982). The primary translation product of the genome is a *ca* 250 kD polyprotein containing sites suceptible to cleavage by L and Pro (Robertson *et al.* 1985). Polyacrylamide gel electrophoresis (PAGE) of disrupted virions separates the capsid proteins (Fig. 1). (Note: VP_1 of Fig. 1 was originally termed VP_3 by us because of its PAGE position, but is now numbered to put it in register on the genome with VP_1s of other picorna viruses.) Several observations indicated that the 24 kD VP_1 is on the surface of the virion: (1) VP_1 on virions is cleaved by trypsin to a 16 kD *in situ*

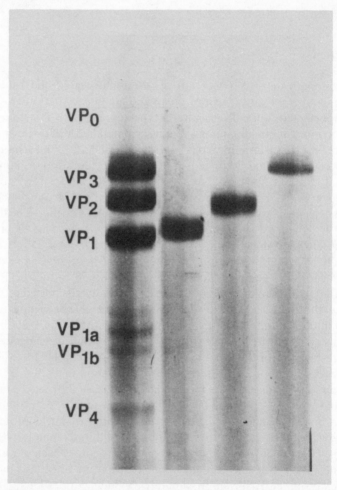

Figure 1. PAGE in SDS/8 M-urea of type A_{12} FMD virus disrupted by boiling in 8M-urea, 2% SDS and 5% mercaptoethanol. Left to right: FMD virus, purified VP_1, VP_2 and VP_3. VP_0 is uncleaved precursor of VP_4 and VP_2. $VP_{1a, 1b}$ are tryptic cleavage products of VP_1 in the virion. Adapted from Bachrach *et al.* (1975).

fragment (Wild *et al.* 1969); (2) ^{125}I-labeling of type A_{12} virus occurs principally on tryosyl residue 136 of VP_1, although the combined tryosyl residue content of VP_2 and VP_3 is twice that of VP_1 (Bachrach *et al.* 1978; Robertson *et al.* 1983); (3) some VP_1s are lost from virions on long exposure to CsCl (Bernard *et al.* 1974).

A vaccine for field use in cattle was produced in 1938. Known as the Schmidt–Waldmann vaccine (Schmidt 1938; Waldmann and Kobe 1938), it consisted of virus in ground epithelium and lymph from lesions on the tongues of cattle that was absorbed on to aluminum hydroxide gel particles and inactivated with formalin. Later, Frenkel (1947) in Holland improved on the source of virus; he grew virus in strips of bovine tongue epithelium suspended in culture fluid. Still used today in Holland, France and the USSR, the Frenkel method produces vaccines of high potency that retain the antigenicities of the field strains of virus used as inocula. Nevertheless, most virus for inactivated vaccines is produced now in stable lines of baby hamster kidney (BHK) cells grown in large fermenters; however, strict protocols must be followed to obtain useful concentrations of virus having field-strain specificity. A huge advantage in FMD vaccine work is that natural hosts such as cattle and swine can be used to test vaccine efficacy. The basic innocuity and potency tests in cattle with no previous exposure to virus were formulated in England from 1939 to 1952 by Henderson (1985) and coworkers. Later, precise relationships between purified virus mass and vaccine potency were determined in both cattle and swine (Polatnick and Bachrach 1964; Bachrach *et al.* 1964). For virus inactivated with acetylethylenimine (AEI) and emulsified with a modified Freund's incomplete adjuvant (FIA), the 50% protective dose (PD_{50}) of purified type A_{12} virus was 40 ng for cattle and 160 ng for swine (Morgan *et al.* 1970; Bachrach and McKercher 1972). In contrast, the PD_{50} of type 0_1 Brugge virus for swine was 3000 ng, demonstrating that type 0_1 virus is intrinsically a much weaker immunogen than type A_{12} virus.

Attenuated live virus vaccines are of little or no use in controlling FMD and are forbidden for use in Western Europe and most other countries. Virus attenuated to the extent needed for use in cattle is generally still too virulent for swine and even for cattle experiencing stresses, such as high-yielding milking cows.

Systematic vaccinations of cattle in Western Europe with Schmidt–Waldmann- and Frenkel-type inactivated vaccines began in the 1940s and a decade or two later in South America. Cattle in most Western European countries are vaccinated with trivalent type A, O, C vaccine twice during their first year of life and once a year thereafter. Swine are not vaccinated systematically, because protection is both brief and difficult to achieve (Bachrach 1968). Any vaccination of this species is generally restricted to stemming outbreaks of FMD in large commercial piggeries.

Ironically, the manufacture and use of inactivated virus vaccines are now a major cause of FMD. From 1968 to 1981, at least 44% of the outbreaks of FMD in Western Europe were caused by live virus in the vaccines or by escape of virus from vaccine factories. A similar situation appears to exist in South America (Bachrach 1982). Alternatives are thus needed, for example: (1) complete inactivation and prevention of virus escape from vaccine factories; (2) eradication as practiced by the United States and England; or (3) the use of protein-subunit or genetically engineered vaccines lacking any possibility of causing F̄MD.

Subunit vaccines

VP₁ and its fragments

Work designated to perfect safe and effective subunit vaccines began in earnest in the mid-1970s when it was discovered that capsid protein VP_1 isolated from FMD virus would induce neutralizing antibodies in swine (Laporte *et al.* 1973, type 0_1 VP_1; Bachrach *et al.* 1975, type A_{12} VP_1) and, more importantly, protective immunity in swine (Bachrach *et al.* 1975). The latter paper represented the first protection of an important natural host with capsid protein stripped from virus particles. We subsequently extended this observation on type A_{12} VP_1 to the protective immunization of cattle (Bachrach *et al.* 1982). Table 1 shows the neutralizing antibody and protective immune responses in these two domestic livestock species following vaccination with 100 μg doses of type A_{12} VP_1 capsid protein antigen. In addition, a 13 kD peptide fragment (amino acid residues 55–179) excised from VP_1 with cyanogen bromide and a 16 kD fragment (amino acid residues 1–144) released from VP_1 by trypsin treatment of virions were found to be similarly immunoprotective for livestock (Table 1).

Cloned subunit vaccines

Because of the immunoprotection afforded livestock by two or more doses of vaccines prepared from VP_1 or from 13 kD and 16 kD fragments of VP_1, we decided to make these, or peptides of similar length, in large amounts by recombinant DNA (rDNA) technology. We first determined *N*- and *C*-terminal amino acid sequences of type A_{12} VP_1 and its 13 kD and 15 kD fragments; the latter fragment derives from VP_1 in virions exposed to a protease present in certain BHK cell cultures. Knowledge of these sequences would permit the selection of correlate genetic sequences for constructing VP_1-specific rDNA. Using oligo dT primer and reverse transcriptase, DNA transcripts were made from a purified viral RNA template and were cloned and amplified in an appropriate pBR322/*Escherichia coli* system. Sequence analyses on restriction endonuclease fragments of this DNA established a partial physical map of the viral genome and identified DNA fragments that coded for VP_1. A recombinant plasmid constructed from pBR322 containing,

Table 1 Neutralizing antibody and protective immunity in swine and cattle vaccinated with type A_{12} FMD vaccines: VP_1, VP_1 fragments, rDNA-derived VP_1 fusion proteins and inactivated virus

Antigen*		Host	Vaccinations		Pre-challenge Neut. Ab	Fraction immune
Kind	MW (kD)		Dose (µg)	No.	(-log PD_{50})†	
VP_1	24	Swine	100	1	ND	1/10
		Swine	100	2	ND	8/10
		Swine	100	3	2.2	2/2
		Cattle	100	2	1.6	0/1
		Cattle	100	2	2.6	5/5
		Cattle	100	3	2.6	2/2
VP_1 frag.	13	Swine	50	2	1.3	3/3
		Cattle	50	2	0.4	2/2
VP_1 frag.	16	Swine	50	2	3.1	3/3
VP_1 fusion	44	Swine	250	2	1.4, 1.5	2/2
		Cattle	250	2	2.1–2.7	6/6‡
VP_1 fusion	26	Cattle	10	2	1.7	5/9
		Cattle	50	2	2.0	7/9
		Cattle	250	2	2.4	8/9
		Cattle	1250	2	2.7	9/9
Virus[AEI]		Swine	10	1	3.1	13/13
		Swine	10	2	4.0	6/6
None		Swine		0	ND	0/30
		Cattle		0	ND	0/23

* Virus inactivated with AEI, and all antigens emulsified with FIA. For VP_1 and VP_1 fragments, swine were revaccinated as shown on days 28 and 60, and were challenge-exposed beginning on day 56 or day 80, respectively; cattle were revaccinated as shown on days 14 and 28, and were challenged on day 72. Revaccinations with the 44 kD VP_1-fusion protein were on day 24 for swine and day 28 for cattle; challenges were on days 32 and 42, respectively (data from Bachrach *et al.* 1975, 1978, 1979, 1982 and Kleid *et al.* 1981). Revaccinations and challenges with the 26 kD VP_1-fusion protein were at 3.5 and 7 months, respectively, for the 10 and 50 µg doses; and at 7.5 and 10.5 months, respectively, for the 250 and 1250 µg doses (data from McKercher *et al.* 1985). For the challenges, half of the unvaccinated animals (bottom two rows) were inoculated with virus and half served as transmission controls. All developed FMD and remained with the vaccinates to expose them continuously to shed virus.
† Neutralizing antibody determined as 50% protective doses for suckling mice.
‡ One steer had a small foot lesion that healed without any other evidence of disease.
ND = Not determined.

in sequence, a *trp* promoter/operator, the first 190 codons of tryptophan synthetase and a DNA sequence corresponding to codons for amino acids 8–211 of the 213 amino acid chain of VP_1 was used to transform *E. coli* K12. After growing the cells in culture and deleting tryptophan, the transformants expressed one to two million copies per cell of a 44 kD VP_1 fusion protein. The extracted and purified fusion protein was shown to elicit neutralizing antibodies and protective immunity against type A_{12} FMD in both swine and cattle (Table 1) (Kleid *et al.* 1981), an achievement described by Secretary of Agriculture John R Block as 'the first production through gene splicing of an effective vaccine against any disease in animals or humans.' Two vaccinations were required with the 44 kD fusion protein vaccine, and challenge was carried out one to one-and-a-half months following the initial vaccination. It was not determined how long this protective immunity would have persisted. However, using a similarly cloned 26 kD fusion protein vaccine containing residues 1–211 of VP_1, immunoprotection of cattle vaccinated on day 1 and again at 3.5 or 7.5 months was still in effect at 7 and 10.5 months, respectively (Table 1) (McKercher *et al.* 1985).

While type A_{12} virus is no longer found in nature, VP_1-specific fusion proteins have now been produced for the current field strains A_{24}, A_{27}, A_{79} and C_3; and the correlate vaccines have been shown to be as effective in cattle as the prototype 44 kD VP_1 fusion protein vaccine (McKercher, personal communication).

Cloned VP_1-specific fusion protein vaccines for type 0_1 FMD are under development; however, those reported thus far evoke neutralizing antibodies in goats (Hofschneider *et al.* 1981) and cattle but less than satisfactory resistance to challenge. This difficulty may involve: (1) the intrinsically weak immunogenicity of type 0_1 virus; (2) possible disulfide bond stabilization of a putative conformational epitope by the two cysteine residues in type 0_1 VP_1 but not in type A_{12} VP_1 which has only one cysteine; or (3) the two regions of type 0_1 VP_1 (residues 138–154 and 200–213) that are on the surface of virions (Strohmaier *et al.* 1982). Whatever the difficulty, a cloned type 0_1 VP_1-specific vaccine should be forthcoming, because a synthetic peptide vaccine has already been reported to induce protective immunity in cattle (DiMarchi *et al.* 1986).

Synthetic peptide vaccines

The chemical synthesis of peptide vaccines for FMD was preceded by the demonstration that livestock could be protectively immunized with type A_{12} VP_1, a 13 kD fragment from VP_1 (amino acid residues 55–179) or a cloned 44 kD VP_1 fusion protein (Bachrach *et al.* 1975, 1982; Kleid *et al.* 1981). Bittle *et al.* (1982) then reported that a single dose of a synthetic type 0_1 icosapeptide (amino acid residues 141–160 of VP_1) linked to carrier protein would evoke neutralizing antibody and protective immunity in guinea pigs; in cattle, however, it induced neutralizing antibody but less than satisfactory protective immunity (Wilson 1984). More recently, however, Di Marchi *et al.* (1986) reported that a 40-residue type 0_1 synthetic peptide which links the 141–158 and 200–213 regions of VP_1 (Cys-Cys-200 . . . 213-Pro-Pro-Ser-141 . . . 158-Pro-Cys-Gly) used with Freund's complete adjuvant but without carrier protein induced both neutralizing antibody and protective immunity in cattle. Controls were not included, however, to demonstrate conclusively that the two regions must be linked covalently, and Freund's complete adjuvant is not acceptable to the livestock industry. Moreover, the two 1 mg or one 5 mg peptide doses used appear to be impractical for field use; they are 30- and 3000-fold less effective on a molar basis than type A_{12} VP_1 fusion proteins and inactivated whole virus vaccines, respectively. Some of these differences may involve the low intrinsic immunogenicity of type 0_1 virions compared to type A_{12} virions.

Antigenic sites

The loci of epitopes on virions, on isolated VP_1 and on 12 S subunit particles (a virion degradation complex of VP_{1-3} lacking VP_4 and RNA) are being determined by several correlate types of information, including: (1) immunogenicity and immunogenicity overlaps of VP_1-specific fragments, fusion proteins and synthetic peptides; (2) reactivity of monoclonal antibodies (mAbs) generated with virus, VP_1 and its 13 kD fragment against virions, 12 S subunits and other VP_1-specific sequences; (3) polyclonal antibody binding of sets of overlapping synthetic hexapeptides spanning the entire VP_1 chain; and (4) amino acid sequence hypervariability between VP_1s of virus types A, O and C. Some of this information and correlations are depicted schematically in Fig. 2. X-ray crystallographic analysis of FMD virus has not yet been reported.

Figure 2a orients immunogenic 13 kD and 16 kD type A_{12} VP_1 fragments and a 32-mer (residues 137–168 in tandem repeat in a fusion protein; Moore 1983) with respect to VP_1. Thus, immunoprotective epitopes could be expected to reside within the Gln-55 through Arg-144 region of total sequence overlap, not to the exclusion, however, of others in the Gly-145 through Met-179 region of partial sequence overlap. These assessments correlate with the apparent surface location of Tyr-136 and Arg-144 (Robertson *et al.* 1983) and with domains defined by the selective reactivities of mAbs (Fig. 2b). All mAbs except 6AE9 neutralized virus; however, 6AE9 did bind to 12 S subunits, VP_1 and to its 13 kD and 16 kD fragments, placing its correlate binding epitope in the 55–144 amino acid sequence of VP_1. Monoclonal antibodies 7SF3 and 6HE4 each bound to virions, 12 S subunits and to the 13 kD fragment, indicating that correlate epitope(s) to these two neutralizing mAbs reside in the 145–168 sequence of VP_1. Monoclonal antibodies 6HC4 and 6EE2 bind virions, 12 S subunits, VP_1 and its 13 kD fragment but not the 32-mer; therefore, the correlate epitope locus for these two neutralizing mAbs appears to reside in the 169–179 sequence of VP_1. Since both correlate neutralization epitope regions 145–168 and 169–179 lie outside the 16 kD immunogenic fragment (Bachrach *et al.* 1979, 1982), additional neutralization-specific epitopes not detected by the above mAbs must exist. Three neutralization-specific domains have been detected on type A_{12} virus

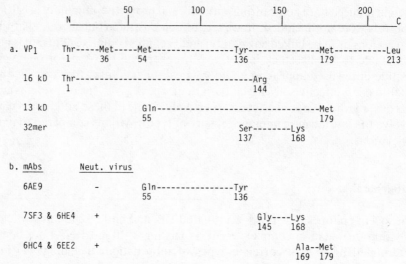

Figure 2. (a) Schematic diagram of type A_{12} VP_1-specific antigens. Tyr-136 is iodinateable and Arg-144 is a point of tryptic cleavage in virions, respectively. (b) Antigenic regions defined by reaction of mAbs with VP_1, 16 kD and 13 kD fragments and the 32-mer shown. Monoclonal antibodies with six prefixes were generated against type A_{12} VP_1; 7SF3 was generated against the 13 kD fragment. Adapted from Robertson *et al.* (1984).

using the four neutralizing mAbs shown in Fig. 2b and two others, 2FF11 and 2PD11, generated with virions (Baxt *et al.* 1984). The two domains defined by the neutralizing mAbs of Fig. 2b are also present on VP_1 and the 12 S subunit, whereas that defined by 2FF11 is a conformational epitope present on intact virions only. Monoclonal antibodies 7SF3, 6HE4 and 2FF11 cause extensive viral aggregation; mAbs 6HC4 and 6EE2 appear to block the site on VP_1 that attaches to cellular receptors; and mAb 2PD11, which is 100-fold more reactive in plaque reduction than the other mAbs, may act by inhibiting viral penetration and/or uncoating.

Regions of amino acid hypervariability between VP_1s of A_{12}, 0_1 and C_1 viruses (Kleid *et al.* 1981; Rowlands *et al.* 1983; Kurz *et al.* 1981; Robertson *et al.* 1983; Beck *et al.* 1983) agree in general with domains defined by immunogenic VP_1 fragments and neutralizing mAbs (Bachrach 1985). Although not indicated using mAbs, a variable region 136–144 could contain a neutralization-specific epitope, because of its apparent surface location on type A_{12} virions and its presence in the 16 kD immunogenic fragment (residues 1–144). However, the evidence for this putative epitope is equivocal at this time. In addition to the evidence summarized in Figs. 2a and 2b, strong evidence for neutralization-specific epitopes in the 145–168 and 169–179 regions of VP_1 stems from the hypervariability of sequences and cross-neutralization reactions involving the type A_{12} variants USA, A, B and C (Rowlands *et al.* 1983). The variants, taken together, have nonconserved residues 147, 152 and 170 within the two putative epitope regions, but retain type A_{12} character even with radical noncontiguous single amino acid substitutions, e.g. Pro, a helix breaker for non-helix breakers at position 152 and negatively charged Glu to neutral Val at position 170. By contrast, multiple contiguous substitutions and insertions/deletions extending rightward from these same positions appear to correlate with changes in immunotype (Bachrach 1985). Sequence variability indicates that region 145–168 could contain two putative epitopes six to seven residues long (*ca* 146–151 and 152–157) and the 169–179 region only one (*ca* 170–175); the epitopes would contain one to two charged amino acid residues.

For type 0_1 VP_1, two regions possess important epitopes, 138–154 (or 141–160) and 200–213 (Strohmaier *et al.* 1982; Bittle *et al.* 1982). Bindings of antibodies specific for 140 S virions, VP_1 or 12 S subunits to short overlapping synthetic peptides spanning the entire 213 amino acid chain of VP_1 are reported to map the former epitope at residues 146–152 (Geysen *et al.* 1984). This epitope, -Gly-Asp-Leu-Gln-Val-Leu-Ala-, is present on virions and VP_1 but not on 12 S subunits; and it is co-sequential with a putative neutralization-specific epitope of type A_{12} VP_1 (Bachrach 1985). In the 0_1 epitope, Leu at positions 148 and 151 is essential for binding to antibody; to a lesser extent, this is also the case for Glu-149 and Ala-152 (Geysen *et al.* 1984).

While the three-dimensional structure of FMD virus has not been reported, proximal alignment of FMD virus VP_1 sequences on VP_1 structures determined for HRV-14 and type 1 poliovirus (Rossmann *et al.* 1985; Hogle *et al.* 1985) indicates that FMD virus VP_1 putative epitope sequences would reside in exposed regions relative to these two correlate picornavirus VP_1 structures (Fig. 3). The type A_{12} and 0_1 FMD virus VP_1 sequences 137–157 fall in the

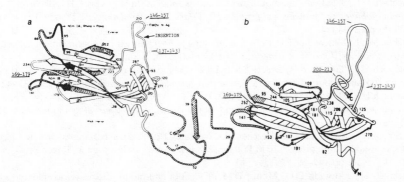

Figure 3. Proximal alignment of FMD virus VP_1 on (a) HRV-14 and (b) poliovirus type 1 VP_1 structures. Four deletion regions (striped) relative to both known structures and one large insertion (arrow) relative to HRV-14 VP_1 are indicated. Underlined numbers depict FMD virus VP_1 continuous epitope regions (see text). A putative discontinuous epitope is possible in type 0_1 VP_1 provided that its C-terminal 200–213 region and major surface loop structure juxtapose as in b. Modified from Rossmann *et al.* 1985 and Hogle *et al.* 1985; the extensive C- and N-termini are not shown on the poliovirus VP_1 chain.

major surface loop structure, whereas residues 169–179 would comprise the fourth looping measured from the N-terminus around the sharp edge of the conserved folding *core* of HRV-14 and poliovirus coat proteins. Four regions of deletion ($C + N$-terminal deletions are considered a single region) relative to HRV-14 and poliovirus VP_1s indicate that epitope equivalents to NIm-IA and IB are lacking in FMD virus VP_1. Of the *ca* 29% cumulative deletions in FMD virus VP_1 versus both HRV-14 and poliovirus VP_1s, *ca* 23% appears to reside in the $C + N$ region. This large $C + N$-deletion correlates with the FMD virions unique loose attachment to VP_1 and *in vitro* dye sensitization to photodynamic inactivation. The juxtapositioning of a proximate C-terminal sequence with the major surface loop in poliovirus VP_1, if repeated in FMD virus type 0_1 VP_1, would account for both an exposed continuous 200–213 epitope region (Strohmaier *et al.* 1982) and apparent discontinuous epitope involving 141–158 and 200–213 regions of FMD virus type 0_1 VP_1 (DiMarchi *et al.* 1986).

References

Bachrach H L 1968. Foot-and-mouth disease, in C E Clifton, S Raffel, M P Starr (eds) *Annual Review of Microbiology*. Annual Reviews Inc, Palo Alto, pp 201–44

Bachrach H L 1977. Foot-and-mouth disease virus: properties, molecular biology and immunogenicity, in J A Romberger (ed) *Beltsville symposium in Agricultural Research I. Virology in agriculture*. Allanheld Osmun, Montclair, New Jersey, pp 3–32

Bachrach H L 1982. Recombinant DNA technology for the preparation of subunit vaccines. *Journal of American Veterinary Medical Association* 181: 992–9

Bachrach H L 1985. Foot-and-mouth disease and its antigens, in M Z Atassi, H L Bachrach (eds) *Immunobiology of proteins and peptides III. Viral and bacterial antigens*. Plenum Press, New York, pp 27–46

Bachrach H L, McKercher P D 1972. Immunology of FMD in swine: experimental inactivated-virus vaccines, *Journal of American Veterinary Medical Association* 160: 521–6

Bachrach H L, Trautman R, Breese S S Jr 1964. Chemical and physical properties of virtually pure foot-and-mouth disease virus, *American Journal of Veterinary Research* 25: 333–42

Bachrach H L, Moore D M, McKercher P D, Polatnick J 1975. Immune and antibody responses to an isolated capsid protein of foot-and-mouth disease virus, *Journal of Immunology* 115: 1636–41

Bachrach H L, Moore D M, McKercher P D, Polatnick J 1978. An experimental protein vaccine for foot-and-mouth disease, in M Pollard (ed) *Perspectives in Virology X*. Raven Press, New York, ch 10, pp 147–59

Bachrach H L, Morgan D O, Moore D M 1979. Foot-and-mouth disease virus immunogenic capsid protein VP_T: N terminal sequences and immunogenic peptides obtained by CNBr and tryptic cleavages, *Intervirology* 12: 65–72

Bachrach H L, Morgan, D O, McKercher P D, Moore D M, Robertson B H 1982. Immunogenicity and structure of fragments derived from foot-and-mouth disease virus capsid protein VP_3 and of virions having intact and cleaved VP_3, *Veterinary Microbiology* 7: 85–96

Baxt B, Morgan D O, Robertson B G, Timpone C A 1984. Epitopes on foot-and-mouth disease outer capsid protein VP_1 involved in neutralization and cell attachment, *Journal of Virology* 51: 298–305

Beck E, Feil G, Strohmaier K 1983. The molecular basis of the antigenic variation of foot-and-mouth disease virus, *EMBO Journal* **2**: 555–9

Bernard S, Wantyghem J, Grosclaude J, Laporte J 1974. Chromatographic separation of purified structural proteins from foot-and-mouth disease virus, *Biochemical and Biophysical Research Communications* **58**: 624–32

Bittle J L, Houghten R A, Alexander H, Shinnick T M, Sutcliffe J G, Lerner R A, Rowland D J, Brown F 1982. Protection against foot-and-mouth disease by immunization with a chemically synthesized peptide predicted from the viral nucleotide sequence, *Nature (London)* **298**: 30–3

DiMarchi R, Brooke G, Gale C, Cracknell V, Doel T, Mowat N 1986. Protection of cattle against foot-and-mouth disease with a synthetic peptide, *Science* **232**: 639–41

Forss S, Schaller H 1982. A tandem repeat gene in a picornavirus, *Nucleic Acids Research* **10**: 6441–50

Frenkel H S 1947. La culture du virus de la fievre aphteuse sur l'epithelium de la langue des bovides, *Bulletin of International Epizootics* **28**: 155–62

Geysen H M, Meloen R H, Barteling S J 1984. Use of peptide synthesis to probe viral antigens for epitopes to a resolution of a single amino acid, *Proceedings of the National Academy of Sciences USA* **81**: 3998–4002

Henderson W 1985. A personal history of the testing of foot-and-mouth disease vaccines in cattle, in *The Massey-Ferguson Papers*. H E Jones Ltd, Birmingham

Hofschneider P H, Burgelt E, Kauzmann M, Mussgay M, Franze R, Ahl R, Bohm H, Strohmaier K, Kupper H, Otto B 1981. Studies on the antigenicity and immunogenicity of foot-and-mouth disease viral protein VP$_1$ expressed in *E. coli*, in P A Bachmann (ed) *Munich symposia on microbiology: Biological products for viral diseases*. Taylor and Frances Ltd, London, pp 105–13

Hogle J M, Chow M, Filman D J 1985. Three-dimensional structure of poliovirus at 2.9 Å resolution, *Science* **229**: 1358–65

Kleid D G, Yansura D, Small B, Dowbenko D, Moore D M, Grubman M J, McKercher P D, Morgan D O, Robertson B H, Bachrach H L 1981. Cloned viral protein vaccine for foot-and-mouth disease: responses in cattle and swine, *Science* **214**: 1125–9

Kurz C, Forss S, Kupper H, Strohmaier K, Schaller H 1981. Nucleotide sequence and corresponding amino acid sequence of the gene for the major antigen of foot-and-mouth disease virus, *Nucleic Acids Research* **9**: 1919–31

Laporte J, Grosclaude J, Wantyghem J, Bernard S, Rouge P 1973. Neutralization en culture cellulaire du pouvoir infectieux du virus de la fievre aphteuse par des serums provenant de porcs immunises a l'aide d'une proteine virale purifiée, *Comptes Rendus de l'Academie des Sciences* **276**: 3399–402

Loeffler F, Frosch P 1897. Kommission erforschung der Maul- und Klauenseuche bei dem Institute fur Infektionskrankheiten in Berlin. *Zentrablatt für Bakteriologie, Mikrobiologie und Hygiene*. 1. ABT. Originale A 22: 257–9

McKercher P D (personal communcation)

McKercher P D, Moore D M, Morgan D O, Robertson B H, Callis J J, Kleid D G, Shire S J, Yansura D G, Dowbenko D, Small B 1985. Dose response evaluation of genetically engineered foot-and-mouth disease virus polypeptide immunogen in cattle, *American Journal of Veterinary Research* **46**: 587–90

Moore D M 1983. Production of a vaccine for foot-and-mouth disease through gene cloning, in L D Owens (ed) *Genetic Engineering: Application to Agriculture. Beltsville Symposium VII*. Rowman and Allanheld, Totowa, New Jersey, ch 7, pp. 89–106

Morgan D O, McKercher P D, Bachrach H L 1970. Quantitation of the antigenicity and immunogenicity of purified FMDV vaccine for swine and steers, *Applied Microbiology* **20**: 770–4

Polatnick J, Bachrach H L 1964. Production and purification of milligram amounts of foot-and-mouth disease virus from baby hamster kidney cell cultures, *Applied Microbiology* **12**: 368–73

Robertson B H, Moore D M, Grubman M J, Kleid D G 1983. Identification of an exposed region of the immunogenic capsid polypeptide VP$_1$ on foot-and-mouth disease virus, *Journal of Virology* **46**: 311–16

Robertson B H, Morgan D O, Moore D M 1984. Location of neutralizing epitopes defined by monoclonal antibodies generated against the outer capsid polypeptide, VP_1, of foot-and-mouth disease virus A_{12}, *Virus Research* **1**: 489–500

Robertson B H, Grubman M J, Weddell G N, Moore D M, Welsh J D, Fischer T, Dowbenko D J, Yansura D G, Small B, Kleid D G 1985. Nucleotide and amino acid sequence coding for polypeptides of foot-and-mouth disease virus type A_{12}, *Journal of Virology* **54**: 651–60

Rossmann M G, Arnold E, Erickson J W, Frankenberger E A, Griffith J P, Hecht H J, Johnson J E, Kamer G, Luo M, Mosser A G, Rueckert R R, Sherry B, Vriend G 1985. Structure of a human common cold virus and functional relationship to other picornaviruses. *Nature (London)* **317**: 145–53

Rowlands D J, Clarke B E, Carrol A R, Brown F, Nicholson B, Bittle J L, Houghten R A, Lerner R A 1983. Chemical basis of antigenic variation in foot-and-mouth disease virus. *Nature (London)* **306**: 694–7

Schmidt S 1938. Adsorption von Maul- und Klauenseuchevirus an Aluminiumhydroxid unter besonder Besucksichtigung der immunisierenden Eigenschaften der Virus-adsorbate. *Zeitschrift für Immunitaetsforschung Immunobiology* **92**: 392–409

Strebel K, Beck E 1986. A second protease of foot-and-mouth disease virus, *Journal of Virology* **58**: 893–9

Strohmaier K, Franze R, Adam K H 1982. Location and characterization of the antigenic portion of the FMDV immunizing protein, *Journal of General Virology* **4**: 313–20

Waldmann O, Kobe K 1938. Die aktive Immunisierung des Rindes gegen Maul- und Klauenseuche, *Deutsche Tierarzliche Wochenschrift (Hannover)* **5**: 523–5

Wild T F, Burroughs J N, Brown F 1969. Surface structure of foot-and-mouth disease virus, *Journal of General Virology* **4**: 313–20

Wilson T 1984. Engineering tomorrow's vaccines, *Biotechnology* **2**: 29–39

A potential cholera vaccine based on hybrid strains expressing *Vibrio cholerae* surface components

Michael W Heuzenroeder; Johannes Pohlner; M B Jalajakumari; Jane Yeadon; Gordon Stevenson; David I Leavesley; Thomas F Meyer; Peter R Reeves; Derrick Rowley; Paul A Manning

Department of Microbiology and Immunology, The University of Adelaide, Adelaide, South Australia 5001, Australia

Introduction

Vibrio cholerae O1 are non-invasive enteric pathogens, which colonize the gut with the watery diarrhea associated with the disease primarily results from an enterotoxin (CT) which is actively excreted. However, the toxin is not the sole virulence determinant and components of the cell envelope and other excreted proteins are involved in the pathogenesis of the disease.

The outer membrane of the cell envelope of *V. cholerae* is typical for Gram-negative bacteria containing both lipopolysaccharide (LPS) and a limited number of proteins. It has been demonstrated in model systems that antibodies to both of these classes of surface antigens are protective (Neoh and Rowley 1970). Antibodies to the protein antigens are more protective on a weight basis than antibodies to the O-antigen. Of these the LPS is by far the more potent immunogen. Presumably antibodies to these components protect by inhibiting adherence and colonization. Little is known about the protective somatic antigens in man except that human convalescent sera contain antibodies to both the LPS and a few proteins (Sears *et al.* 1984). (The term 'protective antigen' will be used here to mean an antigen that is recognized by antibodies which are protective against cholera.)

The fact that the disease is itself an immunizing process has given hope to the concept of live oral vaccines against cholera. Several groups are approaching the problem of attenuating *V. cholerae* by eliminating its toxinogenicity either by chemical mutagenesis (Honda and Finkelstein 1979) or by constructing defined genetic deletions (Mekalanos *et al.* 1983; Kaper *et al.* 1984).

We have taken another approach. It has been demonstrated that avirulent salmonellae capable of colonizing the Peyer's patch lymphoid tissue can stimulate IgA antibodies in the gut (Hohmann *et al.* 1979; Srisart *et al.* 1985).

293

In fact, there is a good correlation between Peyer's patch colonization, IgA response and protection. Consequently the aim is to have *V. cholerae* surface antigens expressed in avirulent salmonellae and to use such strains as oral immunogens. Work with salmonellae expressing determinants of other pathogens suggests that this may be fruitful (Formal *et al.* 1981; Stevenson and Manning 1985).

Outer membrane proteins

The outer membrane of *V. cholerae* contains several major proteins (Fig. 1; Kabir 1980; Kelly and Parker 1981; Manning *et al.* 1982). There are several proteins in the 43–47 kD range and the relative amounts of these are strain- and medium-dependent (Manning *et al.* 1982; P A Manning and R A Alm, unpublished data). These proteins probably represent the major cell porins. In addition, the heat-modifiable 35 kD OmpA-like protein (Alm *et al.* 1986)

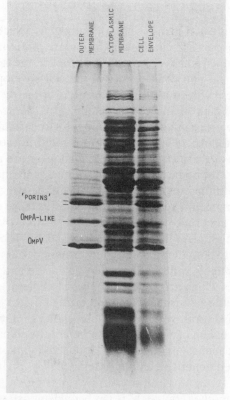

Figure 1. Cell envelope proteins of *Vibrio cholerae*. Cell envelopes were fractionated on sucrose density gradients to separate the inner and outer membranes and analyzed by SDS–PAGE.

and the 26 kD OmpV protein (Stevenson *et al.* 1985) are also major species.

The OmpV protein appears to be strongly immunogenic compared to the other outer membrane proteins (Manning and Haynes 1984). It has been purified and the structural gene cloned from biotypes El Tor and Classical (Stevenson *et al.* 1985). OmpV is found in *V. cholerae* including non-O1 strains but not in other vibrios. Antibodies to OmpV are commonly detected in human convalescent sera (P A Manning, unpublished data).

Because of its properties, effort has been concentrated on OmpV and its gene. The structural gene has been localized within cloned DNA by deletion and transposon insertion analysis (Stevenson *et al.* 1985; Manning *et al.* 1987). However, the gene is poorly expressed in *E. coli* K-12. Analysis of the nucleotide sequence suggests that translational control may be the problem (Pohlner *et al.* 1986a). Thus, in order to perform immunization and absorption experiments, higher levels of expression were required. This has been accomplished as a result of constructing transcriptional and translational fusions (Pohlner *et al.* 1986b).

Construction of OmpV fusions

A series of fusions were constructed in which decreasing amounts of *ompV* DNA were fused to the amino terminal coding region of the MS2 replicase (Fig. 2). Expression is from the P_L promoter of bacteriophage lambda and under the control of a temperature-sensitive cI repressor (Klinkert *et al.* 1986). Examples of proteins produced by such fusions are shown in Fig. 3. Plasmid pOmpV210 mediates the production of high levels of OmpV. Plasmids pOmpV215, pOmpV225 and pOmpV230 lead to the production of a fusion protein which can be processed to mature OmpV, and plasmid pOmpV260 results in a non-processed fusion. The proteins are only produced as a result of cI inactivation at 42 °C.

Nucleotide sequence analysis of the *ompV* DNA present in these fusions demonstrates that all of *ompV* and its Shine–Dalgarno sequence are present in pOmpV210 whereas the other plasmids represent true gene fusions. The fusion junctions in plasmids pOmpV215, pOmpV225 and pOmpV230 are all in the promoter proximal region of the signal sequence and still allow the signal cleavage site to be recognized.

Further gene fusions using smaller fragments have enabled the antigenic determinants recognized on the native and SDS-purified (i.e. denatured) forms of the protein to be localized (see Fig. 2). The epitope(s) on the native form of the protein is at its carboxyl terminus, and the epitope recognized on the purified protein can be localized to a 28 amino acid segment at the amino terminus (Pohlner *et al.* 1986b).

The fusion in pOmpV210 enables the isolation of a fragment containing *ompV* and its Shine–Dalgarno sequence; however, the region which could

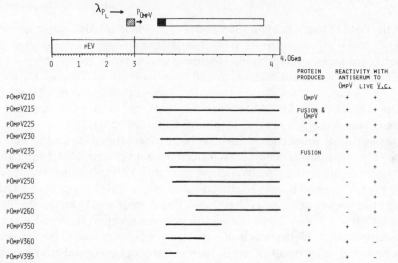

Figure 2. Organization of the DNA in *ompV* gene fusions. *V. cholerae* containing decreasing amounts of *ompV* were cloned into the pEV expression vector adjacent to the amino-terminal coding region of the MS2 replicase (hatched box). Expression is from the λP_L promoter which is controlled by a temperature-sensitive cI repressor: transcription occurs only at 42 °C. The box at the top of the Figure corresponds to the *ompV* coding region with the solid region representing the amino-terminal signal sequence of the precursor and the open region of the mature protein. Both promoters are indicated (λP_L and P_{OmpV}). The lines below correspond to the extent of *V. cholerae* DNA present in each of the plasmids. The proteins produced and their reactivity with antiserum to either purified OmpV or native OmpV on live *V. cholerae* is also shown.

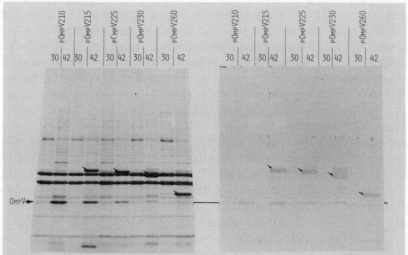

Figure 3. SDS–PAGE of cell envelope of *E. coli* K-12 expressing *ompV* gene fusions followed by either staining with Coomassie Blue or Western blotting using anti-purified OmpV serum. Cells were grown either at 30 °C where no expression occurs or at 42 °C where the fusions are expressed due to inactivation of the temperature-sensitive cI repressor. Arrows indicate the position of the MS2 replicase–OmpV fusion proteins.

form a secondary structure in the mRNA and prevent translation is absent. Thus, this fragment represents a suitable module to be coupled to a constitutive promoter to obtain OmpV protein expression.

O-antigen of the lipopolysaccharide

The LPS of the outer membrane consists of basically three regions: the lipid A region which is hydrophobic and forms part of the lipid bilayer of the outer membrane) the core oligosaccharide and the O-antigen. The outermost region, the O-antigen, provides the major antigenic variability of the cell surface.

In *Vibrio cholerae* strains of the O1 serotype two major subclasses of O-antigen are recognized, Ogawa and Inaba. Strains of the Ogawa serotype have A and B antigens whereas those of the Inaba serotype have A and C antigens (Burrows *et al.* 1946). That is, they both share A while B is Ogawa-specific and C Inaba-specific. However, Ogawa strains may possess small amounts of C (Sakazi and Tamura 1971; Redmond *et al.* 1973). A third, less common serotype, Hikojima, is also found in *V. cholerae* 01 strains (Burrows *et al.* 1946). Hikojima strains produce antigen A and high levels of both B and C.

The O-antigen has been implicated in adhesion in a number of animal experiments (Freter and Jones 1976; Chitnis *et al.* 1982). Also studies with human volunteers showed that serum vibriocidal antibody directed mainly against the LPS rose significantly in challenge trials (Clements *et al.* 1982). Thus the importance of the LPS as a potential protective antigen is clearly demonstrated. Since *V. cholerae* remains in the gut, protection can be provided by preventing adhesion and motility. Thus, as the cell surface and probably the flagellum are coated with LPS, it would not be unreasonable to expect antibodies to the LPS, in particular to the exposed O-antigen region, to be protective.

Molecular cloning and expression of genes for O-antigen biosynthesis

Genomic banks of *V. cholerae* strains 569B and O17 have been constructed using the cosmid cloning vector pHC79 and *in vitro* packaging into bacteriophage λ (Collins and Hohn 1978; Hohn and Collins 1980). Replicas of the cosmid gene banks on nitrocellulose filters were screened by colony blotting using rabbit antiserum to live organisms of either 569B or O17 followed by a goat-anti-rabbit IgG coupled with horseradish peroxidase as described elsewhere (Towbin *et al.* 1979; Hawkes *et al.* 1982; Manning *et al.* 1987). About 20 strong positive reacting colonies from a bank of about 900 clones from 569B and 19 from 650 clones obtained from O17 were further examined (Manning *et al.* 1986).

Cell envelope material from these clones was prepared, solubilized in SDS and analyzed by SDS–polyacrylamide gel electrophoresis followed by silver staining. Of these clones, one derived from 569B and two from O17 showed a pattern typical of O-antigen material (Fig. 4). The plasmids in these clones were designated pPM1001 (Inaba, serotype from 569B), pPM1002 and pPM1003 (Ogawa, serotype from 017) (Manning *et al.* 1986).

Deletion analysis and subclones of pPM1001 suggest that the region of DNA associated with O-antigen biosynthesis is greater than 1 kb.

LPS analysis

LPS has been extracted from *E. coli* K-12 strain DH1 harboring either pHC79, pPM1001 or pPM1003 using the hot-phenol–water method (Westphal and Jann 1965). This material has been compared with LPS extracted from *V. cholerae* in hemagglutination inhibition assays to determine the

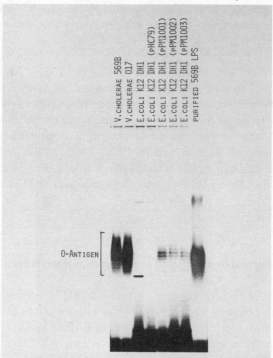

Figure 4. SDS–PAGE followed by silver staining of purified LPS from *V. cholerae* strain 569B and of cell envelopes of *V. cholerae* strains 569B and O17 and *E. coli* K-12 strain DH1 and its derivatives. The gels were fixed so that lipopolysaccharides (and lipoproteins) were stained.

Table 1 Hemagglutination inhibition assays

Source of LPS	Amount (μg) of LPS required to inhibit hemagglutination of sheep erythrocytes sensitized* with LPS from:	
	569B (Inaba)	**O17 (Ogawa)**
V. cholerae 569B (Inaba)	0.012–0.024	0.78
V. cholerae O17 (Ogawa)	0.20	0.20
E. coli K-12 DH1 [pHC79]	>100	>100
E. coli K-12 DH1 [pPM1001]	0.05	3.1
E. coli K-12 DH1 [pPM1003]	0.78	0.78

* Sheep erythrocytes were sensitized with alkali-treated purified LPS (homologous to the antiserum to be used). To 100 μl of diluted antiserum (polyclonal antisera were raised in rabbits against heat-killed organisms) containing four hemagglutinating units of antibody was added 100 μl containing two-fold serial dilutions of purified LPS. Hemagglutination trays were incubated for 60 min at 37 °C and the end points determined.

concentration of LPS capable of inhibiting the agglutination of LPS-sensitized sheep erythrocytes using a constant amount of antibody. The results, summarized in Table 1, show that the plasmids are directing the synthesis of O-antigen of the appropriate serotype and that the homologous serotype is better at inhibiting in both cases.

The presence of plasmid pPM1001 results in the production of O-antigen with the Inaba specificity as judged by the amount of LPS required to inhibit, whereas pPM1003 has the Ogawa specificity. However, it can be seen that there is a considerable cross-reaction, as it is also borne out by Western blot analysis (not shown). This is presumably due to the common A antigen since a polyclonal antiserum to the LPS was used.

Protection tests

Escherichia coli K-12 strains harboring either pHC79 or pPM1001 have been used to immunize rabbits intramuscularly to produce antisera for analysis of their protective activity in the infant mouse animal model system (Chaicumpa and Rowley 1972) using either *V. cholerae* 569B (Inaba) or O17 (Ogawa) as the challenge organism (Manning *et al.* 1986). The results, summarized in Table 2, demonstrate that antisera raised against *E. coli* K-12 harboring pPM1001 compare favorably with antisera similarly raised against *V. cholerae* 569B. That is, the O-antigen produced by *E. coli* K-12 harboring pPM1001 behaves antigenically like that produced by *V. cholerae* 569B and is highly protective in this model system.

Table 2 Infant mouse protection tests*

Antiserum to	Protective index to challenge organism:	
	569B (Inaba)	O17 (Ogawa)
V. cholerae 569B (Inaba)	700–1200	ND†
V. cholerae O17 (Ogawa)	ND	680–850
E. coli K-12 DH1 [pHC79]	<10‡	<10
E. coli K-12 DH1 [pPM1001]	850	223

* Challenge tests were performed using five-day-old infant mice as described (Chaicumpa and Rowley, 1972)). Twenty LD_{50} doses were orally administered simultaneously with dilutions of rabbit antisera. The experiment continued until the last of the controls (fed *V. cholerae* without antiserum) died. The PD_{50} was calculated as the reciprocal of the dilution of antiserum which gave 50% protection.
† ND indicates not done.
‡ Protective indices <10 indicate that no protection was observed with a 1-in-10 dilution of the antiserum.

Construction of a vaccine strain

These studies have implicated the OmpV protein and the O-antigen of the LPS as important antigens. Thus, ideally, the vaccine strain should be capable of expressing both. It is also appreciated that any live oral vaccine strain cannot harbor antibiotic resistance markers because of their potential clinical use; consequently a selection must be developed which does not require any supplements in order to maintain the plasmid. Alternatively, the genes must be incorporated into the chromosome of the host. Both approaches are being taken.

Suitable host strains which are capable of both expressing and delivering the antigen(s) to the Peyer's patch lymphoid tissue are also being examined. These include *S. typhi* mutants such as *galE* (Germanier and Fürer 1975) or *aro* (Hoisketh and Stocker 1981).

Acknowledgements

This research has been supported by the National Health and Medical Research Council of Australia, the Diarrheal Diseases Control Program of the World Health Organization, F H Faulding Pty Ltd, and the Australian National Biotechnology Program.

References

Alm R A, Braun G, Morona R, Manning P A 1986. Detection of an OmpA-like protein in *Vibrio cholerae, FEMS Microbiology Letters* (in press)

Burrows W, Mather A N, McGann V G, Wagner S M 1946. Studies on immunity to Asiatic cholera II. The O and H antigenic structure of the cholera and related vibrios, *Journal of Infectious Diseases* **79**: 168–75

Chaicumpa W, Rowley D 1972. Experimental cholera in infant mice: protective effects of antibody. *Journal of Infectious Diseases* **125**: 480–5

Chitnis D S, Sharma K D, Kamat R S 1982. Role of somatic antigen of *Vibrio cholerae* in adhesion to intestinal mucosa, *Journal of Medical Microbiology* **5**: 53–61

Clements M L, Levine M M, Young C R, Black R E, Lim Y-L, Robins-Browne R M, Craig J P 1982. Magnitude, kinetics and duration of vibriocidal antibody responses in North Americans after ingestion of *Vibrio cholerae, Journal of Infectious Diseases* **145**: 465–73

Collins J, Hohn B 1978. Cosmids: a type of plasmid gene cloning vector that is packageable *in vitro* in bacteriophage λ, *Proceedings of the National Academy of Sciences USA* **75**: 4242–6

Formal S B, Baron L S, Kopecko D J, Washington O, Powell C, Life C A 1981. Construction of a potential bivalent vaccine strain: introduction of *Shigella sonnei* form I antigen genes into the *galE Salmonella typhi* Ty21a typhoid vaccine strain, *Infection and Immunity* **34**: 746–50

Freter R, Jones G W 1976. Adhesive properties of *Vibrio cholerae*: nature of the interaction with intact mucosal surfaces, *Infection and Immunity* **14**: 246–56

Germanier R, Fürer E 1975. Isolation and characterization of *galE* mutant Ty21a of *Salmonella typhi*: a candidate strain for a live, oral typhoid vaccine, *Journal of Infectious Diseases* **131**: 553–8

Hawkes R E, Niday E, Gordon J 1982. A dot immunobinding assay for monoclonal and other antibodies, *Analytical Biochemistry* **119**: 142–7

Hohmann A, Schmidt G, Rowley D 1979. Intestinal and serum antibody responses in mice after oral immunization with *Salmonella, Escherichia coli* and *Salmonella–Escherichia coli* hybrid strains, *Infection and Immunity* **25**: 27–33

Hohn B, Collins J 1980. A small cosmid for efficient cloning of large DNA fragments, *Gene* **11**: 291–8

Hoisketh S K, Stocker B A D 1981. Aromatic-dependent *Salmonella typhimurium* are non-virulent and effective as live vaccines, *Nature (London)* **291**: 238–9

Honda T, Finkelstein R A 1979. Selection and characteristics of *Vibrio cholerae* mutant lacking the A (ADP-ribosylating) portion of the cholera enterotoxin, *Proceedings of the National Academy of Sciences USA* **76**: 2052–6

Kabir S 1980. Composition and immunochemical properties of the outer membrane proteins of *Vibrio cholerae, Journal of Bacteriology* **144**: 382–9

Kaper J B, Lockman H, Baldini M M, Levine M M 1984. Recombinant non-toxigenic *Vibrio cholerae* strains as attenuated cholera vaccine candidates, *Nature (London)* **308**: 655–8

Kelly J T, Parker C D 1981. Identification and preliminary characterization of *Vibrio cholerae* outer membrane proteins, *Journal of Bacteriology* **145**: 1018–24

Klinkert M Q, Herrmann R, Schaller H E 1986. Surface proteins of *Mycoplasma hyopneumoniae* identified from an *Escherichia coli* expression plasmid library, *Infection and Immunity* **49**: 329–35

Manning P A, Haynes D R 1984. A common immunogenic *Vibrio* outer membrane protein, *FEMS Microbiology Letters* **24**: 297–302

Manning P A, Imbesi F, Haynes D R 1982. Cell envelope proteins of *Vibrio cholerae. FEMS Microbiology Letters* **14**: 159–66

Manning P A, Heuzenroeder M W, Yeadon J, Leavesley D I, Reeves P R, Rowley D 1986. Molecular cloning and expression in *Escherichia coli* K12 of the O antigens of the Inaba and Ogawa serotypes of the *Vibrio cholerae* O1 lipopolysaccharides and their potential for vaccine development, *Infection and Immunity* **53**: 272–7

Manning P A, Stevenson G, Heuzenroeder M W 1987. Molecular cloning of a common major outer membrane protein of *Vibrio cholerae*, in Y Takeda, N F Pierce (eds) *Advances in cholera and related diarrheas* **4**. KTK Publications, Japan (in press)

Mekalanos J J, Swartz D J, Pearson D N, Harford N, Groyne F, de Wilde M 1983. Cholera toxin genes: nucleotide sequence, deletion analysis and vaccine development, *Nature (London)* **306**: 551–7

Neoh S H, Rowley D 1970. The antigens of *Vibrio cholerae* involved in vibriocidal action of antibody and complement, *Journal of Infectious Diseases* **121**: 505–13

Pohlner J, Meyer T F, Jalajakumari M B, Manning P A 1986a. Nucleotide sequence of *ompV*, structural gene for a major *Vibrio cholerae* outer membrane protein, *Molecular and General Genetics* **205**: 494–500

Pohlner J, Meyer T F, Manning P A 1986b. Serological properties and processing in *Escherichia coli* K-1 of OmpV fusion proteins of *Vibrio cholerae, Molecular and General Genetics* **205**: 501–6

Redmond J W, Korsch M H, Jackson G D F 1973. Immunochemical studies of the O-antigens of *Vibrio cholerae*. Partial characterization of an acid labile antigenic determinant, *Australian Journal of Experimental Biology and Medical Science* **51**: 229–35

Sakazaki R, Tamura K 1971. Somatic antigen variation in *Vibrio cholerae*, *Japanese Journal of Medical Science and Biology* **24**: 93–100

Sears S D, Richardson K, Young C, Parker C D, Levine M M 1984. Evaluation of the human immune response to outer membrane proteins of *Vibrio cholerae*, *Infection and Immunity* **44**: 439–44

Srisart P, Reynold B L, Rowley D 1985. The correlation between serum IgA antibody levels and resistance to infection with *Salmonella typhimurium* after oral immunization with various salmonellae, *Australian Journal of Experimental Biology and Medical Science* **63**: 177–82

Stevenson G, Manning P A 1985. Galactose epimeraseless (*GalE*) mutant G30 of *Salmonella typhimurium* is a good potential live oral vaccine carrier for fimbrial antigens, *FEMS Microbiology Letters* **28**: 317–32

Stevenson G, Leavesley D I, Lagnado C A, Heuzenroeder M W, Manning P A 1985. Purification of the 25 kDal *Vibrio cholerae* major outer membrane protein and the molecular cloning of its gene: *ompV, European Journal of Biochemistry* **148**: 385–90

Towbin H, Staehelin T, Gordon J 1979. Electrophoretic transfer of proteins from polyacrylamide gels to nitrocellulose sheets: procedure and some applications, *Proceedings of the National Academy of Sciences USA* **76**: 4350–4

Westphal O, Jann K 1965. Bacterial lipopolysaccharides. Extraction with phenol–water and further applications of the procedure, in R L Whistler (ed) *Methods in Carbohydrate Chemistry,* Academic Press, New York, vol 5, pp 83–91

Recombinant vaccinia virus vaccines: an overview

Enzo Paoletti; Marion E Perkus; Antonia Piccini

Laboratory of Immunology, Wadsworth Center for Laboratories and Research, New York State Department of Health, Albany, New York 12201, USA

Introduction

Vaccinia virus, a member of the poxvirus family, is a complex double-stranded DNA virus that replicates in the cytoplasm of infected cells. The virus carries within its coat a large number of enzymes, some of which are involved in the transcription of its genetic material. For recent reviews see Dales and Pogo (1981) and Moss (1985).

Since its introduction by Jenner 190 years ago, vaccinia has been used as a vaccine for smallpox. In 1980 the World Health Organization proclaimed that smallpox, as a human infectious disease, had been globally eradicated. This monumental accomplishment was made feasible by the fact that the smallpox agent did not have an animal reservoir other than man and the availability and properties of the smallpox vaccine, vaccinia virus. Vaccinia is inexpensive to produce and can be administered by a simple dermal abrasion. Significantly, the vaccine can be prepared as a lyophilized preparation, shipped and stored without the requirement for refrigeration, important considerations in under-developed nations.

The ability to express foreign genes in vaccinia virus vectors has raised the exciting possibility of using genetically engineered vaccinia as a live recombinant vaccine directed against a variety of other viral, parasitic or bacterial agents.

Strategy for the construction of recombinant vaccinia virus

A general protocol for constructing recombinant vaccinia viruses is shown in Fig. 1. A defined foreign genetic element is inserted by recombinant DNA technologies into a genetically 'non-essential' locus of the vaccinia DNA. This foreign DNA, now flanked by vaccinia sequences, is transfected into cells that are additionally infected with wild-type vaccinia virus. Recombination

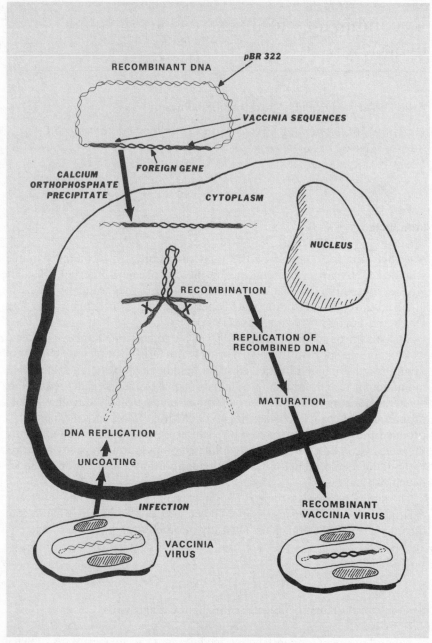

Figure 1. General protocol for constructing recombinant viruses.

occurring between the sequences flanking the foreign DNA and homologous sequences on the DNA of a replicating vaccinia DNA molecule allows the insertion of the foreign DNA into a recombinant vaccinia genome which can in turn be replicated and packaged into progeny virus. Recombinant virus can be identified by a number of techniques and pure viral stocks prepared by plaque cloning.

Foreign genes expressed in vaccinia virus vectors

Table 1 lists the foreign genes expressed in vaccinia viruses to date. What has been learned can be briefly summarized as follows: (a) the expression of the foreign gene is authentic including secondary modifications such as glysosylation; (b) if the foreign gene encodes an 'antigen', the presentation of that antigen is identical to the manner in which that antigen is presented under natural conditions of infection. For example, the hepatitis B virus surface antigen is secreted from the infected cell as a 22 nm particle whereas the herpes simplex glycoprotein D and rabies glycoprotein G are presented as

Table 1 Foreign genes expressed in recombinant vaccinia viruses

	Reference	
Herpes simplex virus thymidine kinase	Panicali *et al.*	1982
	Mackett *et al.*	1982
Influenza virus hemagglutinin	Panicali *et al.*	1983
	Smith *et al.*	1983b
Hepatitis B virus surface antigen	Smith *et al.*	1983a
	Paoletti *et al.*	1984
Herpes simplex virus glycoprotein	Paoletti *et al.*	1984
	Cremer *et al.*	1985
Plasmodium knowlesi sporozoite antigen	Smith *et al.*	1984
Chloramphenicol acetyltransferase	Mackett *et al.*	1984
Rabies virus glycoprotein	Kieny *et al.*	1984
	Wiktor *et al.*	1984
Transmissible gastroenteritis virus gp195	Hu *et al.*	1984
Vesicular stomatitis virus G protein	Mackett *et al.*	1985
Vesicular stomatitis virus N protein	Mackett *et al.*	1985
Influenza virus nucleoprotein	Yewdell *et al.*	1985
Human factor IX (Christmas factor)	de la Salle *et al.*	1985
Neomycin resistance gene	Franke *et al.*	1985
Sindbis virus structural proteins	Rice *et al.*	1985
β-galactosidase	Chakrabarti *et al.*	1985
Epstein–Barr membrane antigen gp340	Mackett and Arrand	1985
Sindbis virus structural proteins	Franke and Hruby	1985
Respiratory syncytial virus glycoprotein G	Ball *et al.*	1986
Tobacco etch virus proteins	Dougherty *et al.*	1986
Friend murine leukemia virus gp70/p15E	Stephens *et al.*	1986

integral components of infected cell membranes; (c) where tested, the vaccinia virus recombinant elicits humoral antibodies against the foreign gene product, elicits cytotoxic T cells and provides significant levels of protection against subsequent challenge with the correlate pathogen.

Potential of recombinant vaccinia viruses as multivalent vaccine vectors

At least three approaches can be considered for using vaccinia virus vectors as live vaccines directed against multiple pathogens. One approach is to construct a number of vaccinia virus recombinants. Each recombinant virus would express a single foreign gene. The individual recombinants could then be mixed prior to vaccination. An example of this approach resulted in the simultaneous immunization of laboratory animals against both herpes simplex virus type 1 and hepatitis B virus (Paoletti *et al.* 1984).

Another approach of utilizing vaccinia virus recombinant to immunize against multiple pathogens is to vaccinate with recombinant viruses expressing novel antigens sequentially as they become available. This approach has been demonstrated in dairy cows (Gillespie *et al.* 1986) and other laboratory animals (Perkus *et al.* 1985). As is demonstrated in Table 2, prior exposure to

Table 2 Anamnestic response to HBsAg on revaccination of rabbits with recombinant vaccinia virus*

Time post-inoculation (weeks)	Anti-HBsAg (RIA units/ ml serum)†	Vaccinia virus plaque reduction (%)‡	
		1600	6400
1	0.08	63	12
3	0.36	69	35
6	18.40	82	12
11	14.40	69	31
40	6.80	57	13
54	6.80	41	0
57	32.70	85	4
59	24.30	95	66
62	24.30	90	67

* A rabbit inoculated intradermally with 1.8×10^7 pfu of a vaccinia virus recombinant expressing the HBsAg was revaccinated with an equivalent dose of a vaccinia virus recombinant expressing the HBsAg 56 weeks after the initial inoculation.
† Anti-HBsAg antibody levels were determined using a commercially available RIA kit from Abbott Laboratories and are noted in RIA units ($\times 10^{-3}$) per ml of serum as defined by the manufacturer. Vaccinia virus was mixed with dilutions of antisera and kept at 4 °C overnight until titrated on CV-1 monolayers.
‡ The percentage reduction of plaques obtained on CV-1 monolayers is indicated as the reciprocal of the serum dilution.

Table 3 Revaccination with recombinant vaccinia virus expressing novel foreign antigens*

Weeks	Anti-HBsAg (RIA units/ml serum)†	Anti-Inf HA‡
3	0.2	<10
6	16	<10
9	72	<10
40	128	<10
54	72	<10
55	72	40
56	63	160
57	43	80
58	63	160
59	63	320
60	63	640

* A rabbit was immunized intradermally with a vaccinia virus recombinant expressing the HBsAg.
† Anti-HBsAg antibodies were assayed using the commercially available radioimmunoassay from Abbott Laboratories and is noted as RIA units ($\times 10^{-3}$)/ml of serum as in Table 2. The same animal was revaccinated at 54 weeks with a novel vaccinia virus recombinant expressing the influenza virus hemagglutinin and anti-influenza HA antibodies were assayed by standard hemagglutination inhibition tests using chicken erythrocytes and 4 HA units.
‡ Reciprocal of serum dilution is shown.

vaccinia virus does not prevent revaccination with the same virus. An anamnestic response to a foreign gene product is observed. As is demonstrated in Table 3, a previous vaccinia virus vaccination does not inhibit subsequent immunization against a second novel foreign antigen carried by another vaccinia virus recombinant.

On revaccination, the period of time before which viral replication is halted by immunological surveillance is probably shortened. This can be compensated by having the foreign gene expressed at a significantly higher level than would be required in a naive individual, thus allowing for the synthesis of sufficient antigenic mass.

The probability that this approach would be useful in the human population is supported by the relatively low level of immunity against vaccinia as measured by humoral antibody levels in vaccinees. Furthermore, when there was an active immunization program against smallpox, the recommendation was that people be revaccinated every three to five years, this process resulted in a significantly high rate of vaccination 'takes'.

The third and perhaps more exciting approach to achieving immunity against multiple foreign pathogens using vaccinia virus recombinants is to express multiple foreign genes within a single vaccinia virus. This was first demonstrated by Perkus *et al.* (1985) with the simultaneous expression in a vaccinia virus recombinant of the herpes simplex virus glycoprotein D, the hepatitis B virus surface antigen and the *Influenza* virus hemagglutinin.

Table 4 Immunological response to vaccination with a recombinant vaccinia expressing multiple foreign genes*

Time post-inoculation (weeks)	Anti-HBsAg (RIA units/ ml serum)†	Anti-HA HI‡	Anti-HSV§	Anti-vaccinia§
Rabbit #257				
1	160	160	640	6400
2	160	160	5120	6400
3	160	320	2560	12800
4	670	320	2560	12800
5	1840	640	1280	12800
Rabbit #288				
1	80	20	<40	<40
2	160	80	320	400
3	360	40	160	400
4	760	80	320	400
5	760	80	160	400

Source: Modified from Perkus *et al.* 1985.
* Rabbits were inoculated with 5×10^7 pfu in 0.5 ml either intravenously (#257) or intradermally (#288) with a vaccinia recombinant expressing the HBsAg, HSV-gD and influenza HA genes and immunological response followed as described.
† Sera were tested for anti-HBsAg antibodies using the commercially available AUSAB radioimmunoassay kit from Abbott Laboratories and titers expressed in RIA units/ml of serum as defined by the manufacturer.
‡ Hemagglutination inhibition tests were performed using 4HA units. Reciprocal of serum dilution is indicated.
§ Plaque-reduction assays monitoring reduction of HSV or vaccinia virus infectivity were performed on CV-1 cells. Reciprocal of serum dilution giving greater than 50% reduction in plaque number is shown.

Inoculation of laboratory animals with this triple recombinant seroconverted them against all three foreign antigens (Table 4).

The ability to express multiple foreign genes in a single vaccinia recombinant arises from the rather plastic nature of the DNA packaging potential of vaccinia virus. As many as 25 kilobases of foreign DNA have been stably inserted into vaccinia virus recombinants (Smith and Moss 1983) and with the availability of viable vaccinia deletion mutants lacking 22 kilobases of DNA (Perkus *et al.* 1986) sufficient space is available for several dozen average-sized foreign genes to be accommodated by vaccinia virus. Whether the immunological system could respond to such a number of foreign antigens expressed by vaccinia recombinants is not known but it is interesting to note that in the example cited above from Perkus *et al.* (1985) serological responses were observed against three foreign antigens when present in a vaccinia virus infection background. Vaccinia itself expresses around 150–200 antigens of its own on infection.

The approach of a multivalent vaccinia recombinant has an additional feature that is attractive. The benefit/risk ratio of such an engineered virus would be skewed to the benefit side since the benefit would be the sum of immunity garnered against the total number of pathogens represented by the expressed foreign genes whereas the risk remains singular, to the single vaccination event.

Prospects

The successful smallpox eradication program was made possible by the availability of the vaccinia vaccine virus. The potential exists that the vaccinia virus, now engineered to vector foreign genes, will be used again as a vaccine for both human and veterinary applications. Although there are measurable risks attendant on use of vaccinia virus, these risks may be overshadowed by the benefit of successful vaccination against serious infectious diseases, for example vaccination against malaria and hepatitis. Future experiments to further attenuate the virus should decrease the risks associated with this vaccination approach. With the molecular technologies available it should be possible to identify the viral genetic functions responsible for adverse reactions and to eliminate these gene(s) if they are non-essential for viral replication or to modify them if these genetic functions are required.

References

Ball L A, Young K K Y, Anderson K, Collins P L, Wertz G W 1986. Expression of the major glycoprotein G of human respiratory syncytial virus from recombinant vaccinia virus vectors, *Proceedings of the National Academy of Sciences USA* **83**: 246–50

Chakrabarti S, Brechling K, Moss B 1985. Vaccinia virus expression vector: coexpression of beta-galactosidase provides visual screening of recombinant virus plaques, *Molecular and Cellular Biology* **5**: 3403–9

Cremer K J, Mackett M, Wohlenberg C, Notkins A L, Moss B 1985. Vaccinia virus recombinant expressing *herpes simplex* virus type 1 glycoprotein D prevents latent herpes in mice, *Science* **228**: 737–40

Dales S, Pogo B G T 1981. Biology of poxviruses, in *Virology Monographs*. Springer-Verlag, New York, vol 18.

de la Salle H, Altenburger W, Elkaim R, Dott K, Dieterle A, Drillien R, Cazenave J-P, Tolstoshev P. Lecocq J-P 1985. Active alpha-carboxylated human factor IX expressed using recombinant DNA techniques, *Nature (London)* **316**: 268–70

Dougherty W G, Franke C A, Hruby D E 1986. Construction of a recombinant vaccinia virus which expresses immunoreactive plant virus proteins, *Virology* **149**: 107–13

Franke C A, Hruby D E 1985. Expression of recombinant vaccinia virus-derived alphavirus proteins in mosquito cells, *Journal of General Virology* **66**: 2761–5

Franke C A, Rice C M, Strauss J H, Hruby D E 1985. Neomycin resistance as a dominant selectable marker for selection and isolation of vaccinia virus recombinants, *Molecular and Cellular Biology* **5**: 1918–24

Gillespie J H, Geissinger C, Scott F W, Higgins W P, Holmes D F, Perkus M, Mercer S, Paoletti

E 1986. Response of dairy calves to vaccinia viruses that express foreign genes, *Journal of Clinical Microbiology* **23**: 283–8

Hu S, Bruszewski J, Boone T, Souza L 1984. Cloning and expression of the surface glycoprotein gp195 of porcine transmissible gastroenteritis virus, in R M Chanock, R A Lerner (eds) *Modern Approaches to Vaccines: Molecular and chemical basis of virus virulence and Immunogenecity*. Cold Spring Harbor Laboratory, New York

Kieny M P, Lathe R, Drillien R, Spehner D, Skory S, Schmitt D, Wiktor T, Koprowski H, Lecocq J P 1984. Expression of rabies virus glycoprotein from a recombinant vaccinia virus, *Nature (London)* **312**: 163–6

Mackett M, Arrand J R 1985. Recombinant vaccinia virus induces neutralising antibodies in rabbits against Epstein–Barr virus membrane antigen gp340, *EMBO Journal* **4**: 3229–34

Mackett M, Smith G L, Moss B 1982. Vaccinia virus: a selectable eukaryotic cloning and expression vector, *Proceedings of the National Academy of Sciences USA* **79**: 7415–9

Mackett M, Smith G L, Moss B 1984. General method for production and selection of infectious vaccinia virus recombinants expressing foreign genes, *Journal of Virology* **49**: 857–64

Mackett M, Yilma T, Rose J K, Moss B 1985. Vaccinia virus recombinants: expression of VSV genes and protective immunization of mice and cattle, *Science* **227**: 433–5

Moss B 1985. Replication of poxviruses, in B N Fields (ed) *Virology*. Raven Press, New York

Panicali D, Paoletti E 1982. Construction of poxviruses as cloning vectors: insertion of the thymidine kinase gene from *herpes simplex* virus into the DNA of infectious vaccinia virus, *Proceedings of the National Academy of Sciences USA* **79**: 4927–31

Panicali D, Davis S W, Weinberg R L, Paoletti E 1983. Construction of live vaccines by using genetically engineered poxviruses: biological activity of recombinant vaccinia virus expressing influenza virus hemagglutinin, *Proceedings of the National Academy of Sciences USA* **80**: 5364–8

Paoletti E, Lipinskas B R, Samsonoff C, Mercer S, Panicali D 1984. Construction of live vaccines using genetically engineered poxviruses: biological activity of vaccinia virus recombinants expressing the hepatitis B virus surface antigen and the *herpes simplex* virus glycoprotein D, *Proceedings of the National Academy of Sciences USA* **81**: 193–7

Perkus M E, Piccini A, Lipinskas B R, Paoletti E 1985. Recombinant vaccinia virus: immunization against multiple pathogens, *Science* **229**: 981–4

Perkus M E, Panicali D, Mercer S, Paoletti E 1986. Insertion and deletion mutants of vaccinia virus, *Virology* **152**: 285–97

Rice C M, Franke C A, Strauss J H, Hruby D E 1985. Expression of Sindbis virus structural proteins via recombinant vaccinia virus: synthesis, processing, and incorporation into mature Sindbis virions, *Journal of Virology* **56**: 227–39

Smith G L, Moss B 1983. Infectious poxvirus vectors have capacity for at least 25 000 base pairs of foreign DNA, *Gene* **25**: 21–8

Smith G L, Mackett M, Moss B 1983a. Infectious vaccinia virus recombinants that express hepatitis B virus surface antigen. *Nature (London)* **302**: 490–5

Smith G L, Murphy B R, Moss B 1983b. Construction and characterization of an infectious vaccinia virus recombinant that expresses the influenza hemagglutinin gene and induces resistance to influenza virus infection in hamsters, *Proceedings of the National Academy of Sciences USA* **80**: 7155–9

Smith G L, Godson G N, Nussenzweig V, Nussenzweig R S, Barnwell J, Moss B 1984. *Plasmodium knowlesi* sporozoite antigen: expression of infectious recombinant vaccinia virus, *Science* **224**: 397–9

Stephens E B, Compans R W, Earl P, Moss B 1986. Surface expression of viral glycoproteins is polarized in epithelial cells infected with recombinant vaccinia viral vectors, *EMBO Journal* **5**: 237–45

Wiktor T J, Macfarlan R I, Reagan K J, Dietzschold B, Curtis P J, Wunner W H, Kieny M-P, Lathe R, Lecocq J-P, Mackett M, Moss B, Koprowski H 1984. Protection from rabies by a vaccinia virus recombinant containing the rabies virus glycoprotein gene, *Proceedings of the National Academy of Sciences USA* **81**: 7194–8

Yewdell J W, Bennink J R, Smith G L, Moss B 1985. Influenza A virus nucleoprotein is a major target antigen for cross-reactive anti-influenza A virus cytotoxic T lymphocytes, *Proceedings of the National Academy of Sciences USA* **82**: 1785–9

Live recombinant vaccinia virus vaccines

Geoffrey L Smith

Division of Virology, Department of Pathology, University of Cambridge, Tennis Court Road, Cambridge CB2 1QP, United Kingdom

Introduction

The practice of vaccination stems from Edward Jenner's successful use of cowpox virus to immunize against smallpox. We now understand that this protection was conferred due to the antigenic cross-reactivity of cowpox virus and variola virus, the etiological agent of smallpox. The virus that was used finally to eradicate smallpox was not cowpox, but vaccinia virus, another orthopoxvirus cross-reactive with both variola and cowpox but distinct from them both. The origins of vaccinia remain obscure and have not been resolved even with the application of modern techniques for detailed analysis of the virus genomes (Mackett and Archard 1979). Several properties of vaccinia virus made it a particularly successful vaccine against smallpox. The virus is able to be transported in tropical countries without refrigeration or loss of potency, it is cheap and simple to manufacture and administer and is effective as a single dose. The scar left at the site of vaccination also provides a rapid method for identifying those who have previously been vaccinated. Smallpox was a disease that was particularly amenable to control by vaccination since it was easily recognizable, it was strictly an acute disease without chronic, latent or persistent infections and the virus possessed no alternative animal reservoir. The combination of a fully available and effective vaccine, the acute nature of the disease and the full commitment and support for the eradication campaign by the World Health Organization (WHO) resulted in the global eradication of smallpox in 1977 (World Health Organization 1980).

With the eradication of smallpox interest in vaccinia virus declined. Nonetheless, research into the molecular biology of vaccinia continued and as a result of these efforts it became possible to modify vaccinia genetically so that genes from other pathogens were expressed by recombinant vaccinia viruses. Since these recombinant viruses retain their infectivity, as they replicate in tissue culture or *in vivo* in animals, the foreign gene is expressed like any other vaccinia gene. In those cases where the foreign gene is a protective antigen from another pathogen the recombinant virus may be directly used as a live vaccine against that pathogen. There are several examples where this potential has been effectively demonstrated. In addition to such direct applications of recombinant vaccinia viruses as live vaccines, the vaccinia expression vector system can be used in vaccine research to identify protective antigens of pathogens and to determine which antigens are recognized by cellular immune defense mechanisms. In this paper examples of these different applications are illustrated.

Biology of vaccinia and construction of recombinant viruses

For a detailed review for the molecular biology of vaccinia virus the reader should refer to Moss (1985). Here the features of vaccinia virus relevant to its use as an expression vector will be described. Vaccinia is a large complex virus with a DNA genome of 185 kilobase pairs (kbp) (Geshelin and Berns 1974). This genome is 66% adenine and thymine and when stripped of proteins it is noninfectious. These properties make direct manipulation of the intact virus genome impracticable and recombinant viruses are consequently constructed by using fragments of the virus genome cloned in plasmid vectors (see below). Within the virus core the DNA genome is associated with virus-encoded transcriptional enzymes that can only transcribe vaccinia virus genes and not those of other eukaryotic viruses or cells. This is despite a large subunit of the vaccinia RNA polymerase having homology to RNA polymerases of bacteria and eukaryotic cells (Broyles and Moss 1986) and the detection of a subunit of the cellular RNA polymerase II in highly purified rabbitpox virions (Morrison and Moyer 1986).

Nucleotide sequences of several early and late vaccinia genes have shown the transcriptional control regions of these genes to be structurally distinct from those of other eukaryotic or prokaryotic genes. Functional analyses of these promoter regions have demonstrated that they are transcribed by the vaccinia but not by cellular RNA polymerase II. Therefore, expression of foreign protein coding sequences in vaccinia is dependent upon linking these sequences to vaccinia virus promoters (Mackett *et al.* 1982).

Construction of recombinant viruses is done in two stages. In the first, the foreign protein coding sequences are joined to a vaccinia promoter in a plasmid vector. Care should be taken to ensure that the transcriptional initiation site is provided by the vaccinia promoter and the translation initiation codon comes from the foreign gene. The foreign gene and vaccinia promoter are then flanked by vaccinia DNA taken from a nonessential locus of the vaccinia virus genome. In the second stage, this plasmid is used to transfer the foreign gene into the vaccinia genome. Cells are infected with wild-type (WT) vaccinia virus and transfected with the plasmid DNA. Within these cells homologous recombination between the nonessential vaccinia DNA of the plasmid and virus genome results in the site-specific insertion of the foreign DNA into the vaccinia genome. The nature of the vaccinia DNA chosen to flank the foreign gene determines the site at which the foreign gene is inserted within the vaccinia genome. Several such sites have been identified (Mackett *et al.* 1982; Panicali and Paoletti 1982; Perkus *et al.* 1985) but a commonly used site is the vaccinia virus thymidine kinase (TK) gene. Not only is this gene nonessential for virus replication but it is possible to select for or against its expression. Since insertion of foreign DNA within the TK gene destroys its activity, recombinants are TK$^-$ and may be distinguished from TK$^+$ WT virus on TK$^-$ cells in the presence of 5-bromodeoxyuridine (BUdR). A selection system for the identification of recombinants is important since the frequency of the homologous recombination means that at best only 0.1% of total progeny virus is recombinant. Other methods of distinguishing recombinant viruses from parental virus are DNA hybridization (Nakano *et al.* 1982), co-expression of selectable markers in vaccinia such as herpes simplex virus TK (Panicali and Paoletti 1982; Mackett *et al.* 1982), the neomycin resistance gene (Franke *et al.* 1985) or co-expression of β-galactosidase permitting visual detection of recombinant virus plaques (Chakrabarti *et al.* 1985). Several plasmid vectors have been constructed to permit the rapid cloning and expression of foreign genes in vaccinia virus (Mackett *et al.* 1984; Boyle *et al.* 1985; Chakrabarti *et al.* 1985).

Once recombinant viruses have been identified by one of the above methods, the virus is plaque purified twice before larger stocks are grown. Analysis of the recombinant virus genomes have indicated that the foreign gene is always inserted at the predicted location, no other DNA alterations occur and the virus is stable upon serial passage. Even when large pieces of foreign DNA are inserted (25 kbp) the recombinant virus is stable and replicates normally *in vitro* (Smith and Moss 1983).

Applications of recombinant viruses

Identification of protective antigens from other pathogens

For many pathogens there are no effective vaccines and the protective antigens upon which vaccines might be based have not been identified. Pathogenic micro-organisms which are surrounded by lipid envelopes often have the protective antigens associated with this envelope. Commonly these antigens are glycoproteins which possess characteristic hydrophobic amino acid sequences that function to transport the protein through the cell membrane and to anchor the protein on the outside of the cell membrane. One approach in the search for such antigens and the genes encoding them is to determine the nucleotide sequence of the genomic DNA and to screen this DNA sequence for open reading frames that have the characteristics of glycoproteins. Rapid DNA sequencing technology has now made this approach feasible for all virus genomes (up to 2.5×10^5 base pairs). Once putative glycoprotein genes are identified they may be rapidly cloned and expressed in vaccinia virus. Vaccinia is a particularly useful expression vector system for eukaryotic glycoproteins because the cells infected with the recombinant virus permit normal processing and transport of the glycoprotein. Additionally, the live recombinant virus may be directly used to immunize animals and so raise an antisera against the foreign protein. This antisera can be tested for its ability to neutralize the infectivity of the corresponding pathogen. If a suitable animal model system exists, the recombinant vaccinia virus may be tested for its ability to immunize against challenge with the appropriate pathogen. This strategy has been successfully used to identify new glycoprotein genes of herpes simplex virus type 1 and human cytomegalovirus that have potential in future vaccines against these viruses (Cranage *et al.* 1986. EMBO Journal **5**: 3057–63).

Identification of viral antigens recognized by cytotoxic T lymphocytes

Cell-mediated and humoral immunity are both important mechanisms in protection against pathogens. For viruses, which replicate inside cells, cell-mediated immune defense mechanisms are particularly important in destroying the infected cell and hence eliminating the infection. For most viruses the antigens recognized by cytotoxic T lymphocytes (CTL) are uncharacterized. Vaccinia virus recombinants expressing individual virus antigens are versatile tools to investigate which particular virus antigens are recognized by CTL. This is illustrated using vaccinia recombinants expressing individual influenza virus genes.

Most CTL produced following influenza A virus infections of man or mouse will lyse autologous target cells infected with both the homologous influenza subtype and other influenza A virus subtypes. This CTL cross-reactivity among all influenza A subtypes was surprising in view of the marked antigenic diversity of the predominant virus surface antigens (hemagglutinin and neuraminidase) between different subtypes. It was possible therefore that more conserved 'internal' antigens might be recognized by CTL and previous reports had claimed some of these antigens were expressed on the cell surface (Virelizier *et al.* 1977). To examine which influenza virus antigens are recognized by CTL a series of vaccinia recombinants were constructed each of which expresses an individual influenza virus antigen. Complementary DNA copies of the M2 and NS2 mRNAs were utilized since vaccinia virus replicates and transcribes in the cytoplasm and does not splice its mRNAs. The results of experiments using recombinants expressing the hemagglutinin (HA) and nucleoprotein (NP) are discussed.

Recombinant vaccinia viruses expressing the HA of influenza A/Japan/57 (H2-VAC) (Smith *et al.* 1983b), HA of influenza A/PR/8/34 (H1-VAC) (Bennink *et al.* 1986) or NP of influenza A/PR/8/34 (NP-VAC) (Yewdell *et al.* 1985) were used. Murine P815 cells were infected with these viruses or WT vaccinia and incubated with CTL from mice primed with an influenza A virus of each of the H1, H2 or H3 subtypes. The results of these cytotoxicity ^{51}Cr release assays showed that NP-VAC infected targets were efficiently lysed by CTL primed with any influenza A virus. In contrast, HA-VAC infected targets were only lysed by CTL primed by the homologous influenza A virus (Yewdell *et al.* 1985; Bennink *et al.* 1984, 1986). CTL directed against HA were therefore subtype-specific while CTL directed against NP were cross-reactive. These conclusions were confirmed by using the recombinant vaccinia viruses to prime CTL responses in immunized mice and using CTL primed in this way as effector cells against targets infected with various influenza A virus subtypes. The ability of recombinant vaccinia virus to stimulate production of CTL specific for the foreign antigen in vaccinated animals also significantly enhances the attractiveness of these recombinant viruses as live vaccines. CTL recognition of other influenza virus antigens expressed by vaccinia recombinants is under evaluation.

Due to the broad host range of vaccinia virus it has also been possible to investigate recognition of influenza antigens by human CTL. Consistent with the murine studies, NP is also recognized by human anti-influenza CTL (McMichael *et al.* 1986).

Although protection from influenza virus is primarily mediated by antibody against the HA, recovery from infection involves CTL. If ways of maintaining high levels of anti-NP CTL can be found this would probably be beneficial in reducing influenza-virus-associated morbidity and enhancing recovery from infection. An understanding of which virus antigens are recognized by CTL is therefore important in design of future anti-viral vaccines.

Vaccinia recombinants as new live vaccines

Vaccinia virus has been established as an effective live vaccine in the eradication of smallpox. Now that recombinant vaccinia viruses can be constructed that express antigens from other pathogens, vaccinia could potentially be used as new live vaccines against other diseases. Recombinant vaccinia viruses have successfully immunized experimental animals against at least six different eukaryotic viruses: influenza virus (Smith *et al.* 1983b; Small *et al.* 1985); herpes simplex virus (Paoletti *et al.* 1984; Cremer *et al.* 1985); hepatitis B virus (Moss *et al.* 1984), rabies virus (Kieny *et al.* 1984; Wiktor *et al.* 1984); vesicular stomatitis virus (Mackett *et al.* 1985) and respiratory syncitial virus (Elango *et al.* 1986). Specific antibody or cell-mediated immune responses have been detected in animals immunized with recombinant vaccinia viruses expressing many other foreign gene products. This type of live vaccine should retain several of the properties which made vaccinia such an effective vaccine against smallpox: (1) its ease of manufacture and administration at low cost; (2) its ability to stimulate both cellular and antibody immune responses; and (3) its stability in freeze-dried form without refrigeration. In addition, the large capacity of vaccinia virus for foreign DNA permits the simultaneous expression of multiple foreign antigens, so creating new polyvalent vaccines (Perkus *et al.* 1985), and the virus has a broad host range enabling use in both veterinary and human medicine.

On the other hand vaccinia does not have an unblemished record as a vaccine. Rarely there were serious complications following vaccination. These were mostly in patients with immunological deficiencies or patients suffering from eczema but very rarely cases of post-vaccination encephalitis occurred in apparently healthy individuals. As smallpox disappeared the disadvantages incurred from vaccination as a result of these rare complications began to outweigh the benefit from vaccination. Naturally, when the eradication was complete vaccination was discontinued. If vaccinia is to be reintroduced as a vaccine delivery system, safer more attenuated viruses may be required. Fortunately, genetic manipulation permits genes from vaccinia to be deleted or inactivated as well as foreign genes added. As the vaccinia genes involved in virus pathogenicity are identified and eliminated or mutated, more attenuated viruses will be constructed. For example, the inactivation of the vaccinia TK gene has been shown markedly to attenuate the virus (Buller *et al.* 1985).

Another possible problem with recombinant vaccinia viruses is the potential that by expressing a foreign antigen which might be incorporated onto the virion surface, the pathogenicity or tropism of the virus may be altered. The expression of the envelope glycoproteins genes of HTLV III/LAV (Chakrabarti *et al.* 1986) or hepatitis B virus (Smith *et al.* 1983a) could conceivably alter vaccinia from a dermotropic virus to a lymphotropic or hepatotropic virus. Although there are no data indicating that this does in fact occur the potential problem needs careful evaluation.

Widespread application of recombinant vaccinia viruses may run into problems due to existing immunity in the population due to prior smallpox vaccination. However, since smallpox vaccination has been stopped in most countries for ten years or so there is already a large population of nonimmune children. Generally it is this age group which need to be vaccinated against infectious diseases. Revaccination can still be performed although the level of immunity resulting from a primary vaccination would be better. Recently, an accidental vaccination of a human by a recombinant vaccinia virus resulted in a good antibody response against the foreign protein despite the person having had a previous smallpox vaccination (Jones *et al.* 1986).

The potential of vaccinia recombinants as new vaccines has been established. Research is now being directed to obtaining higher levels of foreign gene expression by engineering other vaccinia promoter or inserting multiple gene copies. Correct presentation of the antigen to the immune system is also important. This was well illustrated by a blood stage secreted (S) antigen from the human malarial parasite *Plasmodium falciparum*. When expressed in vaccinia in its normal secreted form this antigen was only poorly immunogenic. However, the addition of a membrane anchor domain to the carboxyl terminus resulted in its retention on the infected cell membrane and a dramatic increase in its immunogenicity (Langford *et al.* 1986). Lastly, effort is being directed towards the construction of more attenuated viruses.

Acknowledgements

I thank the conference organisers for their kind invitation and Mary Wright for typing the manuscript.

References

Bennink J R, Yewdell J W, Smith G L, Moller C, Moss B 1984. Recombinant vaccinia virus primes and stimulates influenza virus haemagglutinin-specific cytotoxic T lymphocytes, *Nature (London)* **311**: 578–9

Bennink J R, Yewdell J W, Smith G L, Moss B 1986. Recognition of cloned influenza virus haemagglutinin gene products by cytotoxic T lymphocytes, *Journal of Virology* **57**: 786–91

Boyle D B, Couper B E H, Both G W 1985. Multiple-cloning-site plasmids for the rapid construction of recombinant poxviruses, *Gene* **35**: 169–77

Broyles S S, Moss B 1986. Homology between RNA polymerases of poxviruses, prokaryotes and eukaryotes: nucleotide sequence and transcriptional analysis of vaccinia virus genes encoding 147-kDa and 22-kDa subunits, *Proceedings of the National Academy of Sciences USA* **83**: 3141–5

Buller R M L, Smith G L, Cremer K, Notkins A L, Moss B 1985. Decreased virulence of recombinant vaccinia virus expression vectors is associated with a thymidine kinase-negative phenotype, *Nature (London)* **317**: 813–15

Chakrabarti S, Brechling K, Moss B 1985. Vaccinia virus expression vector: co-expression of β-galactosidases provides visual screening of recombinant virus plaques, *Molecular and Cellular Biology* **5**: 3403–9

Chakrabarti S, Robert-Guroff M, Wong-Staal F, Gallo R C, Moss B 1986. Expression of HTLV-III envelope gene by recombinant vaccinia virus, *Nature (London)* **320**: 535–7

Cranage M P, Kouzarides T, Bankier A T, Satchwell S, Weston K, Tomlinson P, Barrell B, Hart H, Bell S E, Minson A C, Smith G L 1986. Identification of the human cytomegalovirus glycoprotein B gene and induction of neutralizing antibodies via its expression in recombinant vaccinia virus. EMBO Journal **5**: 3057–63.

Cremer K, Mackett M, Wohlenberg C, Notkins A L, Moss B 1985. Vaccinia virus recombinants expressing herpes simplex virus type 1 gylcoprotein D prevents latent herpes in mice, *Science* **228**: 737–40

Elango N, Prince G A, Murphy B R, Venkatesan S, Chanock R M, Moss B 1986. Resistance to human respiratory syncytial virus (RSV) infection induced by immunization of cotton rats with a recombinant vaccinia virus expressing the RSV G glycoprotein, *Proceedings of the National Academy of Sciences USA* **83**: 1906–10

Franke C A, Rice C M, Strauss J H, Hruby D E 1985. Neomycin resistance as a dominant selectable marker for selection and isolation of vaccinia virus recombinants, *Molecular and Cellular Biology* **5**: 1918–24

Geshelin P, Berns K I 1974. Characterization and localisation of the naturally occurring crosslinks in vaccinia virus DNA, *Journal of Molecular Biology* **88**: 785–96

Jones L, Ristow S, Yilma T, Moss B 1986. Accidental human vaccination with vaccinia expressing nucleoprotein gene, *Nature (London)* **319**: 543

Kieny M-P, Lathe R, Drillien R, Spehner D, Skory S, Schmitt D, Wiktor T, Koprowski H,

Lecocq J P 1984. Expression of rabies virus glycoprotein from a recombinant vaccinia virus, *Nature (London)* **312**: 163–6

Langford C J, Edwares S J, Smith G L, Mitchell G F, Moss B, Kemp D J, Anders R F 1986. Anchoring a secreted plasmodium antigen on the surface of recombinant vaccinia virus infected cells increases its immunogenicity, *Molecular and Cellular Biology* **6**: 3191–9

Mackett M, Archard L E 1979. Conservation and variation in the orthopoxvirus genome structure, *Journal of General Virology* **45**: 683–702

Mackett M, Smith G L, Moss B 1982. Vaccinia virus: a selectable eukaryotic cloning and expression vector, *Proceedings of the National Academy of Sciences USA* **79**: 7415–19

Mackett M, Smith G L, Moss B 1984. General method for production and selection of infectious vaccinia virus recombinants expressing foreign genes, *Journal of Virology* **49**: 857–64

Mackett M, Yilma T, Rose J, Moss B 1985. Vaccinia virus recombinants: expression of VSV genes and protective immunization of mice and cattle, *Science* **227**: 433–5

McMichael A J, Michie C A, Gotch F M, Smith G L, Moss B 1986. Recognition of influenza A virus nucleoprotein by human cytotoxic T lymphocytes, *Journal of General Virology* **67**: 719–26

Morrison D K, Moyer R W 1986. Detection of a subunit of cellular *pol*II within highly purified preparations of RNA polymerase isolated from rabbit poxvirus virions, *Cell* **44**: 587–96

Moss B, Smith G L, Gerin J L, Purcell R H 1984. Live recombinant virus protects chimpanzees against hepatitis B. *Nature (London)* **311**: 67–9

Moss B 1985. Replication of poxviruses, in B N Fields, R M Chanock, B Roizman (eds). *Virology*, New York, Raven Press, pp 658–703

Nakano E, Panicali D, Paoletti E 1982. Molecular genetics of vaccinia virus: demonstration of marker rescue, *Proceedings of the National Academy of Sciences USA* **79**: 1593–6

Panicali D, Paoletti E 1982. Construction of poxviruses as cloning vectors: insertion of the thymidine kinase from herpes simplex virus into the DNA of infectious vaccinia virus, *Proceedings of the National Academy of Sciences USA* **79**: 4927–31

Paoletti E, Lipinskas B R, Samsanoff C, Mercer S, Panicali D 1984. Construction of live vaccines using genetically engineered poxviruses: biological activity of vaccinia virus recombinants expressing the hepatitis B virus surface antigen and the herpes simplex virus glycoprotein D. *Proceedings of the National Academy of Sciences USA* **81**: 193–7

Perkus M E, Piccini A, Lipinskas B R, Paoletti E 1985. Recombinant vaccinia virus: immunization against multiple pathogens, *Science* **229**: 981–4

Small P A Jr, Smith G L, Moss B 1985. Intranasal vaccination with recombinant vaccinia containing influenza haemagglutinin prevents both influenza virus pneumonia and nasal infection: intradermal vaccination prevents only viral pneumonia, in G V Quinnan (ed) *Vaccinia Viruses as Vectors for Vaccine Antigens*, New York, Elsevier, pp 175–8

Smith G L, Moss B 1983. Infectious poxvirus vectors have capacity for at least 25 000 base pairs of foreign DNA, *Gene* **25**: 21–8

Smith G L, Mackett M, Moss B 1983a. Infectious vaccinia virus recombinants that express hepatitis B virus surface antigen, *Nature (London)* **302**: 490–5

Smith G L, Murphy B R, Moss B 1983b. Construction and characterization of an infectious vaccinia virus recombinant that expresses the influenza virus hemagglutinin gene and induces resistance to influenza infection in hamsters, *Proceedings of the National Academy of Sciences USA* **80**: 7155–9

Virelizier J L, Allison A, Oxford J, Schild G C 1977. Early presence of ribonucleoprotein antigen on surface of influenza virus-infected cells, *Nature (London)* **266**: 52–3

Wiktor T J, Macfarlan R I, Reagan K J, Dietzschold B, Curtis P J, Wunner W H, Kieny M-P, Lathe R, Lecocq J-P, Mackett M, Moss B, Koprowski H 1984. Protection from rabies by a vaccinia virus recombinant containing the rabies virus glycoprotein gene, *Proceedings of the National Academy of Sciences USA* **81**: 7194–8

World Health Organization 1980. The global eradication of smallpox. Final Report of the Global Commission for the Certification of Smallpox Eradication. Geneva, World Health Organization

Yewdell J W, Bennink J R, Smith G L, Moss B 1985. Influenza A virus nucleoprotein is a major target antigen for cross-reactive anti-influenze A virus cytotoxic T lymphocytes, *Proceedings of the National Academy of Sciences USA* **82**: 1785–9

6 Idiotype and synthetic peptide vaccines

Basic considerations in the use of idiotype vaccines

Ivan M Roitt*; Yasmin M Thanavala†

* Department of Immunology, Middlesex Hospital Medical School, London W1, United Kingdom
† Department of Molecular Immunology, Roswell Park Memorial Institute, Buffalo, New York 14263, USA

The idiotype network

There is considerable evidence that idiotype interaction influences the development of the immunological repertoire. Weaver and colleagues (Weaver et al. 1986) have transfected mice with a new immunoglobulin gene and have shown that a surprisingly high proportion of hybridomas made from these transgenic mice express an idiotype related to the transfected gene although utilizing their endogenous genes for immunoglobulin synthesis; it is difficult to account for such a phenomenon without postulating some intermediary anti-idiotypic regulatory mechanism. Furthermore, Kearney and Vakil (1986) have shown that hybridomas generated early in ontogeny give rise to a high frequency of complementary pairs of idiotype anti-idiotype specificity which is not seen when the experiment is repeated in adult life, suggesting that such high idiotypic connectivity early in life could well be involved in setting the repertoire for later development. The occurrence of a cross-reactive idiotype on antibodies produced to quite distinct epitopes on a given antigen during an immune response, also provides strong evidence for the mediation of some regulatory anti-idiotype, either as antibody or perhaps as T helper cells.

It is generally recognized, at least at the present time(!), that the regulatory idiotype network probably involves germ-line encoded structures which, through the various recombinatorial events leading to diversity, appear on many different antibodies with a variety of possible specificities. These are referred to by Jerne (1973) as nonspecific parallel sets. The collection of paratopes which are stimulated by a given antigenic epitope may also be regulated by anti-idiotypes which would have an internal image-like behavior. In other words, as Jerne also envisaged, there would be receptors bearing idiotypes which resembled in some way the structure of the antigen. The latter system appears to be quite prominent when one looks at the immune responses to hormones and their receptors and there are many studies showing that immunization with hormone or its agonist in such a way as to provoke antibodies results in the generation of anti-idiotypic antibodies which mimic the hormone in its ability to combine with hormone receptor. A similar phenomenon has been observed with viruses where the anti-antibody is capable of combining with the viral receptor on the relevant cell surface, as will be discussed in a subsequent paper by Mark Greene. The frequency of internal image anti-idiotypes which mimic *exogenous* antigens is not well established at the present time.

'Internal image' anti-idiotypes are likely to be important for vaccines

If one is seeking an anti-idiotype to stimulate an immune response as a useful vaccine in outbred populations, it can be argued that the internal image anti-idiotype is more likely to be of benefit than one which is a part of the regulatory idiotype network, as discussed above. The latter would stimulate a series of B cells bearing receptors which express the relevant regulatory idiotype, i.e. it would stimulate the production of the specific antibody required together with very large number of members of the nonspecific parallel set which would have specificities unrelated to those desired in the first place. On the other hand, the internal image anti-idiotype, by definition, would stimulate a variety of receptors which had in common the ability to see the corresponding epitope on the antigen and would therefore be expected to be more effective as a vaccine. This is of particular importance in outbred populations such as humans, where the regulatory idiotopes are frequently under strong genetic constraint.

It is important to recognize that we are looking in functional terms for an anti-idiotypic reagent which will mimic the behavior of the antigen rather than one which necessarily mirrors the precise structure. That is not to say that an internal image-like anti-idiotype may not bear sequences which are identical with those of the epitope on the antigen and Mark Greene will provide evidence that this can in fact be so. However, in dealing with the many epitopes which are conformational rather than linear in structure, it would seem more likely that the structures which mimic the antigen would be individual contact residues, possibly on different complementarity determining regions (i.e. hypervariable loops), and we have discussed this topic in some depth elsewhere (Roitt *et al.* 1985). That close structural similarity is not always required, may be readily seen from the ability of anti-idiotypes to mimic small hormones such as acetylcholine and carbohydrate antigens.

Studies with monoclonal anti-idiotypes which mimic hepatitis B surface antigen

In order to test the feasibility of this approach, we set out to raise monoclonal anti-idiotypes which mimicked the *a* determinant of the hepatitis B surface antigen. The criterion for selection was the ability of the monoclonal anti-idiotype to bear an interspecies idiotype as ascertained by reaction with antibodies to HBsAg raised in several different species. A series of four monoclonal anti-idiotypes were studied in detail, and three were shown to have internal image-like behavior to varying degrees (Thanavala *et al.* 1985a, 1985b).

It should be recognized that, by this procedure, the final anti-idiotype should be mimicking a single epitope on the original antigen. This may be of great value relative to the use of whole antigen in those circumstances where other epitopes may either be cross-reactive with self, or be capable of inducing a strongly suppressor response.

There are two main approaches to the creation of a reagent which mimics a single epitope; one may either produce an appropriate anti-idiotype, or a synthetic peptide. We were fortunate in establishing a collaboration with Professor M W Steward and Dr C Howard of the London School of Hygiene and Tropical Medicine, who had synthesized a peptide of amino acids 139–147 of HBsAg which in their hands was capable of reacting with antisera directed towards the *a* determinant. Since we also assumed that we had an anti-idiotype which resembled the *a* determinant, it was clearly of interest to see to what extent the two surrogate epitopes were capable of mutual interaction.

We showed by quite extensive studies that the anti-idiotype and the synthetic peptide mutually inhibited their binding to a whole range of heterologous antisera to HBsAg, and this has been published (Thanavala *et al.* 1986). The variation in behavior with different antisera raised in various species was ascribed to the ability of the individual species to recognize different amino acid residues on the antigen as a contact residue and we hope to test this view by applying the Geysen technique (Geysen *et al.* 1984) using peptides where individual amino acids are replaced by all the other possible amino acids. This is a technique which Dr Getzoff described more recently in this symposium, and enables one to ascertain which are the important contact residues.

Two important features emerged from these competitive inhibition studies. The first was that the anti-idiotypes had a higher affinity for the anti-hepatitis antibodies than did the peptides. However, the peptide was capable of reacting with a higher proportion of the antibody population making up these antisera. In other words, the anti-idiotype binds more strongly but theoretically might be capable of stimulating a smaller fraction of the available B cells.

The implications of these findings are that the proposed vaccines should contain more than one monoclonal antibody. The monoclonals almost certainly have an advantage over polyclonal reagents in the sense that production on a large scale is easier to achieve and would give rise to a standardized product.

The Chairman asked us to define the criteria which we would use to establish the internal image-like behavior of monoclonals for use in a vaccine, and my view would be that one should choose those anti-idiotypes which react well with polyclonal sera from different individuals of the species to be immunized.

The question of T cell priming using anti-idiotypes raised against B cell products is still uncertain. There have been several studies in which connection with antigen primed T cells has been established, and this area will have to be looked at more intensively.

Advantages of anti-idiotype vaccines

Monoclonal anti-idiotypes should be safe to prepare and available in large quantities. They provide epitope-specific reagents and, in doing so, they provide structures which mimic the behavior of the tertiary configuration of the native antigen in a way which synthetic peptides might not always be able to do. The anti-idiotypes can also mimic nonprotein structures such as carbohydrates which cannot be produced by gene cloning directly. One envisages applications to microbial infections and in particular to carbohydrate antigens. Conceivably, there may be instances where the ability to mimic a specific epitope might be advantageous, as discussed above, where the remainder of the molecule may not be providing an appropriate response, e.g. as in carriers of hepatitis virus. Tumor-specific antigens are frequently weakly immunogenic, particularly those of the embryonic type, and it is conceivable that an anti-idiotype with appropriate adjuvants could be made into a useful surrogate. Lastly, we should mention the possibility of generating auto-antibody responses to human chorionic gonadotrophin (hCG) through this strategy, so providing the basis for an immunological contraceptive, since hCG and the related hormone, LH, are so close in structure that one needs highly selective epitope-specific reagents to produce an immune response which does not have embarrassing cross-reactivity.

References

Geysen H M, Meloen R H, Barteling S J 1984. *Proceedings of the National Academy of Sciences USA* **81**: 3998–4002

Jerne N K 1973, *Scientific American* **229**(1): 52

Kearney J F, Vakil M 1986. *Annales de l'Institut Pasteur, Immunologie (Paris)* **137c**: 77

Roitt I M, Thanavala Y M, Male D K, Hay F C 1985. *Immunology Today* **6**: 265–7

Thanavala Y M, Bond A, Tedder R, Hay F C, Roitt I M 1985a. *Immunology* **55**: 197–204

Thanavala Y M, Bond A, Hay F C, Roitt I M 1985b. *Journal of Immunological Methods* **83**: 227–32

Thanavala Y M, Brown S E, Howard C R, Roitt I M, Steward M W 1986. *Journal of Experimental Medicine* **164**: 227–36

Weaver D, Reis M H, Albanese C, Constantini F, Baltimore D, Imanishi-Kari T 1986. *Cell* **45**: 247

Molecular basis of antigenic mimicry

Mark I Greene

University of Pennsylvania, Department of Pathology and Laboratory Medicine, Philadelphia, Pennsylvania 19104-6082, USA

The mammalian reovirus type 3 induces an oligoclonal antibody response that is dominated by a cross-reactive idiotype (Nepom *et al.* 1982). The development and study of monoclonal antibodies to the reovirus hemagglutinin revealed that the antibodies to the neutralization domain of the hemagglutinin also expressed the major idiotope. We observed that the 9B.G5 monoclonal directed to the neutralization domain of the reovirus 3 hemagglutinin could inhibit the binding of rabbit anti-idiotypic antibodies to polyclonal hemagglutinin-specific immunoglobulin. Using the 9B.G5 monoclonal antibody in a syngeneic immunization protocol led to the development of a monoclonal anti-idiotypic antibody that had several interesting functional as well as structural features (Noseworthy *et al.* 1983). We will review these characteristics and speculate on the relevance to the network theory.

Anti-receptor monoclonals

BALB/c mice that were immunized with the BALB/c derived 9B.G5 monoclonal developed antibodies in the serum that appeared to be anti-idiotypic. After fusion of the spleen cells hybrids were screened for their ability to bind the 9B.G5 monoclonal but not syngeneic and irrelevant antibodies. The binding of the 9B.G5 antibody to the 87.92.6 was inhibitable by free isolated hemagglutinin protein, reflecting that the anti-idiotype interacted with the idiotype at or near the antigen binding site. The 87.92.6 monoclonal was cloned and the immunoglobulin that it secreted was purified by conventional immunochemical techniques to apparent homogeneity. In the first series of studies we found that the 87.92.6 antibody was able to bind to the cellular receptor for the mammalian reovirus expressed on somatic and neuronal cells (Noseworthy *et al.* 1983). Several observations supported this notion. In the first case we were able to show that the antibody bound to a cell surface structure expressed on all cells that were susceptible to reovirus type 3 infection (Kaufmann *et al.* 1983). Furthermore preincubation of the antibody with susceptible cells would prevent virtual complete attachment of the virus. The detailed examination of these cells indicated that in many cases the cells still became infected with reovirus. This was especially true when transformed cells such as thymoma cells were used, but if primary neurones were examined protection from infection was obvious. These results are readily explained from data suggesting that malignantly transformed cells are much more readily infected than nontransformed ones for reasons that are not entirely clear but which may relate to the metabolically active growing state of the targets.

In further studies we examined the ability of anti-receptor antibodies to induce aggregation of the cell surface attachment site for the virus. Addition of the anti-receptor antibodies and a cross-linking second antibody induced movement of the receptor into clusters followed by internalization (Gaulton *et al.* 1985). Polar caps were not readily apparent. Collectively these studies led to the compelling conclusion that the 87.92.6 identified a mobile cell surface structure which served as an attachment site for the reovirus 3 hemagglutinin.

The 87.92.6 antibody as internal image

The development of a syngeneic monoclonal anti-idiotypic anti-receptor antibody permitted the evaluation of its ability to serve as a surrogate antigen. Initial studies were performed to examine whether the 87.92.6 hybrid cell which expressed immunoglobulin on the cell surface might be recognized by reovirus 3 specific killer cells. Initially we used bulk populations of cytolytic killer cells and then later cytolytic lines for these purposes (Sharpe *et al.* 1985). In the course of the experiments with bulk populations we found that 25–40% of the cytolytic T cells could interact with uninfected 87.92.6 cells. Furthermore this interaction could be inhibited with 9B.G5 immunoglobulin. Of interest was the observed H-2 restriction of the lysis indicating that the 87.92.6 immunoglobulin was associating with histocompatibility structures on the cell surface. This functional association of immunoglobulin with class I elements indicated to us that it was likely that two receptor related recognition epitopes were involved. We also felt it unlikely that the immunoglobulin protein was being modified by class I proteins but did not exclude some limited unfolding of the immunoglobulin protein so as to expose some site associated with the antigen binding cleft.

The next series of studies was directed towards analyzing the immunogenicity of the anti-receptor antibody in terms of stimulating cellular immunity and humoral immunity to the virus. The anti-receptor antibody was evaluated in a syngeneic system and was found able in the absence of adjuvant to induce cellular immunity to the virus. The ability to induce cellular immunity including both delayed type hypersensitivity and cell-mediated cytotoxicity to the virus using a monoclonal immunoglobulin protein was unexpected (Sharpe *et al*. 1984).

These studies imply a shared idiotypy for subsets of T helper cells and immunoglobulin bearing hemagglutinin specific B cells. Immunization with the polymerized form of the 87.92.6 resulted in the development of neutralizing antibodies to the reovirus type 3. Furthermore the 87.92.6 antibodies could be administered to pregnant mice whose offspring were found to be generally protected from the lethal effects of the reovirus (Gaulton and Greene 1986). Therefore the ability of this antibody to behave like the virus in terms of its interaction with elements of the immune system indicated that it truly satisfied the criteria of being an internal image.

Molecular analysis of the structure of the 87.92.6 antibody and the reovirus 3 hemagglutinin

Because of the ability of the 87.92.6 to mimic the virus in terms of the immune response it induced, we undertook to establish whether this was due to shared primary structural features. We cloned and sequenced the heavy and light chain genes of the 87.92.6 immunoglobulin, and compared the sequence to that of the reovirus hemagglutinin (Fig. 1). The sequence analysis revealed an

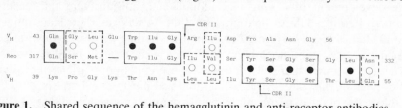

Figure 1. Shared sequence of the hemagglutinin and anti-receptor antibodies.

unexpected high level of homology with the reovirus hemagglutinin. When we examined the second complementary determining domain of the light chain, we observed that there existed a significant level of structural identity over a large region of the sequence. In positions where there was no exact identity there was functional equivalence. The region 5' to the second CDR exists as part of a beta turn and we reasoned that it might be possible to synthesize this peptide which we predicted would maintain some configurational features of the molecule from which it was derived and to examine its effect when used as an immunogen (Bruck *et al*. 1986).

Initial studies were performed using the peptide as an immunogen in BALB/c mice. The mice were primed with peptide coupled with chicken serum albumin, free peptide or irrelevant peptide. The irrelevant peptide shared the same amino acids but randomly arranged. We observed that the peptides were indeed able to induce antibody as well as prime for an immune response as measured by delayed type hypersensitivity.

Implications for the activity of the peptide

Because we were successful in the elicitation and generation of an immune response against the intact virus using the peptide fashioned from the shared sequence of the anti-receptor antibody and the virus hemagglutinin, it is reasonable to expect that this anti-idiotypic antibody induces immunity as a consequence of presenting this particular peptidic region to the immune system. Since both T cell and B cell immunity are stimulated as a consequence of peptide immunization we would consider that the peptide and immunoglobulin from which the peptide is derived are presented by I-A + macrophages. We conclude this latter fact from the observed genetically restricted cellular response that is observed with respect to delayed type hypersensitivity. Since the peptide is as highly effective as the intact virus in stimulating immunity it might be argued that the anti-receptor antibody probably undergoes some level of processing by I-A + macrophages prior to its presentation to T and B cells. If there is no processing there still is undoubtedly I-A restricted antigen presentation.

The fact that anti-idiotypes may be presented to the immune system by I-A + antigen presenting cells (APC) may have some implications for the network theory of the immune system. Perhaps dominant anti-idiotypic regulatory effects are due to the catabolism of antibody idiotypic immunoglobulins by antigen presenting cells, followed by presentation of immunoglobulin break-down remnants including idiotopes by the APC. If so, some systems might be influenced by anti-idiotypic T cells more than are others, and the degree of anti-idiotypic effect might reflect the effective reassociation of idiotopes with class II molecules. One prediction of this notion would be that idiotypic immunoglobulin induced anti-idiotypic suppressor T cells would be most effective at suppressing I-A related immunity, including direct suppression of B cells and interference of I-A restricted T helper cell activation. Results have generally agreed with this prediction (Abbas *et al.* 1982).

The ability to develop peptides which act upon the immune system will allow us to evaluate their activity as pharmaceuticals. It should be noted that the anti-receptor antibody has an effect on the growth of several types of transformed cells by binding to the cellular receptor. Preliminary studies also suggest that the peptides may do so.

References

Abbas A K, Takaoki M, Greene M I 1982. T lymphocyte mediated suppression of myeloma function *in vitro*. IV. Generation of effector suppressor cells specific for myeloma idiotypes, *Journal of Experimental Medicine* **155**: 1216–21

Bruck C, Co M S, Slaoui M, Gaulton G N, Smith T, Mullins J, Fields B N, Greene M I 1986. Nucleic acid sequence of an internal image-bearing monoclonal anti-idiotype and its comparison to that of the external antigen, *Proceedings of the National Academy of Sciences USA* **83**: 65–78

Gaulton G N, Greene M I 1986. Idiotypic mimicry of biological receptors, *Annual Review of Immunology* **4**: 253–80

Gaulton G, Co M S, Greene M I 1985. Anti-idiotypic antibody identifies the cellular receptor of reovirus type 3, *Journal of Cellular Biochemistry* **28**: 69–78

Kauffman R S, Noseworthy J H, Nepom J T, Finberg R, Fields B N, Greene M I 1983. Cell receptors for the mammalian reovirus. II. Monoclonal anti-idiotypic antibody blocks viral binding to cells, *Journal of Immunology* **131**: 2539–41

Nepom J T, Weiner H L, Dichter M, Spriggs D, Powers L, Fields B, Greene M I 1982. Identification of a hemagglutinin specific idiotype associated with reovirus recognition shared by lymphoid and neuronal cells, *Journal of Experimental Medicine* **155**: 155–78

Noseworthy J H, Fields B N, Dichter M A, Sobotka C, Pizer E, Perry L L, Nepom J T, Greene M I 1983. Cell receptors for the mammalian reovirus. I. Syngeneic monoclonal anti-idiotypic antibody identifies a cell surface receptor for reovirus, *Journal of Immunology* **131**: 2533–8

Sharpe A H, Gaulton G N, McDade K K, Fields B N, Greene M I 1984. Syngeneic monoclonal anti-idiotype can induce cellular immunity to reovirus, *Journal of Experimental Medicine* **160**: 1195–205

Sharpe A H, Gaulton G N, Ertl H C G, Finberg R W, Fields B N, Greene M I 1985. Cell receptors for the mammalian reovirus. IV. Reovirus specific cytolic T cell lines which have idiotypic receptors recognize anti-idiotypic B cell hybridomas, *Journal of Immunology* **134**: 2702–6

Synthetic peptides as a basis for anti-influenza and anti-cholera vaccines

Ruth Arnon; Michal Shapira; Chaim O Jacob

Department of Chemical Immunology, The Weizmann Institute of Science, Rehovot 76100, Israel

Introduction

Ever since our finding that a chemically synthesized peptide is capable of eliciting antibodies reactive with a native protein, e.g. lysozyme (Arnon *et al.* 1971), it has been predicted that such peptides could serve for vaccination. Namely, that by adequate molecular engineering it should be possible to design synthetic materials that would elicit anti-viral immunity, leading eventually to multivalent synthetic vaccines (Arnon 1972). The rapid development of DNA cloning and sequencing techniques which facilitate protein sequencing has made the synthetic approach more feasible and practical than before. Primary sequences are available today for many proteins, enabling the synthesis of any selected region, using either chemical laboratory techniques, which are advisable in the case of short peptides, or genetic engineering procedures in the case of longer protein segments, subunits or even whole proteins. Moreover, the synthetic approach should allow the choice of the carrier, as well as the adjuvant, the goal being the production of multivalent vaccines with built-in adjuvanticity.

The antigenic components of vaccines consist usually of macromolecules, mainly proteins and glycoproteins which may carry a large number and variety of epitopes. However, only a limited number of the antigenic sites are immunodominant and only part of these epitopes are involved in inducing neutralizing immunity. Before attempting to synthesize a vaccine one should have some knowledge about the antigenic structure of the target organism and its protein component. This could be achieved either by fragmentation of the native protein antigen and screening of the fragments for antigenic reactivity, or by employing monoclonal antibodies with neutralizing activity for identifying the relevant antigenic sites. Since the spatial conformation has been shown to play a decisive role in determining the antigenic specificity (Crumpton, 1974), crystallographic studies of the three-dimensional structure of proteins serve as an additional source of information in regard to antigenic structure. For most proteins, however, though the primary sequence is known, crystallographic data are not yet available. Hence, several

333

methods based on computational analysis of various regions in the molecule (Hopp and Woods 1981) have been suggested for the prediction of the more likely antigenic determinants. Such cumulative information on segments in protein molecules with the right 'ingredients' have been helpful in the design of synthetic vaccines during the last few years.

Synthetic vaccine against influenza virus

The influenza virus provides a very suitable model for studying the synthetic approach to vaccination for the following reasons: (a) the virus is well characterized and many of its strains have been isolated and analyzed; (b) detailed information is available on the structure and function of this virus, as well as on its serological specificities and genetic variations; (c) there are various reliable assays of the virus for evaluating the effect of the immune response on the different viral functions; (d) the viral proteins which are important for its function have been identified, in particular the hemagglutinin which is mainly responsible for the serological specificity (Laver *et al.* 1981); (e) sufficient information is available on the amino acid sequence of the influenza hemagglutinin of many viral strains, as well as on its three-dimensional structure and immunochemical properties, to allow the synthesis of a peptide that might carry some of its antigenic determinants.

Another advantage of this system is that once such peptides have been synthesized, the immune response they elicit can be assessed on four different levels: (1) the immunochemical reaction, i.e. the capacity of the elicited antibodies to interact with the peptide and to cross react with the intact virus; (2) the inhibitory effect of the antibodies on the biological activity of the hemagglutinin; (3) the *in vitro* neutralization of the virus, as expressed by reduction of virus plaque formation in tissue-cultured cell monolayers; (4) the most crucial criterion is the *in vivo* protection of animals. Since viral strains that infect humans are also infectious in mice, the immune response against the synthetic peptides can be evaluated by the decrease in the incidence and/or severity of infection after active immunization with the synthetic antigens.

The first peptide we synthesized, before the three-dimensional structure was known, consisted of 18 amino acid residues corresponding to the sequence 91–108 of the influenza hemagglutinin (HA) molecule. This region, which is common to at least 12 H3 strains, is a part of a larger cyanogen bromide fragment, previously shown by Jackson *et al.* (1979) to be immunologically active. According to our computer-predicted folded structure of the HA polypeptide chain, this peptide segment should have comprised a folded region with a short α-helical section, and hence an exposed area in the molecular structure. It also contains three tyrosine and two proline residues that had been demonstrated in our early studies to play a dominant role in the antigenicity of several proteins or synthetic antigens. We thus anticipated that the 91–108 peptide which contains these 'ingredients' would be immunologically reactive.

Indeed, a conjugate of this peptide with tetanus toxoid (TT) elicited in both rabbits and mice antibodies that reacted immunochemically with the synthetic peptide, as well as with the intact influenza virus of several strains of type A. These antibodies were capable of inhibiting the capacity of the HA of the relevant strains to agglutinate chicken erythrocytes. They also interfered with the *in vitro* growth of the virus in tissue culture causing up to 60% reduction in viral plaque formation. But, most importantly, mice immunized with the peptide–toxoid conjugate were partially protected against further challenge infection with the virus (Muller *et al.* 1982). Moreover, since the peptide 91–108 was deliberately chosen to be part of a conserved sequence of the HA, it elicited protection against more than one H3 strain (Table 1). This finding indicates that the synthetic approach might lead to multivalent vaccines for cross-strain protection.

According to the three-dimensional structure of the influenza HA (Wiley *et al.* 1981), the region 140–146, which forms antigenic site A, is a 'loop' of seven amino acid residues unusually protruding from the surface of the molecule, and is considered to be one of the epidemiologically most important determinants. Amino acid exchanges in this region result in mutants which differ completely in their serological specificities as well as in their biological activity (Webster *et al.* 1981).

In our studies four peptides have been synthesized (Shapira *et al.* 1984). Two of them corresponded to the sequence 139–146, with either Gly or Asp at position 144. The third peptide corresponded to the sequence 147–164, and the fourth included both segments and corresponded to the sequence 138–164. Conjugates of these peptides with tetanus toxoid elicited high antibody titer against the respective homologous peptides with a significant extent of cross-reactivity among them. The antibodies induced by the four peptides differed in their cross-reactivity with the intact H3 influenza virus. Antibodies against the two octapeptides 139–146 were not cross-reactive, but antibodies raised against the two longer peptides, 147–164 and 138–164 showed significant binding with the intact virus and the anti-138–164 even neutralized it *in vitro*. This peptide was also the only one of this group which induced partial protection in mice against a challenge infection with the A/Eng/42/72 strain (Table 1) with which the sequence of the peptide corresponds.

A third region in the influenza hemagglutinin molecule which is influential in the immunological reactivity in the antigenic site B, comprising the external helical residues 187–196 and a few adjacent residues along the upper edge of a pocket, is tentatively implicated in virus receptor binding (Wiley *et al.* 1981). A synthetic peptide corresponding to the region 181–200, conjugated to tetanus toxoid, elicited antibodies that recognized the intact virus and exhibited neutralizing capacity *in vitro*. It also induced *in vivo* protection in mice (Table 1), although less pronounced than that elicited by the peptide 91–108.

Table 1 Protection of mice against challenge infection with influenza virus

Immunizing conjugate	Infectious strain	Experimental group	Incidence of infection at 10^{-2} dilution‡ into the egg	Mouse lung virus titer ($\log_{10}$)	Statistical significance
(91–108)-TT	A/Tex/77	Immunized*	19/36 (52%)	−1 98 ± 0.28	$p<0.0025$
		Control†	21/23 (11%)	−3.56 ± 0.25	
(91–108)-TT	A/PC/75	Immunized	4/18 (22%)	−0.61 ± 0.30	$p<0.05$
		Control	8/19 (42%)	−1.53 ± 0.40	
(91–108)-TT	A/Eng/42/72	Immunized	8/18 (44%)	−1.61 ± 0.40	$p<0.025$
		Control	15/21 (71%)	−2.9 ± 0.40	
(91–108)-TT	A/PR/8/34 (H1)	Immunized	18/19 (95%)	−3.47 ± 0.25	n.s.§
		Control	20/21 (95%)	−3.95 ± 0.24	
(181–200)-TT	A/Eng/42/72	Immunized	6/8 (75%)	−2.87 ± 0.54	$p<0.0025$
		Control	5/5 (100%)	−4.60 ± 0.24	
(138–164)-TT	A/Eng/42/72	Immunized	4/11 (36%)	−1.18 ± 0.51	$p<0.05$
		Control	7/10 (70%)	−2.6 ± 0.56	
(147–164)-TT	A/Eng/42/77	Immunized	6/11 (55%)	−2.0 ± 0.30	n.s.
		Control	7/10 (70%)	−2.6 ± 0.56	
(139–146(144-Asp))-TT	A/Eng/42/77	Immunized	7/8 (87.5%)	−4.25 ± 0.64	n.s.
		Control	7/8 (87.5%)	−4.5 ± 0.7	
(139–146(144-Gly))-TT	A/Eng/42/77	Immunized	7/8 (87.5%)	−4.0 ± 0.62	n.s.
		Control	7/8 (87.5%)	−4.5 ± 0.7	

* Immunized with the respective conjugate in complete Freund's adjuvant.
† Control groups were injected with tetanus toxoid alone in complete Freund's adjuvant.
‡ The lowest dilution of lung homogenate that is infective in eggs (average for all the mice in each group).
§ Nonsignificant.

These findings are of interest in view of the report by Wabuke-Bunoti *et al.* (1984) that a similar synthetic peptide corresponding to the sequence 181–204 of the HA induces in mice cytolytic T lymphocytes.

Synthetic anti-influenza vaccine with built-in adjuvanticity

The choice of adjuvant for vaccine preparation is of crucial importance, particularly when synthetic vaccines are being considered, since the synthetic materials are usually water-soluble and, therefore, less immunogenic than particulate substances. All the results reported above were achieved by immunization with the various conjugates using complete Freund's adjuvant (CFA) for augmenting their immune reactivity. This adjuvant, consisting of a water-in-oil emulsion containing killed mycobacteria, is very effective and evokes a high level of antibodies and long-lasting immunity. However, it is not suitable for human use since it induces local reactions and granulomas, inflammation and fever due to both the low metabolizable mineral oil and mycobacteria. Efforts are being made to replace it by other adjuvants, preferably by eliminating the mineral oil and/or replacing the mycobacteria by less damaging materials.

The minimal structure that can substitute for mycobacteria was identified as *N*-acetylmuramyl-L-analyl-D-isoglutamine, denoted MDP for muramyl dipeptide (Adam *et al.* 1972). This material and some of its synthetic analogs have already been used in combination with synthetic antigens (Arnon *et al.* 1980; Audibert *et al.* 1982). We have employed MDP in combination with the 91–108 peptide of HA for induction of anti-influenza response and demonstrated protection that was achieved by immunizing with the MDP-containing conjugate (Shapira *et al.* 1985).

Cholera toxin (CT) and heat-labile toxin of *E. coli* (LT)

The synthetic approach to vaccination has been employed also in the case of bacterial toxins. This has been first demonstrated by Audibert and her colleagues (1982) who have reported a synthetic peptide analogous to a region of diphtheria toxin (188–201) that led to the production in guinea pigs of antibodies capable of neutralizing the dermonecrotic activity of diphtheria toxin. A similar approach was used to provoke antibodies that are reactive with cholera toxin and capable of partially neutralizing its biological activity. The toxin of *Vibrio cholerae* is composed of two subunits A and B. Subunit A activates adenylate cyclase which triggers the biological activity, whereas subunit B is responsible for binding to cell receptors (GM1 ganglioside) and also expresses most of the toxin's antigenic reactivity (Lai, 1980).

Six peptides corresponding to various segments of the B subunit of cholera toxin have been synthesized and employed in appropriate conjugates for immunization of rabbits and mice. Of most interest among these peptides were those denoted CTP 1 (residues 8–20) and CTP 3 (residues 50–64). Antibodies to CTP 3 gave the strongest cross-reactivity with the intact B subunit as well as with the holotoxin. Furthermore, this was the only peptide reactive with antibodies against the native toxin. Antibodies to CTP 1 reacted not only with the B chain but also with the A chain of the toxin.

More interestingly, antisera against these two peptides exerted significant inhibition of the biological activity of cholera toxin. The toxic effect of CT can be demonstrated by skin vascular permeation and by fluid accumulation in ligated intestinal loops, as well as on the biochemical level, by the induction of adenylate cyclase. The inhibitory effect of the anti-peptide sera was manifested in all the assays of the biological activity, with very good correlation between the biochemical level and the end biological effect of the toxin. In both cases the inhibition reached a value of approximately 60% (Jacob *et al.* 1983, 1984a).

The heat-labile toxin (LT) of pathogenic strains of *Escherichia coli* is the causative agent of diarrhea in many tropical countries and, due to its wide spread, presents probably a more serious health problem than cholera. There is a high level of sequence homology between the B subunits of the LT and the CT. Moreover, an immunological relationship was demonstrated between the two toxins with the existence of both shared and specific antigenic determinants. It was, therefore, of interest to investigate whether the synthetic peptides derived from CT might cross-react with the LT and/or provide a comparable degree of protection against the heterologous toxin. Indeed, we have demonstrated that the antiserum elicited by CTP 3 is highly cross-reactive with the LT. This is not surprising, since in this region the sequence homology between the two toxins is complete.

The antiserum against CTP 1 was also cross-reactive with the two toxins, although to a much lower extent. However, antisera to both CTP 1 and CTP 3, which are inhibitory towards CT, were found equally effective in neutralizing the biological activity of the *E. coli* LT (Jacob *et al.* 1984b). This was manifested by significant inhibition of both adenylate cyclase induction and the fluid secretion into ligated loops of rats. The inhibition by the anti CTP 3 was expected in view of the high level of immunological cross-reactivity, as well as the sequence identity. As for the anti-CTP 1, its high efficacy in the inhibition of the biological activity contrasted by the very low serological cross-reactivity, may imply that the inhibition it confers is due to a possible interaction with subunit A, and not necessarily with subunit B, in spite of the lack of homology in sequence in the A subunit of the two toxins. The immunological relationship in this case could stem from similarities in conformation rather than sequence. Interestingly, anti-CTP 3 (but not anti-CP 1) is also reactive with LT from *E. coli* of porcine origin. These findings are indicative of one of the potential advantages of synthetic peptides, their capacity to elicit antibodies with cross-reactive properties, i.e. of broader specificity.

Combining recombinant DNA and synthetic approaches for vaccine development

A novel approach we recently employed was to explore whether the expression of CTP 3 by bacteria other than *Vibrio cholerae* may provide an appropriate agent for induction of immunity towards both cholera and *E. coli* toxins, and whether this could be approached by recombinant DNA techniques. To allow *E. coli* to synthesize CTP 3, we constructed two plasmids containing a synthetic DNA sequence encoding this peptide (a 54 base pair duplex) fused in phase to a truncated *LacZ* gene. The resulting fusion protein, which was expressed by the two vectors, was enzymatically active, and reacted with antibodies against β-galactosidase. It also reacted with antibodies against CTP 3, and to a lesser extent with antibodies against intact cholera toxin. Immunization with this protein as such did not lead to a significant titer of antibodies recognizing CT. However, when followed by a booster injection of a minute amount (1 μg) of CT, too small to provide any immune response by itself, it led to a substantial level of neutralizing anti-CT antibodies. Similar results were obtained after boosting with LT (Jacob *et al.* 1985), Thus, the fusion protein is capable of inducing an effective priming immunization against both CT and LT. These findings demonstrate that when relevant epitopes are defined, their corresponding synthetic oligonucleotides, which encode relatively small peptides, can be utilized, thus combining genetic-engineering and peptide chemistry for the future synthesis of vaccines.

Concluding remarks

In the results described above we have demonstrated that it is feasible to use synthetic peptide 'vaccines' to induce protective immunity in two systems, influenza and cholera. In both cases, it seems that the approach offers several advantages, in particular the potential capacity to induce cross-reactivity and cross-protection. In the case of influenza this might lead to a wide range cross-strain protection, and in the case of cholera toxin the synthetic peptides could serve as a basis for a future general vaccine against the coli-cholera family diarrheal diseases. Evidently, any realistic approach for future prospects must take into consideration the development of adjuvants that are acceptable for human use, preferably as built-in adjuvanticity. Equally important is the possibility to induce cell-mediated immunity as well as effective local immunity, when applicable, for better protection. All these parameters have to be further investigated; however, the progress made in the last few years in this area of research and the cumulative data obtained on the effectivity of synthetic peptides as immunogens for various viral and even parasitic diseases make the synthetic approach to vaccination a promising venture.

References

Adam A, Ciorbaru R, Ellouz F, Petit J F, Lederer E 1972. Isolation and properties of a macromolecular, water soluble, immunoadjuvant fraction from the cell of *Mycobacterium smegmatis*, *Proceedings of the National Academy of Sciences USA* **69**: 851–4

Arnon R 1972. Synthetic vaccine – dream or reality? in A Kohen, A M Klinberg (eds) *Immunity of Viral and Rickettsial Diseases*. Plenum Press, New York, pp 209–22

Arnon R, Maron E, Sela M, Anfinsen C E 1971. Antibodies reactive with native lysozyme elicited by a completely synthetic antigen, *Proceedings of the National Academy of Sciences USA* **68**: 1450–5

Arnon R, Sela M, Parant M, Chedid L 1980. Antiviral response by a completely synthetic antigen with built-in adjuvanticity, *Proceedings of the National Academy of Sciences USA* **77**: 6769–72

Audibert F, Jolivet M, Chedid L, Arnon R, Sela M 1982. Successful immunization with a totally synthetic diphtheria vaccine, *Proceedings of the National Academy of Sciences USA* **79**: 5042–6

Crumpton M L 1974. M Sela (ed) *The Antigens 1974 2: Protein antigens: The molecular basis of antigenicity and immunogenicity*. Academic Press, New York, pp 1–78

Hopp T P, Woods K R 1981. Prediction of protein antigenic determinants from amino acid sequences, *Proceedings of the National Academy of Sciences USA* **78**: 3824–8

Jackson D C, Brown L E, White D O, Dopheide T A A, Ward C W 1979. Antigenic determinants of influenza virus hemagglutinin. IV. Immunogenicity of cyanogen bromide fragments isolated from the hemagglutinin of A/Mem/72, *Journal of Immunology* **123**: 2610–17

Jacob C O, Sela M, Arnon R 1983. Antibodies against synthetic peptides of the B subunit of cholera toxin: cross-reaction and neutralization of the toxin, *Proceedings of the National Academy of Sciences USA* **80**: 7611–15

Jacob C O, Sela M, Pines M, Hurwitz S, Arnon R 1984a. Adenylate cyclase activation by cholera toxin as well as its activity are inhibited with antibody against related synthetic peptides, *Proceedings of the National Academy of Sciences USA* **81**: 7893–7

Jacob C O, Pines M, Arnon R 1984b. Neutralization of heat labile toxin of *E. coli* by antibody to synthetic peptides derived from B subunit of cholera toxin, *EMBO Journal* **3**: 2889–93

Jacob C O, Arnon R, Sela M 1985. Effect of carrier on the immunogenic capacity of synthetic cholera vaccine, *Molecular Immunology* **22**: 1333–9

Lai C Y 1980. Cholera toxin. *CRC Critical Reviews in Biochemistry* **9**: 171–207

Laver W G, Air G M, Webster R G 1981. Mechanism of antigenic drift in influenza virus, *Journal of Molecular Biology* **145**: 339–61

Muller G M, Shapira M, Arnon R 1982. Anti-influenza response achieved by immunization with a synthetic conjugate, *Proceedings of the National Academy of Sciences USA* **79**: 569–73

Shapira M, Jibson M, Muller G, Arnon R 1984. Immunity and protection against influenza virus by synthetic peptide corresponding to antigenic sites of hemagglutinin, *Proceedings of the National Academy of Sciences USA* **81**: 2461–5

Shapira M, Jolivet M, Arnon R 1985. A synthetic vaccine against influenza with built-in adjuvanticity. *International Journal of Immunopharmacology* **7**: 719–23

Wabuke-Bunoti M A N, Taku A, Fan D P, Kent S, Webster R G 1984. Cytolytic T lymphocytes and antibody responses to synthetic peptides of influenza virus hemagglutinin, *Journal of Immunology* **133**: 2194–2201

Webster R G, Hinshaw V J, Berton M T, Laver W G, Air G M 1981. Antigenic drift in influenza viruses and association of biological activity with topography of the hemagglutinin molecule, in D B Nayak (ed) *Genetic Variation among Influenza Viruses*. Academic Press, New York, pp 309–22

Wiley D C, Wilson I A, Skehel J J 1981. Structural identification of the antibody binding sites of the Hong Kong influenza hemagglutinin and their involvement in antigenic variation, *Nature (London)* **289**: 373–8

Enhancement of anti-influenza response by anti-idiotype antibodies

Thomas M Moran; Raoul Mayer; Constantin A Bona

Department of Microbiology, Mount Sinai School of Medicine, New York, New York 10021, USA

Introduction

One of the practical implications of the network theory is based on the concept of idiotypes as the internal image of the antigen (Jerne 1974). This concept appears as a statistical necessity in network theory, since if somehow we can average the three-dimensional structures of all epitopes of the foreign antigenic dictionary and of V domains of receptors of lymphocytes, their average must be similar. Among idiotypes of immunoglobulin molecules the idiotypes of anti-idiotypic antibodies probably have the highest probability of mimicking foreign antigen. Indeed, if the paratype of an antibody specific for a given antigen can be envisioned as the negative imprint of the epitope, then the anti-idiotype can express an idiotope which will be the positive imprint of the antigen. The first experimental evidence supporting this concept was provided by experiments carried out by Sege and Peterson (Sege and Peterson 1978) which demonstrated that an anti-idiotype against an anti-insulin antibody binds to insulin receptors and behaves like insulin.

Ensuing years have produced vast amounts of evidence demonstrating that anti-idiotype antibodies can mimic biologically active substances such as hormones, vitamins, drugs (data reviewed by Farid in press), viral, bacterial and parasitic antigens (data reviewed by Bona and Moran 1985; McNamara *et al.* 1984; Ertl *et al.* 1986; Kennedy and Dreesman 1986; Stein and Soderstrom 1984; Sachs 1984) or tumor antigens (Herlyn and Koprowski in press). However, it should be pointed out that only a small fraction of anti-idiotypes carry the internal image of the antigen. Actually anti-idiotypic antibodies represent a heterogenous population of antibodies, composed of three major populations:

1. Ab_2 alpha are the conventional anti-idiotype antibodies which recognize an idiotope associated with the combining site or the framework of the immunoglobulin variable region (Jerne 1982). Depending on the dose parenterally administered or the amount spontaneously produced *in vivo*,

these anti-idiotypes can either enhance or suppress the immune response (reviewed in Bona 1981).
2. Ab$_2$ beta are the anti-idiotypic antibodies expressing the internal image of the antigen. Their binding to immunoglobulin receptors induces the proliferation of clones in lieu of antigen.
3. Ab$_2$ epsilon (epibodies) are a particular category of anti-idiotype which bind to idiotype of antibody as well as to the initial antigen (Bona *et al.* 1982). These antibodies have been observed only in autoimmune diseases and perhaps play a role in pathogenesis. A large fraction of cryoglobulins from type II mixed cryoglobulinemia exhibit epibody-like activities (Geltner *et al.* 1980; Renversez *et al.* 1984).

One of the most attractive applications of the internal image concept is the utilization of anti-idiotypes as vaccines (Kieber-Emmons *et al.* 1986). This is particularly important in diseases in which attenuated vaccines do not exist or purified antigen used to prepare the vaccines are not yet available. Of particular interest for the utilization of idiotype vaccines are the viruses or parasites which exhibit extensive natural variation. In these cases, conventional vaccines can be used to protect the population against only the circulating viruses. However, an anti-idiotype vaccine can in principle stimulate the clones producing antibody for the circulating viruses as well as for the clones which will recognize antigenic variants, emerging subsequent to antigenic drift. Influenza virus and HTLV-3 viruses actually exhibit this type of genetic variations as a result of continuous nucleotide changes in the genes encoding the hemagglutinin or GP120 envelope protein, respectively. Oudin and Cazenave (1971) showed that antibodies with different antigenic specificity share idiotopes, and this phenomenon has been observed in various antigenic systems. Therefore, it is conceivable that immunoglobulins specific for antigenic determinants of circulating viruses or those emerging subsequent to genetic variation may share idiotopes. If such idiotype connectivity exists between antibodies specific for different viral variants, conceptually an anti-idiotype vaccine may elicit immunity against both.

In the case of influenza virus, two envelope glycoproteins, hemagglutinin and neuraminidase, are the major antigenic determinants. Both are capable of significant antigenic variation and the antibodies which react with one form of these glycoproteins often do not react with the variants. This unique capacity for antigenic variation permits the virus to circumvent the protective effects of population immunity. Thus, anti-idiotypic antibodies recognizing cross-reactive idiotypes on antibodies specific for various subtypes of hemagglutinin or neuraminidase or variants of these antigens can represent a candidate for an idiotype vaccine.

Antibodies specific for sequential induced variants share cross-reactive idiotypes

The antibody response to the hemagglutinin of influenza virus is extremely heterogeneous. Staudt and Gerhard (1983) estimated the repertoire of BALB/c antibodies directed to the H1 hemagglutinin of influenza A/PR/8/34 virus to consist of at least 1500 different paratypes. The diversity of this repertoire is a reflection of the variety of V_H and V_L genes families, J_H, D and J_L gene segments which combine to produce the active V genes encoding hemagglutinin specific antibodies. Additional diversity is imparted by random pairing of heavy and light chains and somatic mutational events (Clarke *et al.* 1985; McKean *et al.* 1984). With this enormous potential for diversity it was very important to determine if antibody to sequential viral mutants could share idiotypy, that is, to prove that connectivity could exist between antibodies with unique specificities. Reale *et al.* (1986) prepared in our laboratory monoclonal antibodies in different, individual BALB/c mice against sequentially selected variants of PR8 influenza virus. These monoclonal antibodies are specific for antigenic changes in the SA epitope. Indeed, the nucleotide sequence in hemagglutinin genes of PR8 wild type and two sequential variants indicate that variant 1 differs from PR8 by a point mutation in position 555, and variant 2 shows a back mutation in position 555 and a new mutation in position 580. The specificity of monoclonal antibodies to sequential PR8 variants was determined by hemagglutination inhibition assay (Reale *et al.* 1986) and the results are illustrated in Table 1. Molecular studies aimed to characterize the V genes encoding the specificity of these antibodies show that Py102, specific for the PR8 hemagglutinin, uses a V_H gene from the 7183 family and a light chain from the V_k21 ADEF subgroup, while VM113, specific for variant virus Py102-V1, also uses a V_k21 ADEF light chain and an unknown heavy chain. Among the VM113-V1 virus specific antibodies VM201 uses a heavy chain derived from the S107 family with a V_k21 ADEF light chain, while VM202 derives its active heavy chain gene from the V_H 7183

Table 1 Specificity of monoclonal antibodies to sequential PR8 variants

	Monoclonal antibodies			
Virus	PY102	VM113	VM201	VM202
PR8	+*	−	+	+
PY102-V1†	−	+	−	−
VM113-V1‡	+	−	+	+

* Positive or negative as determined by hemagglutination inhibition.
† PY102-V1 was selected subsequent to incubation of PR8 with PY102 antibodies.
‡ VM113-V1 was selected subsequent to incubation of PY102-V1 with VM113 antibodies.

family and uses a light chain which is not derived from the V_k21 ADEF subgroup.

The most striking observation arising from this study was that two antibodies specific for a single amino acid substitution in the hemagglutinin of the VM113-V1 variant use genes from completely different families (i.e. VM201 V_H S107/V_k21^+, VM202 V_H 7183/V_k21^-), indicating that the same paratope can be created by the pairing of totally different V_H and V_L genes. This is further supported by the experimental results depicted in Table 2 which show

Table 2 Inhibition of binding of I^{125}-labeled VM202 to virus by various monoclonal antibodies

Inhibitor	Concentration (μg/ml):			
	0.625	1.25	2.5	5.0
Saline	3224 ± 745^a			
VM201		860 ± 130	794 ± 90	580 ± 52	583 ± 102
VM202		1458 ± 198	982 ± 192	630 ± 38	490 ± 54
XY101		3252 ± 400	2912 ± 558	3490 ± 270	3492 ± 150

* Counts per minute of I^{125}-labeled VM202 bound to VM113-V1 influenza virus coated plate (25 μg/ml).

that the binding of I^{125}-labeled VM202 to VM113-V1 virus was completely inhibited by VM201 antibody. It was therefore important 'to study the expression of cross-reactive idiotypes on clones producing antibodies specific for variant viruses. This was carried out by using polyclonal and monoclonal anti-idiotypic antibodies against the four monoclonal antibodies to the viral variants.

The data sumarized in Table 3 show that anti-idiotype antibodies against Py102 recognize the cross-reactive idiotype shared by VM113, specific for

Table 3 Specificity, V genes and idiotypy of monoclonal antibodies

MAb	Specificity	V_H	V_k21	PY102 (IdX)	VM113 (IdI)	VM201 (IdX)	VM202 (IdI)
PY102	H1*	7183	ADEF	+	−	−	−
VM113	H1	ND‡	ADEF	+	+	−	−
VM201	H1	S107	ADEF	−	−	+	−
VM202	H1	7183	−	+	−	−	+
H36-5-3	H1	S107	C	−	−	+	−
H36-7-3	H1	S107	C	−	−	+	−
PT109	H1(HA-2)†	7183	ADEF	+	−	−	−
XY101	H3	7183	ADEF	+	−	−	−

* Hemagglutinin subtype.
† Carboxy-terminal cleavage product of hemagglutinin.
‡ Not done.

variant 1 and one of two antibodies (VM202) specific for the second variant. The idiotypic studies also show that these four clones are different since each of them expresses unique individual idiotopes. Indeed, Py102 did not share the VM113 IdI defined by rabbit anti-VM113, the IdI of VM202 antibody recognized by the syngeneic monoclonal antibody TM-1 and an IdX expressed on VM201 and shared with other H1 specific monoclonal antibodies using genes from the $V_H S107$ and $V_k 21$ families. Interestingly the Py102 cross-reactive idiotype was also identified on antibodies specific for the HA2 portion of H1 and on antibodies specific for H3. Taken together these results show that antibodies specific for wild type virus and sequential variants or subtypes of type A hemagglutinin can share idiotopes.

Effect of syngeneic anti-idiotypic antibodies on the anti-influenza response

Among a panel of syngeneic monoclonal anti-idiotypic antibodies specific for antibodies to influenza hemagglutinin, SP3-5A and SN3-1A were chosen to test their ability as idiotype vaccines. These antibodies were chosen for the following reasons:

1. They recognize a cross-reactive idiotype expressed on monoclonal antibodies specific for the H1 and H3 hemagglutinin and on antiviral antibodies produced during primary and secondary immune responses of BALB/c mice immunized with PR8, X-31, A/Singapore, A/Houston and A/Chicken (Moran *et al.* 1987). They have also been demonstrated on human antibodies to PR8 (Sigal *et al.* in press).
2. The binding of SN3-1A was antigen inhibitable (Moran *et al.* 1987).
3. Using a Western blot, SP3-5A was shown to recognize the idiotype exclusively on the heavy chain.

Therefore these antibodies fill most of the criteria proposed to define an Ab_2 beta, namely binding to a interspecies cross-reactive idiotype, binding to idiotypes shared by antibodies with various specificities, binding to an antigen inhibitable (i.e. combining site related) idiotype, and binding to an idiotype located exclusively on one chain. The effectiveness of these Ab_2 antibodies as idiotype vaccines was tested in a syngeneic (BALB/c) and allogeneic (C3H) system and evaluated by determining hemagglutination inhibiting antibodies in sera as well as viral titers in lungs. The animals treated with anti-idiotype were challenged by i.p. injection and PR8 or X-31 influenza viruses or by aerosol infection. Multiple parameters were studied: (a) priming of animals with anti-idiotypes in saline, alum precipitated or linked to KLH; (b) doses ranging from 100 ng to 50 µg per mouse; (c) challenge with optimal or suboptimal virus dose; (d) various intervals between priming with anti-idiotype and viral challenge.

Table 4 Hemagglutinin inhibition titers and idiotype levels in animals preimmunized with anti-idiotype

Immunization*		Challenge	Serum titers	Day 0	Day 3	Day 7	Day 21
1°	2°						
Saline	Saline	PR8	HI*	0	3 + 0	6 + 0	5 ± 0.63
			IdX†	<1	8.72 ± 2.36	1.84 ± 3.68	0.2 ± 0.4
PR8	Saline	PR8	HI	4.8 ± 1.46	4.2 ± 1.16	7.4 ± 1.01	7 ± 0.89
			IdX	<1	8.22 ± 5.6	1.6 ± 1.4	0.9 ± 1.8
SP35A(5 µg)	SP35A	PR8	HI	0 + 0	2.8 + 0.4	6.8 + 0.74	7 ± 0.89
			IdX	<1	3.74 ± 4.2	7.68 ± 9.5	25.14 ± 9.6
SP35A(5 µg)	SP35A	Saline	HI	1.2 ± 0.74	1.2 ± 0.75	0	1.8 ± 2.4
			IdX		<1	ND	ND
Saline	Saline	X-31	HI	0	0.4 ± 0.49	5 ± 0	5 ± 0.63
			IdX	<1	<1	7.06 ± 3.6	9.24 ± 6.29
X-31	Saline	X-31	HI	3.6 ± 0.49	4 + 0	5.8 ± 0.75	7.6 ± 0.8
			IdX	<1	<1	23.84 ± 4.7	12.2 ± 4.1
SP35A(5 µg)	SP35A(5 µg)	X-31	HI	0	0.2 + 0.4	5.5 ± 0.5	5.75 ± 0.43
			IdX	<1	<1	21.54 ± 5.1	7.74 ± 2.7
SP35A(5 µg)	SP35A(5 µg)	Saline	HI	0	0	0	0
			IdX	<1	<1	ND	ND

* Animals were immunized with anti-Id, saline or virus on day −42 (1°) or day −21 (2°) and challenged with the indicated virus.
† Hemagglutinin inhibition in $\log_2$ units.
‡ Percentage inhibition of PY206 bindings to SP3-5A by a 1:10 dilution of serum.

After evaluation of these parameters the following scheme of immunization was adopted:

Day 0 : priming with 5 μg alum precipitated anti-idiotype per mouse.
Day 21 : repeat priming, 5 μg anti-idiotype in saline per mouse.
Day 42 : i.p. challenge 1 μg or 2.5 μg virus or aerosol infection per mouse.

Hemagglutination-inhibiting antibodies were measured in blood samples 3, 7, 14 and 21 days after virus injection i.p. HA titers and lung viral titers from homogenates were determined on day 3, 7 and 14 in animals infected with viruses. In the same blood samples used to determine the HI titer, the level of idiotype was also evaluated by competitive inhibition radioimmunoassay.

Table 4 shows the results of one experiment using the anti-idiotype SP35A as the priming Ab_2. A two log_2 units increase above the animals primed with saline was observed on day 21 after challenge with PR8. A concomitant increase in serum idiotype was also observed. In the animals challenged with X-31 no significant increase in HA titer could be detected while the idiotype level was equal to animals primed with virus. Subsequent experiments did not yield even this small amount of enhancement and more importantly animals primed with anti-idiotype had lung viral titers equal to those of animals primed with saline. Therefore priming with these anti-idiotypes did not provide any protection against viral infection.

Effect of anti-idiotype antibodies on anti-neuraminase immune response

While antibodies against the hemagglutinnin of influenza virus play an important role in protection against reinfection by preventing binding of virus to target cells, antibodies specific for neuraminidase decrease the capacity to transmit the virus to susceptible contracts yet allow sub-clinical infections. Mayer *et al.* (in preparation) prepared a syngeneic monoclonal antibody against Py203, a monoclonal antibody specific for PR8 H1N1 neuraminidase. This anti-idiotypic antibody recognizes a cross-reactive idiotype expressed on N1 and N2 specific monoclonal antibodies as well as on antibodies elicited in BALB/c mice immunized with PR8 (H1N1) and X-31 (H3N2) virus subtypes. The effect of this antibody (RM1) was studied on the anti-neuraminidase response of BALB/c mice primed with 10 or 100 ng RM1 and boosted one month later with 5 μg of purified virus. The amount of anti-neuraminidase antibody was determined by neuraminidase inhibition assay on blood samples harvested 3, 7, 14 and 21 days after challenge. A significant increase of the anti-NA response was observed in the mice injected with 100 ng RM1 and boosted with PR8 as compared to those injected with IDA 10, a monoclonal antiidiotype specific for an irrelevant idiotype (A48) (Table 5). Similarly, the effect was noted on days 7 and 14 following the immunization with X-31 in the

Table 5 Enhancement of anti-neuraminidase response by monoclonal anti-idiotype RM1

Experimental animal group*	Concentration (μg/ml):	
	Py203-Id bearing Ig	**NA-specific Ig**
PR8–PR8	276 ± 53	653 ± 21
IDA10–PR8	203 ± 23	498 ± 23
RM1–PR8	522 ± 37	627 ± 19
X31–X31	357 ± 41	629 ± 33
IDA10–X31	235 ± 29	487 ± 31
RM1–X31	519 ± 32	615 ± 26

* Immunized day 0 with 100 ng PR8 or X31 or 100 ng IDA or RM1 and day 42 challenged with PR8 or X31.

animals pretreated with 100 ng RM1 compared to IDA 10. The increase in the NA specific response was paralleled by an increase in the Py203 idiotype level in the animals pretreated with RM1 and boosted with X-31. However, no anti-neuraminidase activity was observed in the animals primed and boosted with RM1. This result clearly indicates that RM1 by itself was unable to induce the differentiation of N1 and N2 precursors into antibody-forming cells, in spite of an increased level of immunoglobulin, bearing the Py203 idiotype ('parallel set'). These results suggest that RM1 behaves as an Ab_2 alpha, able to prime the cells which subsequently can differentiate into antibody-forming cells by antigen challenge.

In conclusion, our results show that:

1. We have identified syngeneic monoclonal anti-idiotype antibodies specific for cross-reactive idiotypes shared by clones specific for various hemagglutinin or neuraminidase viral subtypes.
2. The administration of these anti-idiotypic antibodies followed by antigenic boost increased the clones specific for viral HA and NA determinants bearing cross-reactive idiotopes. The enhancement of the anti-neuraminidase response was more significant than the anti-hemagglutinin response, a fact which may be related to the smaller heterogeneity of paratopes of anti-NA antibodies versus anti-HA antibodies.
3. Alone, the anti-idiotype antibodies were unable to elicit any anti-viral response, indicating clearly the difficulties in selecting anti-idiotypes carrying the internal image of the antigen which can be used as idiotype vaccines in the influenza system.

Acknowledgements

This work was supported by US Public Health Service Research Grant no. AI 18316-06 from the National Institutes of Health.

References

Bona C 1981. *Idiotypes and Lymphocytes*. Academic Press, New York.

Bona C, Moran T 1985. Idiotype vaccines. *Annales d'Immunologie (Paris)* **136C**: 299–312

Bona C A, Finley S, Waters S, Kunkel H G 1982. Anti-immunoglobulin antibodies III. Properties of sequential anti-idiotypic antibodies to heterologous anti-γ-globulins. Detection of reactivity of anti-idiotype antibodies with epitopes of Fc fragments (homobodies) and with epitopes and idiotopes (epibodies), *Journal of Experimental Medicine* **156**: 986–9

Clarke S H, Huppi K, Ruezinsky L, Staudt L, Gerhard W, and Weigert M 1985. Inter and intraclonal diversity in the response to influenza hemagglutinin, *Journal of Experimental Medicine* **161**: 687–704

Ertl H C J, Skinner M A, Finberg R W 1986. Induction of anti-viral immunity by an anti-idiotypic antibody directed to a Sendai virus specific T helper cell clone, *International Review of Immunology* **1**: 41–66

Farid N R 1987. Anti-idiotype antibodies mimicking active biological substances, in C A Bona (ed) *Elicitation and Use of Anti-Idiotypic Antibodies and Their Biological Applications* CRC Press, Boca Raton, Florida (in press)

Geltner D, Franklin E C, Fragione B 1980. Anti-idiotypic activity in the IgM fractions of mixed cryoglobulins, *Journal of Immunology* **125**: 1530–6

Herlyn D, Koprowski H 1987. Anti-idiotypic antibodies in cancer therapy, in C A Bona (ed) *Elicitation and Use of Anti-Idiotypic Antibodies and Their Biological Applications*. CRC Press, Boca Raton, Florida (in press)

Jerne N K 1974. Towards a network theory of the immune system, *Annales d'Immunologie (Paris)* **125C**: 373–89

Jerne N K, Roland J, Cazenave P A 1982. Recurrent idiotopes and internal images, *EMBO Journal* **1**: 243–7

Kennedy R C, Dreesman G R 1986. Anti-idiotypic antibodies as idiotope vaccines that induce immunity against infectious agents, *International Review of Immunology* **1**: 67–79

Kieber-Emmons T, Ward R E, Raychaudhuri S, Rein R, Kohler H 1986. Rational design and application of idiotope vaccines, *International Review of Immunology* **1**: 1–26

Mayer R, Moran T, Johansson B, Bona C Effect of anti-idiotypic antibody on anti-neuraminidase response, *Journal of Immunology* (in preparation)

McKean D, Huppi K, Bell M, Staudt L I, Gerhard W, Weigert M 1984. Generation of antibody diversity in the immune response of Balb/c mice to influenza virus hemagglutinin, *Proceedings of the National Academy of Sciences USA* **81**: 3180–4

McNamara M K, Ward R E, Kohler H 1984. Monoclonal idiotope vaccine against *Streptococcus pneumoniae* infection, *Science* **226**: 1325–6

Moran T M, Monestier M, Lai A C K, Norton G, Reale M A, Thompson M A, Schulman J L, Riblet R, Bona C A 1987. Characterization of variable region genes and shared cross-reactive idiotypes of antibodies specific for antigens of various influenza viruses, *Viral Immunology* **1**(1): 1–17

Oudin J, Cazenave P A 1971. Similar idiotypic specificities in immunoglobulin fractions with different antibody functions or even without detectable antibody function, *Proceedings of the National Academy of Sciences USA* **68**: 2616–20

Reale M A, Manheimer A J, Moran T M, Norton G, Bona C A, Schulman J L 1986. Characterization of monoclonal antibodies specific for sequential influenza A/PR/8/34 virus variants, *Journal of Immunology* **137**: 1352–9

Renversez J C, Roussel S, Vallee M J, Brighouse G, Lambert P H 1984. *Blood Transfusion and Immunohematology* **27**: 737–55

Sachs D L 1984. Induction of protective immunity using anti-idiotypic antibodies: immunization against experimental trypanosomiasis, in H Kohler, J Urbain, P A Cazenave (eds) *Idiotypes in Biology and Medicine*. Academic Press, New York, pp 401–16

Sege K, Peterson P A 1978. Use of anti-idiotypic antibodies as cell-surface receptor probes, *Proceedings of the National Academy of Sciences USA* **75**: 2443–7

Sigal N, Reale M, Moran T, Bona C 1987. Cross species idiotype found on human monoclonal antibodies to influenza virus in M Zanetti, F Celada, C Bona (eds) *Idiotypes in disease*, Karger, Basel (in press)

Staudt L M, Gerhard W 1983. Generation of antibody diversity in the immune response of BALB/c mice to influenza virus hemagglutinin, *Journal of Experimental Medicine* **157**: 687–705

Stein K, Soderstrom J 1984. Neonatal administration of idiotype or anti-idiotype primes for protection against *E. coli* K13 injection in mice, *Journal of Experimental Medicine* **160**: 1001–11

Properties of a protective anti-idiotype vaccine for viral hepatitis B

Gordon R Dreesman; Richard D Henkel; En-Min Zhou;
Ronald C Kennedy

Department of Virology and Immunology, Southwest Foundation for Biomedical Research, San Antonio, Texas 78284, USA

The idiotype (Id) network for immune regulation proposed by Jerne (1974) suggested that the immune response to a given antigen was regulated via a series of Id-anti-Id reactions. In its most simplistic form, the antigen-induced antibodies (Ab-1) not only recognize antigens, but they also display new antigenic determinants (Id) that are recognized by a second set of antibodies (anti-Id) or Ab-2. The Id determinants define the variable region of the antibody molecule. The specific area or site of the antibody variable region which makes contact and combines with a given epitope on the antigen is called the paratope of the antibody. If a defined Id determinant, referred to as an idiotope, and its paratope are one and the same site on the antibody, then the anti-Id and antigen should bear a similar conformation. Anti-Id which have this specificity will be referred to as internal image anti-Id in this paper. Two independent research groups initially proposed that the idiotope on the anti-Id might have vaccine potential (Nisonoff and Lamoyi 1981; Roitt *et al.* 1981).

Recent studies have confirmed the above concepts that anti-Ids can serve as potential vaccines for a large number of infectious agents (for reviews see Dreesman and Kennedy 1985; Kennedy and Dreesman 1986). The systems where anti-Id appear useful as possible vaccines against virus infections are summarized in Table 1.

Our laboratories have been involved with studies characterizing the Id associated with human antibodies to hepatitis B surface antigen (anti-HBs) (Kennedy *et al.* 1982; Kennedy and Dreesman 1983). Hepatitis B virus (HBV) represents a significant worldwide health problem in that approximately 175 million people are infected with this virus yearly. The major concern of this infected population is a group containing 200 million people who have developed chronic HBV infections, many of whom develop chronic liver disease or hepatocellular carcinoma (Maupas and Melnick 1981).

HBV contains two distinct antigenic determinants, hepatitis B core antigen (HBcAg) and hepatitis B surface antigen (HBsAg) (for reviews see Melnick *et al.* 1976; Dreesman 1984). HBcAg is associated with the viral nucleocapsid

Table 1 Summary of systems where anti-Ids have been used to induce an immune response against viral agents

System	Authors	Disease	Anti-Id source
Hepatitis B surface antigen	Kennedy and Dreesman (1984)	Serum hepatitis	Rabbit
Reovirus hemagglutinin	Sharpe *et al.* (1984)	Encephalitis	Mouse monoclonal
Sendai virus T-cell clone	Ertl and Finberg (1984)	Systemic infection	Mouse monoclonal
Rabies surface glycoprotein	Reagan *et al.* (1983)	Rabies	Rabbit
Poliovirus VP1	Uytdehaag and Osterhaus (1985)	Polio	Mouse monoclonal
Herpes simplex virus glycoprotein	Gell and Moss (1985)	Encephalitis, latent diseases	Rabbit
Herpes simplex virus glycoprotein	Lathey *et al.* (1987)	Encephalitis, latent diseases	Rabbit
Feline leukemia virus glycoprotein	Uytdehaag *et al.* (1986)	Immune deficiency diseases	Mouse monoclonal

and HBsAg composes the surface or envelope of the virion. HBsAg contains within its structure a cross-reacting group antigen termed *a* and two sets of mutually exclusive subtype antigens designated *d* or *y* and *w* or *r* (LeBouvier 1971; Bancroft *et al.* 1972). It has been shown that antibodies to the group-specific or common *a* determinant(s) provide protection against infection with HBV (Szmuness *et al.* 1980).

We have previously described a common human Id on anti-HBs molecules derived from individuals infected with HBV (Kennedy and Dreesman 1983). Our subsequent studies indicated that group *a* determinant is responsible in the induction of the anti-HBs Id (Kennedy *et al.* 1982). In addition, it was shown that the Id-anti-Id reaction detects an interspecies Id that is produced by active immunization of a number of experimental animals with HBsAg (Kennedy *et al.* 1983a). These observations indicated that the anti-Id preparation might contain an internal image (Ab2β) bearing population that had the ability to recognize a three-dimensional conformation on the anti-HBs molecules expressing the interspecies Id (Kennedy *et al.* 1982, 1983a, 1983c). More specifically, HBsAg induced an Ab-1 V region containing a conformation that has complementarity to HBsAg and can be identified with an anti-Id reagent.

The internal image anti-Id antibodies were further characterized by testing their ability to bind to anti-HBs-secreting hybridomas. Both cell surface binding as well as cytoplasmic staining of fixed hybridoma cells was noted (Kennedy *et al.* 1986b). The binding of anti-Id to anti-HBs-secreting hybridomas was inhibited by prior incubation with purified intact HBsAg particles. Immunoprecipitation studies demonstrated that anti-Id bound to immunoglobulin molecules on the cell surface. These studies added to our prior observations (Kennedy *et al.* 1983a) showed that the anti-Id reacts with an interspecies Id (Kennedy *et al.* 1986b).

Anti-Id reagents have originally been described to serve as a powerful tool to identify cell receptors for reovirus (Nepom *et al.* 1982; Noseworthy *et al.* 1983). This approach was of particular interest for HBV because no-one has successfully propagated the virus *in vitro*. We used the anti-Id to attempt to identify potential viral receptors on chimpanzee hepatocytes. Specific binding of the anti-Id to chimpanzee hepatocytes was detected by immune electron microscopy employing electron dense colloidal gold particles (Kennedy *et al.* submitted for publication). Binding of anti-Id to membrane receptors on chimpanzee hepatocytes was completely inhibited by prior incubation with purified HBsAg. To substantiate the validity of these findings, it was observed that hepatocytes derived from a baboon, a species not susceptible to human HBV infection, failed to react with the anti-Id reagent. These data suggest that the anti-Id can identify viral receptors on hepatocytes derived from animals susceptible to HBV infections.

The above observations strongly indicate that the anti-Id prepared to human anti-HBs has an internal image specificity in that: (1) the Id-anti-Id is equally inhibited with three antigenic subtypes of HBsAg, as well as with a cyclic HBsAg synthetic peptide; (2) it is directed to an interspecies Id; and (3) it combines with cell receptors on susceptible chimpanzee hepatocytes. Based on these results we postulated that immunization with anti-Id should induce an antibody response similar to that invoked with HBsAg.

Our first experiments were designed to examine the effect of priming with anti-Id and the anti-HBs response. Groups of mice were pretreated with either rabbit anti-Id, Ab-2 (made against purified human anti-HBs, Ab-1) or control non-immune rabbit IgG preparations. Each group of animals was subsequently injected with HBsAg. We analyzed the antibody response of these mice by determining the number of spleen cells secreting anti-HBs (Kennedy *et al.* 1983b). A significantly higher number of anti-HBs plaques were detected in the group of mice receiving anti-Id prior to HBsAg indicating that Ab-2 had the ability to prime the immune response. These data suggested that the immune response to HBsAg was regulated via an idiotype network, and perhaps manipulation of this network by anti-Id reagents would enhance the anti-HBs response. To confirm the studies described above, we next tested the immune response to HBsAg by anti-Id treatment and tested sera of mice for the presence of anti-HBs activity (Kennedy *et al.* 1984a; Kennedy and Dreesman 1984). These experiments confirmed our previous data in that sera obtained from mice pretreated with anti-Id prior to HBsAg or from mice injected with anti-Id only contained significantly higher amounts of anti-HBs when compared to sera of mice receiving control non-immune antibodies. We also generated antibodies comparable to those obtained with HBsAg alone by inoculating a combination of anti-Id and a cyclic synthetic HBsAg peptide (Kennedy *et al.* 1984b). These data indicate that anti-Ids appear to be useful in enhancing the immunogenic potential of a relatively weak antigen. In addition, anti-HBs activity was produced in mice by injection of anti-Id alone, without any prior HBsAg exposure.

A possible pitfall associated with potential anti-Id vaccines has been observed in an initial report which noted genetic restriction in various inbred strains of mice inoculated with anti-Id reagents against *Trypanosoma* (Sacks and Sher 1983). This failure to cross genetic barriers was related to the fact that the anti-Id used in these studies did not possess internal image components. To test this property we injected rabbits with anti-Id to induce an anti-HBs response. The anti-Id induced anti-HBs response produced in rabbits recognized the *a* group HBsAg determinants (Kennedy *et al.* 1986c). These findings indicated that genetic restriction was not a limitation of internal image based anti-Id vaccines.

The critical question that must be addressed in the development of a new vaccine is whether it will provide protection against challenge with the respective infectious agent. In the case of HBV infections, chimpanzees provide the relevant model of a human response to HBV immunization and infection. Consequently, the internal image anti-Id adsorbed to alum was used to immunize two non-immune chimpanzees. A third chimpanzee was inoculated with a similar concentration of non-immune rabbit IgG adsorbed to alum. The two animals that were injected with four injections of affinity-purified rabbit anti-Id developed detectable anti-HBs one week after the fourth dose. Peak serum antibody activity in both animals was noted approximately eight weeks after the fourth immunization. Sera pooled from blood obtained after the final immunization was analyzed to test its specificity against the rabbit anti-Id. After removal of anti-isotypic and anti-allotypic antibodies by affinity chromatography on normal rabbit IgG columns, the two chimpanzee antisera preferentially bound to both rabbit anti-Id and to HBsAg. Thus, it was established that both animals had produced an anti-anti-Id (Ab-3) response (Kennedy *et al.* 1986a).

The ability of an anti-Id vaccine to protect against infection was tested by challenging the two immunized animals, the control animal immunized with normal rabbit IgG and an untreated chimpanzee with 3000 chimpanzee infectious doses of HBV. The anti-Id immunized chimpanzees were solidly protected since they developed no serological, enzymatic or clinical signs of infection during a subsequent year of observation (Kennedy *et al.* 1986a). In contrast, both control animals developed disease markers consistent with those observed with hepatitis type B infections.

A question has been posed regarding the persistence of detectable immunity induced by anti-Id inoculations. The above chimpanzees have been followed after challenge and each presents long-lasting immunity as evidenced by constant levels of serum anti-HBs for one year. Thus, anti-Id induced immunity does not appear to be transient.

The above studies indicate that internal image anti-Id preparations present logical vaccine candidates against HBV and other infectious agents.

Acknowledgements

Supported by grants AI-22307-01, AI-22380-01, AI23619-01 and AI23472-01 from the National Institutes of Health. En-Min Zhou is a visiting scholar from the Peoples' Republic of China.

References

Bancroft W R, Mundon F K, Russell P K 1972. Detection of additional antigenic determinants of hepatitis B surface antigen, *Journal of Immunology* **109**: 842–8

Dreesman G R 1984. Polypeptide and synthetic peptide vaccines for hepatitis B virus, in F U Chisari (ed) *Advances in Hepatitis Research*. Masson Publishing, New York, pp 216–22

Dreesman G R, Kennedy R C 1985. Anti-idiotypic antibodies: implications of internal image-based vaccines for infectious diseases, *Journal of Infectious Diseases* **151**: 761–5

Ertl H C J, Finberg R W 1984. Sendai virus-specific T-cell clones: induction of cytolytic T cells by anti-idiotypic antibody directed against a helper T-cell clone, *Proceedings of the National Academy of Sciences USA* **81**: 2850–4

Gell P G H, Moss P A H 1985. Production of cell-mediated immune response to herpes simplex virus by immunization with anti-idiotypic heteroantisera, *Journal of General Virology* **66**: 1801–4

Jerne N K 1974. Towards a network theory of the immune system, *Annales d'Immunologie (Paris)* **125C**: 373–89

Kennedy R C, Dreesman G R 1983. Common idiotypic determinant associated with human antibodies to hepatitis B surface antigen, *Journal of Immunology* **130**: 385–9

Kennedy R C, Dreesman G R 1984. Enhancement of the immune response to hepatitis B surface antigen; *in vivo* administration of anti-idiotype induced anti-HBs that expresses a similar idiotype, *Journal of Experimental Medicine* **159**: 655–65

Kennedy R C, Dreesman G R 1986. Anti-idiotypic antibodies as idiotype vaccines that induce immunity against infectious agents, *International Reviews of Immunology* **1**: 67–78

Kennedy R C, Sanchez Y, Ionescu-Matiu I, Melnick J L, Dreesman G R 1982. A common human anti-hepatitis B surface antigen idiotype is associated with the group *a* conformation-dependent antigenic determinant, *Virology* **122**: 219–21

Kennedy R C, Ionescu-Matiu I, Sanchez Y, Dreesman G R 1983a. Detection of interspecies idiotypic cross-reactions associated with antibodies to hepatitis B surface antigen, *European Journal of Immunology* **13**: 232–5

Kennedy R C, Adler-Storthz K, Henkel R D, Sanchez Y, Melnick J L, Dreesman G R 1983b. Immune response to hepatitis B surface antigen: enhancement by prior injection of antibodies to the idiotype, *Science* **221**: 853–5

Kennedy R C, Dreesman G R, Sparrow J T, Culwell A R, Sanchez Y, Ionescu-Matiu I, Hollinger F B, Melnick J L 1983c. Inhibition of a common human anti-hepatitis B surface antigen idiotype by a cyclic synthetic peptide, *Journal of Virology* **46**: 653–5

Kennedy R C, Melnick J L, Dreesman G R 1984a. Antibody to hepatitis B virus induced by injecting antibodies to the idiotype, *Science* **223**: 930–1

Kennedy R C, Sparrow J T, Sanchez Y, Melnick J L, Dreesman G R 1984b. Enhancement of viral hepatitis B antibody (anti-HBs) response to a synthetic cyclic peptide by priming with anti-idiotype antibodies, *Virology* **136**: 247–52

Kennedy R C, Eichberg J W, Lanford R E, Dreesman G R 1986a. Anti-idiotypic antibody vaccine for type B viral hepatitis in chimpanzees, *Science* **232**: 220–3

Kennedy R C, Henkel R D, Dreesman G R 1986b. Further characterization of internal image-bearing anti-idiotype antibodies: specific binding to immunoglobulin receptors on murine hybridoma cell secreting antibodies to hepatitis B surface antigen, *Scandinavian Journal of Immunology* **23**: 481–9

Kennedy R C, Eichberg J W, Dreesman G R 1986c. Lack of genetic restriction by a potential anti-idiotype vaccine for type B hepatitis, *Virology* **148**: 369–74

Kennedy R C, Smith G C, Zhou E M, Eichberg J W, Dreesman G R. Anti-idiotypic antibodies identify possible receptors for hepatitis B virus on hepatocytes from chimpanzees (submitted for publication)

Lathey J L, Courtney R J, Rouse B T 1987. Production, binding characteristics, and immunogenicity of heterologous anti-idiotypic antibody to herpes simplex virus glycoprotein C, *Viral Immunology* **1**: 13–23

LeBouvier G L 1971. The heterogeneity of Australia antigen, *Journal of Infectious Diseases* **123**: 671–5

Maupas P, Melnick J L (eds) 1981. Hepatitis B virus and primary hepatocellular carcinoma, *Progress in Medical Virology* vol 27. S Karger, New York.

Melnick J L, Dreesman G R, Hollinger F B 1976. Approaching the control of viral hepatitis type B, *Journal of Infectious Diseases* **133**: 210–29

Nepom J T, Weiner H L, Dichter M A, Tardieu M, Spriggs D R, Gramm C F, Powers M L, Fields B N, Greene M I 1982. A hemagluttinin-specific idiotype associated with reovirus recognition shared by lymphoid and neural cells, *Journal of Experimental Medicine* **155**: 155–67

Nisonoff A, Lamoyi E 1981. Implications of the presence of an internal image of the antigen in anti-idiotypic antibodies: possible application to vaccine production, *Clinical Immunology and Immunopathology* **21**: 397–406

Noseworthy J H, Fields B N, Dichter M A, Sobotka C, Pizer E, Perry L L, Nepom J T, Greene M I 1983. Cell receptors for the mammalian reovirus. I. Syngeneic monoclonal anti-idiotypic antibody identifies a cell surface receptor for reovirus, *Journal of Immunology* **131**: 2533–8

Reagan K J, Wunner W H, Wiktor T J, Koprowski H 1983. Anti-idiotypic antibodies induce neutralizing antibodies to rabies virus glycoprotein, *Journal of Virology* **48**: 660–6

Roitt I M, Cooke A, Male D K, Hay F C, Guarnotta G, Lydyard P M, DeCarvalho L P, Thanavala Y, Ivany J 1981. Idiotypic networks and their possible exploitation for manipulation of the immune response, *Lancet* **i**: 1041–4

Sacks D L, Sher A, 1983. Evidence that anti-idiotype induced immunity to experimental African trypansomiasis is genetically restricted and requires recognition of combining site-related idiotypes, *Journal of Immunology* **131**: 1511–15

Sharpe A H, Gaulton G N, McDade K K, Fields B N, Greene M I 1984. Syngeneic monoclonal anti-idiotype can induce cellular immunity to reovirus, *Journal of Experimental Medicine* **160**: 1195–1205

Szmuness W, Stevens C E, Harley E J, Zang E A, Oleszko W R, William D C, Sadovsky R, Morrison J M, Kellner A 1980. Hepatitis B vaccine. Demonstration of efficacy in a controlled clinical trial in a high-risk population in the United States, *New England Journal of Medicine* **303**: 833–41

Uytdehaag F G C M, Osterhaus A D M E 1985. Induction of neutralizing antibody in mice against Poliovirus type II with monoclonal anti-idiotypic antibody, *Journal of Immunology* **134**: 1225–9

Uytdehaag F G C M, Bunschoten H, Weijer K, Osterhaus A D M E 1986. From Jenner to Jerne: towards idiotypic vaccines, *Immunological Reviews* **90**: 93–114

Immunogenicity of anti-idiotypes directed to Sendai virus specific T cell clones

Hildegund C J Ertl; Linda Woo; Robert W Finberg

Dana–Farber Cancer Institute and Harvard Medical School, 44 Binney Street, Boston, Massachusetts 02115, USA

Introduction

The variable regions of immunologically relevant receptors such as those expressed on antibody molecules or T cell receptors are immunogeneic (Urbain *et al.* 1977; Cazenave 1977; Takemori and Rajewsky 1984). They may either induce or, alternatively, suppress immune cells with complementary receptors. Each immunogenic site of a variable region is called an idiotope and collectively the set of idiotopes found on a particular variable region is called an idiotype. The concept of complementary idiotypes–anti-idiotypes was initially defined for B cell receptors (Jerne 1974). T cell receptors are genetically distinct but as they show idiotypic cross-reactivity with antibodies (Eichmann *et al.* 1980) they might be governed by similar rules.

It has been shown in several microbial systems that anti-idiotypic antibodies (especially those which carry an internal image) may have a potential as vaccines (Sacks *et al.* 1982; McNamara *et al.* 1984; UytdeHaag and Osterhaus 1985; Reagan *et al.* 1983; Grzych *et al.* 1985; Kennedy *et al.* 1983; Sharpe *et al.* 1984). Anti-idiotypic antibodies made against antigen reactive antibodies have been used to generate neutralizing antibodies and in addition T cells which mediate a delayed-type hypersensitivity response (DTH) (class II restricted T cells, Sharpe *et al.* 1984). Soluble anti-idiotypic antibodies made against B cell receptors seem to be unable to induce class I region restricted, cytolytic T cells (though this has only been tested in one system, Sharpe *et al.* 1984). Such T cells seem to be crucial in the defense of an organism against infections with intracellular pathogens (Yap *et al.* 1978; Ada *et al.* 1981). B cell defined anti-idiotypes thus seem to act similarly to inert vaccines such as inactivated pathogens or peptide vaccines which are in general poor inducers of class I restricted T cells, and could thus conceivably be used to induce protective immunity to pathogens whose successful removal is mediated by antibodies or class II region restricted T cells.

It was shown several years ago (Frischknecht *et al.* 1978) that anti-idiotypic antisera to T cell populations could induce class I as well as class II restricted T cells. Using T cell specific antibodies might thus be an alternative approach for the development of anti-idiotype vaccines to intracellular pathogens.

Material and methods

Mice

Female B10.D2, DBA/2 (H-2^d), C57Bl/6 (H-2^b), AJ (H-2^a), B10.BR and AKR (H-2^k) mice were purchased from The Jackson Laboratory, Bar Harbor, Maine, USA, kept in the mouse colony of the Dana–Farber Cancer Institute and used at the age of 8–12 weeks. Sentenial mice were routinely screened serologically to exclude contamination with Sendai virus.

Virus

Sendai virus and influenza A/PR8 virus were propagated in embryonated chicken eggs as described by Ertl *et al.* (1976).

Tumor cell lines

P815 mastocytoma cells, P3-NS11-Ag4-1 (NS-1) myeloma cells and 1B4.E6/H6 hybridoma cells were grown *in vitro* in Dulbecco's modified Eagle's medium (DMEM) supplemented with 10% fetal bovine serum (FBS). L929 mouse fibroblasts were most kindly provided by B Fields' Laboratory, Harvard Medical School.

Sendai virus specific T cell clones

T cell clones were either induced *in vivo* with Sendai virus or 1B4.E6/H6 antibody and subsequently restimulated *in vitro* with Sendai virus. The detailed methods to generate, maintain and characterize Sendai virus specific T cell clones has been described in detail elsewhere (Ertl and Finberg 1984a).

Generation of the 1B4.E6/H6 hybridoma

B10.D2 mice were immunized every other week with (1–2) $\times$ 10^6 syngeneic cloned T helper cells (clone 2H3.E8) over a period of six months. One week after the last immunization, immune splenocytes were fused with NS-1 myeloma cells. Hybrid supernatants were screened for binding to the 2H3.E8 T cell lines by indirect immunofluorescence and subsequent analysis in a fluorescence-activated cell sorter. Cells of one well which was found to exhibit binding were subcloned; two subclones, 1B4.E6 and 1B4.H6, which are presumably identical, were expanded and used for further studies.

Immunization of mice

Mice were injected intraperitoneally with 1B.E6/H6 or, as a positive control, 10^3 hemagglutinin units (HAU) of ultraviolet-light inactivated Sendai virus.

In vitro *stimulation of T cells*

Splenocytes (6×10^6) of naive or immune splenocytes were incubated with 10^2 HAU UV-light inactivated Sendai virus in 1.6 ml DMEM supplemented with 2% FBS and 0.1 mm-2-mercaptoethanol (2-ME) in Costar 24-well tissue culture plates. To stimulate splenocytes in limiting dilution a low number of splenocytes of Sendai virus or 1B4.E6 immune mice were cocultured with 1×10^6 irradiated (2000 rad) Sendai virus presenting syngeneic splenocytes and conditioned medium (rat Concanavalin A supernatant or $2°$ mixed leukocyte culture supernatant) as lymphokine source in 48–96 wells of round-bottom microtiter plates in DMEM supplemented with 10% FBS. Control wells received stimulator cells and lymphokines only.

Mediation of a delayed-type hypersensitivity response

One week after immunization $(0.8–1) \times 10^8$ immune splenocytes were transferred intravenously into naive recipient mice which were injected immediately afterwards with 10^3 HAU infectious Sendai virus into the left foot. Control mice were injected with virus only. Footpad thickness was measured 24 hr later. The percentage increase of footpad thickness was calculated using the formula:

$$\frac{\text{Thickness of left footpad} - \text{thickness of right footpad}}{\text{thickness of right footpad}} \times 100$$

^{51}Cr-release assay

Effector cells were harvested after five days, passed through a Ficoll gradient, counted and diluted in DMEM supplemented with 10% FBS. A graded number of responder cells were added in $100\,\mu$l medium to $(2–5) \times 10^3$ ^{51}Cr-labeled uninfected or Sendai virus infected target cells in V-bottom microtiter plate wells. After a 4–5 hr incubation time at $37°$C, $75\,\mu$l of supernatant were harvested and analyzed in a gamma-counter. The percentage specificity lysis was calculated using the formula:

$$\frac{^{51}\text{Cr release in presence of effector cells} - {}^{51}\text{Cr release in presence of medium}}{\text{maximally possible } {}^{51}\text{Cr release} - {}^{51}\text{Cr release in presence of medium}} \times 100$$

The cytolytic activity of lymphocytes stimulated under limiting dilution conditions was tested six days after induction. Equal fraction of cells from each well were transferred onto $(1-2) \times 10^3$ ^{51}Cr-labeled Sendai virus infected or uninfected target cells. ^{51}Cr release was measured 5–6 hr after incubation. Cells of wells which showed ^{51}Cr release more than three standard deviations above ^{51}Cr release in the presence of cells from control wells (which received 0 responder cells) were regarded as being positive.

Proliferation of T cell clones to antigen

Cloned T cells $((1-2) \times 10^4)$ were cocultured with 1×10^6 irradiated splenocytes with or without antigen in flat-bottom microtiter plates as described by Ertl and Finberg (1984a).

Induction of protective immunity

Groups of 5–6 B10.D2 mice were injected intraperitoneally three times in four-day intervals with 200 μl 1B4.E6 or once with 10^3 HAU UV-light inactivated Sendai virus or A/PR8 virus. Six days later, immune mice and naive control mice were inoculated intranasally with a lethal dose of infectious Sendai virus.

Results

Characteristics of the 2H3.E8 T helper cell clone

The 2H3.E8 T cell clone was derived from splenocytes of B10.D2 mice which had been immunized with UV-light inactivated Sendai virus. The 2H3.E8 T cell clone which was phenotypically Ly-1.2$^-$, Lyt-2.2$^-$ and Thy-1.2$^+$ proliferated and secreted lymphokines in response to Sendai virus presented on H-2 I region compatible splenic stimulator cells. *In vivo* the clone mediated an inflammatory response to Sendai virus which histologically resembled a DTH response. Under certain experimental conditions this clone, which failed to lyse Sendai virus infected target cells *in vitro*, augmented a cytolytic T cell response to a subimmunogenic dose of Sendai virus *in vivo*. In spite of these *in vivo* functions, the 2H3.E8 T cell clone failed to transfer protective immunity to mice which has been infected with a lethal dose of Sendai virus (Ertl and Finberg 1984a).

362

Characteristics and specificity of the 1B4.E6/H6 antibody

The 1B4.E6/H6 antibody was generated in B10.D2 mice by multiple immunizations with the 2H3.E8 T cell clone. The antibody, which was classified as an IgM molecule by radial immunodiffusion, bound to a high percentage of Sendai virus specific T cells as shown by indirect immunofluorescence on T cell clones and T cell populations, which had been enriched for Sendai virus specific effector cells (by *in vivo* immunization and *in vitro* restimulation with viral antigen). T cells which expressed the 1B4.E6/H6 idiotope could be found in mouse strains of both different H-2 haplotypes and IgH allotypes. The antibody bound predominantly (but not exclusively) to Sendai virus specific Thy-1.2$^+$, Ly-1.2$^+$, L3.T4$^+$, Lyt-2.2$^-$ T cells. As far as has been tested, the antibody failed to bind to T cells directed to other antigens or to splenic or thymic T cells of naive mice (Ertl and Finberg 1984b). The antibody exhibited no detectable binding to soluble or cell-bound Sendai virus. The 1B4.E6/H6 antibody failed to immunoprecipitate any detectable surface proteins from T cells which showed positive binding by immunofluorescence and fluorescent activated cell sorter (FACS) analysis. Nevertheless, according to its binding specificity it presumably represents an anti-idiotypic reagent which recognizes a dominant idiotope of the Sendai virus specific T cell repertoire.

In vitro *functions of the 1B4.E6/H6 antibody*

The anti-idiotype specificity of the 1B4.E6/H6 antibody was furthermore confirmed by its *in vitro* functions: the antibody induced proliferation of 1B4.E6/H6$^+$, Sendai virus specific T cells of the helper cell phenotype in absence of antigen (Ertl *et al.* 1986).

In vivo *functions of the 1B4.E6/H6 antibody: induction of T cell mediated immunity*

In vivo the 1B4.E6/H6 antibody was shown to induce T cells which mediated a DTH response to Sendai virus (Table 1 (Ertl *et al.* 1984)) as well as Lyt-2.2$^+$ T cells which upon *in vitro* restimulation with viral antigen lysed Sendai virus infected target cells (Ertl and Finberg, 1984b), or the 1B4.E6/H6 hybridoma cell line which expresses the antibody as surface immunoglobulin (Table 2). Both T cell functions were antigen-specific and could be generated in mice of different H-2 haplotypes and IgH allotypes. Both responses could be induced with 1B4.E6/H6 but had to be elicited by Sendai virus; i.e. splenocytes of mice immunized with Sendai virus or 1B4.E6/H6 failed to cause an inflammatory response to subcutaneously injected antibody (data not shown). Similarly, cytolytic T cells which were induced *in vivo* with virus or 1B4.E6/H6 and subsequently restimulated *in vitro* with antibody rather than viral antigen failed to mediate significant levels of virus-specific target cell lysis (data not shown).

363

Table 1 Induction of a delayed-type hypersensitivity response by an anti-T cell antibody*

Donor	Immunogen	Increase in footpad thickness (%)			
		Recipient A		Recipient B	
Experiment I + (II)		B10.D2		C57Bl/6	
—	—	3	(5)	4	(0)
B10.D2	None	8	(n.t.)	4	(n.t.)
B10.D2	SV	25	(22)	2	(4)
B10.D2	1B4.E6	20	(26)	11	(5)
C57Bl/6	None	1	(n.t.)	2	(2)
C57Bl/6	SV	1	(20)	51	(23)
C57Bl/6	1B4.E6	19	(32)	27	(31)
Experiment III		B10.D2		AKR	
—	—	20		25	
B10.D2	SV	74		20	
B10.D2	1B4.E6	101		25	
AKR	SV	25		86	
AKR	1B4.E6	48		86	
Experiment IV		DBA/2		C57Bl/6	
—	—	6		7	
DBA/2	SV	47		3	
DBA/2	1B4.E6	43		5	
C57Bl/6	SV	7		32	
C57Bl/6	1B4.E6	11		32	

* Donor mice (B10.D2, DBA,2 [$H\text{-}2^d$], C57Bl/6 [$H\text{-}2^b$] or AKR [$H\text{-}2^k$]) were immunized intraperitoneally with Sendai virus (SV) or 1B4.E6. One week after immunization $(0.8-1) \times 10^8$ naive (None) or immune splenocytes were transferred intravenously into naive recipient mice which were injected immediately afterwards with 10^3 HAU infectious Sendai virus into the left foot. Control mice were injected with virus only. Footpad thickness was measured 24 hr later.
n.t. = not tested.

Both T cells which mediated a DTH response and T cells which caused target cell lysis were characterized by an apparent loss of H-2 restriction as opposed to a virally induced T cell response. As shown in Table 1, $H\text{-}2^k$ (AKR) and $H\text{-}2^b$ (C57Bl/6) effector cells mediated a DTH response across H-2 barriers in most experiments (two out of three for C57Bl/6 mice) while $H\text{-}2^d$ (B10.D2 and DBA/2) effector cells only mediated a DTH response in H-2 compatible mice. Cytolytic T cells which are tested by a more sensitive *in vitro* assay system showed an even more pronounced cross-reactivity between target cells of different H-2 haplotypes. Effector cells of $H\text{-}2^d$ origin lysed

Table 2 Induction of cytolytic cells by an anti-T cell antibody*

Effector cells	Antigen	Specific lysis of SV infected and uninfected target cells (%)									
		P815.SV		**P815.N**		**1B4.E6**		**L929.SV**		**L929.N**	
Experiment I											
B10.D2	SV	68	71	4	1	11	8	n.t.		n.t.	
B10.D2	1B4.E6	39	30	17	11	57	43	n.t.		n.t.	
DBA/2	None	31	20	7	4	25	13	n.t.		n.t.	
DBA/2	SV	53	41	2	1	8	8	n.t.		n.t.	
DBA/2	1B4.E6	46	30	17	12	63	50	n.t.		n.t.	
AJ	None	18	8	0	<0	1	2	5	3	0	<0
AJ	SV	37	25	11	5	19	16	35	24	6	3
AJ	1B4.E6	35	29	17	8	61	37	37	23	10	5
B10.BR	None	29	16	7	4	17	7	32	22	12	6
B10.BR	SV	27	18	9	5	40	29	43	27	1	1
B10.BR	1B4.E6	43	30	18	12	58	37	54	40	16	9
C3H	SV	9	8	2	1	3 c. 3		21	12	2	1
C3H	1B4.E6	26	20	11	10	56	37	24	14	7	3
Experiment II											
DBA/2	None	3	3	4	9	0	<0	n.t.		n.t.	
DBA/2	SV	49	37	2	12	6	4	9	8	0	<0
DBA/2	1B4.E6	22	17	9	12	27	17	35	29	11	3

* Mice (B10.D2, DBA,2 [H-2^d]; AJ [H-2^a]) B10.BR or C3H [H-2^k]) were immunized intraperitoneally with 1B4.E6 or Sendai virus (SV). Seven days later 6 × 10^6 splenocytes of naive (None) or immune (SV, 1B4.E6) splenocytes were restimulated *in vitro* with Sendai virus. Effector cells were harvested after five days, and added to uninfected (N) or Sendai virus infected (SV) tumor target cells (P815–H-2^d, L929–H-2^k) or uninfected 1B4.E6 hybridoma cells in V-bottom mircrotiter plate wells at an effector-to-target-cell ratio of 40:1 (first column) and 20:1 (second column). After a 4 hr incubation at 37 °C, 75 μl of supernatant were harvested and analyzed in a gamma-counter.
<0 below spontaneous ^{51}Cr release.
n.t. = not tested.

Sendai virus infected H-2^k target cells and vice versa. Lysis of the 1B4.E6/H6 hybridoma cell by 1B4.E6/H6 induced effector cells was not H-2 restricted and was generally higher than lysis of Sendai virus infected target cells, which might reflect that only a portion of 1B4.E6/H6$^+$ effector cells exhibits specificity for Sendai virus. In addition, these data might indicate that 1B4.E6/H6 induced effector cells have a higher affinity for the antibody than the viral epitope. Differences at the level of the target cells (i.e. infected tumor cells as compared to hybridoma cells), such as differences in susceptibility to lysis or density of target antigens, would provide an alternative explanation for the increased lysis of the 1B4.E6/H6 hybridoma cell.

The lack of H-2 restriction which clearly distinguished the 1B4.E6/H6 induced T cell response from a response generated to virus was further investigated using clonally derived T effector cells. Splenocytes of BALB/c mice which had been immunized *in vivo* with Sendai virus or 1B4.E6/H6 were restimulated *in vitro* under limiting dilution conditions on Sendai virus pre-treated stimulator cells and subsequently tested for cytolytic activity on Sendai virus infected target cells of different H-2 haplotypes (Table 3). As expected, the majority of Sendai virus induced cytolytic T cells were H-2 restricted (76%) and only lysed the H-2 compatible Sendai virus infected target. Never-theless a significant percentage of these T cell clones showed cross-reactivity between infected target cells of $H-2^d$ and $H-2^b$ origin. Antibody-induced clones showed a more complex pattern: (1) less than one-third of the positive wells exhibited H-2 restriction; (2) a comparable number of clones recognized viral antigen on either of the allogeneic target cells without lysing the H-2 compatible target cells; (3) the majority of the clones lysed the infected H-2 compatible target and either one or both of the H-2 incompatible targets.

To further analyze the restriction and antigen specificity pattern, T cell clones of B10.D2 origin which had been induced *in vivo* with 1B4.E6/H6 antibody were generated and selected for Sendai virus specificity by *in vitro*

Table 3 Specificity of 1B4.E6 induced cytolytic T cells (tested by limiting dilution analysis)*

	No. of positive wells/total no. of wells tested†	
Target cells	**BALB/c anti-SV effector cells**	**BALB/c anti-1B4.E6 effector cells**
P-815 ($H-2^d$)–SV	11/46	14/92
EL4 ($H-2^b$)–SV	0/46	7/92
BW-5147 ($H-2^k$)–SV	0/46	6/92
($H-2^d$ + $H-2^b$)–SV	0/46	6/92
($H-2^d$ + $H-2^k$)–SV	3/46	9/92
($H-2^d$ + $H-2^b$) + $H-2^k$–SV	0/46	6/92
$H-2^k$ + $H-2^b$–SV	0/46	0/92
EL4–N†	2/48	4/96
Total no. of positive wells	14/46	48/92

* BALB/c mice were immunized with Sendai virus or 1B4.E6. Seven days later splenocytes were stimulated under limiting-dilution conditions (48 wells received 2 × 10^3 Sendai virus-immune responder cells; 96 wells received 1 × 10^3 1B4.E6-immune responder cells). Seven days later, aliquots of each well were incubated with either 10^3 SV-infected P815, EL4, or BW5147 target cells or 10^3 uninfected EL4 cells. Supernatants were harvested 5 hr later. Cells of wells that caused lysis three standard deviations above the mean ^{51}Cr release of target cells in the presence of cells from control wells were regarded as being positive.
† Cells of wells that lysed uninfected target cells were considered as nonspecific and were subtracted from the analysis.

Table 4 Proliferation of 1B4.E6 induced T cell clones to antigen + H-2

	Thymidine uptake (cpm)							
	ID.B7.A8[1]				2D3.F1.G10[1]			
	antigen −[2]		antigen +[2]		antigen −		antigen +	
	medium	M5 114.15.2	medium	M5 114.15.2	medium	M5 114.15.2	medium	M5 114.15.2
B10.D2	453	784	1637	310	1136	1129	5496	419
DBA/2	2503	749	6902	1682	5923	1156	21025	2281
C57Bl/6	1171	1135	4612	994	3351	843	5896	1450

* [1]ID.B7.A8 and 2D3.F1.G10 T cell clones which had been generated from 1B4.E6 immune B10.D2 mice, were tested for proliferation on irradiated splenocytes of B10.D2, DBA/2 or C57B1/6 origin, which were either unmodified [2](Antigen −) or had been pretreated with UV-light inactivated Sendai virus [2](Antigen +). Either medium or monoclonal anti-IA antibody (M5 114.15.2 directed to IA^{d,b,q,u},IE^{l,k}, kindly donated by T Springer) was added.

culture and cloning on Sendai virus presenting stimulator cells. T cell clones were phenotypically Thy-1.2$^+$, Ly-1.2$^+$, Lyt-2.2$^-$, L3.T4$^+$, and 1B4.E6/H6$^+$ and belonged thus to the T helper cell subset which is generally restricted to class II antigens. The anti-idiotype induced T cell clones exhibited specificities which were markedly different from those of conventional Sendai virus induced T cells clones (Ertl and Finberg 1984a). The anti-idiotype induced T cell clones proliferated consistently upon coculture with splenocytes from naive H-2^d (B10.D2 and DBA/2) and H-2^b (C57B1/6) mice (but not from H-2^k or H-2^a mice; data not shown) in absence of viral antigen (Tables 4, 5).

Table 5 Proliferation of 1B4.E6 induced T cell clones to antigen presented on splenocytes of naive or immune mice*

T cell clones	Thymidine uptake (cpm)				
	B10.D2 n.N	B10.D2 n.SV	B10.D2 i.N	B10.D2 i.SV	Medium
ID.B7.C8	2777	3919	1475	43855	473
2D3.F1.G10	3352	2937	1807	24182	813
Control	807	717	759	1570	—

* T cell clones ID.B7.C8 (which was derived from the same parental line as ID.B7.A8; see Table 4) and 2D3.F1.G10 were tested for proliferation upon coculture with irradiated splenocytes of naive (n) or Sendai virus immune (i) B10.D2 mice which did (SV) or did not (N) present Sendai virus as described in detail in Table 4. In addition T cell clones were tested for thymidine uptake in absence of irradiated splenocytes (Medium).
† Control: stimulator cells only.

Addition of viral antigen increased proliferation only marginally, if at all. Proliferation to unmodified or Sendai virus pretreated stimulator cells could be inhibited by addition of a monoclonal anti-Ia antibody which cross-reacts between class II molecules of several haplotypes (d, b, q, u, l, k; Table 4) as was described previously for Sendai virus induced T cell clones (Ertl and Finberg 1984a). In order to obtain significant proliferation to antigen, Sendai virus had to be presented on splenocytes of mice which had been immunized previously (more than four weeks beforehand) with Sendai virus. Increase in proliferation on immune stimulator cells was unlikely to be due to IL-2 release by Sendai virus specific T cells present in the stimulator cell population as the HT-2 line, an IL-2 sensitive T cell line, when tested in parallel, showed no significant increase in uptake of thymidine as compared to background incorporation in presence of medium. The requirement for immune splenocytes might reflect release of factors other than interleukin 2 by immune cells present in the stimulator cell population. Alternatively it might reflect differences in antigen uptake and presentation.

Induction of protective immunity

To test if the immunity which was induced by the 1B4.E6/H6 antibody was adequate to protect the recipient against a subsequent infection with Sendai virus, mice were hyperimmunized with 1B4.E6/H6 and subsequently inoculated with a lethal dose of Sendai virus. All of the immune mice survived the infection, which killed four out of five naive control mice (Ertl and Finberg 1984b).

Discussion

Data presented here clearly demonstrate that a monoclonal antibody to a T cell idiotope can induce a T cell mediated response *in vivo* and serve as a vaccine to induce protective immunity. Similar results were obtained using an anti-idiotypic serum to a Listeria monocytogenes specific T helper cell clone (Kaufmann *et al.* 1985).

An anti-T cell antibody was generated to a Sendai virus specific T helper cell clone. The anti-T cell antibody not only bound to the parental T cell clone (2H3.E8) but, in addition, to approximately 30% of all Sendai virus specific class II restricted T helper cell clones/lines tested so far. Naive T cells such as thymocytes or splenic T cells or T cells directed against other unrelated antigens failed to bind this antibody, thus confirming its specificity. The expression of the 1B4.E6/H6 idiotope was genetically not restricted. We assume that this antibody recognizes an idiotope of the T cell receptor which dominates the response of class II restricted T cells to Sendai virus. In addition the 1B4.E6/H6 idiotope can be detected serologically on class I region restricted T cells to Sendai virus (data not shown). The anti-idiotype specificity of the 1B4.E6/H6 antibody was confirmed by its *in vitro* functions. The parental 2H3.E8 T cell clone or other 1B4.E6/H6$^+$ T cell clones proliferated in response to culture supernatant of the 1B4.E6/H6 hybridoma cell line in presence of unmodified (i.e. untreated with Sendai virus) syngeneic stimulator cells (Ertl *et al.* 1986).

In vivo the 1B4.E6/H6 antibody was shown to induce T cells which, in an adoptive transfer system, mediated a DTH response to Sendai virus as well as Lyt-2.2$^+$ T cells which, upon *in vitro* restimulation with viral antigen, lysed virus infected target cells. Neither response was genetically restricted but could be elicited in any mouse strain tested.

What is the advantage of using a T cell defined anti-idiotypic reagent rather than an antibody specific for a B cell idiotope? B cell defined anti-idiotypic antibodies have been successfully used to induce a humoral response (Urbain *et al.* 1977; Cazenave *et al.* 1977), as well as T cells which mediate a DTH response (Sharpe *et al.* 1984). Anti-idiotypic antibodies to a B cell defined idiotope have even been shown to induce cytolytic T cells if presented in the form of surface immunoglobulins on H-2 compatible cells to the immune system (Sharpe *et al.* 1984). The same antibody failed to induce a cytolytic T cell response if injected as a soluble protein, (i.e. without H-2 (Sharpe *et al.* 1984), thus indicating that differences in antigen presentation are crucial for the stimulation of distinct T cell subsets (Ada *et al.* 1981).

B cell defined anti-idiotypic antibodies might thus have merits as vaccines to combat infections which are controlled by neutralizing antibodies. Infections which require cytolytic T cells for successful removal of the invading organisms such as viruses or intracellular bacteria might better be prevented by T cell defined anti-idiotypic antibodies which, as shown here, induce a cytolytic T cell response.

To understand how anti-idiotypes induce an immune response a precise knowledge of the antigen binding sites of the immune receptors involved is needed. The antigen binding site of immunoglobulin molecules has been characterized by sequencing (Wu and Kabat 1970) and X-ray crystallography (Segal *et al.* 1974). Very little is known about the antigen combining sites of the T cell receptors. The T cell receptor only recognizes cell-bound antigen in association with self cell surface molecules encoded for by genes of the major histocompatibility complex (Zinkernagel and Doherty 1974) and thus, as opposed to B cells, fails to recognize soluble antigen. Anti-idiotypic antibodies which so far have been generated to T cell receptor have been selected for high binding affinity to the parental T cell clone. They are thus fundamentally different from soluble antigen and (presumably) processed antigen presented in context with H-2 molecules.

How can an anti-idiotype with high affinity to the receptor mimic an antigen which fails to bind the receptor? Assuming that the T cell receptor forms a trimolar complex with foreign antigen and MHC determinants (Ashwell and Schwartz 1986; Watts *et al.* 1986) one could assume that the anti-idiotype might resemble both antigen and self cell surface molecule. If an anti-idiotype (with either one large or two small combining regions) would mimic an MHC + antigen complex, it would have to be restricted in its binding to H-2 identical T cell clones. 1B4.E6/H6 bound to Sendai virus specific T cells of any haplotype tested. We assume that the 1B4.E6/H6 recognizes an idiotope of a T cell receptor which has low affinity for an epitope of Sendai virus. Stimulation of T cells which express the 1B4.E6/H6 idiotope might thus either occur by direct binding of the anti-idiotypic antibody or, alternatively, upon processing and presentation by antigen presenting cells. Alternatively 1B4.E6/H6 might bind a regulatory idiotope commonly used by Sendai virus specific T cell clones.

Another question which requires further investigation is whether T cells induced by an antibody to the T cell receptor are identical to T cells which are induced by conventional antigen. Our data indicate that Sendai virus specific 1B4.E6/H6 induced T cells, i.e. cytolytic T cells, T cells which mediate a DTH response and long-term T cell clones derived from 1B4.E6/H6 immune mice which had been selected for Sendai virus speicificity by *in vitro* culture methods, showed (as opposed to Sendai virus induced T cells) a remarkable lack of H-2 restriction. Though we do not know if the apparent lack of H-2 restriction reflects a high affinity of the T cell receptor to Sendai virus, recognition of the antigen in association with framework determinant of H-2 molecules, or both, these data clearly indicate that the anti-idiotypic antibody induces Sendai virus specific T cell clones which are not induced upon infection with virus.

Acknowledgements

We wish to thank Eileen Sheehan for excellent secretarial help. This work was supported by grants NIH AI20541, AI20382, AI34503, Milton Fund and AHA 83959. Robert Finberg is a scholar of the Leukemia Society.

References

Ada G L, Leung, K-N, Ertl H C J 1981. An analysis of effector T cell generation and function of mice exposed to Influenza A or Sendai virus, *Immunological Reviews* **58**: 5–24

Ashwell J D, Schwartz R H 1986. T cell recognition of antigen and the Ia molecule as a ternary complex, *Nature (London)* **320**: 176–9

Cazenave P A 1977. Idiotypic–anti-idiotypic regulation of antibody synthesis in rabbits, *Proceedings of the National Academy of Sciences USA* **74**: 5122–5

Eichmann K, Ben-Neriah Y, Hetzelberger D, Polke C, Givol D, Lonai P 1980. Correlated expression of Vh framework and Vh idiotypic determinants on T helper cells and on functionally undefined T cells binding group A streptococcal carbohydrate, *European Journal of Immunology* **10**: 105–12

Ertl H C J, Finberg R W 1984a. Characteristics and functions of Sendai virus specific T cell clones, *Journal of Virology* **50**: 425–31

Ertl H C J, Finberg R W 1984b. Sendai specific T cell clones IV. Induction of cytolytic T cells by an anti-idiotypic antibody directed against a T helper cell clone, *Proceedings of the National Academy of Sciences USA* **81**: 1720–7

Ertl H, Gerlich W, Koszinowski U 1976. Detection of antibodies for Sendai virus by enzyme-linked immunosorbent assay, *Journal of Immunological Methods* **28**: 163–76

Ertl H C J, Homans E, Tournas S, Finberg R W 1984. Sendai virus-specific T cell clones V. Induction of a virus specific response by anti-idiotypic antibodies directed against a T helper cell clone, *Journal of Experimental Medicine* **159**: 1778–83

Ertl H C J, Skinner M A, Finberg R W 1986. Induction of anti-viral immunity by an anti-idiotypic antibody directed to a Sendai virus specific T helper cell clone, *International Review of Immunology* **1**: 41–65

Frischknecht H H, Binz H, Wigzell H 1978. Induction of specific transplantation immune reaction using anti-idiotypic antibodies, *Journal of Experimental Medicine* **147**: 500–14

Grzych J M, Capron P H, Lambert C, Dissous S, Torres S, Capron D 1985. An anti-idiotype vaccine against experimental schistosomiasis, *Nature (London)* **316**: 74–6

Jerne N K 1974. Towards a network theory of the immune system, *Annales d'Immunologie (Paris)* **125C**: 373–82

Kaufmann S H E, Eichmann K, Muller J, Wrazel L J 1985. Vaccination against the intracellular bacterium *Listeria monocytogenes* with a clonotypic antiserum, *Journal of Immunology* **134**: 4123–7

Kennedy R C, Adler-Stortz K, Henkel R D, Sanchez Y, Melnick J L, Dreesman G R 1983. Immune response to hepatitis B surface antigen: enhancement by prior injection of anti-idiotype antibodies, *Science* **221**: 853–5

McNamara M K, Ward R E, Koehler H 1984. Monoclonal idiotope vaccine against *Streptococcus pneumonia* infection, *Science* **226**: 1325–6

Reagan K J, Wunner W H, Wiktor T J, Koprowski H 1983. Anti-idiotypic antibodies induce neutralizing antibodies to rabies virus glycoprotein, *Journal of Virology* **48**: 660–6

Sacks D L, Esser K M, Sher A 1982. Immunization of mice against African trypanosomiasis using antiidiotypic antibodies, *Journal of Experimental Medicine* **155**: 1108–19

Segal D M, Padlan E A, Cohen G H, Rudikoff S, Potter M, Davies D R 1974. The three-dimensional structure of a phosphocholine-binding mouse immunoglobulin Fab and the nature of the antigen binding site, *Proceedings of the National Academy of Sciences USA* **71**: 4298–302

Sharpe A H, Gaulton G N, McDade K K, Fields B B, Greene M I 1984. Syngeneic monoclonal antiidiotype can induce cellular immunity to reovirus. *Journal of Experimental Medicine* **160**: 1195–206

Takemori T, Rajewsky K 1984. Mechanism of neonatally induced idiotype suppression and its relevance for the acquisition of self-tolerance, *Immunological Reviews* **79**: 103–18

Urbain J, Wikler M, Franssen J D, Collignon C 1977. Idiotypic regulation of the immune system by the induction of antibodies against anti-idiotypic antibodies, *Proceedings of the National Academy of Sciences USA* **74**: 5126–9

UytdeHaag F G C M, Osterhaus A D M E 1985. Induction of neutralizing antibody in mice against poliovirus type II with monoclonal anti-idiotypic antibody, *Journal of Immunology* **134**: 1225–9

Watts T H, Gaub H E, McConnel H M 1986. T cell mediated association of peptide antigen and major histocompatibility complex protein detected by energy transfer in an evanescent wave-field, *Nature (London)* **320**: 179–81

Wu T T, Kabat E A 1970. An analysis of the sequences of the variable regions of Bence–Jones protein and myeloma light chains and their implications for antibody complementarity, *Journal of Experimental Medicine* **132**: 211–23

Yap K L, Ada G L, McKenzie I F C 1978. Transfer of specific cytotoxic T lymphocytes protects mice inoculated with *influenza* virus. *Nature (London)* **273**: 238–40

Zinkernagel R M, Doherty P C 1974. Restriction of *in vitro* T cell mediated cytotoxicity in lymphocytic choriomeningitis within a syngeneic or semi-allogeneic system, *Nature (London)* **251**: 547–9

Anti-idiotypic vaccines in parasitic diseases

Giuseppe Del Giudice*; Jean-Marie Grzych†; Monique Capron†; André
Capron†; Paul-Henri Lambert*

* World Health Organization – Immunology Research and Training Centre,
Department of Pathology, University of Geneva, 1 rue Michel Servet, 1211
Geneva 4, Switzerland
† Centre d'Immunologie et de Biologie Parasitaire, Institut Pasteur, 15 rue
Camille Guérin, 59019 Lille, France

Parasitic diseases affect a majority of the world population and represent a
most important public health problem in many tropical countries. Efforts to
control these diseases have been mainly oriented in the past towards the
limitation of vector density with insecticides and the promotion of chemo-
prophylaxis. However, the increasing appearance of resistant insects or
parasites has hampered the efficiency of those approaches and led to the
development of new strategies aiming at the obtention of vaccines against
parasitic diseases. Indeed, in the last ten years there was an explosion of our
knowledge in relation to parasite antigens and anti-parasitic host effector
mechanisms. It also appeared that, during their evolution, parasites have
learned to cope with most of these effector mechanisms and, thus, to escape
the host immune response. Therefore the development of efficient anti-
parasite vaccines should be based on the triggering of selective immune
mechanisms with a higher degree of efficiency than the immune response
resulting from natural exposure to the parasites themselves.

Along that line, anti-idiotypes may be of particular interest to overcome
some tricks used by the parasite to circumvent the effect of antigen-induced
immune response.

Parasite escape mechanisms limiting the efficiency of anti-parasite vaccines

Importance of the nature of parasite surface antigens

Surface antigens of the infecting form of the parasites have been usually
selected as first candidates for vaccine development. Several factors limit the
effectiveness of this approach. Thus, it is well known that protozoan parasites, e.g. trypanosomes or plasmodia, can exhibit considerable antigenic
variation of their major surface antigens (Vickerman and Barry 1982;

Hommel 1985) and be always one step ahead of the corresponding immune response. Adult schistosomes can also disguise themselves by integrating a variety of host antigenic constituents in their coat (Sher *et al.* 1978).

Some parasite products have also been shown to induce a state of general immunosuppression either directly or through polyclonal lymphocyte activation (Rosenberg 1978; Colley 1981; Kobayakawa *et al.* 1979). The existence of repetitive epitopes in major antigens of protozoan parasites (Anders 1985; Rodriguez *et al.* 1985; Peterson *et al.* 1986) also appears to be beneficial for the parasite in its fight against the host. Such repetitive epitopes might favor the production of low-avidity antibodies and their nature may sometimes limit the immune responsiveness of the host. A restricted immunogenicity of a repetitive epitope of a major antigen coating *Plasmodium falciparum* sporozoites, seriously considered as a potential malaria vaccine, has been observed recently.

Importance of genetic restriction in limiting the effectiveness of anti-parasite vaccines: the example of malaria

The production of monoclonal antibodies directed against plasmodial antigens and the progress achieved in molecular biology led to the characterization of several antigens able to confer some degree of immune protection against malaria infection (Drager-Dayal and Lambert 1987).

One of the most extensively studied malaria antigens is the circumsporozoite (CS) protein. Individuals living in malaria-endemic areas produce antibodies against these proteins after natural malaria infections and the antisporozoite antibody titers increase as a function of age (Nardin *et al.* 1979; Hoffman *et al.* 1986; Del Giudice *et al.* 1987a, 1987b).

The CS proteins consist of an amino acid sequence tandemly repeated several times and flanked by unrepeated sequence (Nussenzweig and Nussenzweig 1985). The repetitive epitope of *P. falciparum* CS protein consists of four amino acids (Asn-Ala-Asn-Pro = NANP) repeated 37 times. Using synthetic peptides, it has been shown that three (NANP) repeats represent the minimal size of the molecule able both to be recognized efficiently by specific antibodies (Zavala *et al.* 1985) and to prime specifically murine T cells *in vivo* and *in vitro* (Togna *et al.* 1986). The large $(NANP)_{40}$ synthetic peptide was used as coating antigen for ELISA in a longitudinal study carried out in a rural community of Tanzania (Del Giudice *et al.* 1987a). It was found that, at ten years of age, about half of the children who have been heavily exposed to malaria infections did *not* develop anti-NANP antibodies. Furthermore, considerable differences in antibody levels against $(NANP)_{40}$ were observed in children living in different households but exposed to the same epidemiological conditions, although their antibody titers to asexual blood stage antigens were similar. These data suggested that the antigenic background may be of particular importance for the regulation of anti-sporozoite response.

$(NANP)_n$ synthetic and recombinant peptides conjugated to carrier proteins were shown to be highly immunogenic in mice and rabbits: the antibodies raised against them recognized specifically *P. falciparum* sporozoites and inhibited the penetration of sporozoites into cultured hepatic cells and their maturation into exoerythrocytic forms (Mazier *et al.* 1986).

The immunogenicity of $(NANP)_n$ sequences could be directly studied in our laboratories, both at T and B cell levels, using the $(NANP)_{40}$ synthetic peptide without any carrier. C57BL/6 mice $(H-2^b)$ responded strongly to $(NANP)_{40}$, producing high titers of IgG and IgM antibodies which also recognized specifically extracts of *Anopheles stephensi* mosquitoes infected with *P. falciparum* sporozoites. (C57BL/6 × BALB/c) F1 hybrid mice responded in the same manner. However neither athymic C57BL/6 *nu/nu* nor congenic C57BL/6.H-2^k mice produced anti-$(NANP)_{40}$ antibodies (Del Giudice *et al.* 1986). These results suggested that the production of antibodies to carrier-free $(NANP)_n$ peptides (i) was T-cell dependent and (ii) was possibly linked to particular haplotypes of murine major histocompatibility complex (MHC) H-2.

Fourteen mouse strains bearing nine different H-2 haplotypes were also immunized with $(NANP)_{40}$ without carrier, but surprisingly only H-2^b mice were able to mount a strong antibody response against the peptide, all non-H-2^b mouse strains tested being completely unresponsive (Fig. 1). The anti-(NANP) antibody response was shown to be strictly linked to the presence of the *b* allele in the I-A region of the H-2 gene complex (Del Giudice *et al.* 1986). In fact, only I-A^b recombinant B10.A(5R) mice produced such antibodies. Furthermore, the antibody response against $(NANP)_{40}$ was extremely weak in B6CH-2^{bm12} mutant mice, which carry a gene conversion leading to the substitution of three amino acids of the beta 1 domain of the I-A^b beta chain (McIntyre and Seidman 1984). These findings were confirmed by experiments employing (NANP)-specific T cell clones derived from lymph node cells of C57BL/6 mice immunized with carrier-free $(NANP)_{40}$ (Togna *et al.* 1986). The L3T4 T cell clones proliferated only in the presence of irradiated spleen cells from C57BL/6 or B10.A(5R) mice as antigen presenting cells (APCs), not in the presence of APCs from B10.A(4R) nor from B6CH-2^{bm12} mice. T-cell clone proliferation was specifically inhibited by adding an anti-I-A^b monoclonal antibody to the cultures. A similar genetic restriction of the immune response to NANP was recently confirmed (Good *et al.* 1986). The inability to respond to $(NANP)_{40}$ could be overcome in non-H-2^b mice when they were immunized with the peptide conjugated to a carrier protein (Del Giudice *et al.* 1986).

This exceptional restriction of the immune response against the $(NANP)_n$ epitope is surprising since, usually, mice of more than one H-2 haplotype are able to respond to a given epitope (Schwartz 1986). An analogous genetic control of the antibody response to $(NANP)_n$ peptides could also exist in man, and may limit the effectiveness of the vaccination with the $(NANP)_n$ peptides. On the other hand, such a genetic control could also exist for the antibody

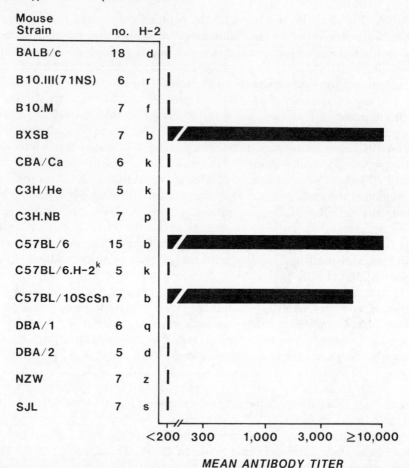

Figure 1. IgG antibody response against $(NANP)_{40}$ in 14 mice bearing nine different H-2 haplotypes. Mice were immunized at the base of the tail with $50\,\mu l$ volumes containing $20\,\mu g$ of $(NANP)_{40}$ in complete Freund's adjuvant. Four weeks later, they were boosted in the same way with the peptide in incomplete Freund's adjuvant. Sera were taken seven days later and were tested individually by ELISA employing $(NANP)_{40}$, $1\,\mu g/ml$, for the coating. Solid bars represent the geometrical mean of the titer obtained in each group. Titers less than 1:200 were considered negative.

response to whole *P. falciparum* sporozoites. This could also explain the observation that a significant percentage of young subjects living in malaria-endemic areas do not develop anti-NANP antibodies (Nardin *et al.* 1979; Hoffman *et al.* 1986; Del Giudice *et al.* 1987a, 1987b). Further studies are required in order to determine the actual role played by MHC gene products in man in controlling the ability of different individuals to respond to sporozoites and/or to sporozoite peptides.

Importance of triggering appropriate T cell subsets

Several protozoal species which are major pathogens of man have a predominantly intracellular location. Such organisms are shielded from the action of specific antibody and their elimination depends on the recognition of parasite antigens on the host cell surface, particularly by specific T cells. Therefore, it is essential that vaccines developed against such infections would contain epitopes involved in T cell recognition. In addition, it was shown recently that the nature and the number of specific T cells may be critical in order to achieve the elimination of the parasites. For instance, it appears that an excess of $L3T4^+$ versus $Ly2^+$ T lymphocytes may be detrimental in the evolution of cutaneous leishmaniasis in mice (Titus *et al.* 1984).

Importance of inducing appropriate antibody isotypes

The protective role of IgE and of some other particular antibody isotypes was just demonstrated in parasitic diseases. In schistosomiasis, defense mechanisms have been defined in a rat model of infection with *Schistosoma mansoni*. Three major target antigens have been identified: gp38, p28 and p22–26. Antibodies against these particular antigens can lead to the destruction of the larval stage of the parasite, the schistosomula, through antibody-dependent cell-mediated cytotoxicity (ADCC) mechanisms involving various effector cell populations (Capron and Dessaint 1985). Macrophages, eosinophils and platelets have been shown to kill schistosomula in the presence of antibody of the anaphylactic isotypes: IgE in man, IgE and IgG2a in rats. However, the development of immunity to schistosomes is impaired by the appearance of blocking antibodies. For instance, in rats, the production of IgG2a antibodies against the gp38 schistosome antigen is soon followed by the appearance of IgG2c antibodies which react with the same glycanic epitope. These IgG2c antibodies compete with the corresponding IgG2a antibodies and inhibit the killing of schistosomula (Grzych *et al.* 1984). Similar blocking antibodies have been found in human patients with schistosomiasis.

Anti-idiotype vaccines against parasites

Anti-idiotypes may be considered as potential alternatives to parasite antigens for the development of vaccines either when major parasite epitopes cannot be easily obtained or when an appropriate immune response cannot be induced by a conventional approach.

Schistosomiasis

In schistosomiasis, although a very significant degree of protection could be transfered *in vivo* using IgG2a monoclonal antibodies (Grzych *et al.* 1982) against a glycanic epitope of schistosomula gp38 antigen (Dissous *et al.* 1982), such an epitope appears difficult to synthesize and purification from the parasite cannot be envisaged for the preparation of vaccines. For those reasons, an anti-idiotypic approach was attempted to induce protection against schistosomiasis.

Monoclonal IgG2a anti-gp38 antibodies were produced in rats. Anti-idiotypic (Ab-2) monoclonal antibodies were then prepared by immunization of syngeneic rats with one of these anti-gp38 antibodies. (Ab-1) and Ab-2 clones were selected on the basis of the capacity of culture supernatants to inhibit the binding of Ab-1 to gp38. One of these Ab-2 IgM clones, JM8-36, was repeatedly injected (1 mg/injection, without adjuvant) into syngeneic rats.

In a first set of experiments, the serum of those rats was tested for anti-*Schistosoma mansoni* antibodies. After four to six weeks of injections, anti-parasite antibodies were detected by indirect immunofluorescence on schisto-somula sections and their efficiency was demonstrated *in vitro* in cytotoxicity assays in the presence of rat eosinophils. These Ab-3- or Ab-1-like antibodies were mainly of the IgG2a subclass. The biological relevance of these *in vitro* findings was confirmed *in vivo* with the observation that passively transferred Ab-3 sera could lead to a 50% reduction of the number of adult worms recovered from a syngeneic rat challenged with 800 *S. mansoni* cercariae (Grzych *et al.* 1985). In such infections, there is no replication of the infecting parasite in the final host and the burden of adult worms directly reflects the number of infecting larvae which survive the first few days after infection.

In a second set of experiments, rats were also immunized with Ab-2 monoclonal antibodies, then directly challenged with 800 cercariae. A marked protective effect was observed with reduction of the worm burden ranging from 50 to 76% (Grzych *et al.* 1985). Thus, a remarkable protective effect of anti-idiotype vaccines was obtained in the rat model of *S. mansoni* as compared to the results achieved by immunization with parasite antigens.

Trypanosomiasis

Trypanosomiasis was the first parasitic disease where the potential applicability of anti-idiotypes as vaccines was demonstrated (Sacks *et al.* 1982).

In this model, polyclonal anti-idiotype antibodies have been raised in SJL mice against three protective monoclonal antibodies specific for variable antigens of *Trypanosoma rhodesiense* (VAT). These authors demonstrated that the treatment of mice with a purified IgG-1 fraction of anti-idiotypic antibodies collected from SJL mice serum was able to modify the course of the primary parasitemia in the animals by comparison to the appropriate control. The immunity induced in these conditions was manifested either by a reduction of the first peak of parasitemia or by a selection against parasite expressing the corresponding VAT.

Recently, Sacks *et al.* have extended their observations to an intracellular trypanosome, *Trypanosoma cruzi*. These authors have produced polyclonal rabbit Ab-2 antibodies against the WIC 29–26 monoclonal antibody specific for the carbohydrate moieties of a 72 kD glycoprotein (gp72) present on the surface of *Trypanosoma cruzi* epimastigotes and metacyclic trypomastigotes (Snary *et al.* 1981). This glycoprotein is able to induce a partial immunity in mice infected with metacyclic trypomastigotes (Snary 1983). Immunization of BALB/c mice, guinea pigs and rabbits with the rabbit anti-idiotypic antibodies induced the production of antibodies reacting with the gp72 trypanosome antigen but no protection was obtained in that system.

Conclusion

The use of anti-idiotypes as surrogate vaccines against parasitic diseases represents an interesting approach in the fight against these diseases but, obviously, this is still limited to experimental models and its applicability to human diseases is still questionable.

Indeed, several factors hamper the use of anti-idiotype as vaccines. First, their production is mainly based on mouse hybridoma technology and the use of heterologous monoclonal anti-idiotypic antibodies as a vaccine in man may be considered as unethical. However, hybrid man–mouse molecules can be envisaged and progress made in the synthesis of anti-idiotypic peptides may provide the means to circumvent such problems. Another limitation of anti-idiotypes is the selection of certain idiotopes and of certain epitopes as unique targets with the risk of generating suppression or inefficiency resulting from genetic restriction.

In addition, one cannot exclude that some of the injected anti-idiotypes would react as anti-cell receptor autoantibodies, particularly when such anti-idiotypes would have been raised against Ab-1 reacting with parasite epitopes involved in binding to host cell membrane receptors. Similarly, immunopathology can result from the generation of idiotype–anti-idiotype complexes.

However, the use of anti-idiotype vaccines can also offer some advantages as compared to conventional approaches for anti-parasite vaccines. Thus, it may be the only possibility when complex glycanic epitopes, difficult to synthesize, represent the ideal target for protective antibodies. Such anti-idiotypic vaccines may in fact be essential for the induction of immunity against carbohydrate epitopes at early stages of B cell ontogeny, such as in young children. It also allows some selection in the type of antibodies (idiotypes or isotypes) generated after immunization with or without parasitic antigens.

Finally, anti-idiotypes have been shown in several instances to be operational in the absence of adjuvants and this advantage cannot be neglected.

Acknowledgements

This work was supported by the World Bank/UNDP/WHO Special Programme for Research and Training in Tropical Diseases, by the Swiss National Foundation, grant no. 3.803.0.86, and by INSERM U167-CNRS 624.

References

Anders R F 1985. Candidate antigens for an asexual blood stage vaccine, *Parasitology Today* **1**: 152–5

Capron A, Dessaint J P 1985. Effector and regulatory mechanisms in immunity to schistosomes: a heuristic view, *Annual Review of Immunology* **3**: 455–76

Colley D G 1981. Immunoregulatory aspects of parasitic diseases, *Federation Proceedings* **40**: 1440–2

Del Giudice G, Cooper J A, Merino J, Verdini A, Togna A R, Engers H D, Corradin G, Lambert P H 1986. The antibody response in mice to carrier-free synthetic polymers of *Plasmodium falciparum* circumsporozoite repetitive epitope is I-A^b restricted: implications for malaria vaccines, *Journal of Immunology* **137**: 2952–5

Del Giudice G, Engers H D, Tougne C, Biro S S, Weiss N, Verdini A S, Pessi A, Degremont A A, Freyvogel T A, Lambert P-H, Tanner M. 1987a. Antibodies to the repetitive epitope of *Plasmodium falciparum* circumsporozoite protein in rural Tanzanian community: a longitudinal study of 132 children, *American Journal of Tropical Medicine and Hygiene* **36**: 203–12

Del Giudice G, Verdini A S, Pinori M, Pessi A, Verhave J-P, Tougne C, Ivanoff C, Lambert P-H, Engers H D 1987b. Detection of human antibodies against *Plasmodium falciparum* sporozoites using synthetic peptides. *Journal of Clinical Microbiology* **25**: 91–6

Dissous C, Grzych J-M, Capron A 1982. *Schistosoma mansoni* surface antigen defined by a rat monoclonal IgG2a, *Journal of Immunology* **129**: 2232–4

Drager-Dayal R, Lambert P-H 1987. Plasmodial antigens implicated in the protective immune response, in I McGregor, W Wernsdorfer (eds) *Textbook of Malaria*. Churchill Livingstone, Edinburgh (Scotland). In press.

Good M F, Berzofsky J A, Maloy W L, Hayashi Y, Fijii N, Hockemeyer N T, Miller L H 1986. Genetic control of the immune response in mice to a *Plasmodium falciparum* sporozoite vaccine. Widespread nonresponsiveness to single malaria T epitope in highly repetitive vaccine, *Journal of Experimental Medicine* **164**: 655–60

Grzych J-M, Capron M, Bazin H, Capron A 1982. *In vitro* and *in vivo* effector function of rat IgG2a monoclonal anti-*S. mansoni* antibodies, *Journal of Immunology* **129**: 2739–43

Grzych J-M, Capron M, Dissous C, Capron A 1984. Blocking activity of rat monoclonal antibodies in experimental schistosomiasis, *Journal of Immunology* **133**: 998–1004

Grzych J-M, Capron M, Lambert P-H, Dissous C, Torres S, Capron A 1985. An anti-idiotype vaccine against experimental schistosomiasis, *Nature (London)* **316**: 74–6

Hoffman S L, Wistar R Jr, Ballou W R, Hollingdale M R, Wirtz R A, Schneider I, Marwoto H A,

Hockmeyer W T 1986. Immunity to malaria and naturally acquired antibodies to the circumsporozoite protein of *Plasmodium falciparum*, *New England Journal of Medicine* **315**: 601–6

Hommel M 1985. Antigenic variation in malaria parasites, *Immunology Today* **6**: 28–33

Kobayakawa T, Louis J, Izui S, Lambert P-H 1979. Autoimmune response to DNA, red blood cells and thymocyte antigens in association with polyclonal antibody synthesis during experimental African trypanosomiasis, *Journal of Immunology* **122**: 296–301

Mazier D, Mellouk S, Beaudoin R L, Texier B, Druilhe P, Hockmeyer W, Trosper J, Paul C, Charoenvit Y, Young J, Miltgen F, Chedid L, Chigot J P, Galley B, Brandicourt O, Gentilini M 1986. Effect of antibodies to recombinant and synthetic peptides on *P. falciparum* sporozoites *in vitro*, *Science* **231**: 156–9

McIntyre K R, Seidman J G 1984. Nucleotide sequence of mutant I-Abeta^{bm12} gene is evidence for genetic exchange between mouse immune response genes, *Nature (London)* **308**: 551–3

Nardin E H, Nussenzweig R S, McGregor I A, Bryan J H 1979. Antibodies to sporozoites: their frequent occurrence in individuals in areas of hyperendemic malaria, *Science* **206**: 597–9

Nuzzenzweig V and Nussenzweig R S 1985. Circumsporozoite proteins of malaria parasites, *Cell* **42**: 401–3

Peterson D S, Wrightman R A, Manning J E 1986. Cloning of a major surface antigen gene of *Trypanosoma cruzi* and identification of a nonapeptide repeat, *Nature (London)* **322**: 566–8

Rodriguez E, Afchain D, Capron A, Dissous C, Santoro F 1985. Major surface protein of *Toxoplasma gondii* (p30) contains an immunodominant region with repetitive epitopes, *European Journal of Immunology* **15**: 747–9

Rosenberg Y J 1978. Autoimmune and polyclonal B cell responses during murine malaria, *Nature (London)* **274**: 170–2

Sacks D L, Esser K M, Sher A 1982. Immunization of mice against African trypanosomiasis using anti-idiotype antibodies, *Journal of Experimental Medicine* **155**: 1108–19

Sacks D L, Kirchmoff L V, Hieny S, Sher A 1985. Molecular mimicry of a carbohydrate epitope on a major surface glycoprotein of *Trypanosoma cruzi* by using anti-idiotypic antibodies, *Journal of Immunology* **135**: 4155–9

Schwartz R H 1986. Immune response (Ir) genes of the murine major histocompatibility complex, *Advances in Immunology* **38**: 31–201

Sher A, Hall B F, Vadas M A 1978. Acquisition of murine major histocompatibility gene products by schistosomula of *Schistosoma mansoni*, *Journal of Experimental Medicine* **148**: 46–57

Snary D 1983. Cell surface glycoproteins of *Trypanosoma cruzi*: protective immunity in mice and antibody levels in human chagasic sera, *Transactions of the Royal Society of Tropical Medicine and Hygiene* **77**: 126–9

Snary D, Ferguson M A J, Scott M T, Allen A K 1981. Cell surface antigens of *Trypanosoma cruzi*: use of monoclonal antibodies to identify and isolate an epimastigote specific glycoprotein, *Molecular Biochemistry and Parasitology* **3**: 343–56

Titus R G, Lima G C, Engers H D, Louis J A 1984. Exacerbation of murine cutaneous leishmaniasis by adoptive transfer of parasite-specific helper T cell populations capable of mediating *Leishmania major*-specific delayed-type hypersensitivity, *Journal of Immunology* **133**: 1594–1600

Togna A R, Del Giudice G, Verdini A, Bonelli F, Pessi A, Engers H D, Corradin G 1986. Synthetic *P. falciparum* circumsporozoite peptide elicits heterogenous L3T4$^+$ T cell proliferative responses in H-2^b mice, *Journal of Immunology* **137**: 2956–60

Vickerman K, Barry J D 1982. African trypanosomiasis, in S Cohen, K S Warren (eds) *Immunology of Parasitic Infections*, 2nd edn, Blackwell Scientific Publications, Oxford, p 204

Zavala F, Tam J P, Hollingdale M R, Cochrane A H, Quakyi I, Nussenzweig R S, Nussenzweig V 1985. Rationale for development of a synthetic vaccine against *Plasmodium falciparum* malaria, *Science* **228**: 1436–40

Idiotype vaccines for infections and cancer

Syamal Raychaudhuri; Yukihiko Saeki; Hiroshi Fuji; Heinz Kohler

Department of Molecular Immunology, Roswell Park Memorial Institute, Buffalo, New York 14263, USA

Introduction

The efficacy of immunotherapy of human cancers has still to be proven. Although the idea of stimulating the immunological defense mechanisms to attack the tumor is not new, it has worked inconsistently, and only in occasional cases could tumor rejection be achieved in cancer patients (Lamon *et al.* 1972). This failure of the immune system to destroy the tumor cells is actually unexpected since unique tumor-associated antigens have been described in many tumors of viral origins (Stutman 1975). In tumors where expression of tumor neoantigens was demonstrated, therapeutic immunity could not be achieved even by vigorous immunization regimens using tumor cells or tumor-derived vaccines. Thus it remains to be explained why tumor antigens are weak and why the tumor antigen in the face of concomitant immunity fails to mount an effective anti-tumor response.

A common explanation for the absence of an anti-tumor immunity is that the immune system has been compromised or tolerized by the tumor mass at both the B and T cell level. If this were to be correct, steps could be undertaken to break the existing anti-tumor tolerance. An effective method to break experimentally induced tolerance is to present the critical epitope in a different molecular environment than the tolerized host (Weigle 1961). While this can be done easily with haptens and other well-defined antigens, it is impossible for most tumor antigens because they are chemically ill-defined and difficult to purify.

The network hypothesis of Neils Jerne offers an approach to transform epitope structures into idiotypic determinants expressed on the surface of antibodies (Jerne 1974). According to this theory, for each external antigen, including self antigen, an internal idiotope image exists. The repertoire of mirror-image antigens arises as statistical necessity from the large structural diversity in the antibody repertoire. Already several such internal image antigens have been used as surrogate antigens to induce specific and protective immunity (for review see Kohler *et al.* 1985; Kennedy *et al.* 1985). These experiments include the use of anti-idiotypic antibodies which mimic tumor-associated antigens. However, the work with such surrogate tumor antigens has not been completely successful since in no instance could complete protection against the tumor be achieved. Thus, an in-depth analysis of the immune reactions of B and T cells induced by stimulation with idiotope images may help to improve the idiotype tumor approach.

In this paper we report our findings from an experimental tumor system in which we induced anti-tumor immunity by conventional and idiotypic immunization protocols. We compared the anti-tumor immunity induced by conventional and idiotypic immunizations at the level of cytotoxic T cells. The results show that immunization with radiated tumor cells or monoclonal anti-idiotypic antibody induces cytotoxic T cells specific for the L1210/GZL

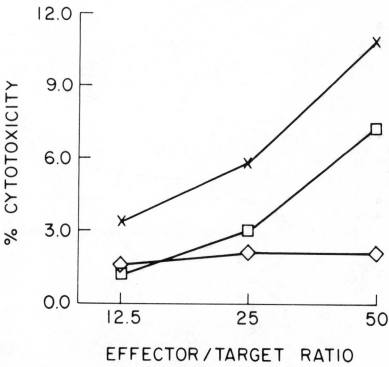

Cytoxicity of Ab2 Hybridomas

Figure 1. DBA/2 mice were immunized with a high dose (10^8) of radiated tumor cells in IFA followed by inoculation of live tumor (10^5 cells/mouse) a week later. The mice were sacrificed when the tumor size attained approximately 0.5 cm and lymph node cells were prepared and stimulated *in vitro* with irradiated tumor for six days. At the end of incubation, live cells were harvested and tested against ^{51}Cr-labeled hybridoma targets 3A4 (×), 2F10 (□) and 4C11 (◇) in a 4 hr chromium release assay at different effector-to-target ratios. A high level of cytotoxicity was obtained against L1210/GZL target (data not shown).

tumor. Furthermore, we provide evidence that the tumor growth and the survival of tumor-bearing mice is prolonged in mice which had been immunized with anti-idiotype antigens.

Results

Specificity of cytotoxic T cells

Immunization with tumor cells can induce cytotoxic T cell responses specific for the immunizing tumor (Matis *et al.* 1985; Rosenberg *et al.* 1985). If

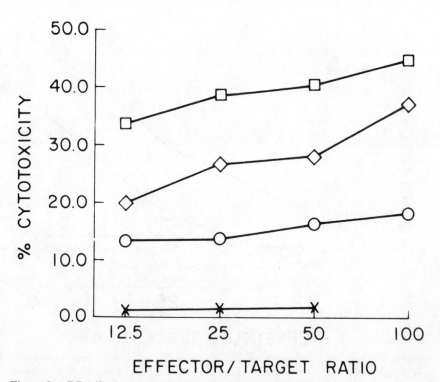

Figure 2. DBA/2 mice were immunized with 50 μg of KLH-conjugated 2F10 or 3A4 s.c. at biweekly intervals. As controls, the mice were also immunized with 4C11 and irradiated L1210/GZL. Seven days later lymph node cells from normal (×), 2F10 immunized (○), 3A4 immunized (◇) and tumor immunized (□) mice were restimulated *in vitro* with irradiated L1210/GZL. Effector cells were tested at three different effector-to-target cell ratios ^{51}Cr-labeled L1210/GZL in a 4 hr ^{51}Cr-release assay.

anti-idiotype hybridomas bear the tumor image antigen, it should be possible to induce T cell cytotoxicity in mice immunized with tumor cells against the internal antigen producing Ab2beta hybridoma. Since the Ab2 hybridomas were raised in A strain, (DBA/2 × A/J) F1 mice were immunized with radiated L1210/GZL cells and their lymph node cells were tested for killing of ^{51}Cr-labeled hybridoma cells. The data in Fig. 1 show that tumor-immunized F1 mice can lyse 3A4 and 2F10 hybridoma cells but they cannot control 4C11 cells. These results indicate that anti-idiotypic hybridoma cells which produce internal image antibodies are targets for anti-tumor cytotoxicity.

Since cytotoxic T cells induced by immunization with tumor cells recognize internal image hybridoma cells, it can be assumed that immunization with such hybridomas would generate cytotoxic T cells against tumor cells. DBA/2 mice were immunized with KLH conjugates of 2F10, 3A4 and 4C11 hybridomas as described, and lymph node cells were challenged *in vitro* with radiated L1210/GZL cells. After six days of culture, cells were harvested and used as effector cells against ^{51}Cr-labeled L1210/GZL and P815 tumor cells. The data (Fig. 2) show that immunization with 2F10 or 3A4 induces cytotoxic cells which can lyse L1210/GZL tumor cells. Immunization with an unrelated anti-idiotypic hydridoma does not induce tumor-specific cytotoxicity. No lysis was observed with either cell population on labeled P815 cells (data not shown).

Analysis of CTL precursors

In order to obtain more quantitative information about the cytotoxic T cells induced by internal images, a precursor analysis of cytotoxic T cell was performed. DBA/2 mice were immunized with either 2F10–KLH, 3A4–KLH or radiated L1210/GZL cells. Lymph node cells from immunized groups or normal controls were restimulated *in vitro* with radiated L1210/GZL under limiting dilution conditions and analyzed for killing of either ^{51}Cr-labeled L1210/GZL or P815 cells. The results are shown in Fig. 3. It was found that the frequency of tumor-specific cytotoxic T cells in anti-idiotype immunized mice is comparable to that of mice immunized with irradiated tumor.

Discussion

The studies on the murine L1210 tumor are relevant to human cancer because mouse mammary tumor virus (MMTV) that is present in L1210 tumor line and the expressed gp52 surface antigen is related to the human mammary tumor virus. Antigenic cross-reaction between the mouse and human envelope proteins have been described (Segev *et al.* 1985). Thus it is an attractive assumption that some of the idiotype internal image antigens can be exploited for their effectiveness in humans.

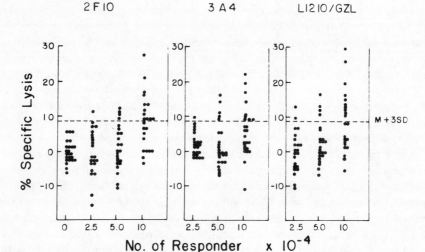

Figure 3. Groups of DBA/2 mice were immunized twice with 50 μg of either KLH-conjugated 2F10, 3A4 or 4C11. As controls, mice were also injected with 10×10^6 irradiated L1210/GZL in IFA. Seven days later, lymph node cells were restimulated with irradiated L1210/GZL. Six days later, cells of each well were tested on either L1210/GZL or P815 in a 4 hr ^{51}Cr-release assay. Very few wells showed lysis against P815. Target wells that showed lysis more than three standard deviations above the mean ^{51}Cr release of control wells (^{51}Cr target incubated with cold target) were considered positive. Each dot represents lytic activity of a single well.

The utilization of idiotype network in immunotherapy of tumors opens new perspectives and enriches the therapeutic armamentarium. Basically two approaches are feasible. The first takes advantage of the existence of internal antigen images in the idiotype repertoire. This approach has already been used successfully by several investigators (see for reference Rosenberg *et al.* 1985; Segev *et al.* 1985). The use of internal image antigens has the advantage of not being genetically restricted, and these antigens are effective across the species barrier. The other method of using the idiotype network rests on the existence of so-called regulatory idiotypes (Gleason and Kohler 1982; Victor-Korbin *et al.* 1985). These idiotypic specificities are recurrent idiotypes which are linked to important immune responses preventing life-threatening infections. They also may be linked to the network in anti-cancer responses. Discovering these linkages in anti-tumor responses would be important and could be the first step towards using these regulatory idiotypes to control tumor growth by immunological measures. While these ideas are at present speculative, they deserve to be explored.

In our studies on the B and T cell idiotype response to the murine L1210 tumor we have begun to dissect the involved network. We noted an interesting and obvious disparity of demonstrable T cell response and effectiveness *in vivo* in inhibiting tumor growth. While mice immunized with two internal image idiotypes elicit virtually identical T cell responses and similar idiotypic antibodies, only the 2F10 group shows increased tumor survival (data not shown). We suspect that regulatory T cells may be induced by immunization with 3A4 that neutralizes the *in vitro* effective CTLs. The different induction of the 11C1 Ab1 idiotype in the anti-gp52 response by the two internal images may be indicative for stimulation of regulatory idiotypes.

The finding that two internal image antibodies induce different B cell idiotype profiles and have different effects on tumor growth *in vivo* emphasizes the role of regulatory network interaction in the response to internal image antigens. In this respect internal antigens do not differ from nominal antigens which are subject to network regulation. For the purpose of developing an anti-tumor idiotype vaccine our data indicate that the regulatory component in the immune response to internal antigens plays a decisive role which determines the *in vivo* effectiveness of such vaccines and must be taken into consideration in attempts to develop idiotype tumor vaccines for use in humans.

Conclusion

The validity of the idiotype vaccine approach was tested in an experimental tumor model, the L1210 DBA/2 tumor. Hybridoma anti-idiotypic antibodies were generated against a monoclonal anti-tumor antibody. Mice immunized with anti-idiotypic antibodies have an increased number of cytolytic T cells reacting with L1210 tumor cells. This finding indicates that the anti-idiotypic vaccine approach could be utilized in immunotherapy of tumors.

Acknowledgements

This work was supported in part by Grant no. IM405 from the American Cancer Society and Grant no. CTR1565R2 from The Council for Tobacco Research – USA, Inc.

References

Gleason K, Kohler H 1982. Regulatory idiotypes. T helper cells recognize a shared Vh idiotope on phosphorylcholine-specific antibodies, *Journal of Experimental Medicine* **156**: 539–49
Jerne N K 1974. Towards a network theory of the immune system, *Annales d'Immunologie (Paris)* **125C**: 373–9
Kennedy R C, Dreesman G R, Kohler H 1985. Vaccines utilizing internal image anti-idiotypic antibodies that mimic antigens of infectious organism, *Biotechniques* **3**: 4040–9
Kohler H, Muller S, Bona C 1985. Internal antigen and the immune network, *Proceedings of the Society of Experimental Biology and Medicine* **178**: 189–95

Lamon E W, Skurzak H M, Klein E 1972. The lymphocyte response to a primary viral neoplasm (MSV) through its entire course in Balb/c mice, *International Journal of Cancer* **10**: 581–8

Matis L A, Ruscetti S K, Longo D L, Jacobson S, Brown E J, Zinn S, Kruisbeek A M 1985. Distinct proliferative T cell clonotypes are generated in response to a murine retrovirus-induced syngeneic T cell leukemia: viral gp70 antigen-specific MT4$^+$ clones and Lyt-2$^+$ cytolytic clones which recognize a tumor-specific cell surface antigen, *Journal of Immunology* **135**: 703–13

Rosenberg S A, Mule J J, Spiess P J, Reichert C M, Schwarz S L 1985. Regression of established pulmonary metastases and subcutaneous tumor mediated by the systemic administration of high-dose recombinant interleuken 2, *Journal of Experimental Medicine* **161**: 1169–88

Segev N, Hizi A, Kirenberg F, Keydar I 1985. Characterization of a protein released by T47D cell line, immunologically related to the major envelope protein of mouse mammary tumor virus, *Proceedings of the National Academy of Sciences USA* **82**: 1531–5

Stutman O 1975. Immunodepression and malignancy, *Advances in Cancer Research* **22**: 261–422

Victor-Korbin C, Bonilla F A, Bellon B, Bona C A 1985. Immunochemical and molecular characterization of regulatory idiotopes expressed by monoclonal antibodies exhibiting or lacking beta2–6 fructosan binding activity, *Journal of Experimental Medicine* **162**: 647–62

Weigle W O 1961. The immune response of rabbits tolerant to bovine serum albumin to the injection of other heterogeneous serum albumins, *Journal of Experimental Medicine* **114**: 111–25

7 Human and veterinary vaccines

New era vaccinology

Maurice R Hilleman

Merck Institute for Therapeutic Research, Merck Sharp & Dohme Research Laboratories, West Point, Pennsylvania 19486, USA

Vaccinology, or the science of vaccines, had its beginning near the end of the eighteenth century with Jennerian prophylaxis of smallpox using attenuated pox virus grown in calf skin. From that time on, for viral vaccines, it has been a long-term pursuit to create systems for producing viral antigens or for growing attenuated live viruses. During the timespan of nearly two centuries, the sequence of substrates employed for propagating viruses progressed from mammalian organs to embryonated hens' eggs, to cell cultures, and finally to recombinant technology employing a variety of producer host cells. What the future holds is uncertain, but surely subunit antigens prepared by recombinant technology in prokaryotic and eukaryotic cells in culture or synthesized chemically must find an important if not the dominant role in new-era vaccinology. Human hepatitis B virus vaccine, prepared initially from viral surface antigen purified from the plasma of carriers of human hepatitis B (Hilleman *et al.* 1982), and now from recombinant yeast (McAleer *et al.* 1984; Hilleman *et al.* 1985) has served as a model for preparing subunit viral antigens and for establishing the precedents for new-era vaccines. As expected, it has also provided important technologic approaches to the development of a vaccine against acquired immune deficiency disease (AIDS).

Hepatitis B vaccines

The virus of hepatitis B does not grow in cell culture. First-generation hepatitis B vaccine has been prepared using purified surface antigen of hepatitis B virus that circulates in abundance in bloods of certain carriers of hepatitis B virus infection (Hilleman *et al.* 1982). The purified and inactivated surface antigen incorporated into an alum adjuvant has proved safe, highly immunogenic and protective against hepatitis B virus infection. This vaccine was licensed for general use in 1981 and has been used in about three million persons to date.

Limitation in supply of suitable plasma and the need to apply highly technical procedures to purify the antigen and to assure safety led us (McAleer *et al.* 1984; Hilleman *et al.* 1985) to develop a new vaccine prepared using hepatitis B surface antigen produced by recombinant technology in yeast. The plasmid construct used in the yeast was developed by Valenzuela *et al.* (1982). This new vaccine of recombinant origin has proved equally as safe, immunogenic and protective in tests in human subjects as the plasma-derived vaccine. The recombinant vaccine was licensed for general use in West Germany in May 1986 and in the USA in July 1986. This new vaccine is the first licensed vaccine of any sort produced by recombinant technology. It provides the technology and precedent for preparing similar subunit vaccines and may find special application to the problem of developing a vaccine ıgainst AIDS.

Acquired immune deficiency disease or AIDS of man

Acquired immune deficiency syndrome or AIDS and the Retrovirus that causes it are commanding worldwide attention (Curran *et al.* 1985; World Health Organization 1985; Biggar 1986; Rich 1985). There have been more than 20,000 identified cases of AIDS in the USA with about 50% mortality to date. Mounting concern is being expressed because of approximate annual doubling of numbers of AIDS cases and the estimated present reservoir of between 1 million and 1.5 million infected persons in the USA. Additionally, the high prevalence of AIDS virus infections in parts of Africa and the awesome spread of the virus throughout the world emphasize the urgent need for an effective means of control. The best present hope for preventing AIDS is by an effective vaccine given prior to exposure to infection. The question is whether, how and when such a vaccine might be developed. AIDS virus is new and there is no significant data base that would permit judgment to be made for a vaccine against AIDS based on experiences with the virus itself. However, some clues, both positive and negative, for preventive control of human Retrovirus infections by vaccines can be obtained by examination of the previous findings with animal Retroviruses, particularly those of mice, cats, horses and sheep.

Retroviruses

Classification

The Retroviruses are a family of enveloped single-stranded RNA viruses that produce a reverse transcriptase whereby the viral RNA codes for DNA that

Table 1 Simplified guide to retrovirus classification

Subfamily	Principal pathology/disease	Best studied species
Oncovirus (subtype C) (primarily cell proliferation)	Human T-lymphotropic viruses	Man
	HTLV-I adult T-cell leukemia	Man
	HTLV-II hairy cell leukemia	
	Leukemia, lymphoid cell tumors, and immunodepression	Mice, cats, chickens, bovines, monkeys
Spumavirus (vacuolation of cells)	Miscellaneous, relatively unimportant	Various mammalian species
Lentivirus (primarily slow cell destruction)	Human AIDS virus, HTLV-III (LAV) (T-helper cell suppression)	Man
	Human AIDS-like virus, HTLV-IV (? non-pathogenic for man)	Man
	Human AIDS virus, LAV-2	Man
	African Green Monkey T-cell lymphotropic virus (STLV-III$_{AGM}$)	African Green Monkey
	Macaca monkey SAIDS virus (STLV-III$_{MAC}$)	*Macaca* monkey
	Equine infectious anemia	Horse
	Visna/maedi (lung, CNS)	Sheep
	Caprine arthritis/encephalitis	Goats

can be inserted into the host cell genome (Wong-Staal and Gallo 1985; Gallo 1985; Reitz and Gallo 1985). The Retroviruses, as shown in Table 1, are divided into three subfamilies. These are the Oncoviruses that primarily cause cell proliferation; the Lentiviruses that primarily cause cell destruction; and the Spumaviruses that are of no great importance.

Human T-cell leukemia and hairy cell leukemia are caused by human T-cell lymphotropic viruses HTLV-I and HTLV-II, respectively. These agents are closely related to the leukemia/lymphoma viruses of a wide variety of animal species.

AIDS appears to be caused by a virus of the Lentivirus subfamily that, within the overall group, might be related most closely to Retroviruses found in African Green Monkeys (Kanki *et al.* 1985) that do not develop disease, and to a virus of *Macaca* monkeys that causes AIDS-like disease in that species (Letvin *et al.* 1985). The exact position of HTLV-III delta virus of macaques, possibly derived initially from mangabey monkeys, is not presently known (Murphey-Corb *et al.* 1986). The origin of human AIDS virus is not known with certainty, but it might have derived from the African Green Monkey virus, STLV-III$_{AGM}$ (Kanki *et al.* 1986). Alternatively, AIDS virus might have originated from an apparently non-disease-producing virus, HTLV-IV (Kanki *et al.* 1986) recently isolated from healthy persons in West Africa, that bears close resemblance to the African Green Monkey virus. The possible relationship of HTLV-IV, in turn, to the LAV-II agent (Walgate 1986; Palca 1986b), recovered recently from patients with AIDS in Portugal, remains to be clarified.

More distantly, AIDS virus shares characteristics with the maedi/visna virus of sheep, caprine arthritis/encephalitis virus of goats and the equine infectious anemia virus of horses (Stephens *et al.* 1986; Casey *et al.* 1985; Chiu *et al.* 1985). It seems likely that a wider variety of Retroviruses infecting man than are presently known will be discovered as suggested by presence of such an agent in cases of multiple sclerosis (Koprowski *et al.* 1985) and possibly in non-A,non-B hepatitis (Iwarson *et al.* 1985). The AIDS Retrovirus kills or reduces the function of T4 (CD4) helper cells, impairs the immune system and renders the host highly susceptible to opportunistic infections that would otherwise cause no great harm (Popovic *et al.* 1984a). Infection of other cells of the immune system including macrophages and B cells has been reported (Wong-Staal and Gallo 1985). Infection of cells of the brain may also occur (Black 1985), possibly by transport of infected cells (macrophages) across the blood–brain barrier (Palca 1986a). Effective vaccines have been developed against certain animal Oncoviruses (Hunsmann 1985) but not against Lentiviruses. AIDS virus has recently been named HIV virus (human immunodeficiency virus) (Coffin *et al.* 1986) but will be called AIDS virus in this review since the HIV terminology has not been accepted by all workers.

Morphology

Structurally, as shown in Fig. 1, in the Bolognesi *et al.* (1978) model, a Retrovirus consists of: (a) an outer lipid envelope with its associated glycoproteins; (b) an inner coat protein; and (c) a core that contains the nucleocapsid, RNA, reverse transcriptase and core-associated proteins. The envelope glycoproteins of the virus are encoded by the viral *env* or envelope gene; the internal proteins by the *gag* or group antigen gene; and the reverse transcriptase by the *pol* or polymerase gene. Additional gene products may be encoded by additional genes (Reitz and Gallo 1985) in the Lentiviruses, or by alternative initiation sites in the reading frames.

The envelope glycoproteins of AIDS virus (Veronese *et al.* 1985; Fischinger *et al.* 1985) consist of a major glycoprotein, gp120, and a less glycosylated glycoprotein, gp41. gp41 has a hydrophobic segment by which it is inserted into the lipid membrane. The means for attachment of the major glycoprotein, gp120, to the transmembrane glycoprotein is not firmly established but may be by disulfide linkage or by hydrogen bonding (Fischinger *et al.* 1985). The ready loss of gp120 from mature virions suggests that simple noncovalent bonding may be the more likely (Gelderblom *et al.* 1985). The major external glycoproteins of the Retroviruses are characteristically highly type-specific while the transmembrane protein appears to be more broad-spectrum (Fischinger *et al.* 1985). The internal proteins, because of their location, appear to be of little or no importance in inducing anti-viral immunity but might play a role in immunity directed against virus-infected cells of the host if these antigens are present in the cell membrane (cf. van der Hoorn *et al.* 1985; Pillemer *et al.* 1986).

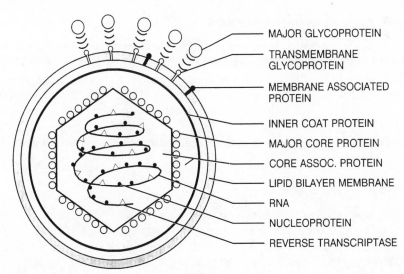

Figure 1. Stylized structure of retroviruses (after Bolognesi *et al.* 1978, with liberties).

Human AIDS virus vaccine considerations

Animal vaccine precedent

The driving force for developing an AIDS virus vaccine is based more on urgent need than on any meaningful leads with human virus at the present time. Some optimism has been generated by the past development of effective vaccines against feline and mouse leukemia Oncoviruses (Hunsmann 1985; Lewis *et al.* 1981; Osterhaus *et al.* 1985). Though human AIDS virus is a Lentivirus, the animal Oncoviruses, especially feline leukemia virus, are being used as principal models for human vaccines, primarily because there is nothing better.

Aggregates of major glycoprotein of Friend mouse leukemia virus attached to the transmembrane protein and, given to mice in Freund adjuvant, induce substantial resistance against challenge with the homologous virus (Hunsmann 1985). Feline leukemia virus vaccines, apparently composed of aggregates of major and transmembrane glycoproteins that are shed from cells transformed by leukemia virus, have been reported to be highly effective in preventing leukemia in cats when given in Freund's emulsified mineral oil adjuvant (Lewis *et al.* 1981) or on glycosydic structures called ISCOMS (immunostimulatory complex) (Osterhaus *et al.* 1985). A feline leukemia virus vaccine was recently licensed for commercial distribution based on the surface membrane antigen vaccine in Freund's adjuvant (Lewis *et al.* 1981), but disappointing results have been reported in field use (Pedersen *et al.* 1985).

Possible subunit vaccine against AIDS

Based on the animal virus experience, it is currently believed that a vaccine made of outer membrane glycoprotein of human AIDS virus that is linked to its transmembrane protein and presented in suitable micellar aggregates or immunostimulating complexes is worthy of a try (Lewis *et al.* 1981; Osterhaus *et al.* 1985). The observation that only a fraction of persons who are infected with AIDS virus actually develop disease, gives credence to the idea that there might be some form of immunologic control in the natural infection.

Antibody in natural infection

AIDS virus-infected individuals do develop antibody, but neutralizing antibody either does not appear or is present in low titer (Fischinger *et al.* 1985; Robert-Guroff *et al.* 1985; Sarngadharan *et al.* 1984; Weiss *et al.* 1985). Gelderblom (Gelderblom *et al.* 1985) has suggested that release of gp120 from the virus particles may bind to neutralizing antibody and mask its presence. AIDS virus or AIDS viral antigens can be detected in a majority of persons with circulating antibody (Fischinger *et al.* 1985; Popovic *et al.* 1984b; Shaw *et al.* 1984; Levy and Shimabukuro 1985), the same as in other persistent viral infections such as herpes simplex. Humoral antibodies usually do little to suppress viruses in well-established infections; they are poorly therapeutic. The principal function of vaccines is to induce antibodies that prevent or at least greatly limit the extent of infection on first exposure to the virus. The opportunity to do this is greatest when the invading virus is cell-free, in contrast to cell-associated virus that may escape neutralization through the mechanism of cell-to-cell transfer. A cell-free state of the invading virus might be a pre-condition for vaccine efficacy; AIDS virus appears to be strongly cell-associated when present in blood and body secretions.

Antigenic hypervariability

An even greater concern for a practical AIDS vaccine is the hypervariability (Wong-Staal and Gallo 1985; Fischinger *et al.* 1985; Wong-Staal *et al.* 1985; Benn *et al.* 1985), in AIDS virus isolates, of the gene that encodes the major envelope glycoprotein, gp120. Because of expected significant antigenic differences between strains, there is reason to question whether antibodies raised against the antigens of any one viral isolate could protect against a significant number of different virus strains. The concern for antigenic variability is accentuated by the relationship (Wong-Staal and Gallo 1985; Stephens *et al.* 1986; Casey *et al.* 1985; Chiu *et al.* 1985; Clements *et al.* 1980; Montelaro *et al.* 1984), though distant, of AIDS virus to the Lentiviruses of sheep and horses. In maedi/visna infection of sheep, and in equine infectious anemia of horses, there is continuing evolution of new antigenic variants during the course of infection against which previously formed antibody is totally nonaffective. This cycle of neutralization, mutation and immunologic escape creates such diversity of antigenically different strains of horse and sheep viruses as to make vaccine development impossible at the present time. Though genomic variability in the envelope region of AIDS viruses is presently established, the extent of the differences in this antigen is not known and it is also unknown whether there is antigenic drift in human virus that is analogous to that of the horse and sheep viruses. Measurement of the magnitude of antigenic diversity among AIDS viruses in man must be of highest research priority and will be critical to predicting how soon a vaccine solution to AIDS might be evolved.

Search for conserved group antigens

If it be found that the antibodies that are ordinarily expressed against major surface glycoprotein 120 are too highly strain-specific to be practically useful for preventing AIDS virus infection, then other immunodeterminants must be sought that are group-reactive. There are two sources for such group determinants. One is in the conserved regions of gp120 that may be more hydrophobic, more sequestered and hence not expressed immunologically in ordinary infection. The other is the transmembrane glycoprotein 41, the equivalent of which in Oncoviruses is highly conserved and is antigenically similar in different viral strains (Thiel *et al.* 1981). A systematic search of the gp120 sequences will most likely reveal a number of immunodeterminants that might be targets for vaccine preparation. Whether antibodies directed against them will be neutralizing and protective will need to be determined. Studies of animal leukemia viruses have demonstrated the induction of potent neutralizing and cytotoxic antibodies on artificial immunization with major glycoprotein that have a far more broad reactivity with distantly related viruses than are seen to follow natural infection (Schäfer and Bolognesi 1977). Additionally, deglycosylation of gp120 might expose group-specific determinants in the amino acid backbone structure that might induce useful antibodies of greater cross-reactivity. Antibody in high titer might also be induced by artificial immunization against the highly conserved transmembrane antigen gp41 (Thiel *et al.* 1981; Fischinger *et al.* 1976) that could provide a broad-spectrum immunity against the multiplicity of AIDS virus variants. There might be a second possible benefit of antibody against transmembrane protein since this antigen, in animal leukemias at least, is immunosuppressive for a variety of cells that are involved in the immune response to viral infection, thereby permitting evasion of immune surveillance (Cianciolo *et al.* 1985). Thus, antibody against gp41 might provide an additional benefit in preventing the immunosuppressive action of this particular antigen. Of possible importance is the recent demonstration of *gag* gene encoded antigens in the membranes of cells infected with mouse leukemia virus (van der Hoorn *et al.* 1985; Pillemer *et al.* 1986). The *gag* encoded antigens are generally associated with critical viral functions and tend therefore to be highly conserved. Vaccines employing such identified antigens might be able to stimulate humoral or cellular immunity against infected cells while maintaining immunologic homogeneity. Finally, the genome of AIDS virus has the potential to encode at least three gene products in addition to those specified by the *gag*, *pol* and *env* genes. These are products of the *sor*, *3′orf*, *tat*$_{III}$ and *art* genes, and are worthy of investigation of possible immune responses to them (Sodroski *et al.* 1986a, 1986b).

Contemporary vaccine approaches

A substantial research effort for vaccine development (Kennedy *et al.* 1986; Wright 1986; Hu *et al.* 1986; Chakrabarti *et al.* 1986; see Fischinger *et al.* 1985) is being made in the scientific community for alternative approaches with attention being given to attenuated live virus vaccines and to recombinants of AIDS virus genes inserted into vaccinia virus genome. Most importantly, there is a concerted effort, using monoclonal antibody and synthetic antigen approaches, to find meaningful immunologic determinants or epitopes to incorporate into vaccines. Antigen production is also being sought employing recombinant yeast or mammalian cells into which various segments of AIDS virus genome is inserted. Anti-idiotype antibodies that present an image of the original antigen are also being explored since it is possible that the important epitopes may be discontinuous, requiring the bringing together into close association of more than a single continuous amino acid sequence.

Vaccine perspective

An attenuated live virus vaccine against AIDS virus would present almost insuperable problems of tests for safety in man and there are no examples of effective synthetic or anti-idiotype vaccines. Principal hope in the practical sense, therefore, is being placed in production of appropriate subunit antigens by genetic recombinant technology.

Just what host cell will prove optimal for producing surface antigen and other antigens of AIDS virus remains to be determined. Yeast currently provides fewest problems from the standpoints of possible toxicity and freedom from concerns for safety. If, however, highly specific glycosylation is a requirement for antigenicity, then cells of mammalian origin might be required. Immunopotentiation of candidate subunit vaccines might be approached using alum alone, virosomes, micellar aggregation, or ISCOMS (Morein and Simons 1985).

The development and preparation of candidate AIDS subunit vaccines may well parallel those for recombinant hepatitis B vaccine, as already discussed. Tests to establish safety, immunogenicity and protective efficacy for man may also benefit from the hepatitis B vaccine experience. Preclinical laboratory tests to measure immunogenicity and protective efficacy will be assisted by meaningful animal models, especially if a susceptible primate that develops AIDS-like disease can be found. The Retroviruses of African Green and *Macaca* monkeys are different from AIDS virus of man. Chimpanzees, though infectible with human AIDS virus, develop only a mild disease that resembles the AIDS-related lymphadenopathy syndrome (Alter *et al.* 1984) and are of very limited availability.

Comment

The development of hepatitis B virus vaccines has provided a success story that will pave the way to new-era vaccines. Among contemporary vaccine needs, there can be none more important than a vaccine against AIDS.

Present evidence suggests that the development of an AIDS vaccine is possible, by a number of different vaccine approaches, once the antigens and their epitopes that are meaningful in immunity have been found. As with earlier vaccines, answers to seemingly unsurmountable problems have a way of appearing and solutions to problems are often provided in the absence of an understanding of the problem in the first place.

The Congress is evidently betting on the technologic solution and is backing its bet with more than 200 million dollars in research money for 1986. It will be an exciting race to follow – to see whether the virus can be controlled before there is wipeout of a substantial proportion of the human population. A risky situation, to say the least!

References

Alter H J, Eichberg J W, Masur H, Saxinger W C, Macher A M, Lane H C, Fauci A S 1984. Transmission of HTLV-III infection from human plasma to chimpanzees: an animal model for AIDS, *Science* **226**: 549–52

Benn S, Rutledge R, Folks T, Gold J, Baker L, McCormick J, Feorino P, Piot P, Quinn T, Martin M 1985. Genomic heterogeneity of AIDS retroviral isolates from North America and Zaire, *Science* **230**: 949–51

Biggar R J 1986. The AIDS problem in Africa, *The Lancet* **i**: 79–83

Black P H 1985. HTLV-III, AIDS, and the brain, *New England Journal of Medicine* **313**: 1538–40

Bolognesi D P, Montelaro R C, Frank H 1978. Assembly of type C oncornaviruses: a model, *Science* **199**: 183–6

Casey J M, Kim Y, Andersen P R, Watson K F, Fox J L, Devare S G 1985. Human T-cell lymphotropic virus type III: immunologic characterization and primary structure analysis of the major internal protein, p24, *Journal of Virology* **55**: 417–23

Chakrabarti S, Robert-Guroff M, Wong-Staal F, Gallo R C, Moss B 1986. Expression of the HTLV-III envelope gene by a recombinant vaccinia virus, *Nature (London)* **320**: 535–7

Chiu I-M, Yaniv A, Dahlberg J E, Gazit A, Skuntz S F, Tronick S R, Aaronson S A 1985. Nucleotide sequence evidence for relationship of AIDS retrovirus to lentiviruses, *Nature (London)* **317**: 366–8

Cianciolo G J, Copeland T D, Oroszlan S, Synderman R 1985. Inhibition of lymphocyte proliferation by a synthetic peptide homologous to retroviral envelope proteins, *Science* **230**: 453–5

Clements J E, Pedersen F S, Narayan O, Haseltine W A 1980. Genomic changes associated with antigenic variation of visna virus during persistent infection, *Proceedings of the National Academy of Sciences USA* **77**: 4454–8

Coffin J, Haase A, Levy J A, Montagnier L, Oroszlan S, Teich N, Temin H, Toyoshima K, Varmus H, Vogt P, Weiss R 1986. What to call the AIDS virus? *Nature (London)* **321**: 10

Curran J W, Morgan W M, Hardy A M, Jaffe H W, Darrow W W, Dowdle W R 1985. The epidemiology of AIDS: current status and future prospects, *Science* **229**: 1352–7

Fischinger P J, Schäfer W, Bolognesi D P 1976. Neutralization of homologous and heterologous oncornaviruses by antisera against the p15(E) and gp71 polypeptides of Friend murine leukemia virus, *Virology* **71**: 169–84

Fischinger P J, Robey W G, Koprowski H, Gallo R C, Bolognesi D P 1985. Current status and strategies for vaccines against diseases induced by human T-cell lymphotropic retroviruses (HTLV-I, -II, -III), *Cancer Research* **45**: 4694s–9s

Gallo R C 1985. The human T-cell leukemia/lymphotropic retroviruses (HTLV) family: past, present, and future, *Cancer Research* **45**: 4524s–33s

Gelderblom H R, Reupke H, Pauli G 1985. Loss of envelope antigens of HTLV-III/LAV. A factor in AIDS pathogenesis, *The Lancet* **ii**: 1016–17

Hilleman M R, Buynak E B, McAleer W J, McLean A A, Provost P J, Tytell A A 1982. Hepatitis A and hepatitis B vaccines, in W Szmuness, H Alter, J Maynard (eds) *Viral Hepatitis. 1981 International Symposium*. The Franklin Institute Press, Philadelphia, pp 385–97

Hilleman M R, Weibel R E, Scolnick E M 1985. Recombinant yeast human hepatitis B vaccine, *Journal of the Hong Kong Medical Association* **37**: 75–85

Hu S-L, Kosowski S G, Dalrymple J M 1986. Expression of AIDS virus envelope gene in recombinant vaccinia viruses, *Nature (London)* **320**: 537–40

Hunsmann G 1985. Subunit vaccines against exogenous retroviruses: overview and perspectives, *Cancer Research* **45**: 4691s–3s

Iwarson S, Schaff Z, Seto B, Norkrans G, Gerety R J 1985. Retrovirus-like particles in hepatocytes of patients with transfusion-acquired non-A,non-B hepatitis, *Journal of Medical Virology* **16**: 37–45

Kanki P J, Alroy J, Essex M 1985. Isolation of T-lymphotropic retrovirus related to HTLV-III/LAV from wild-caught African Green Monkeys, *Science* **230**: 951–4

Kanki P J, Barin F, M'Boup S, Allan J S, Romet-Lemonne J L, Marlink R, McLane M F, Lee T-H, Arbeille B, Denis F, Essex M 1986. New human T-lymphotropic retrovirus related to simian T-lymphotropic virus type III (STLV-III$_{AGM}$), *Science* **232**: 238–43

Kennedy R C, Henkel R D, Pauletti D, Allan J S, Lee T H, Essex M, Dreesman G R 1986. Antiserum to a synthetic peptide recognizes the HTLV-III envelope glycoprotein, *Science* **231**: 1556–9

Koprowski H, DeFreitas E C, Harper M E, Sandberg-Wollheim M, Sheremata W A, Robert-Guroff M, Saxinger C W, Feinberg M B, Wong-Staal F, Gallo R C 1985. Multiple sclerosis and human T-cell lymphotropic retroviruses, *Nature (London)* **318**: 154–60

Letvin N L, Daniel M D, Sehgal P K, Desrosiers R C, Hunt R D, Waldron L M, MacKey J J, Schmidt D K, Chalifoux L V, King N W 1985. Induction of AIDS-like disease in Macaque monkeys with T-cell tropic retrovirus STLV-III, *Science* **230**: 71–4

Levy J A, Shimabukuro J 1985. Recovery of AIDS-associated retroviruses from patients with AIDS or AIDS-related conditions and from clinically healthy individuals, *Journal of Infectious Diseases* **152**: 734–8

Lewis M G, Mathes L E, Olsen R G 1981. Protection against feline leukemia by vaccination with a subunit vaccine, *Infection and Immunity* **34**: 888–94

McAleer W J, Buynak E B, Maigetter R Z, Wampler D E, Miller W J, Hilleman M R 1984. Human hepatitis B vaccine from recombinant yeast, *Nature (London)* **307**: 178–80

Montelaro R C, Parekh B, Orrego A, Issel C J 1984. Antigenic variation during persistent infection by equine infectious anemia virus, a retrovirus, *Journal of Biological Chemistry* **259**: 10539–44

Morein B, Simons K 1985. Subunit vaccines against enveloped viruses: virosomes, micelles and other protein complexes, *Vaccine* **3**: 83–93

Murphey-Corb M, Martin L N, Rangan S R S, Baskin G B, Gormus B J, Wolf R H, Andes W A, West M, Montelaro R C 1986. Isolation of an HTLV-III-related retrovirus from macaques with simian AIDS and its possible origin in asymptomatic mangabeys, *Nature (London)* **321**: 435–7

Osterhaus A, Weijer K, Uytdehaag F, Jarrett O, Sundquist B, Morein B 1985. Induction of protective immune response in cats by vaccination with feline leukemia virus ISCOM, *Journal of Immunology* **135**: 591–6

Palca J 1986a. Infection mechanism? *Nature (London)* **319**: 470

Palca J 1986b. AIDS Research. New human retroviruses: (one causes AIDS) . . . and the other does not, *Nature (London)* **320**: 385

Pedersen N C, Johnson L, Ott R L 1985. Evaluation of a commercial feline leukemia virus vaccine for immunogenicity and efficacy, *Feline Practice* **15**: 7–20

Pillemer E A, Kooistra D A, Witte O N, Weissman I L 1986. Monoclonal antibody to the amino-terminal L sequence of murine leukemia virus glycosylated *gag* polyproteins demonstrates their unusual orientation in the cell membrane, *Journal of Virology* **57**: 413–21

Popovic M, Flomenberg N, Volkman D J, Mann D, Fauci A S, Dupont B, Gallo R C 1984a. Alteration of T-cell functions by infection with HTLV-I or HTLV-II, *Science* **226**: 459–62

Popovic M, Sarngadharan M G, Read E, Gallo R C 1984b. Detection, isolation, and continuous production of cytopathic retroviruses (HTLV-III) from patients with AIDS and pre-AIDS, *Science* **224**: 497–500

Reitz M S, Gallo R C 1985. Retroviruses of human T cells: their role in the aetiology of adult T-cell leukaemia/lymphoma and the acquired immune deficiency syndrome, *Cancer Surveys* **4**: 313–29

Rich V 1985. Soviets admit AIDS cases, *Nature (London)* **318**: 502

Robert-Guroff M, Brown M, Gallo R C 1985. HTLV-III-neutralizing antibodies in patients with AIDS and AIDS-related complex, *Nature (London)* **316**: 72–4

Sarngadharan M G, Popovic M, Bruch L, Schupach J, Gallo R C 1984. Antibodies reactive with human T-lymphotropic retroviruses (HTLV-III) in the serum of patients with AIDS, *Science* **224**: 506–8

Schäfer W, Bolognesi D P 1977. Mammalian C-type oncornaviruses: relationships between viral structural and cell-surface antigens and their possible significance in immunological defense mechanisms, in M G Hanna Jr, F Rapp (eds) *Contemporary Topics in Immunobiology*, vol 6, *Immunobiology of oncogenic viruses*. Plenum Press, New York and London, pp 127–67

Shaw G M, Hahn B H, Arya S K, Groopman J E, Gallo R C, Wong-Staal F 1984. Molecular characterization of human T-cell leukemia (lymphotropic) virus type III in the acquired immune deficiency syndrome, *Science* **226**: 1165–71

Sodroski J, Goh W C, Rosen C, Tartar A, Portetelle D, Burny A, Haseltine W 1986a. Replicative and cytopathic potential of HTLV-III/LAV with *sor* gene deletions, *Science* **231**: 1549–53

Sodroski J, Goh W C, Rosen C, Dayton A, Terwilliger E, Haseltine W 1986b. A second post-transcriptional *trans*-activator gene required for HTLV-III replication, *Nature (London)* **321**: 412–17

Stephens R M, Casey J W, Rice N R 1986. Equine infectious anemia virus *gag* and *pol* genes: relatedness to Visna and AIDS virus, *Science* **231**: 589–94

Thiel H-J, Broughton E M, Matthews T J, Schäfer W, Bolognesi D P 1981. Interspecies reactivity of type C and D retrovirus p 15E and p 15C proteins, *Virology* **111**: 270–4

Valenzuela P, Medina A, Rutter W J, Ammerer G, Hall B D 1982. Synthesis and assembly of hepatitis B virus surface antigen particles in yeast, *Nature (London)* **298**: 347–50

van der Hoorn F A, Lahaye T, Müller V, Ogle M A, Engers H D 1985. Characterization of gP85*gag* as an antigen recognized by Moloney leukemia virus-specific cytolytic T cell clones that function *in vivo*, *Journal of Experimental Medicine* **162**: 128–44

Veronese F D, DeVico A L, Copeland T D, Oroszlan S, Gallo R C, Sarngadharan M G 1985. Characterization of gp41 as the transmembrane protein coded by the HTLV-III/LAV envelope gene, *Science* **229**: 1402–5

Walgate R 1986. AIDS research. New human retroviruses: one causes AIDS . . . (and the other does not), *Nature (London)* **320**: 385

Weiss R A, Clapham P R, Cheingsong-Popov R, Dalgleish A G, Carne C A, Weller I V D, Tedder R S 1985. Neutralization of human T-lymphotropic virus type III by sera of AIDS and AIDS-risk patients, *Nature (London)* **316**: 69–71

Wong-Staal F, Gallo R C 1985. Human T-lymphotropic retroviruses, *Nature (London)* **317**: 395–403

Wong-Staal F, Ratner L, Shaw G, Hahn B, Harper M, Franchini G, Gallo R 1985. Molecular biology of human T-lymphotropic retroviruses, *Cancer Research* **45**: 4539s–44s

World Health Organization 1985. The acquired immunodeficiency syndrome (AIDS): Memorandum from a WHO meeting, *Bulletin of the World Health Organization* **63**: 667–72

Wright K 1986. AIDS protein made, *Nature (London)* **319**: 525

Vaccines against animal parasites

K D Murrell; H P Marti; H R Gamble

Helminthic Diseases Laboratory, Animal Parasitology Institute, Agricultural Research Service, United States Department of Agriculture, Beltsville Agricultural Research Center, Beltsville, Maryland 20705, USA

Interest in the development of immunological controls for parasitic diseases of veterinary importance is growing as a result of concern over the problems of safety, expense and resistance associated with chemotherapy. Although vaccines have been pursued for more than 50 years, progress has been slow. In the effort to produce vaccines have come some clues as to why progress has been limited. It is now clear that the strategy for most parasites is not simply to gain entry into their host, but also to establish a chronic 'partnership' with the host in order to achieve their reproductive goals. To do this, selection has favored the evolution of host–parasite relationships which allow mutual survival. Among the potential mechanisms that may contribute to the establishment of such relationships are parasite influences on the host's immune response (Mitchell 1982), although few yet have convincing data to support them. Among the examples in which modulation of immunological processes is the best explanation for the parasite's success are:

1. Immunosuppression in periparturient livestock, especially sheep and cattle. This is indicated by increased susceptibility to infection by gastrointestinal nematodes during pregnancy and lactation, and significant decreases in host lymphoid cell responses to specific antigen at parturition (Chen and Soulsby 1976). Also, hypobiotic or arrested larvae in these animals are activated at the time of parturition (Gibbs 1968). The involvement of endocrine changes, especially in prolactin, has been suggested (Lloyd 1983).
2. Immunological unresponsiveness to parasites in young animals. Control is particularly difficult because this age group is usually at high risk of infection. Why such parasitic worms as *Haemonchus contortus* infect young lambs without engendering an immune response is perplexing because the same animals can respond to microbial antigens. Further, at three to six months of age lambs develop protective resistance to *H. contortus*. The mechanism(s) responsible for this early susceptibility is not understood, although neonatal tolerance and colostral transfer of soluble

suppressor factors, tolerizing antigen, and maternal blocking antibody have been suggested (Soulsby 1985). In sheep, maternal antibody may also suppress the synthesis of endogenous antibody and hence delay maturation of the fetal immune system (Sterzl and Silverstein 1967).

3. Immunomodulation during parasitism. This may be more important than has been recognized. Immunoparasitologists are now benefiting immensely from the insights provided by basic research on lymphocyte interactions and cell mediators, especially the lymphokines. Although much of the immunosuppression of lymphocyte responses observed under experimental conditions may be a consequence of abnormally high infection levels, there is increasing evidence that modulation of the immune response in livestock during gastrointestinal nematode infection occurs at levels frequently observed in naturally infected hosts (Gasbarre 1986). For example, peripheral blood lymphocytes from cattle infected with *Ostertagia ostertagi* show a transient, suppressed response to parasite antigens (Klesius *et al.* 1984). Although the abomasal lymph nodes show tremendous hypercellularity, they contain few antigen-specific lymphocytes. In contrast, direct immunization with *O. ostertagi* antigens does produce abundant specific T-cells (Gasbarre 1986). Among the explanations for this natural infection-induced hyporesponsiveness are polyclonal lymphocyte activation and interference in lymphokine-mediated growth of active cells. The humoral antibody response to *O. ostertagi* infection is also weak (Klesius *et al.* 1987). These observations, if shown to be responsible for the very slow development of resistance in cattle (or lack thereof), may also provide clues to the approaches needed to overcome this poor protective response.

4. Antigenic modulation and complexity. This poses another serious problem. Although the antigenic diversity of parasitic protozoa is not as great as that of most helminths, many of them use antigenic variation, an immune evasion mechanism that can be devastating to vaccine development efforts. This feature is best exemplified by the trypanosomes, which have a repertoire of surface antigens that enable relapse variants to express new antigens. The number of genes that can be expressed may be 300–1000 (Parsons *et al.* 1984).

Among helminth parasites, there may be a multiplicity of antigenic epitopes, only a few of which may induce protective immunity. Hence, the search for protective antigens has been, until the recent advent of monoclonal antibodies, an extremely difficult immunochemical task, usually compounded by the lack of convenient bioassay procedures that can distinguish directly between relevant and irrelevant antigens. Because of the need to carry out experimental work in laboratory models, a persistent danger exists that the research results will not be applicable to the target host–parasite relationship (see swine trichinellosis, discussed below, as an example).

It is obvious that the identification and isolation of antigens with vaccine potential will be impacted by the selective pressure on parasites with chronic host relationships to reduce or alter their immunogenicity or antigenicity, and/or to modulate the host's immune response. General pessimism in this regard, however, should not obscure the important progress that has been made in some instances; a few vaccines have reached the marketplace (Table 1). Although vaccines that employ live, attenuated parasites have had some

Table 1 Commercial and experimental vaccines for animal parasites

Vaccine	Disease	Vaccine type
Commercial		
Dictol*	Bovine lungworm	Live-irradiated
Coccivax†	Poultry coccidiosis	Controlled exposure
Canine Hookworm vaccine‡	Dog hookworm	Live-irradiated
Dilfil§	Ovine lungworm	Live-irradiated
Experimental		
	Poultry coccidiosis	Live-attenuated
	Ovine trichostrongylocis	Live-irradiated
	Bovine facioliasis	Live-irradiated
	Swine ascariasis	Live-irradiated
	Equine verminous arteritis	Live-irradiated
	Bovine schistosomiasis	Live-irradiated
	Bovine piroplasmosis	Live-attenuated; Culture-derived antigens
	Bovine and ovine cysticercosis	Culture-derived antigens
Cattle Tick vaccine‖	Cattle ticks	Recombinant

* Allen & Hanburys
† Sterwin Labs.
‡ Jensen–Salsbery (withdrawn from production).
§ Produced by government laboratories in user countries.
‖ Development is a joint collaboration between the Australian Commonwealth Scientific and Industrial Research Organization and Biotechnology Australia.

success to date, there are as yet no commercially produced, antigenically defined vaccines. This may reflect the need to present to the host a variety of antigens, especially those associated with several stages of parasite development. Parasites that do invoke strong host immunity usually exhibit multiple developmental stages within the host, often associated with migration through one or more host organs or tissues. However, similar characteristics are also found in parasites that induce only weak host immunity. The greater immunogenicity of live parasites versus parasite extracts may also be due to poor stability or low concentration in extracts of the protective parasite antigens. If this is an important variable, then improvements in immunization could be achieved by developing improved procedures for isolating parasite antigens.

Many of the past efforts at developing parasite vaccines have been made in the absence of a thorough understanding of the nature of the protective immune response. As the vaccine development examples chosen illustrate, such information can be decisive. The two examples illustrate current conceptual approaches and hazards encountered in this effort.

Avian coccidiosis vaccine

An example of benefits from the revolution in biotechnology is the effort to produce a vaccine for avian coccidiosis. These intestinal protozoa, related to malaria, cost the poultry industry in the United States approximately $300 million annually, in spite of the availability of a wide variety of anti-coccidial drugs. Therefore, important efforts are underway to develop antigen-derived vaccines, the most advanced of these being directed at *Eimeria tenella*.

The antigens of the initial infective stage, the sporozoite, the main target of the bird's protective immune response, have been detected with monoclonal antibodies (Danforth 1982). It was observed that some of these monoclonal antibodies inhibited cell penetration *in vitro*. Although there is evidence that these surface antigens may not be relevant to the protective immune response (Augustine and Danforth 1985), the monoclonal antibodies directed against them, as well as the polyclonal antibodies in immune infected chicken sera, have played important roles in the production of sporozoite antigens by recombinant DNA methods (Danforth *et al.* 1985). Messenger RNA was isolated from sporulating oocysts and used to generate cDNA which was inserted into bacteriophage λgt 11. The bacteriophage transfected *Escherichia coli* and bacterial clones expressing coccidial antigens were identified with these monoclonal and polyclonal antibody probes. The cDNA was then removed from the bacteriophage vector and inserted into a plasmid which was in turn inserted into *E. coli*. Clones of *E. coli* expressing coccidial antigen were identified with antibody and the selected clones propagated. Coccidial proteins recovered from bacterial lysates have been examined. One antigen, 5401, stimulated production of chicken antibodies to soluble sporozoite antigen and, at a dose of 2.4 μg/bird, provided partial protection against infection (Danforth 1986); the immunized birds had better feed conversion, and fewer intestinal lesions than controls. Although this research is far from complete, it may serve as a model for the employment of biotechnology in vaccine development for other parasites.

Swine trichinellosis vaccine

Considerable effort is now underway in the United States to eradicate the helminth parasite *Trichinella spiralis* from the pork supply, an effort that involves government, industry and university research (Murrell 1985a). Epidemiological research shows that the transmission of *T. spiralis* in the farm ecosystem varies, not always (or usually) due to the feeding of uncooked garbage. Among the more important routes of transmission are hog cannibalism, consumption by hogs of infected rats and, perhaps, infected wild animal tissue (Hanbury *et al.* 1986; Schad *et al.* 1987; Murrell *et al.* 1987). A serious impediment for control is the difficulty in interrupting such transmission through changes in farm management practices because of resistance by many farm operators to the often drastic changes required. A control strategy more appealing to both farmer and government agency is the application of a vaccine, since most hog farmers are accustomed to the use of vaccines for the control of infectious diseases.

Fortunately, a great deal of basic research has already been carried out on the immunochemistry and protective properties of the antigens of *T. spiralis*. It is clear from these investigations that antigens from the muscle larvae (L1) are especially immunogenic in rodents (Silberstein and Despommier 1984; Gamble 1985). Isolation of individual antigens by immunoaffinity technics using monoclonal antibodies has demonstrated that antigens secreted by the worm's secretory organ (stichosome) are highly immunogenic in mice (Silberstein and Despommier 1984; Gamble 1985). The immune responses induced by these antigens appear to mimic the enhanced intestinal expulsion of worms observed in rodents immunized by live infection. Although the nature of this intestinal immune response is not completely defined, immediate hypersensitivity appears to play an important role (Alizadeh and Murrell 1984; Durham *et al.* 1984; Wakelin and Denham 1983).

Following successful immunization of rodents with larval stage stichosome antigens, we evaluated the soluble fraction of the large stichosome particles, S3, and its antigenic components isolated by antibody affinity chromatography (PAW) in pigs (Murrell and Despommier 1984). The S3 preparation was indeed protective in pigs, although at a level lower than that achieved in mice (Fig. 1). Increasing the amount of S3 or PAW administered did not increase protection beyond the 50% level.

Because of the possibility that protective stichosome antigens were degraded or destroyed during preparation of S3, a second series of pig trials were carried out using a secretory antigen preparation (ES), derived by *in vitro* parasite maintenance; this antigen preparation is highly immunogenic in mice (Gamble 1985). Again, the maximal levels of protection induced by ES antigen in pigs were only moderate, reaching about 50% at the 300 mg dose.

Concurrent research on the nature of acquired immunity to *T. spiralis* in swine suggested that a straightforward extension of immunization protocols derived from rodent models might be inappropriate because the pig did not develop a rapid intestinal expulsion response comparable to that usually seen in rodents, especially rats (Murrell 1985b). Intestinal immunity could not account for the nearly complete resistance infected pigs exhibited to the

407

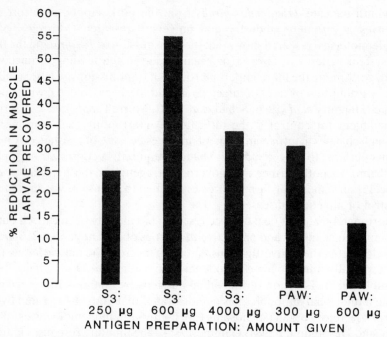

Figure 1. Immunization of pigs with *T. spiralis* stichosome antigen (S$_3$) and an immunoaffinity preparation of S$_3$ (PAW). Percentage reduction in challenge muscle larvae burden determined by comparing recoveries from control pigs with recoveries from immunized pigs (data from Murrell and Despommier 1984).

establishment of the progeny (muscle larvae) of the secondary infection, especially in low-level infections (Fig. 2). Although the production of new-born larvae (NBL) by the female worm (fecundity) is severely inhibited in immune rodents (Denham and Martinez 1970), the antifecundity effect in immune pigs proved to be inadequate to account for the reduction in the establishment of challenge infection-derived NBL (Marti and Murrell 1986). These observations implicated an important postintestinal protective effector mechanism directed at the NBL in swine. The existence of such stage-specific immunity had been reported previously in rodents (Maloney and Denham 1979; Perrudet-Badoux *et al*. 1981). NBL opsonized with specific monoclonal antibody were shown to have reduced infectivity upon injection into rats (Ortega-Pierres *et al*. 1984). Immunochemical studies have also demonstrated that the NBL surface is antigenic (Philipp *et al*. 1981) and, in the presence of antibody, very attractive to granulocytes and mononuclear cells (Kazura and Grove 1978; Ruitenberg *et al*. 1983).

The importance of anti-NBL immunity in the pig was investigated by a series of passive antibody transfer experiments. The injection of nursing piglets with immune pig serum provided strong resistance to the establishment of muscle larvae after challenge inoculation with *T. spiralis* (Marti and Murrell 1986). Significantly, transferred immune sera had little or no effect on

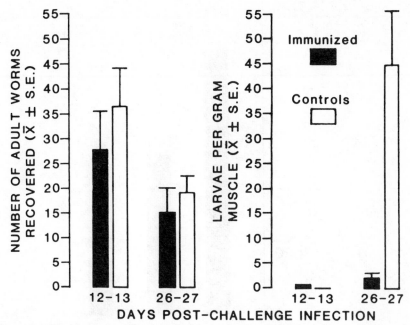

Figure 2. Development of resistance in pigs by live infection with *T. spiralis*. Pigs inoculated initially with 112 muscle larvae and reinoculated six weeks later with 500 muscle larvae; adult and larval worm recoveries made at various intervals post-challenge (data from Murrell 1985).

the establishment or fecundity of the challenge worms. By indirect fluorescent antibody assay, immune pig serum was demonstrated to contain antibodies to the NBL surface.

These results indicated that NBL antigens were capable of inducing a strong protective immunity in swine. To test this directly, pigs were immunized with killed NBL emulsified in CFA (Marti *et al.* 1987), and then challenged. Pigs receiving NBL had 80% fewer muscle larvae at necropsy than did the controls (Fig. 3). These results have stimulated a concerted effort to isolate and characterize the NBL antigens responsible for this effect. Because of the difficulty in producing the NBL stage, monoclonal antibodies are being prepared to the NBL antigens in an attempt to isolate and characterize individual antigens from extracts. If successful, the potential exists to produce these antigens by recombinant DNA methods similar to those described for the chicken coccidian, *Eimeria tenella*. It is also clear that alternatives to recombinant DNA procedures are emerging for the production of vaccines for antigens that are scarce or difficult to produce. One of these is the synthesis of peptides that simulate the antigenic epitope; peptides can be selected from amino acid sequences for the specific antigen or chosen from an amino acid sequence that has been predicted from the DNA sequence. This approach has recently yielded success in the production of antibodies against an important sequence in the envelope glycoprotein of HTLV-III virus

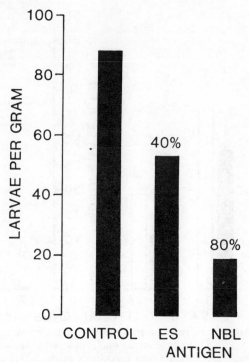

Figure 3. Muscle larvae recoveries from immunized and control pigs six weeks after challenge. NBL, whole, killed newborn larvae; ES, larval excretory secretory antigen. (data from Marti *et al.* 1986.)

(Kennedy *et al.* 1986a). Still another potentially useful strategy is the induction of protective antibodies with anti-idiotype antibodies that mimic the relevant antigenic epitope. In this approach, detailed knowledge of the antigenic structure is unnecessary. The first success in vaccination against viral hepatitis with an anti-idiotypic vaccine was recently announced (Kennedy *et al.* 1986b). It is probable that new technologies or strategies for vaccine production will keep pace or even exceed the development of the immunochemical understanding of parasite antigens and that when candidate parasite antigens are produced, investigators will have several options for utilizing them as vaccines.

It is hoped that this review of efforts to develop a vaccine for swine trichinellosis illustrates some of the points made in the introduction, namely that efforts to develop vaccines against parasites, especially helminths, may be seriously hindered without an adequate understanding of the immunobiology of the specific host–parasite interaction. Our experience also illustrates the hazard of relying too heavily on laboratory models for these efforts. The nature of the host–parasite compromise in the 'natural' host may often be substantially different, both qualitatively and quantitatively, than that existing in more convenient laboratory models.

References

Alizadeh H, Murrell K D 1984. The intestinal mast cell response to *Trichinella spiralis* infection in mast cell-deficient w/w^v mice, *Journal of Parasitology* **70**: 767–73

Augustine P C, Danforth H D 1985. Effects of hybridoma antibodies on invasion of cultured cells by sporozoites of *Eimeria*, in *Avian Diseases* **29**: 1212–23

Chen P, Soulsby E J L 1976. *Haemonchus contortus* infection in ewes: blastogenic responses of peripheral blood leucocytes to third stage larval antigen, *International Journal of Parasitology* **6**: 135–41

Danforth H D 1982. Development of hybridoma-produced antibodies directed against *Eimeria tenella* and *E. mitis, Journal of Parasitology* **68**: 392–7

Danforth H D 1986. Use of hybridoma antibodies combined with genetic engineering in the study of protozoan parasites: a review. L R McDougald, L P Joyner, P L Long (eds), in *Research in Avian Coccidiosis*, University of Georgia Press, Athens (Georgia), pp 514–90

Danforth H D, McCandliss R, Libel M, Augustine P C, Ruff M D 1985. Development of an avian coccidial antigen by recombinant DNA technology, *Poultry Science* **64**: 85–94

Denham D A, Martinez P R 1970. Studies with methyridine and *Trichinella spiralis* II. The use of drugs to study the rate of larval production in mice, *Journal of Helminthology* **44**: 357–63

Durham C P, Murrell K D, Lee C M 1984. *Trichinella spiralis*: immunization of rats with an antigen fraction enriched for allergenicity, *Experimental Parasitology* **57**: 297–306

Gamble H R 1985. *Trichinella spiralis*: immunization of mice using monoclonal antibody affinity-isolated antigens, *Experimental Parasitology* **59**: 398–404

Gasbarre L C 1986. Limiting dilution analysis for the quantification of cellular immune responses in bovine ostertagiasis, *Veterinary Parasitology* **20**: 133–47

Gibbs H C 1968. Some factors in the 'spring-rise' phenomenon in sheep, E J L Soulsby (ed) in *The reaction of the host to parasitism, Veterinary Medical Reviews*, pp 160–73

Hanbury R, Doby P B, Miller H O, Murrell K D 1986. Trichinosis in a herd of swine: cannibalism as a major mode of transmission, *Journal of the American Veterinary Medical Association* **188**: 1155–9

Kazura J W, Grove D I 1978. Stage-specific antibody-dependent eosinophil mediated destruction of *Trichinella spiralis, Nature (London)* **274**: 588–9

Kennedy R C, Henkel R D, Pauletti D, Allan J S, Lee T H, Esex M, Dreesman G R 1986a. Antiserum to a synthetic peptide recognizes the HTLV-III envelope glycoprotein, *Science* **231**: 1556–9

Kennedy R C, Eichberg J W, Lanford R E, Dreesman G R 1986b. Anti-idiotypic antibody vaccine for type B viral hepatitis in chimpanzees, *Science* **232**: 220–3

Klesius P H, Washburn S M, Ciordia H, Haynes T B, Snyder T G III 1984. Lymphocyte reactivity to *Ostertagia ostertagi* L$_3$ antigen in Type I ostertagiasis, *American Journal of Veterinary Research* **45**: 230–3

Klesius P H, Washburn S M, Haynes T B 1987. Serum antibody response to soluble extract of the third-larvae stage of *Ostertagia ostertagi* in cattle, *Veterinary Parasitology* (in press)

Lloyd S 1983. Effect of pregnancy and lactation upon infection, *Veterinary Immunology and Immunopathology* **4**: 153–76

Maloney A, Denham D A 1979. Effects of immune serum and cells on newborn larvae of *Trichinella spiralis, Parasite Immunology* **1**: 3–12

Marti H P, Murrell K D 1986. *Trichinella spiralis*: antifecundity and anti-newborn larvae immunity in swine, *Experimental Parasitology* **62**: 370–5

Marti H P, Murrell K D, Gamble H R 1987. *Trichinella spiralis*: immunization of swine with newborn larval antigen, *Experimental Parasitology* **63**: 68–73

Mitchell G F 1982. Host-protective immune response to parasites and evasion by parasites: generalizations and approaches to analysis, in G F Mitchell (ed) *Biology and Control of Endoparasites*. Academic Press, Sydney (Australia), pp 331–41

Murrell K D 1985a. Strategies for the control of human trichinosis transmitted by pork, *Food Technology* **39**: 65–70

Murrell K D 1985b. *Trichinella spiralis*: acquired immunity in swine, *Experimental Parasitology* **59**: 347–54

Murrell K D, Despommier D D 1984. Immunization of swine against *Trichinella spiralis*, *Veterinary Parasitology* **15**: 263–70

Murrell K D, Stringfellow F, Dame J B, Leiby D A, Duffy C, Schad G A 1987. *Trichinella spiralis* in an agricultural ecosystem: II. Evidence for natural transmission to local wildlife, *Journal of Parasitology* (in press)

Ortega-Pierres M G, MacKenzie C D, Parkhouse R M 1984. Protection against *Trichinella spiralis* induced by a monoclonal antibody that promotes killing newborn larvae by granulocytes, *Parasite Immunology* **6**: 275–84

Parsons M, Nelson R G, Agabian N 1984. Antigenic variation in African trypanosomes: DNA rearrangements program immune evasion, *Immunology Today* **5**: 43–50

Perrudet-Badoux A, Binaghi R A, Boussac-Aron Y, Ruitenberg E J 1981. Antibody dependent mechanisms of immunity against migrating larvae of *Trichinella spiralis*, *Veterinary Parasitology* **8**: 89–94

Philip M, Taylor P M, Parkhouse R M E, Ogilvie B M 1981. Immune response to stage-specific surface antigens of the parasitic nematode, *Trichinella spiralis*, *Journal of Experimental Medicine* **154**: 210–15

Ruitenberg E J, Buys J, Teppema J S, Elgersma A 1983. Rat mononuclear cells and neutrophils are more efficient than eosinophils in antibody-mediated stage-specific killing of *Trichinella spiralis in vitro Zeitschrift für Parasitenkunde* **69**: 807–15

Schad G A, Duffy C H, Leiby D A, Murrell K D, Zirkle E W 1987. *Trichinella spiralis* in an agricultural ecosystem: transmission under natural and experimentally modified on-farm conditions, *Journal of Parasitology* (in press)

Silberstein D S, Despommier D 1984. Antigens from *Trichinella spiralis* that induce a protective response in the mouse, *Journal of Immunology* **132**: 898–904

Soulsby E J L 1985. Advances in immuno-parasitology, *Veterinary Parasitology* **18**: 303–19

Sterzl J, Silverstein A M 1967. Developmental aspects of immunity: *Advances in Immunology* **6**: 337–84

Wakelin D, Denham D A 1983. The immune response, in W C Campbell (ed) *Trichinella and Trichinosis*. Plenum Press, New York, pp 265–308

Molecular mimicry: streptococci and myosin

Madeleine W Cunningham; Karen K Krisher; Robert A Swerlick; Lou Ann Barnett; Patricia F Guderian

Department of Microbiology and Immunology, College of Medicine, University of Oklahoma Health Sciences Center, Oklahoma City, Oklahoma 73190, USA

Introduction

Rheumatic carditis is a sequela of group A streptococcal infection and although the exact mechanisms of pathogenesis are unknown, it has been suggested to be due to an autoimmune mechanism related to biological mimicry between the streptococcus and human heart (Zabriskie 1966; Kaplan 1963). Heart-reactive antibodies have appeared in the sera of rabbits immunized with *Streptococcus pyogenes* or their membranes (Zabriskie and Freimer 1966), and sera from patients with acute rheumatic fever (ARF) were four times more reactive with human heart than were sera from other streptococcal diseases (Zabriskie *et al.* 1970). The presence of heart reactive antibodies in the ARF sera and the deposition of immunoglobulin and complement in heart tissue of patients with ARF supports the hypothesis that ARF has an autoimmune origin (Zabriskie *et al.* 1970; Kaplan 1963).

The streptococcal components which have been implicated in immunological cross-reactions with heart tissue include purified membranes (van de Rijn *et al.* 1977), M proteins, particularly types 1, 5 and 19 (Dale and Beachey 1982; Lyampert *et al.* 1968, 1976), and group A carbohydrate (Goldstein *et al.* 1968). Heart-reactive antibodies in ARF sera were shown to react with streptococcal membrane polypeptides, and the cross-reactive antigen was found to be associated with all group A streptococcal membranes (van de Rijn *et al.* 1977). Other studies implicated cell wall components and M protein in the immunologic cross-reactions between heart-reactive antibodies and streptococcal antigens (Dale and Beachey 1982). Recent analysis of homogeneous M protein preparations revealed that M types 5 and 19 possess heart cross-reactive epitopes, and preparations of the cloned M protein gene product retained the epitopes which bind heart-reactive antibodies (Poirer *et al.* 1985). These past studies have shown that at least some of the M proteins, especially M type 5, share epitopes or structures with host antigens. Structural analysis of M proteins has led to the conclusion that they are α-helical coiled-coil structures with a seven amino acid residue periodicity (Fischetti and Manjula 1982). The M proteins have been compared to tropomyosin and more recently to myosin and the desmin-keratin family of α-helical proteins (Manjula *et al.* 1985). Pepsin has been shown to divide the M protein molecule in half separating the amino-terminal half containing type specific epitopes from the carboxy terminus containing amino acid residues in a sequence conserved among the M types of group A streptococci (Phillips *et al.* 1981; Jones *et al.* 1985). The regions of cross-reactivity are yet to be determined.

In our studies we have demonstrated the first evidence of serological cross-reactivity between anti-streptococcal monoclonal antibodies and myosin (Krisher and Cunningham 1985). These antibodies, which first were shown to react with streptococcal membrane components (Cunningham *et al.* 1984), also were found to react with M protein, the major virulence determinant of group A streptococci (Cunningham and Swerlick 1986). Table 1 shows

Table 1 Antigen binding of cross-reactive monoclonal antibodies

MAb 36.2.2	MAb 49.8.9	MAb 54.2.8
M protein, types 5 and 6	M protein, type 5	M protein, types 5 and 6
Myosin, LMM	?	Myosin, LMM*, HMM*
Actin		DNA
Keratin		PolyI
		PolydT
		(Blocked by anti-vimentin sera)
		Cardiolipin (weak)

* LMM, light meromyosin (Sigma); HMM, heavy meromyosin (Sigma).

an overview of the specificities of our cross-reactive monoclonal antibody probes. Monoclonal antibody 36.2.2 reacted with a family of α-helical proteins, while another antibody 54.2.8 reacted with DNA and myosin (Cunningham and Swerlick 1986). Monoclonal antibody 49.8.9 was cross-reactive but the host antigens remain unidentified. This evidence supports the hypothesis that by some mechanism, group A streptococci activate certain autoantibody-producing B cell clones.

Heart cross reactive streptococcal antigens identified by monoclonal antibody probes

Cross-reactive monoclonal antibody probes were obtained following immunization of BALBc/BYJ mice with purified membranes from M type 5 *S. pyogenes*. Hybridomas were initially screened for antibody using whole streptococci and whole heart extracts as antigens in the enzyme-linked immunosorbent assay (ELISA) (Cunningham and Russell 1983). Once the hybrids were cloned, the antibodies were characterized and all found to be of the IgM isotype (Cunningham *et al.* 1984).

The monoclonal antibodies were found to react with proteins in purified streptococcal membranes and in sodium dodecyl sulfate (SDS) extracts of whole streptococci. Figure 1 shows the Western immunoblot of *S. pyogenes* M type 5 proteins from membranes and whole cells reacted with monoclonal antibodies 36.2.2, 49.8.9 and 54.2.8. In whole cell extracts, proteins in the

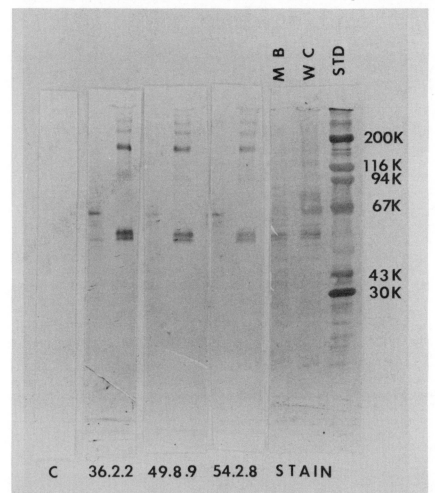

Figure 1. Western immunoblot of SDS-extracted, M type 5 *S. pyogenes* membranes (MB or left lane) and whole cells (WC or right lane) after separation in a 10–20% slab gel gradient by SDS–PAGE. Electroblotted MB and WC proteins were reacted separately with Amido Black (STAIN), monoclonal antibodies 36.2.2, 49.8.9, 54.2.8, and a medium control containing mouse IgM (18 μg/ml). Antibody reactions were detected using goat anti-mouse IgM horseradish peroxidase conjugated antibody with development in 4-chloro-1-naphthol substrate. Stained molecular weight standards (STD) included myosin 200×10^3, β-galactosidase 116×10^3, phosphorylase B 94×10^3, bovine serum albumin 67×10^3, egg albumin 43×10^3, and carbonic anhydrase 30×10^3. Reproduced with the permission of Rockefeller University Press (Cunningham and Swerlick 1986).

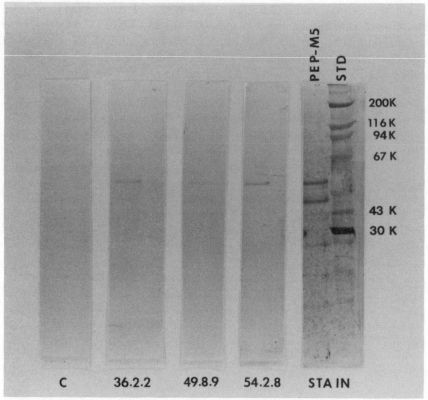

Figure 2. Western immunoblot of M type 5 protein extracted with pepsin (Pep M-5) after separation in a 10–20% slab gel gradient by SDS–PAGE. Pep M-5 protein was reacted separately with Amido Black (STAIN), monoclonal antibodies 36.2.2, 49.8.9 and 54.2.8 and a medium control containing mouse IgM (18 μg/ml). Antibody reactions were detected using goat anti-mouse IgM horseradish peroxidase conjugated antibody with development in 4-chloro-1-naphthol substrate. Stained molecular weight standards (STD) included myosin 200×10^3, β-galactosidase 116×10^3, phosphorylase B 94×10^3, bovine serum albumin 67×10^3, egg albumin 43×10^3, and carbonic anhydrase 30×10^3. Reproduced with the permission of Rockefeller University Press (Cunningham and Swerlick 1986).

$(50-60) \times 10^3$ range and high molecular weight range reacted with the antibodies. When pepsin-extracted type 5 M protein (Pep M-5) was reacted in Western immunoblots with the monoclonal antibodies, only 54.2.8 and 36.2.2 reacted with a protein piece near 58×10^3 while 49.8.9 did not react (Fig. 2). Another Pep M-5 preparation was obtained for comparison with our preparations from the laboratory of Dr Edwin Beachey, VA Medical Center, Memphis, Tennessee, USA. Monoclonal antibody 54.2.8 also reacted with a protein piece near 58×10^3 and weakly with smaller peptides $\leq 30 \times 10^3$ in this Pep M-5 preparation.

In addition to the reaction of Pep M-5 protein with monoclonal antibodies

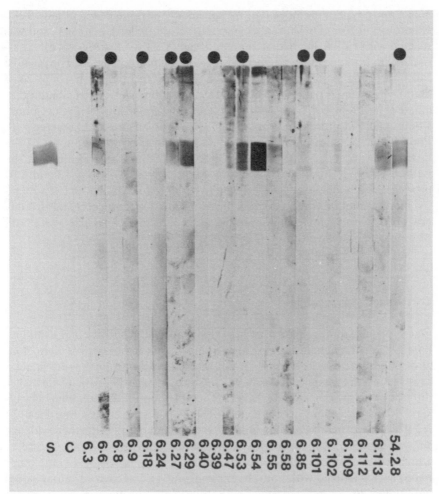

Figure 3. Western immunoblot of the cloned type 6 *Streptococcus pyogenes* M protein produced in *Escherichia coli*. The M-6 protein product was a generous gift from Dr Vincent A Fischetti, Rockefeller University, New York, USA. After separation of M-6 protein by electrophoresis in a 12% SDS–polyacrylamide gel, protein was electroblotted onto nitrocellulose and reacted with monoclonal antibody probe 54.2.8 and with a panel of new hybridoma antibodies 6.3, 6.6, 6.8, 6.9, 6.18, 6.24, 6.27, 6.29, 6.40, 6.39, 6.47, 6.54, 6.55, 6.58, 6.85, 6.101, 6.102, 1.109, 6.112, 6.113 prepared from spleens of BALB/c mice immunized with purified streptococcal membranes and subsequently boosted intravenously with type 5 M protein. Antibody reactions were developed after reaction with horseradish peroxidase goat anti-mouse polyvalent immunoglobulins and 4-chloro-1-naphthol substrate. M-6 protein was stained with Amido Black (S) and was reacted with cell culture medium containing 20% fetal bovine serum (C). Dots at the top of the blot indicate the antibodies which were also positive in immunoblots with rabbit skeletal muscle myosin.

36.2.2 and 54.2.8, the cloned type 6 M protein gene product was obtained as a generous gift from Dr Vincent A Fischetti, Rockefeller University, and was reacted with 54.2.8 and with a number of new heart and streptococcal cross-reactive hybridoma antibodies in Western immunoblots (Fig. 3). The positive reaction of monoclonal antibody 54.2.8 with M-6 protein is shown as compared with the new panel of cross-reactive hybridoma antibodies. Antibodies 6.6, 6.27, 6.29, 6.47, 6.53, 6.54, 6.55 and 6.113 were positive with the cloned, whole type 6 M protein molecule (Fig. 3). Only 6.54 and 6.113 reacted with Pep M-5 in Western immunoblots (data not shown), although most of the heart and streptococcal cross-reactive antibodies had been positive in the ELISA with Pep M-5 and cloned M-6. Hybridomas 6.3, 6.8, 6.18 and 6.39 produced antibodies which were negative with M proteins in both ELISA and the immunoblot but were very specific for group A streptococci and strongly cross-reactive with myosin. Antibodies 6.27, 6.29 and 6.53 reacted with both M-6 protein and myosin.

Cross-reactive autoantigens

Our previous studies of heart or host tissue antigens (Krisher and Cunningham 1985; Cunningham *et al.* 1986) have shown that cross-reactive monoclonal antibody probes 36.2.2 and 54.2.8 reacted with purified rabbit skeletal muscle myosin (Sigma Chemical Co., St Louis, Missouri, USA), while 49.8.9 did not react with myosin (Fig. 4). Monoclonal antibody 49.8.9 has always served as an excellent negative control since it produces IgM but does not react with myosin or M protein in the Western immunoblot. Further evidence showed that 36.2.2 reacted with skeletal muscle myosin but failed to react with purified human cardiac myosin (Cunningham *et al.* 1986). On the other hand, 54.2.8 reacted with both the skeletal and cardiac myosin. Monoclonal antibodies 36.2.2 reacted only with the light meromyosin subfragment (LMM) of the myosin heavy chain, while 54.2.8 reacted with light and heavy meromyosin (HMM) subfragments (Cunningham *et al.* 1986). Positions of the light and heavy meromyosin subfragments are shown in a diagram of myosin (Fig. 5). When the new hybridoma antibody panel was screened with myosin, 9/21 antibodies were positive with myosin (data not shown).

The specificities of the monoclonal antibody probes 36.2.2, 49.8.9, and 54.2.8 were investigated further by indirect immunofluorescence after their reaction with human fibroblasts (Cunningham and Swerlick 1986). Reaction of 54.2.8 with the nucleus was an interesting finding which was followed by competitive inhibitions with DNA and synthetic nucleotide homopolymers. Monoclonal antibody 54.2.8 was inhibited strongly by DNA, poly I and poly dT, and weakly by cardiolipin. Competitive inhibition ELISAs of 36.2.2, 49.8.9, and 54.2.8 with α-helical coiled-coil proteins revealed that 36.2.2 and 54.2.8 reacted with different proteins which inhibited their reactions with type

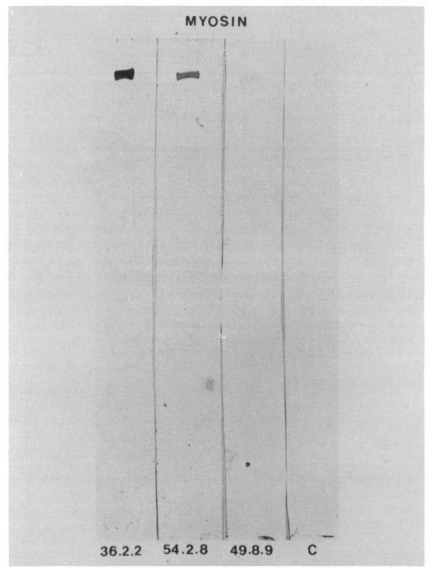

Figure 4. Reactivity of monoclonal antibodies 36.2.2, 54.2.8 and 49.8.9 with rabbit skeletal muscle myosin. C is the medium and antibody conjugate control. Immunoblots were developed with horseradish peroxidase labeled anti-mouse IgM conjugate and 4-chloro-1-naphthol substrate. Reproduced with the permission of Reedbooks Ltd (Cunningham *et al.* 1985).

5 group A streptococci (Cunningham and Swerlick 1986). Monoclonal antibody 36.2.2 reacted with a family of α-helical coiled-coil proteins including myosin, actin and keratin, but it did not react with DNA. However, 54.2.8 reacted with myosin and DNA and was blocked by anti-vimentin sera

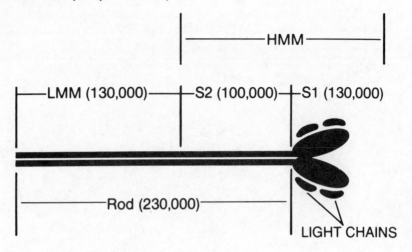

Diagram of the myosin molecule.

Figure 5. Diagram of the myosin molecule. Reproduced with the permission of the *Journal of Immunology* (Cunningham *et al.* 1986).

(Cunningham and Swerlick 1986). None of the antibodies were rheumatoid factors nor were they inhibitible by collagen, bovine serum albumin, lysozyme or histones.

Conclusion

The evidence demonstrates that monoclonal antibodies against streptococci and heart react with a number of heart and streptococcal antigens. Well characterized heart cross-reactive monoclonal antibody probes 54.2.8 and 36.2.2 reacted with Pep M-5 and with the cloned M-6 protein gene product. Reaction of a 58×10^3 protein in Pep M-5 preparations suggests that a larger piece of M protein may be required for reactivity, especially if conformational determinants are involved in the cross-reactivity with myosin. An alternative explanation may be that it is another protein sharing epitopes with M protein since the 58×10^3 protein reacted with anti-5 sera from CDC (gift of Dr Richard Facklam). Neither the 36.2.2 nor the 54.2.8 antibody probe was opsonic nor thought to be specific for the serospecific type 5 M protein epitopes. Study of a new panel of hybridoma antibodies revealed that several of the myosin and M-6 positive antibodies did not react with Pep M-5 in Western immunoblots. These data suggest that the presence of the carboxy terminus of M protein is necessary for the heart cross-reactive antibodies to react with the M protein molecule in the immunoblots. The carboxy-terminal region has been shown to have a conserved sequence among M serotypes (Scott *et al.* 1986). Therefore, the heart cross-reactive sequence or conformational structure might be expected to be shared among M types.

Reactions of the monoclonal antibody probes with myosin show that the cross-reactive epitopes reside in both the light meromyosin fragment and the α-helical coiled-tail region of myosin. Whether or not an epitope is in S-1 or the globular headpiece is yet to be determined. Figure 5 shows a diagram of the myosin molecule and subfragments. The observation that the monoclonal antibody 36.2.2 reacted only with the skeletal muscle myosin and 54.2.8 with both skeletal and cardiac myosin suggests that there are probably cross-reactive antibodies to cardiac myosin alone as well.

Our data support recent work (Manjula *et al.* 1985) on the α-helical structure of M protein. The amino acid sequence of M protein revealed a seven amino acid residue periodicity similar in comparison with tropomyosin, myosin and the desmin-keratin family of the α-helical proteins. Our monoclonal antibodies 36.2.2 and 54.2.8 react with these α-helical coiled-coil proteins and M protein.

A most intriguing finding was the reaction of monoclonal antibody probe 54.2.8 with the cell nucleus and DNA (Cunningham and Swerlick 1986). Although there are very few studies of the presence of anti-DNA antibodies in ARF, one study reported that 29% of the ARF patients tested were anti-nuclear antigen positive (Das *et al.* 1972). Anti-DNA murine monoclonal antibodies produced from mice susceptible to systemic lupus erythematosus reacted with endogenous bacteria including *Streptococcus faecalis* (Carroll *et al.* 1985). These antibodies also reacted with the nucleus, polyI, polydT, and cardiolipin (Andrezejiroski *et al.* 1981; Lafer *et al.* 1981). The antibodies found in mice susceptible to systemic lupus erythematosus appeared to be similar in activity to 54.2.8, and it could be speculated that they come from the same types of B cell clones. Since anti-DNA and anti-nuclear antibodies have been reported in autoimmune disorders (Shoenfeld and Schwartz 1984), the amplification of antibody producing clones directed at self antigens by infectious agents or micro-organisms is a possible mechanism for the production of some of the autoantibodies (Das *et al.* 1972; Shoenfeld and Schwartz 1984).

The polyspecific nature of these antibodies may explain the multiple antigen binding activities of anti-streptococcal sera with host tissues (Zabriskie and Freimer 1966; Lyampert *et al.* 1976; Husby *et al.* 1976), and the confusion over heart cross-reactivity associations with both streptococcal membrane and cell wall antigens such as M protein. The further investigation of the autoantibodies and antigens involved in the cross-reactivity between host antigens and streptococci is important in understanding the role of the streptococcus in autoantibody production and in the development of rheumatic heart disease.

Acknowledgements

The authors express gratitude to Carol Crossley for technical assistance and to Cricket Baughman for typing of the manuscript.

This work was supported by American Heart Association Grant no. 841337 funded in part by the American Heart Association Oklahoma Affiliates.

References

Andrezejiroski C Jr, Rauch J, Lafer E, Stollar B D, Schwartz R S 1981. Antigen-binding diversity and idiotype cross reactions among hybridoma autoantibodies to DNA, *Journal of Immunology* **126**: 226–31

Carroll P, Stafford D, Schwartz R S, Stollar B D 1985. Murine monoclonal anti-DNA autoantibodies bind to endogenous bacteria, *Journal of Immunology* **135**: 1086–90

Cunningham M W, Graves D C, Krisher K 1984. Murine monoclonal antibodies reactive with human heart and group A streptococcal membrane antigens, *Infection and Immunity* **46**: 34–41

Cunningham M W, Russell S M 1983. Study of heart reactive antibody in antisera and hybridoma culture fluids against group A streptococci, *Infection and Immunity* **42**: 531–8

Cunningham M W, Swerlick R A 1986. Polyspecificity of anti-streptococcal murine monoclonal antibodies and their implications in autoimmunity, *Journal of Experimental Medicine* **164**: 998–1012

Cunningham M W, Krisher K, Graves D C 1985. Immunological similarities: human heart and group A streptococci, in Y Kimura, S Kotami, Y Shiokawa (eds) *Proceedings of the 9th Lancefield International Symposium on Streptococci and Streptococcal Diseases; Recent Advances in Streptococci and Streptococcal Diseases.* Reedbooks Ltd, pp 275–7

Cunningham M W, Hall N K, Krisher K K, Spanier A M 1986. A study of anti-group A streptococcal monoclonal antibodies cross reactive with myosin, *Journal of Immunology* **136**: 293–8

Dale J B, Beachey E H 1982. Protective antigenic determinant of streptococcal M protein shared with sarcolemmal membrane protein of human heart, *Journal of Experimental Medicine* **156**: 1165–76

Das S K, Cassidy J T, Petlz R E 1972. Antibodies against heart muscle and nuclear constituents in cardiomyopathy, *American Heart Journal* **83**: 159–66

Fischetti V A, Manjula B N 1982. Biologic and immunologic implications of the structural relationship between streptococcal M protein and mammalian tropomyosin, in L Weinstein, B N Fields (eds) *Seminars in Infectious Disease*, vol 4, J B Robbins, J C Hill, J C Sadoff (eds) *Bacterial vaccines*, pp 411–18. Thieme-Stratton Inc., New York

Goldstein I, Reybeyrotte P, Parlebas J, Halpern B 1968. Isolation from heart valves of glycopeptides which share immunological properties with *Streptococcus hemolyticus* group A polysaccharides, *Nature (London)* **219**: 866–8

Husby G, van de Rijn I. Zabriskie J B, Abdin Z H, Williams R C Jr 1976. Antibodies reacting with cytoplasm of subthalmic and caudate nuclei neurons in chorea and acute rheumatic fever, *Journal of Experimental Medicine* **144**: 1094–110

Jones K F, Manjula B N, Johnston K H, Hollingshead S K, Scott J R, Fischetti V A 1985. Location of variable and conserved epitopes among the multiple serotypes of streptococcal M protein, *Journal of Experimental Medicine* **161**: 623–8

Kaplan M H 1963. Immunologic relation of streptococcal and tissue antigens. I. Properties of an antigen in certain strains of Group A streptococci exhibiting immunologic cross-reaction with human heart tissue, *Journal of Immunology* **90**: 595–606

Krisher K, Cunningham M W 1985. Myosin: a link between streptococci and heart, *Science* **227**: 413–15

Lafer E M, Rauch J, Andrezejewski C Jr, Mudd D, Furie B, Schwartz R S, Stollar B D 1981.

Polyspecific monoclonal lupus autoantibodies reactive with both polynucleotides and phospholipids, *Journal of Experimental Medicine* **153**: 897–909

Lyampert I M, Borodiyuk N A, Ugryumova G A 1968. The reaction of heart and other organ extracts with the sera of animal immunized with group A streptococci, *Immunology* **15**: 845–54

Lyampert I M, Beletskrya L V, Borodiyuk N A, Gnezditskaya E V, Rassokhina I I, Danilova T A 1976. A cross-reactive antigen of thymus and skin epithelial cells common with the polysaccharide of group A streptococci, *Immunology* **31**: 47–55

Manjula B N, Trus B L, Fischetti V A 1985. Presence of two distinct regions in the coiled-coil structure of streptococcal pep M5 protein: relationship to mammalian coiled-coil proteins and implications to its biological properties, *Proceedings of the National Academy of Sciences USA* **82**: 1064–68

Phillips G N Jr, Flicker P F, Cohen C, Manjula B N, Fischetti V A 1981. Streptococcal M protein: α-helical coiled-coil structure and arrangement on the cell surface, *Proceedings of the National Academy of Sciences USA* **78**: 4689–93

Poirer T P, Kehoe M A, Dale J B, Timmis K N, Beachey E H 1985. Expression of protective and cardiac tissue cross-reactive epitopes of type 5 streptococcal M protein in *Escherichia coli*, *Infection and Immunity* **48**: 198–203

Scott J R, Hollingshead S K, Fischetti V A 1986. Homologous regions within M protein genes in group A streptococci of different serotypes, *Infection and Immunity* **52**: 609–12

Shoenfeld Y, Schwartz R S 1984. Immunologic and genetic factors in autoimmune diseases, *New England Journal of Medicine* **311**: 1019–29

van de Rijn I, Zabriskie J B, McCarty M 1977. Group A streptococcal antigens cross-reactive with myocardium. Purification of heart-reactive antibody and isolation and characterization of the streptococcal antigen, *Journal of Experimental Medicine* **146**: 579–99

Zabriskie J B 1966. Mimetic relationships between the group A streptococci and mammalian tissues, *Advances in Immunology* **7**: 147–88

Zabriskie J B, Freimer E H 1966. An immunological relationship between the group A streptococcus and mammalian muscle, *Journal of Experimental Medicine* **124**: 661–78

Zabriskie J B, Hsu K C, Seegal B C 1970. Heart reactive antibody associated with rheumatic fever: characterization and diagnostic significance, *Clinical and Experimental Immunology* **7**: 147–59

Antigens shared by *Streptococcus mutans* and cardiac muscle – a reevaluation

Murray W Stinson; Franklin J Swartzwelder; Russell J Nisengard; Boris Albini

Schools of Medicine and Dental Medicine, State University of New York at Buffalo, Buffalo, New York 14214, USA

Introduction

Dental caries has been a troublesome infectious disease of man since prehistoric times. Worldwide, it is far more prevalent today than ever before and is one of the most common diseases of bacterial etiology. The progressive demineralization and destruction of tooth enamel that is characteristic of caries is due primarily to lactic acid elaborated by the mass of bacteria growing on the tooth as dental plaque. The principal cariogenic bacterium is *Streptococcus mutans*, a viridans group streptococcus that can also cause subacute bacterial endocarditis (Harder *et al.* 1974).

Colonization of tooth surfaces by *S. mutans* and subsequent development of dental plaque can be effectively inhibited in experimental animals by the presence of specific sIgA in saliva (reviewed by McGhee and Michalek 1981; Hamada *et al.* 1986). Whereas this indicates that immunization of humans with *S. mutans* antigens is a feasible approach to caries protection, there are several obstacles to the development of a practical vaccine. The most formidable is the likelihood of adverse side-effects. Serum antibodies produced in rabbits as a result of parenteral administration of *S. mutans* antigens have been found to bind *in vitro* to cardiac muscle components (discussed below). This observation can be interpreted to mean that certain streptococcal antigens share epitopes with components of host tissue and that immunization may induce serious immunopathological changes similar to those seen in acute rheumatic fever. It should be emphasized at the outset that while the existence of heart-reactive antibodies in rabbit anti-*S. mutans* sera is well documented, their cross-reactivity with bacterial antigens has not been proved unequivocally. For this reason, we will refer to them as heart-reactive antibodies rather than the more commonly used designation, cross-reactive antibodies. In this paper, we will discuss three possible mechanisms by which *S. mutans* may induce the production of heart-reactive antibodies (Table 1).

Table 1 Mechanisms by which *S. mutans* may induce formation of heart-reactive antibodies

1. Epitopes shared by components of bacteria and cardiac muscle may stimulate production of cross-reactive antibodies.
2. Nonspecific stimulation of self-reactive B lymphocytes by bacterial components may result in production of autoantibodies.
3. Damage to muscle by *S. mutans* components may cause exposure of hidden self antigens and subsequent autoantibody production.

Streptococcus mutans-induced heart-reactive antibodies

The immunological properties of *S. mutans* components have been examined using the rabbit as an experimental model. van de Rijn *et al.* (1976) first reported that intravenous injection of *S. mutans* resulted in the production of heart-reactive antibodies that could be detected by indirect immunofluorescence (IIF) assays on thin sections of cardiac muscle. These antibodies were detected in 1:5 dilutions of sera raised to six bacteria representing serogroups *a*, *b*, *c* and *d*. Cross-reactivity of these antibodies with streptococci was decided on the basis of the ability of *S. mutans* to absorb heart-reactive antibodies from these sera; IIF reactions were reduced from a level of 3+ to 1+ within the same serum dilution. Hughes *et al.* (1980), using IIF, indirect radioimmunoassay (IRIA) and crossed-immunoelectrophoresis (CIE), also detected low quantities of heart-reactive antibodies in the sera of rabbits immunized with *S. mutans* Ingbritt. Although the actual serum dilutions were not reported, IRIA results indicated that heart-reactive IgG increased only 83% during the immunization period of four to eight months. Absorption of anti-*S. mutans* sera with intact bacteria abolished the ability of these sera to precipitate heart components in CIE. When extracts of *S. mutans* were tested against an antiserum raised to human cardiac muscle, two precipitin peaks were formed, designated ID and IF. Antigen IF of *S. mutans* was subsequently identified by Russell (1979) as a protein of M_r 190,000. The very low concentrations of heart-reactive antibodies produced in rabbits following immunization with *S. mutans* was further emphasized by Ferretti *et al.* (1980). To obtain precipitation of the heterologous antigens in CIE, it was necessary to concentrate the serum before its incorporation into the agarose; final dilution was approximately 1:2.

Quantitative analyses of the antibody response in *S. mutans*-immunized rabbits and the ability of bacterial components to absorb heart-reactive antibodies was reported by Stinson *et al.* (1983) and Nisengard *et al.* (1983). Because the reproducibility of the IIF and IRIA in our laboratories was within one doubling dilution of serum, a difference of two serial doubling dilutions (400%) between the reactivities of the antiserum and preimmunization serum was considered significant. Similarly, absorption of serum with antigen should reduce antibody activity at least two dilutions or 75%. Using these criteria, only three of the 14 *S. mutans* strains tested elicited heart-reactive antibodies in rabbits during the six to ten month immunization period. A concentrated study on two of these, *S. mutans* MT703 and *S. mutans* K1R (now *S. sobrinus* K1R), revealed that 23 of 34 antisera (67%) reacted with monkey cardiac muscle components in IIF assay; 100% were positive by IRIA. Titers ranged from 20 to 40 in IIF and from 320 to 1280 in IRIA. The heart-reactive antibodies reached maximum titers between three and six months after the start of immunization. The difference between the activities of preimmunization and hyperimmune sera ranged between three and six serial doubling dilutions. Based upon IRIA, heart-reactive antibodies were effectively absorbed by alkali-solubilized *S. mutans* antigens but only weakly by equivalent amounts of whole bacteria, cytoplasmic membranes and cell-free extracts. The first of these preparations also removed much larger quantities of *S. mutans*-reactive antibodies. A consistent observation in each of these studies was the unexpected difficulty in absorbing heart-reactive antibodies with *S. mutans*. Explanations proposed to explain this include that the bacterial antigen is present in very low concentrations or is relatively inaccessible to antibodies because of its normal location.

The tempting conclusion of serum absorption experiments is that some antibodies cross-react with bacteria and cardiac muscle. The very low quantities of heart-reactive antibodies in these sera and the difficulty in accurately measuring them necessitates some caution in their interpretation. In the experiments described by Stinson *et al.* (1983), the extensive immune precipitation obtained with *S. mutans* antigens may have caused a nonspecific reduction of heart-reactive antibodies. Ferretti *et al.* (1980) addressed this problem by incorporating an internal standard (antibodies to bovine serum albumin (BSA) in the antiserum to be absorbed. The reactivities of the serum before and after absorption with streptococci were compared by rocket immunoelectrophoresis. Precipitation of BSA was achieved with both absorbed and unabsorbed sera, whereas heart components were precipitated by only the unabsorbed serum. The conclusion that the removal of heart-reactive antibodies was the result of cross-reactivity with *S. mutans* can still be debated because the BSA pecipitin peak in the absorbed serum was 30% taller than that obtained in the unabsorbed serum. This indicates that 30% of the anti-BSA immunoglobulins were removed as a result of nonspecific absorption. From our experience, a 30% loss of heart-reactive antibodies could cause this precipitin peak to disappear because the peak, obtained with heart components verses unabsorbed serum, was very faint and incomplete.

To resolve the question on the specificity of serum absorption, we have expanded upon the approach of Ferretti *et al.* (1980). A rabbit anti-*S. mutans* MT703 serum that also contained heart-reactive antibodies was mixed with a small quantity of rabbit anti-BSA serum so that its final titer was identical to the heart-reactive antibodies. A portion of the composite serum was then absorbed with intact *S. mutans* MT703, grown in chemically defined medium. Both the absorbed and unabsorbed serum fractions were assayed by Bio-Dot immunoassay; antibody reactivities were reduced 99.9% on *S. mutans*, 75% on BSA, rabbit cardiac muscle and myosin. This indicates that very low-titer heterologous antibodies in hyperimmune serum are susceptible to nonspecific absorption by the homologous antigens or resulting immune complexes. Consequently, absorption data in support of antibody cross-reactions with *S. mutans* and cardiac muscle cannot be considered reliable.

Definitive evidence of the cross-reactions of the antibodies in rabbit anti-*S. mutans* sera would be provided simply and most directly by fused precipitin lines in agar gel double diffusion assays or tandem rocket immunoelec-trophoresis in which appropriate extracts of bacteria and cardiac muscle are placed in adjacent wells. These techniques have been tried many times without success. Lines of immunological identity, if formed, are obscured by the multitude of precipitin lines seen with the homologous system and the diffuse, fuzzy lines obtained with many components of animal tissue. More-over, it is not known if the relevant antigens are even precipitated by reaction with antibodies. Still, these assay procedures should be used again if prospec-tive antigens are obtained in purified form.

Interaction of heart-reactive antibodies with cardiac muscle tissue

Analyses of rabbit anti-*S. mutans* sera by IIF on thin sections of cardiac muscle have been undertaken by several research groups with somewhat different results. van de Rijn *et al.* (1976) used longitudinally cut human tissue sections that were extracted with acetone and found diffuse sarcoplas-mic staining with increased staining intensity along the sarcolemmal sheaths. Hughes *et al.* (1980) saw prominent cross-striational patterns as well as sheath staining on sections of human cardiac muscle that was air-dried prior to assay. IIF assays on monkey and human cardiac muscle that was maintained at −70 °C until the time of assay showed almost exclusively cross-striational staining with anti-*S. mutans* sera (Nisengard *et al.* 1983; Stinson *et al.* 1980, 1983). Our laboratories also determined in preliminary experiments that the different methods of tissue preservation may be responsible for the various IIF staining. When acetone fixation was used, these antisera gave diffuse staining patterns similar to that described by van de Rijn *et al.* (1976). It is not clear whether the sarcolemmal sheath staining seen on solvent-treated tissue sections is the result of unmasking of tissue components by extraction of lipids or a condensation of sarcoplasmic components along the internal surface of the sheath as a result of extreme dehydration of the muscle fiber.

Identification of muscle components reactive with *S. mutans*-induced antibodies

The crossed-immunoelectrophoresis studies of Hughes *et al.* (1980) and Ferretti *et al.* (1980) detected two components (HL1 and HL2) in extracts of human cardiac muscle that precipitated with anti-*S. mutans* sera. The precipitin peaks showed immunological identity. Two immunologically distinct antigens were detected in monkey muscle by Stinson *et al.* (1983) using similar CIE techniques. The monkey heart components showed electrophoretic mobilities unlike those reported for human heart components. In each of these studies, the heart components were precipitated by rabbit anti-*S. mutans* sera but not by pooled normal sera or preimmunization sera. Although this serological assay system has provided some valuable insight into the complexity of the interaction of antibodies with cardiac muscle components, its usefulness is severely limited by its relative insensitivity.

Most recently, Western blot assays have been used to resolve both cardiac muscle and *S. mutans* components. This assay combines the high resolution of sodium dodecyl sulfate–polyacrylamide gel electrophoresis with the extreme sensitivity of radioimmunoassay. Ayakawa *et al.* (1985) found that rabbit anti-*S. mutans* BHT (now *S. rattus* BHT) serum bound to several components of human cardiac muscle, M_r 69,000, 54,000, 41,000 and 32,000. Also, rabbit anti-human heart serum contained antibodies that bound to *S. rattus* components of M_r 82,000, 62,000, 46,000 and 42,000 as well as several minor bands. None of these antibodies were detected in sera of nonimmunized rabbits when tested at the same dilutions. This study clearly shows that antibodies reactive to heterologous antigens are produced concurrently with those to the immunogen; however, it is not clear whether the antibodies are separate and unrelated or cross-react with bacteria and heart.

In our laboratories (Swartzwelder *et al.* 1986), Western blot assays with rabbit anti-*S. mutans* MT703 sera have revealed 10 or more components in sodium dodecyl sulfate extracts of human, monkey and rabbit cardiac muscle. The strongest antibody reactions were with components of M_r 205,000, 160,000, 135,000 and 70,000. Similar dilutions of preimmunization sera from these animals showed no antibody reactivities on tissue extracts; however, lower dilutions (e.g. 1:10) gave banding patterns that were nearly identical to those seen with the immune sera. Importantly, a few of these normal rabbit sera with heart-reactive antibodies did not contain detectable antibodies to *S. mutans* components as determined by IIF, Western blot and Bio-Dot immunoassay. This indicates that an immunological relationship between *S. mutans* MT703 and the heart-reactive antibodies in these sera is highly unlikely.

We have determined that the M_r 205,000 heart component detected in Western blot assays is myosin and that 14 of 18 normal rabbit sera (78%) showed anti-myosin activities at serum dilutions of 1:10 to 1:80. Of the immune sera, 100% have antibodies to myosin with dilutions as high as 1:320.

We have been unable to obtain convincing proof for an immunological relationship between myosin and *S. mutans*. Absorption of the serum with intact bacteria reduced reactivity to myosin by 75%. On the other hand, antibodies that were carefully affinity-purified on a column of rabbit muscle myosin–Sepharose 4B, bound strongly to myosin in human, monkey, rabbit cardiac muscle in Western blot assays, but did not bind to *S. mutans* components in Western blots, or to intact or disrupted bacteria in Bio-Dot immunoassays. Nor has it been possible for us to show that antibodies that were affinity-purified on a mixture of bacterial proteins, precipitated from culture medium with ammonium sulfate, react with myosin in these various serological assays. These results indicate that naturally occurring antibodies to cardiac muscle components are present in the sera of most unimmunized rabbits. Immunization with streptococci does not appear to stimulate production of new antibody to cardiac muscle but rather appears to boost the antibody response of pre-existing clones of B lymphocytes to the cardiac muscle components. It is possible that components of the bacterial cell wall are responsible for this effect. Serotype polysaccharides, peptidoglycan and lipoteichoic acid of *S. mutans* have been shown to possess mitogenic activities for murine and rat lymphoid cells (Torii *et al.* 1986; Morisaki *et al.* 1986). Since these substances were present in all vaccines used to immunize rabbits, the appearance of heart-reactive antibodies may be the result of polyclonal B cell activation.

The presence of low levels of naturally occurring, circulating autoantibodies has been well documented in man (for reviews see Grabar 1983; Mackay 1983; Beutner and Kumar 1985). Specific autoantibodies to heart, liver and brain were detected in 18 of 18 normal human sera by Daar and Fabre (1981). Shu *et al.* (1975) also detected antinuclear antibodies in the sera of 45% of healthy blood donors. Autoantibodies to smooth muscle, gastric parietal cells and thyroid cytoplasm were also found at lower incidences. Guilbert *et al.* (1982) and Dighiero *et al.* (1982) reported extensive studies on the ubiquity of naturally occurring autoantibodies in sera of normal donors; using specific immunoabsorbents, autoantibodies were found to tubulin, actin, thyroglobulin, myoglobin, fetuin, transferrin, albumin, cytochrome *c* and collagen. It has been proposed that these autoantibodies serve a positive physiological role in the animal by promoting phagocytosis and clearing damaged or senescent components of tissue (Grabar 1983; Beutner and Kumar 1985). The quantity of these antibodies in a given serum may reflect the antigenic burden in the animal; i.e. when hidden self antigens are released in quantities that are not promptly degraded enzymatically, these intact components remain in circulation and stimulate autoantibody formation. Thus, injection of streptococcal components that damage muscle tissue by direct toxicity or *in situ* immune complex formation may indirectly induce antibody formation to cardiac muscle. Physical injury to cardiac muscle is known to elicit autoantibody formation in man; 50% of postcardiotomy patients produce anti-heart antibodies (DeScheerder *et al.* 1984). Moreover, polyclonal B cell activation by peptidoglycan and lipoteichoic acid (LTA) may cause production of autoantibodies (Weigle *et al.* 1972).

Interaction of heart-reactive antibodies *in vivo*

Myocardial lesions in hearts of rabbits infected with *S. mutans* components have been reported. Hughes *et al.* (1980) detected lesions in 3 of 6 rabbits that were characterized by a subacute infiltration of macrophages with smaller numbers of lymphocytes and polymorphonuclear cells, surrounding a small focus of degenerating muscle fibers. Stinson *et al.* (1983) found that 4 of 16 *S. mutans*-immunized rabbits contained IgG and IgA deposits in cardiac muscle. Immunofluorescence revealed granular patterns in the sarcolemma and along the capillaries (Fig. 1A). Hematoxylin and eosin stain revealed perivascular infiltrations by polymorphonuclear and plasma cells in the hearts of these rabbits (Fig. 1B). The relationship of these myocardial lesions to the Aschoff nodules of acute rheumatic fever has not been determined. Nor is it clear whether the immunoglobulins are bound directly to heart components or to *S. mutans* components bound to heart (Stinson *et al.* 1984).

Interaction of *S. mutans* components with cardiac muscle

Interpretation of early studies of *S. mutans*-induced heart-reactive antibodies are complicated by the nature of the medium used to grow the bacteria. Todd–Hewitt broth, an infusion of bovine heart, has traditionally been the medium of choice because of the luxuriant growth it supports. Surface components of *S. mutans* have been found to bind selectively to low and high molecular weight cardiac muscle components from Todd–Hewitt broth during their growth (Stinson and Jones 1983). These adsorbed medium components can remain on the surface of the bacteria and react with heart-reactive antibodies in subsequent serological assays. Although actual contribution of these tissue components in the immune response to the streptococci has not been defined, the implication for serious complications are clear. Substitution of a chemically defined medium for the growth of *S. mutans* has been reported recently (Ferretti *et al.* 1980; Stinson *et al.* 1983). Interestingly, these bacteria also caused the formation of heart-reactive antibodies in rabbits.

An alternative hypothesis for the mechanisms by which *S. mutans* causes production of heart-reactive antibodies was proposed by Stinson *et al.* (1980). Cell surface adhesins, present in the injected vaccine, may be carried via the blood to cardiac muscle where it accumulates through direct binding interactions. Muscle fibers may be injured by toxicity of the adhesin or through inflammation induced by *in situ* reaction of the adhesin with antibody and

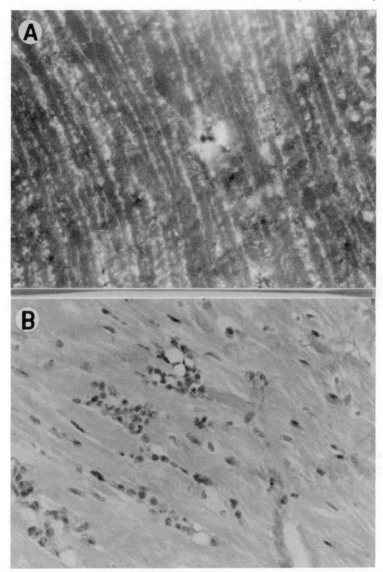

Figure 1. Micrographs of rabbit cardiac muscle obtained after 24 weeks of immunization with *S. mutans* MT703. (A) Direct staining with FITC-antibodies to rabbit IgG showing perivascular immune deposits (×125). (B) Hematoxylin and eosin stain showing focal infiltration by PMN and plasma cells (×200).

complement. The release of hidden self antigens would then lead directly to autoantibody formation. Indeed, surface components extracted from several serotypes of oral streptococci bind *in vitro* to sarcolemmal sheaths and blood vessels of monkey and human cardiac muscle. Our recent studies show that five bacterial proteins (M_r 170,000, 57,000, 47,000, 40,000 and 32,000) were consistently eluted from homogenized cardiac muscle that had been preincubated with alkali-extracted components of *S. mutans* MT703 (Stinson *et al.* 1986). Analysis of culture medium indicated that these proteins are released by the streptococci during their growth (unpublished data). In addition, lipoteichoic acid from streptococci has been reported by Simpson *et al.* (1982) to bind to human heart cells in culture and exhibit potent cytotoxicity. Although the pathogenic activities of all these *S. mutans* components have yet to be determined in an animal model, the implication of their presence in streptococcal vaccines used to immunize rabbits cannot be overemphasized.

Summary

The injection of *S. mutans* components into rabbits often results in the production of heart-reactive antibodies in the blood. These antibodies are in very low concentrations and bind *in vitro* to cross-striations of muscle fibers of freshly collected, native cardiac muscle. Heart-reactive antibodies can be removed from anti-*S. mutans* sera by absorption with *S. mutans* cells and extracts; however, it appears that this effect is most likely nonspecific. Conclusive proof of serological cross-reactivity is still lacking. Western blot immunoassays indicate that nonimmunized rabbits have naturally occurring antibodies to several heart components and that their concentration is increased by immunization with *S. mutans*. We now believe that this effect is most likely due to either polyclonal B cell activation or injury to muscle fibers by *S. mutans* components that exposes hidden self antigens and stimulates increased autoantibody formation. The relationship, if any, between the production of heart-reactive antibodies and pathological states in *S. mutans*-immunized animals remains to be determined.

Acknowledgements

This work was supported by Public Health Service Grant DE05696 from the National Institute of Dental Research. We thank our previous and present coworkers for their contributions to this work.

References

Ayakawa G Y, Siegel J L, Crowley P J, Bleiweis A S 1985. Immunochemistry of the *Streptococcus mutans* BHT cell membrane: detection of determinants cross-reactive with human heart tissue, *Infection and Immunity* **48**: 280–6

Beutner E H, Kumar V 1985. Autoantibodies in health and disease, in F Milgrom, C J Abeyounis, B Albini (eds) *Antibodies: Protective, Destructive, and Regulatory Role*. Karger, Basel, p. 158–63

Daar A S, Fabre J W 1981. Organ-specific IgM autoantibodies to liver, heart and brain in man: generalized occurrence and possible functional significance in normal individuals and studies in patients with multiple sclerosis, *Clinical and Experimental Immunology* **45**: 37–47

DeScheerder I, Wulfrank D, van Renterghem L, Sabbe L, Robbrecht D, Clement D, Derom F, Plum J, Verdonk G 1984. Association of anti-heart antibodies and circulating immune complexes in the post-pericardiotomy syndrome, *Clinical and Experimental Immunology* **57**: 423–8

Dighiero G, Guilbert B and Avrameas S 1982. Naturally occurring antibodies against nine common antigens in humans sera. II. High incidence of monoclonal Ig exhibiting antibody activity against actin and tubulin and sharing antibody specificities with natural antibodies, *Journal of Immunology* **128**: 2788–92

Ferretti J J, Shea C, Humphrey M W 1980. Cross-reactivity of *Streptococcus mutans* antigens and human heart tissue, *Infection and Immunity* **30**: 69–73

Grabar P 1983. Autoantibodies and the physiological role of immunoglobulins, *Immunology Today* **4**: 337–40

Guilbert B, Dighiero G, Avrameas S 1982. Naturally occurring antibodies against nine common antigens in human sera: detection, isolation and characterization, *Journal of Immunology* **128**: 2779–87

Hamada S, Michalek S M, Kiyono H, Menaker L, McGhee J R (eds) 1986. *Molecular Microbiology and Immunology of Streptococcus mutans*. Elsevier, Amsterdam

Harder E J, Wilkowske C J, Washington J A II, Geraci J E 1974. *Streptococcus mutans* endocarditis, *Annals of Internal Medicine* **80**: 364–8

Hughes M, MacHardy S M, Sheppard A J, Woods N C 1980. Evidence for an immunological relationship between *Streptococcus mutans* and human cardiac tissue, *Infection and Immunity* **27**: 576–88

Mackay I R 1983. Natural autoantibodies to the fore – forbidden clones to the rear, *Immunology Today* **4**: 340–2

McGhee J R, Michalek S M 1981. Immunology of dental caries: microbial aspects and local immunity, *Annual Review of Microbiology* **35**: 595–638

Morisaki I, Torii M, Kimura S, Koga T, Yamamoto T, Hamada S, Kiyono H, Michalek S M, McGhee J R 1986. Lymphoid cell response to cell wall components of *Streptococcus mutans*. II. Peptidoglycan and lipoteichoic acid, in S Hamada, S M Michalek, H Kiyono, L Menaker, J R McGhee (eds) *Molecular Microbiology and Immunobiology of Streptococcus mutans*. Elsevier, Amsterdam, pp 237–48

Nisengard R J, Stinson M W, Pelonero L 1983. Immunologic cross-reactivity between *Streptococcus mutans* and mammalian tissues, in E H Beutner, R J Nisengard, A Albini (eds) *Defined Immunofluorescence and Related Cytochemical Methods. Annals of the New York Academy of Sciences* **420**: 401–9

Russell R R B 1979. Wall-associated protein antigens of *Streptococcus mutans*, *Journal of General Microbiology* **114**: 109–15

Shu S, Nisengard R J, Hale W L, Beutner E H 1975. Incidence and titers of antinuclear, antismooth muscle and other autoantibodies in blood donors, *Journal of Laboratory and Clinical Medicine* **86**: 259–65

Simpson W A, Dale J B, Beachey E H 1982. Cytotoxicity of the glycolipid region of streptococcal lipoteichoic acid for cultures of human heart cells, *Journal of Laboratory and Clinical Medicine* **99**: 1180–6

Stinson M W, Albini B, Nisengard R J 1986. Adverse effects of *Streptococcus mutans* antigens on host tissues, in S Hamada, S M Michalek, H Kiyono, L Menaker, J R McGhee (eds) *Molecular Microbiology and Immunobiology of Streptococcus mutans*. Elsevier, Amsterdam, pp 307–18

Stinson M W, Jones C A 1983. Binding of Todd–Hewitt Broth antigens by *Streptococcus mutans*, *Infection and Immunity* **40**: 1140–5

Stinson M W, Nisengard R J, Bergey E J 1980. Binding of streptococcal antigens to muscle tissue *in vitro*, *Infection and Immunity* **27**: 604–13

Stinson M W, Nisengard R J, Neiders M E, Albini A 1983. Serology and tissue lesions in rabbits immunized with *Streptococcus mutans*, *Journal of Immunology* **131**: 3021–7

Stinson M W, Barua P K, Bergey E J, Nisengard R J, Neiders M E, Albini B 1984. Binding of *Streptococcus mutans* antigens to heart and kidney basement membranes, *Infection and Immunity* **46**: 145–51

Swartzwelder F J, Albini B, Stinson M W 1986. Naturally-occurring antibodies to cardiac muscle components, *Abstracts of the Annual Meeting of the American Society for Microbiology*, p 29, B33

Torii M, Kumura S, Kiyono H, Michalek S, Hamada S, McGhee J R 1986. Lymphoid cell responses to cell wall components of *Streptococcus mutans*. I. Serotype carbohydrate, in S Hamada, S Michalek, H Kiyono, L Menaker, J R McGhee (eds) *Molecular Microbiology and Immunobiology of Streptococcus mutans*, Elsevier, Amsterdam, pp 227–36

van de Rijn I, Bleiweis A S, Zabriskie J B 1976. Antigens in *Streptococcus mutans* cross-react with human heart muscle, *Journal of Dental Research* **55c**: 59–64

Weigle W O, Chiller J M, Habicht G S 1972. Effect of immunological unresponsiveness on different cell populations, *Transplantation Reviews* **8**: 3–25

8 Abstracts of Poster Presentations

Immunogenicity of Measles Virus Glycoproteins Associated to Liposomes and Iscoms

O Bakouche*; B Mougin†; D M Gerlier*

* *INSERM U. 218, Centre Léon Bérard, 69373 Lyon Cedex 08, France*
† *INSERM U. 51, 1 pl J Renaut, 69371 Lyon Cedex 08, France*

The immunogenicity of measles virus hemagglutinin (HA) and fusion (F) glycoproteins presented as soluble antigens, liposomes, Iscoms or as whole virus was studied in syngeneic rats. HA and F presented in artificial or natural vehicles induced *in vitro* a primary cellular proliferative response and primed *in vivo* for the generation of an *in vitro* anamnestic response. Soluble HA and F induced a radiosensitive immunosuppression both *in vivo* and *in vitro*. Therefore, the use of a vector for an antigen could improve its immunogenicity by bypassing a suppressive mechanism and this was shown to be dependent on accessory cells. Preliminary data indicate that the vector may act by modifying the uptake and processing of HA and F by macrophages.

Immune responses of Melanoma Patients Undergoing Vaccinia Melanoma Oncolysate (VMO) Immunotherapy

J A Bash*; E S Darnell*; M K Wallack*; E Leftheriotis†

* *Department of Surgery, Mount Sinai Medical Center, Miami Beach, Florida, USA*
† *Institut Merieux, Lyon, France*

A vaccine prepared from vaccinia-infected melanoma cell lines (VMO) was administered intradermally in weekly or bimonthly injections to stage I and II melanoma patients. Blood samples drawn before treatment and at three-month intervals during treatment provided both serum and lymphocytes for *in vitro* assays. Serological assays included a protein A-binding (rosette) assay and a leukocyte-dependent antibody (LDA) cytolytic (^{51}Cr release) assay. Cellular assays included blastogenic ^{3}H-thymidine incorporation responses to phytohemagglutinin, VMO, or mitomycin-C-treated stimulator cells as well as cytolysis (^{51}Cr release) of target cells before and after culture with interleukin-2. The majority of patients developed melanoma-reactive antibody, although lytic activity did not correlate with binding activity. Cellular mechanisms were suppressed during the initial 3–6 months of treatment but then increased during the final 9–12 months. The interrelationship of these immunological parameters and clinical courses remains to be determined.

Immunoprotective Capacity of a *Candida albicans* Ribosomal Vaccine in Mice

A Bebely; A M Pinel; G Normier; L Dussourd d'Hinterland

Centre d'Immunologie et de Biologie P. FABRE, Castres, France

The aim of this study was to demonstrate the protective capacity of a ribosomal vaccine against *Candida albicans* infection in mice. Vaccine was prepared with ribosomes from *Candida albicans* plus membrane proteoglycans (MPG) from *Klebsiella pneumoniae* as adjuvant. Its immunoprotective capacity was studied in NMRI mice as a function of dose and route of administration. Six days after subcutaneous or oral immunization with four different doses, groups of mice were infected i.v. with *Candida albicans* serotypes A or B. More than half the mice immunized subcutaneously at the two-dose level survived. With oral vaccination maximum survival was achieved with the four-dose level. This study indicates that oral or subcutaneous immunization with a ribosomal vaccine induces significant protection in mice against lethal infection of *Candida albicans*.

Potentiation of Immune Response to a Melanoma Antigen Vaccine

J-C Bystryn; R Oratz; M Harris; R Roses; J Speyer

New York University School of Medicine and the Kaplan Cancer Center, New York 10016, USA

To identify methods of enhancing the immunogenicity of tumor vaccines in man, a polyvalent melanoma vaccine prepared from shed material was used to immunize 55 patients with malignant melanoma. The ability of different immunization schedules, alum, or low-dose cyclophosphamide to augment humoral and/or cellular immune responses to melanoma was compared after two months of immunization. Immunization every two weeks with an intermediate dose of vaccine was more immunogenic than weekly immunization with escalating doses. Immune responses were induced more frequently in stage II than in stage III patients. Alum or pretreatment with $300 \, mg/m^2$ cyclophosphamide three days prior to each immunization did not augment immunogenicity. There was a reciprocal relationship between induction of humoral and cellular immune responses.

Lipopolysaccharide (LPS) Antibody (Ab) Induced by *E. coli* J5 Vaccination Enhances Complement (C)-Mediated Bacteriolysis of *N. gonorrhoeae*

P A Dale; P A Rice

Maxwell Finland Laboratory for Infectious Diseases, Boston City Hospital, Boston University School of Medicine, Boston, Massachusetts, USA

The LPSs of enteric Gram-negative bacteria and *N. gonorrhoeae* may share antigenic determinants which are targets of bactericidal Ab. Normal human IgM directed against LPS is bactericidal for serum-sensitive (SS) gonococci. Immune IgG against LPS is often bactericidal for gonococci that resist killing (SR) by normal human serum. We utilized ^{51}Cr-loaded liposomes, sensitized with LPS from SS or SR gonococci (SS- or SR-LPS liposomes), and examined whether anti-LPS IgM or IgG, induced by *E. coli* J5 vaccination, facilitates C-mediated liposomolysis (^{51}Cr release).

After vaccination, serum IgG ($\mu g/ml$) increased >20-fold against SR-LPS. Bactericidal activity against the whole SR gonococci also developed and immune lysis of SR-LPS-liposomes increased >50-fold. IgM against SS-LOS increased (>10-fold) as well, but immune lysis of SS-LPS-liposomes was not enhanced.

Immune Ab, induced by *E. coli* J5 vaccination, recognizes determinants on the LPSs of both SS and SR gonococci. However, it discriminates for bacteriolytic epitopes expressed solely by the LPS of SR gonococci.

Safety and Efficacy of Two Pseudorabies Vaccines Produced by Genetic Engineering

C Dees*; M Bartoski*; S Kit†

* *Biologics Corporation/TechAmerica, Inc., Omaha, Nebraska, USA*
† *Baylor College of Medicine, Houston, Texas 77030, USA*

Omnivac PRV®, a thymidine kinase pseudorabies (PRV) deletion mutant (tk^-), is the first licensed vaccine produced by genetic engineering. The safety and efficacy of Omnivac PRV® in laboratory animals was compared to commercially available tk^+ PRV vaccines and a new PRV ($gIII^-/tk^-$) vaccine. Both tk^- vaccines protected outbred mice against challenge with virulent PRV. $10^{4.59}$ TCIDs of tk^+ vaccine given intraperitoneally killed 3/5 outbred mice. The second tk^+ vaccine killed 3/5 mice at $10^{3.59}$. No mice were killed by tk^+ or $gIII^-/tk^-$ when given $10^{10.59}$ TCIDs. 5/5 nude mice (nu/nu) were killed when given tk^+ vaccine, whereas all nude mice survived when given tk^- vaccines. The tk^- vaccines produced by genetic engineering are efficacious and many times safer than commercially available tk^+ vaccines produced by conventional methods.

Genetic Control of the Antibody Response to Carrier-free Synthetic Malaria Peptides in Mice

G Del Giudice*; A S Verdini†; H D Engers*; G Corradin‡; P-H Lambert*

* *WHO–IRTC, Department of Pathology, University of Geneva, Switzerland*
† *Eniricerche, Monterotondo, Italy*
‡ *Institute of Biochemistry, University of Lausanne, Switzerland*

A novel synthetic peptide consisting of 40 (Asn-Ala-Asn-Pro) repeats of *P. falciparum* circumsporozoite protein [$(NANP)_{40}$] was used to immunize mice of 14 strains with nine different H-2 haplotypes. *Only* H-2^b mice produced antibodies against the carrier-free $(NANP)_{40}$ peptide. However, C57BL/6 (H-2^b) *nu/nu* mice did not produce anti-$(NANP)_{40}$ antibodies. Using H-2 recombinant mice, the response mapped to the I-A region of the H-2 complex. This finding was confirmed by the experiments in B6CH-2^{bm12} I-A^b-mutant mice. Non-responder mice produced antibodies to $(NANP)_{40}$ after immunization with the peptide conjugated to a carrier protein. Based on these observations, peptide-specific T cell responses in individuals receiving sporozoite vaccines might be difficult to achieve. If so, the desired booster effects following natural exposure to *P. falciparum* sporozoites may not be observed.

Antibodies to Synthetic Carbohydrate Antigens

K R Diakun; S Yazawa; S A Abbas; R Jain; K L Matta

Roswell Park Memorial Institute, Department of Gynecologic Research, Buffalo, New York, USA

Antibodies to the chemically synthesized carbohydrates, Fuc α 1–3 Gal (a colon tumor-associated antigen), Gal β 1–3 GalNAc (a breast tumor-associated antigen) and Gal β 1–3 (GlcNAc β 1–6) GalNAc (part of an ovarian tumor-associated antigen) were developed. The diazophenyl derivatives were used as immunogens. Analysis of the antibodies via inhibition of enzyme immunoassays using chemically synthesized related oligosaccharides was performed. Information concerning the structural antigenic requirement and the side of antibody approach was obtained.

The antibodies were tested against tissues known to contain the antigen in question, and, in the case of Fuc α 1–3 Gal, the antibodies were used to screen other tissues.

(This investigation was supported by PHS Grant CA 36021, awarded by the National Cancer Institute, DHHS.)

Expression of *Schistosoma mansoni* Antigens in *E. coli*

M El-Sherbeini; K A Bostian; D Lustgarten; P Suri; P M Knopf

Division of Biology and Medicine, Brown University, Providence, Rhode Island 02912, USA

Some of the proteins produced by four-week-old worms of *S. mansoni* are natural immunogens in laboratory rats. Determining which of these are relevant to protective immunity will facilitate development of a vaccine which significantly protects laboratory hosts against infection by this parasite. To achieve this objective an expression library of *S. mansoni* cDNA sequences (provided by D Lanar, NIH), cloned in the lysogenic bacteriophage λgt11, has been immunoscreened. Immune serum from twice-infected Fisher rats (F-2x), which confers resistance in a passive immunization assay, and immune serum from twice-infected Wistar Furth rats (W-2x), which does not confer resistance, were used. Of approximately $(4–5) \times 10^5$ plaques screened, 87 F-2x$^+$ clones expressing *S. mansoni* epitopes fused to β-galactosidase were identified. When these clones were further immunoscreened with W-2x, some nine clones were found to be F-2x specific (F-2x$^+$, W-2x$^-$). Those clones were analyzed by SDS–PAGE and shown to express polypeptides larger than β-galactosidase. These clones are candidates for vaccine development.

Aspects of a Synthetic Peptide Vaccine Against *P. falciparum* Sporozoites

H M Etlinger*; E P Heimer†; A Trzeciak‡; A M Felix†; D Gillessen‡

* *Pharmaceutical Research Division*
† *Peptide Research Department, Hoffman–La Roche Inc., Nutley, New Jersey 07110, USA*
‡ *Central Research Units, F Hoffman–La Roche & Co. Ltd Basel, Switzerland*

A synthetic dodecapeptide, (NANP)$_3$, the main determinant of *P. falciparum* circumsporozoite protein, was conjugated to tetanus toxoid (TT). Two injections of alum-adsorbed conjugate evoked high anti-(NANP)$_3$ antibody responses in mice. The molar ratio of (NANP)$_3$ to TT did not appear critical, since conjugates containing 23 or 6 mol (NANP)$_3$/mol TT evoked good antibody responses. Preimmunization with TT inhibited anti-(NANP)$_3$ responses to one but not two boosts with conjugate. Offspring from mothers immunized with TT presented slightly reduced levels of anti-(NANP)$_3$ antibody when injected with conjugate. One-week-old mice evidenced good priming with conjugate, suggesting that young children will respond well. Fifteen out of 15 mouse strains produced anti-(NANP)$_3$ antibody, indicating that the genetically diverse human population will be responsive.

Binding of Streptococci to Rabbit Kidney

I Glurich; M W Stinson; B Albini

Departments of Microbiology and Medicine, State University of New York at Buffalo, Buffalo, New York, USA

Repeated i.v. injections of disrupted *Streptococcus mutans* or *S. pyogenes* T12 into New Zealand White rabbits leads to nephritis. Perfusion of isolated rabbit kidneys with streptococcal preparations resulted in various patterns of deposition involving glomeruli, tubules, and the interstitium. Infusion of these preparations into the left renal artery resulted in focal and segmental, predominantly linear and patchy deposits in glomeruli and the interstitium. Upon administration of antibodies to streptococci to the rabbit, the extent of deposits increased over the next five to eight days. *In vitro* experiments using a modified EIA demonstrated binding of *S. pyogenes* to collagen IV, laminin and proteoglycans, but not fibronectin. The proteoglycan-binding component was identified as of low molecular weight (around 10 kD).

Studies on the characterization of streptococcal-binding proteins should contribute to the understanding of the pathogenesis of kidney diseases arising in the wake of infectious diseases.

(Supported by NIDR Grant DE05696.)

Quantitative Analysis of Anti-Idiotypic Mimicry of Streptococcal Group A Carbohydrate (GAC)

N S Greenspan; William J Monafo; J M Davie

Departments of Microbiology and Immunology and Pathology, Washington University School of Medicine, St Louis, Missouri 63110, USA

We previously investigated the abilities of five rat monoclonal anti-Ids specific for a prototype anti-GAC monoclonal antibody (mAb), HGAC 39, to mimic patterns of binding of GAC to a large panel of anti-GAC mAbs. One of the anti-Ids previously shown to bind to an Id intimately associated with the HGAC 39 hapten-binding site, was found to bind to about two-thirds of the anti-GAC mAbs with a wide range of affinities. A single immunization with a

KLH-conjugate of this anti-Id in complete Freund's adjuvant induces anti-GAC antibody in C57BL/6J mice. Neither of two isotype-matched anti-Ids (derived from the same donor rat) elicited anti-GAC antibody under the same conditions of immunization.

Temperature-Sensitivity as a Method of Attenuation for Bacterial Vaccine Development

---

A M Hooke*; D O Sordelli*; M C Cerquetti*; J D Foulds†; P J Arroyo*; J A Bellanti*; M P Oeschger‡

* *Georgetown University School of Medicine, Washington, DC, USA*
† *NIDDK, Bethesda, Maryland, USA*
‡ *Louisiana State University Medical Center, New Orleans, Louisians, USA*

Temperature-sensitivity has been exploited as a means of attenuation for bacterial vaccine development. We have established methods to produce strains unable to sustain replication in the vaccinee, but, at the same time, capable of synthesizing antigens only expressed *in vivo*. We have also established methods to enhance the genetic stability of such mutants, making them safe for vaccine use. Animals immunized with these mutant strains are protected from challenge with the virulent parental wild-types.

Side-Product-Free, Quantitative Phenyl Isothiocyanate (PITC) Derivatization of an Insoluble Tumor Surface Octapeptide T Cell Epitope Gave the Peptide a Chromophore, Extended HPLC Analysis of the Peptide, and Increased the Peptide's Solubility

C A Hooper; R H Reid

Department of Gastroenterology, Walter Reed Army Institute of Research, Washington, DC 20307-5100, USA

At the *N*-terminus of a surface glycoprotein on human ductal carcinoma (breast) cells, the octapeptide G N T I V A V E comprises a T cell epitope with, except in trifluoroacetic acid (TFA), $<25\,\mu M$ solubility. HPLC of the solid-phase-synthesized octapeptide, on a C_{18} column with 0.1% TFA in an aqueous acetonitrile (MeCN) gradient, eluted a single, 210 nm absorbing peak. Needing water, an insoluble 20 nmol of peptide refluxed at 50 °C for 5 min in 90 μl of aqueous MeCN-methanol containing 360 nmol triethylamine (TEA) and 65 nmol PITC to give a soluble product. An ethyl acetate azeotrope removed excess PITC. These TEA and PITC amounts gave a peptide derivative HPLC background of <1%, revealing one major 254 nm absorbing peak. The increased solubility of the derivative indicates that the octapeptide cohesion results from hydrophobic and strong ionic interpeptide attractions.

The Design of Hepatitis B Synthetic Peptide Vaccines

C R Howard; J Allen; S-H Chen; S E Brown; M W Steward

Department of Medical Microbiology, London School of Hygiene and Tropical Medicine, London WC1E 7HT, UK

Synthetic peptides mimicking antigenic determinants on the major surface polypeptide of hepatitis B virus (HBsAg) have been studied. The affinity of antibody responses in mice immunized with a cyclical peptide representing amino acids 139–147 showed that high molecular weight polymers gave the most consistent results with affinity values for HBsAg similar to those found in individuals immune to hepatitis B. Peptides mimicking the so-called pre-S determinants induced high titers of antibodies against HBsAg in animals immunized with peptide–protein conjugates. These antisera identify determinants important for virus attachment and are considered essential components of a synthetic vaccine. Various antigen-presenting procedures incorporating both peptides are described.

Clinical Evaluation of Recombinant Hepatitis B Vaccine in Healthy Adults and Dialysis Patients

---

W Jilg*; M Schmidt; B Weinel; J Bommer; R Müller; F Deinhardt

* Max von Pettenkofer Institute, University of Munich
† City Hospitals, Ludwigshafen
‡ Department of Medicine, University of Heidelberg
§ Medical School Hannover, Federal Republic of Germany

Healthy young adults (283) were vaccinated three times with $10\,\mu g$ of HBsAg produced in recombinant yeast (Merck, Sharp & Dohme). Seroconversion rates, geometric mean anti-HBs concentrations, subtype specificity of anti-HBs and antibody-decay curves, followed for two years, were similar to those obtained after $10\,\mu g$ of plasma-derived HBsAg. Immune responses of 49 dialysis patients vaccinated three times with $40\,\mu g$ of recombinant HBsAg were considerably lower than those of controls after $10\,\mu g$ recombinant HBsAg. A schedule using six monthly doses of either $20\,\mu g$ or $40\,\mu g$ HBsAg tested in 39 patients did not show any advantage over the three-dose regimen. The new vaccine was well tolerated; no serious adverse reactions were observed.

Protective Activity of Non-Conformation-Specific Antibodies

M E Jolivet*; F Audibert*; L Chedid*; A Tartar†; H Gras-Masse†;
E H Beachey‡

* *University of South Florida, College of Medicine, Tampa, Florida 33612,
USA*
† *Laboratoire de Chimie Organique, Faculté de Pharmacie, 59045 Lille
Cedex, France*
‡ *The Veterans Administration Medical Center and the University of
Tennessee, College of Medicine, Memphis, Tennessee 38104, USA*

It is generally agreed that anticonformational antibodies are a critical requirement for protective activity. We investigated whether linear epitopes can induce protective antibodies. The antibodies studied were obtained against either the streptococcal M24 protein (Pep M24) or a synthetic peptide which was copied as part of its sequence.

Circular dichroism showed that two peptides are structured (1–34 and heteropeptide composed of 19–34 plus 20 foreign amino acids) and two others are not (19–34 and 24–35 sequences). Like Pep M24, all these peptides were capable of inducing protective antibodies. However, ELISA competition studies demonstrated that only the structured peptides provoked anticonformational antibodies.

Future studies are required to know whether these results are unique in relation to the streptococcal model or to what extent thay may be generalized.

Effect of Glycoprotein D Subunit Vaccines on Primary and Recurrent Genital *Herpes simplex* Virus Type 2 (HSV-2) Infections of Guinea Pigs

E R Kern*; P E Vogt*; T Gregory†; L A Lasky†; P W Berman†

* *University of Utah School of Medicine, Salt Lake City, Utah, USA*
† *Genentech Inc., South San Francisco, California, USA*

Intravaginal inoculation of 200 g guinea pigs with 10^5 pfu of HSV-2 results in a primary infection with vaginal viral replication and external vesicular lesions followed by spontaneous recurrent episodes. Vaccination with recombinant glycoprotein D from either HSV-1 or HSV-2 prior to infection markedly altered vaginal viral replication, reduced or prevented the development of external lesions, prevented the establishment of latent HSV-2 infections in dorsal root ganglia, and reduced the frequency of recurrent episodes. Glycoprotein D from HSV-2 was more effective than the protein derived from HSV-1. Vaccination after primary infection had no effect on the frequency or duration of recurrent HSV-2 episodes. These results suggest that vaccines of this type could potentially play a role in the management of primary genital herpes in humans.

Towards the Development of a Vaccine for the Human Blood Fluke *Schistosoma mansoni*

H van Keulen*; S Modavi*; M Simurda*; D M Rekosh†; P T LoVerde*

Departments of *Microbiology and †Biochemistry, State University of New York, Buffalo, New York 14214, USA

Natural immunity against schistosomes is induced by an active infection but directed against the invading larvae (schistosomula) of challenge infections. More than 40 antigens were identified by isolation of RNA from either adult worm pairs or cercariae/schistosomula stage followed by *in vitro* translation and immunoprecipitation of the translated products with pooled sera from chronically infected patients. An adult worm cDNA library was screened with cDNA probes derived from known fractions of (poly A$^+$) RNA. The clones were screened by positive selection and immunoprecipitation with patient sera. The clones encoding different antigens were then rescreened with polyclonal sera made to defined antigens. The polyclonal sera were made by immunizing mice with silver-stained spots removed from 2-dimensional gels of schistosomular extracts. A cDNA clone identified by this procedure encodes a putative protective antigen.

Role of *Neisseria lactamica* Lipo-oligosaccharides in the Development of Natural Immunity to *Neisseria meningitidis*

J J Kim; R E Mandrell; J McL Griffiss

Veterans Administration Medical Center and Departments of Laboratory Medicine and Medicine, University of California, San Francisco, California 94121, USA

Neisseria lactamica (NL), an unencapsulated nonpathogen and early pharyngeal colonizer of infants, induces antibody directed against subcapsular components of *Neisseria meningitidis* (NM).

We studied lipo-oligosaccharides (LOS) of 26 NL and 20 group A NM. Silver-stained SDS–PAGE gels showed LOS of from one to four components of M_r between 4300 and 5400. LOS antigenic similarities between NL and NM were studied using mouse monoclonal antibodies (MAb) previously shown to bind neisserial LOS using a solid-phase radioimmunoassay, immunoblot and/or dor-blot assay. One MAb recognized an epitope on 10/20 NM and 23/26 NL. A second MAb bound LOS of all group A NM and 2/26 NL.

These shared LOS epitopes may contribute to the development of natural immunity to the meningococcus.

Antigen-Antibody Interaction in ELISA

E A Klasen; Q Vos; N D Zegers; C Deen; M J Fasbender; J J Haaijman

TNO Medical Biological Laboratory, 2280 AA Rijswijk ZH, The Netherlands

The performance of the direct ELISA is influenced by antigen concentration during coating, dissociation of antigen during the assay, epitope density per antigen molecule, antibody concentration, antibody affinity and the characteristics of the anti-immunoglobulin reagent. Antigen presentation in ELISA was investigated by analyzing the interaction of human IgG and Hb with monoclonal antibodies (MAb) elicited against short, IgG-specific amino acid sequences and polyclonal antibodies elicited against native Hb. MAb specific for the haptens FITC and 2-acetylaminofluorene have been used to analyze the prozone phenomenon, observed when increasing concentrations of antibody are incubated in wells coated with a fixed concentration of antigen, and the hook effect which may be observed when a fixed concentration of antibody is incubated in wells coated with increasing concentrations of antigen.

Designing Peptide Vaccines: The Effects of Hydrophobic Feet, Cysteine Dimerization and Replicate Epitopes With and Without Carrier Proteosomes

G H Lowell; L F Smith; W D Zollinger

Department of Bacterial Diseases, Walter Reed Army Institute of Research, Washington, DC 20307, USA

Making synthetic peptide vaccines has been complicated by a paucity of efficient carrier proteins and adjuvants acceptable for human use. We have found that without proteins or adjuvants, a small peptide can be made immunogenic in mice by adding a lauric acid hydrophobic foot to the peptide's amino terminus, a cysteine residue (to promote dimerization of the hybrid lipopeptide), replicating the peptide epitope three to five times and selectively dialyzing away detergent. Hydrophobic complexing (via dialysis) of the cysteine-containing lipopeptides to 'proteosomes' (meningococcal outer membrane proteins) made even single-epitope peptides highly immunogenic and increased the immunogenicity of replicate-epitope peptides. Since proteosomes have safely been given to people, these methods may serve as models for designing immunogenic synthetic peptide vaccines for human use.

Human Immune Response to Monoclonal Antibody-Defined Epitopes of *Neisseria gonorrhoeae* Lipooligosaccharides

R E Mandrell*; J Sugai*; J Boslego†; R Chung†; P Rice‡; J McL Griffiss*

* *Veterans Administration Medical Center and Departments of Laboratory Medicine and Medicine, University of California, San Francisco, California, USA*
† *Walter Reed Army Institute of Research, Washington, DC, USA*
‡ *Boston University School of Medicine, Boston, Massachusetts, USA*

Five and seven strains of *Neisseria gonorrhoeae* isolated from local (LI) and disseminated (DGI) infections, respectively, were screened with a battery of 10 monoclonal antibodies (MAb) specific for components of neisserial lipo-oligosaccharides (LOS). The MAb binding and SDS–PAGE silver stain profile of each strain's LOS were unique. Homologous pre-infection, acute and convalescent sera were tested as competitors of the binding of MAbs to LOS epitopes. Sixteen of 35 (46%) total epitope reactions were competed by DGI convalescent sera, compared to 2 of 28 (7%) for LI convalescent sera. This result was supported by the presence of higher levels of total LOS antibody in the DGI convalescent sera compared to LI sera. We conclude that humans respond to multiple MAb-defined LOS epitopes on multiple LOS components.

Molecular Analysis of Genes for Surface Antigens of *Vibrio cholerae* O1

P A Manning; M W Heuzenroeder; R Morona; J Pohlner; M B Jalajakumari; J Yeadon; P R Reeves; D Rowley

Department of Microbiology and Immunology, The University of Adelaide, Adelaide, S.A. 5001, Australia

Vibrio cholerae O1, the causative agent of cholera in man, is a noninvasive pathogen which remains localized in the intestine and produces an entero-toxin responsible for the diarrhea. Protection against infection would appear to be mediated by antibodies in the gut to specific surface components associated with adherence. Our aim was to clone the genes encoding the biosynthesis of these components and introduce them into avirulent *Salmonella typhi* strains to be used as oral immunogens against cholera (and typhoid).

The genes encoding synthesis of the O-antigen of both the major serotypes (Inaba and Ogawa) have been cloned. The O-antigen is substituted on to the core oligosaccharide of the LPS of *E. coli* K-12 and antibodies raised against such *E. coli* are highly protective.

The gene *ompV*, for a major outer membrane protein, has been cloned and the nucleotide sequence determined. Gene and protein fusions have enabled the major antigenic domains of the protein to be localized. The gene *ompV* is subject to translational control.

Murine T Cell Responses Detected after Immunization with Vectors Containing the Cloned *Herpes simplex* virus (HSV) Gene Coding for Glycoprotein D (gD)

S Martin*; P W Berman†; B Moss‡; B T Rouse*

* *University of Tennessee, Knoxville, Tennessee 37996–0845, USA*
† *Genetech Inc., San Francisco, California 94080, USA*
‡ *National Institutes of Health, Bethesda, Maryland 20205, USA*

We used a transfected L cell and a vaccinia vector carrying the HSV-1 gene coding for gD to characterize anti-HSV T cell responses. Mice immunized with either vector developed class II MHC-restricted T cell-responses which helped produce anti-HSV antibodies, produced IL-2 and gamma interferon upon HSV stimulation, and lysed HSV-1-infected cells expressing histocompatible Ia antigens.

Such mice also developed potent suppressor T cells which prevented HSV-specific lymphoproliferation and cytotoxic T cell (Tc) generation *in vitro*.

Surprisingly, neither vector was capable of forming a target cell complex which was recognized by class I MHC-restricted anti-HSV specific Tc.

The studies suggest tht gD-specific class I MHC-restricted anti-HSV Tc do not develop during HSV infection possibly because of active suppression.

Monoclonal Antibodies Detect Bovine Herpes Virus-1, Parainfluenza-3 and Diarrhea Viruses in Mixed Infections

H C Minocha; A Ghram; D Tyrell

Department of Laboratory Medicine, Kansas State University, Manhattan, Kansas 66506

Monoclonal antibodies to bovine herpesvirus-1 (BHV-1), parainfluenza-3 (PI-3) and bovine virus diarrhea (BVD) viruses were purified by DEAE Affi-gel® Blue column chromatography. The antibodies detected virus glycoproteins in multiply infected cultures by competition ELISA, and neutralized $>10^5$ plaque-forming units of viruses. High virus multiplicities ($>1.0\,\text{cell}^{-1}$) decreased virus synthesis in doubly infected cultures; however, maximum propagation of both viruses occurred when cells were inoculated with virus multiplicity of less than $0.1\,\text{cell}^{-1}$. Prior infection of bovine peripheral lymphocytes with PI-3 enhanced BHV-1 production and suppressed blastogenic activity measured by ^{3}H-thymidine incorporation. No correlation was observed between lymphocyte blastogenic response to phytohemagglutinin and interleukin-2 production in virus-infected cell cultures.

Molecular Cloning of *Haemophilus influenzae* Type b Outer Membrane Protein P1

R S Munson Jr

Washington University School of Medicine, St Louis, Missouri 63110, USA

Outer membrane protein P1 of *Haemophilus influenzae* type b is a heat-modifiable protein. It has an apparent molecular weight of 35 000 on SDS–PAGE, if the sample is solubilized at room temperature and an apparent molecular weight of 50 000 when the sample is heated at 100 °C. The protein has been purified and polyclonal sera generated in rabbits. A genomic library of type b *Haemophilus* was prepared in the lambda vector EMBL3. Plaques were screened with αP1 and three immunologically reactive plaques were detected. Synthesis of P1 was confirmed by Western blots of sonicates from infected cells. Both the heat-modified and non-heat-modified forms of the protein were observed. The recombinant clones synthesized a protein with the same apparent molecular weight as the *Haemophilus* protein. Each clone had an insert of approximately 15 kb. Subcloning and localization of the protein in *E. coli* are in progress.

Identification of a 16 600 Dalton Outer Membrane Protein on Nontypable *Haemophilus influenzae* as a Target for Human Serum Bactericidal Antibody

T F Murphy*; L C Bartos*; P A Rice†; M B Nelson*; K C Dudas*; M A Apicella*

* *State University of New York at Buffalo, Buffalo, New York, USA*
† *Boston University, Boston, Massachusetts 02118, USA*

A 16 600 Dalton outer membrane protein is present in all strains of *Haemophilus influenzae* and antibodies to this protein are present in human serum. The present study was designed to assess the role of this outer membrane protein (P6) in nontypable *H. influenzae* as a target for human serum bactericidal antibody. P6 was isolated and coupled to an affinity column. Depleting normal human serum of antibodies to P6 by affinity chromatography resulted in reduced bactericidal activity of that serum for nontypable *H. influenzae*. Immunopurified antibodies to P6 from human serum were bactericidal. Finally, preincubation of bacteria with a monoclonal antibody which recognizes a surface epitope on P6, inhibited human serum bactericidal killing. Taken together, these experiments establish that P6 is a target for human bactericidal antibodies. This observation provides evidence that P6 plays an important role in human immunity to infection by nontypable *H. influenzae*.

Use of Monoclonal Antibodies to Investigate the Immunity Induced by a *Streptococcus pyogenes* Group A Ribosomal Vaccine

G Normier*; A M Pinel*; D A Levy*; L Dussourd d'Hinterland*;
C Lindqvist†; H Wigzell†

* *Centre d'Immunologie et de Biologie P Fabre, Castres, France*
† *Karolinska Institute, Department of Immunology, Stockholm, Sweden*

Ribosomes of *Streptococcus pyogenes* group A induce protective immunity against infection with the homologous bacteria in mice (Schalla and Johnson, 1975, *Infection and Immunity* **11**: 1195–202). To study the specificity of this protection, hybridoma technology was used to raise monoclonal antibodies against antigenic determinants on ribosomes isolated from the corresponding virulent strain. Only ribosomes derived from the virulent strain gave significant active protection against infection of mice with the homologous strain. Two monoclonal antibodies (MAbs) directed against the virulent strain failed to protect mice passively against the virulent strain and did not react with the M protein produced only by the virulent strain. A MAb (C3G12) raised against M protein conferred significant passive protection in mice. Using ELISA, this MAb reacted with ribosomes from the virulent strain but not with ribosomes from the non-virulent strain, showing that M protein epitopes were linked to ribosomes from the virulent strain. These data suggest that the immunoprotective capacity of *Streptococcus pyogenes* group A ribosomes is at least closely related to their ability to induce a strong specific immune response to cell surface antigens such as M protein, and that small amounts of the corresponding epitopes must be strongly linked to the ribosomes.

Antigenic Properties of Pseudomonas Proteases Revealed by Monoclonal T Cells

M J Parmely; R T Horvat

University of Kansas Medical Center, Kansas City, Kansas 66103, USA

Since evidence suggests that T lymphocytes may be involved in limiting the growth of *Pseudomonas aeruginosa*, we isolated and characterized a large series of human T cell clones specific for Pseudomonas antigens. 80% of the clones recognized either alkaline protease (AP) or elastase (E), the two principal proteases of the organism. Panel analyses, limiting dilution analyses and immunochemical studies revealed that: (a) both antigenic molecules bear common (conserved) as well as allomorphic (strain-specific) determinants; (b) the determinants could be separated biochemically; (c) T cells specific for most of the determinants produced gamma interferon; and (d) protease-specific T cells producing gamma interferon were present at relatively high frequencies in the blood of immune donors. This model should help identify protease epitopes that stimulate T cell-mediated responses to the organism.

Immune Responses of Chickens Trickle Immunized with *Eimeria tenella*

S H Parry; M E J Barratt; M Morgan; P J Davis

Immunology Department, Unilever Research, Colworth House, Sharnbrook, Bedfordshire, UK

Trickle immunization (TI) of chicks with very low numbers of encapsulated coccidial oocysts, administered in feed over the first three weeks of life, provides a practical and remarkably effective means of vaccination. TI is superior to single-shot immunization in that solid immunity can be achieved with as few as 300 oocysts without concomitant clinical or pathological signs. A spectrum of protective cellular and antibody responses is stimulated at the gut mucosa while potentially damaging inflammatory response are minimal. In contrast to single-shot vaccination, TI birds have low levels of circulating IgG and low levels of IgG plasma cells in the cecal mucosa. This correlates with the absence of type III responses and a lack of inflammatory response at the mucosal level.

Suppression of the Immune Response of Carp, *Cyprinus carpio*, by *Aeromonas salmonicida*: A Problem for Vaccine Development

C N Pourreau*; D Evenberg†; W M de Raadt*; R G F R Hendriks*;
R C J Kimanai*; W B van Muiswinkel*

** Department of Experimental Animal Morphology and Cell Biology,
Agricultural University, 6700 AH Wageningen, The Netherlands
† Institute of Molecular Biology and Department of Molecular Biology,
University of Utrecht, TB Utrecht, The Netherlands*

Aeromonas salmonicida is a significant bacterial pathogen of salmonid and cyprinid fishes against which oral and immersion vaccines (crude bacterins, surface antigens, or toxoids) are still inefficient. Observations in carp, *Cyprinus carpio*, suggest that virulent *A. salmonicida* perturb the immune system of the fish: (1) injection of formalin-killed bacteria in fish leads to production of specific serum antibodies that are not protective against subsequent lethal challenges; (2) total serum proteins including immunoglobulins drop dramatically; (3) efficiency at mounting a secondary humoral immune response to sheep erythrocytes (number of PFC, serum antibody titres) decreases; (4) culture supernatants containing bacterial extracellular products are lethal to fish when injected intraperitoneally; and (5) supernatants suppress the mitogen response of normal carp leucocytes to PHA *in vitro*. Presently, our research focuses on nonimmunosuppressive bacterial products that evoke protective immunity.

Influence of Epitope Structure and Conformation on Antibody Recognition: A Model Study Using the Cyclic Peptide Cyclosporine

V Quesniaux*†; M H Schreier*; R M Wenger*; M H V Van Regenmortel‡

* *Sandoz Ltd, CH-4002 Basel, Switzerland*
† *On leave from IBMC, F-67084 Strasbourg, France*
‡ *IBMC, Strasbourg, France*

More than 180 monoclonal antibodies (MAbs) have been prepared against the rigid cyclic undecapeptide cyclosporin (Cs). The fine antigenic recognition patterns of these MAbs were determined using 100 different Cs-derivatives. Small clusters of amino acid residues on different sides of the Cs molecule were recognized by different families of MAbs. Slight conformational changes (as determined by ^{13}C-NMR or X-ray crystallography) induced by the modification of residues located outside an epitope were detected by the corresponding MAb. At the sub-amino acid level, the fine specificity of MAbs for the new nine-carbon amino acid 1 was studied using a series of derivatives modified in residue 1. Some MAbs were shown to recognize specifically either the beginning or the end of the nine-carbon chain.

Epstein–Barr Virus, Its DNA Replication and the Immune Response

P J Siegel Randolph

Department of Biology, Boston University, Boston, Massachusetts 02215, USA

We have studied viral DNA production of Epstein–Barr virus (EBV) for several years (Siegel *et al.* 1980, *Journal of Virology* **38**: 880). Nascent linear viral DNA is produced via bidirectional replication of a relaxed circular intermediate. *Hind*III restriction digests of the 65S precursor show the left end (A) to be joined to the right (D_1 or D_{1het}). Unwindase inhibitors present a new source of anti-EBV agents; AIDS victims who are immune-suppressed by EBV and CMV, as well as by HTLV-III/LAV, could benefit.

Faulty replication at two lytic DNA replication origins generate one-third genomes; these contain early gene regions and cause overproduction of early antigen (EA). The latter could contribute to pathogenesis and be useful for mapping and production of early viral proteins and antigens.

Developments in Foot-and-Mouth Disease Vaccine Production and Disease Control in India

B U Rao

Southern Regional Station, Indian Veterinary Research Institute, Bangalore-560 024, Karnataka, India

Foot-and-mouth disease is widespread and endemic in the subcontinent with 400 million of the domestic livestock population infected. The conventional inactivated virus vaccine is produced by continuous suspension cell cultures in fermenters in millions of doses annually. The scope of live attenuated vaccine has not been explored.

Research is being conducted on recombinant DNA technique for development of immunogens, hybridoma technique for production of monoclonal antibodies, freeze-drying of vaccine and crystallization of virus. Laboratory techniques like ELISA, electrofocusing, Western and Southern blotting, nucleotide sequencing and nucleic acid hybridization were adopted and hexokinase activity was studied as a marker for virus harvesting.

The disease control program is based on immunoprophylaxis with mass vaccination of valuable productive animals and creation of selected disease-free zones.

GM$_1$ Ganglioside-Binding Peptide of Cholera Toxin B Chain Serves as a Carrier for Synthetic Octapeptide During *In Vitro* Immunization of Rabbit Spleen B-Cells

R H Reid; L Y Tseng; C A Hooper; T G Brewer

Department of Gastroenterology, Walter Reed Army Institute of Research, Washington, DC 20307–5100, USA

A synthetic 21 amino acid (AA) peptide representing the 30–50 AA peptide fragment of cholera toxin B chain has been found to bind to multilamellar liposomes containing GM$_1$ ganglioside. To determine if the 21 AA peptide could function as a carrier for an added *N*-terminal octapeptide, rabbit spleen mononuclear cells in microculture were immunized *in vitro* with the 29 AA peptide. Maximum ELISA responses were seen on day 12 with specific antibody against the 29 AA peptide and against the *N*-terminal octapeptide. The antibody response was mainly IgM. In conclusion, the synthetic GM$_1$ ganglioside-binding peptide of cholera toxin B chain can function as a carrier for an added *N*-terminal octapeptide during *in vitro* primary immunization of rabbit spleen B-cells.

Immunity to American Cutaneous Leishmaniasis: Possible Role of K/NK Cells in the Local Control of Infection

P-R Ridel; J-P Dedet; P Esterre; R Pradinaud

Institute Pasteur de la Guyane Francaise, 97306 Cayenne Cedex, France

Mechanisms which limit American cutaneous leishmaniasis to its localized skin form appear of primary importance and merit investigation because the level of protection afforded by sensitized T cells is not fully efficient, since lesions last for months or years and since vaccination protects only 30% of immunized subjects. Using monoclonal antibodies and immunoperoxidase techniques, skin biopsies showed a high percentage of K/NK cells, highly variable percentages of T4, TAC-positive cells and, in contrast to the histological examination, only seldom monocytic cells. Our results indicate that the local control of leishmaniasis could be mediated by K/NK cells. This observation could be of primary importance in terms of development of new strategies for disease control.

Analysis of Immune Responses to *Streptococcus mutans*

M W Russell; C Czerkinsky; Z Moldoveanu; S M Michalek; J R McGhee; J Mestecky

Department of Microbiology, University of Alabama at Birmingham, Birmingham, Alabama 35294, USA

The enzyme-linked immunospot (ELISPOT) assay has been used to assess immune responses to *S. mutans* at the cellular level. In mice injected with *S. mutans* cells, the spleen cell response was predominantly against protein antigen I/II. These results correlated with the development of serum antibodies, and similar results were obtained in rabbits. Weak polyclonal responses and rheumatoid factor (RF) were also induced by immunization with *S. mutans*. Purified antigen I/II was highly immunogenic, and tended to induce polyclonal and RF responses. Human sera frequently revealed high levels of IgM, IgG and IgA antibodies to antigen I/II. After oral immunization of volunteers with capsules containing killed *S. mutans*, cells capable of synthesizing IgA antibodies to antigen I/II appeared in the circulation, and salivary IgA antibodies were developed.

(Supported by US–PHS grants DE-06746, DE-02670 and DE-06669.)

Quantitation of Antibody to *E. coli* 0111:B4 (J5) Lipopolysaccharide (LPS) by Two Variations of ELISA

T A Schwartzer; D V Alcid; D J Gocke

Departments of Medicine and Microbiology, UMDNJ–Rutgers Medical School, New Brunswick, New Jersey, USA

Interest in therapeutic applications of LPS-specific antibodies has led to widespread use of ELISA for antibody quantitation with highly variable results. We compared measurement of anti-J5 LPS using a standard curve prepared with affinity-purified anti-J5 LPS versus measurements expressed as equivalence units from a polyclonal Ig standard curve. Although acceptable precision could be obtained within each method, results for IgG- and IgM-specific anti-J5 LPS in five different human sera differed about 300-fold between methods. These data indicate that ELISA is not a gravimetric measure of antibody content and results obtained with different ELISA methods are not directly comparable.

Immunochemical Reactivities and Size Distribution of Carbohydrate Haptens of *Brucella abortus* Endotoxins (Fraction 5A)

A M Wu*; N E Mackenzie†

* Department of Veterinary Pathology and †Departments of Veterinary Chemistry and Microbiology, Texas A&M University, College Station, Texas, USA

The O-haptens of the major fraction of the *B. abortus* (strain 2308 and strain 19) smooth lipopolysaccharide were prepared by hydrolysis of native sLPS (Fraction 5A) in 1% acetic acid at 100°C for 2 hr. O-haptens were separated from Lipid A and protein by centrifugation, and small fragments by ultrafiltration (MWCO[1] 1.0×10^3). These carbohydrate haptens were found to be immunoactive by precipitin-inhibition assay, and were further fractionated by both membrane filtration and dialysis. The size distribution of carbohydrate hapten of endotoxins ranged from several oligosaccharides up to 1.0×10^4. Three major fractions of molecular sieves $(8.0-10) \times 10^3$, $(3.5-5.0) \times 10^3$ and $<1.0 \times 10^3$, were dominant, and consisted of 85% of total immunoactive materials. Major fractions of haptens were found to be a repeat unit of *N*-formylperosamine.

(This work was aided by grants from the Texas Agricultural Experiment Station (TAES H6194), USDA/SEA/ARS Coop, Agreement No.58-6125-5-4, and USDA/SEA Formula Animal Health Funds (Project 6648).)

---

[1] MWCO = molecular weight cut-off

T Cell Recognition of Synthetic Peptide Subunits of Herpes simplex Virus Glycoprotein D Corresponding to Antibody Determinants

J H Wyckoff III*; R J Eisenburg†‡; G H Cohen†§;; B T Rouse*

* *Department of Microbiology, College of Veterinary Medicine, University of Tennessee, Knoxville, Tennessee 37996, USA*
† *Department of Pathology, School of Veterinary Medicine, and ‡Center for Oral Research, §Department of Microbiology, School of Dental Medicine, University of Pennsylvania, Philadelphia, Pennsylvania 19104, USA*

Four synthetic peptides were evaluated for *in vitro* stimulatory activity for Herpes simplex virus (HSV)-primed murine T cells. Peptides corresponded to antibody determinants (some of which are neutralization sites) defined on HSV glycoprotein D within amino acid residues 1–23, 268–287 and 340–356. Responses evaluated included lymphoproliferation, interleukin 2 secretion, and suppressor factor generation. Stimulation of splenic T cells from mice immunized four to six weeks previously with HSV resulted in both helper and suppressor T cell responses. However, draining lymph node cells from mice immunized one week prior to stimulation with peptides gave almost exclusively helper T cell responses. These results suggest these peptides may be viable vaccine candidates in that they correspond to both virus neutralization antibody determinants and helper T cell epitopes.

Immunological Characteristics of Lipopolysaccharide Fractions from *Salmonella typhimurium*

H-Y Yeh; D M Jacobs

Department of Microbiology, State University of New York at Buffalo, Buffalo, New York 14214, USA

Characteristics of lipopolysaccharide (LPS) subunits of different sizes have been analyzed. *Salmonella typhimurium* LPS was separated into three fractions (1–3 in order of elution) on Sephadex G-200® in the presence of deoxycholate (DOC). Samples in each peak were pooled, dialyzed exhaustively to remove DOC, and tested in a mitogenic assay. Fraction 3 was the most potent mitogen. On silver-stained SDS–PAGE gels fractions 2 and 3 had ladder-like patterns, with the fastest migrating bands in fraction 3. Fraction 1 barely entered the gel. Transblots were exposed to anti-0.4 mAb and detected with ^{125}I-labeled protein A. Fraction 1 was not detected. The fastest migrating bands of fraction 3 and unfractionated LPS detected on stained gels were not detected in the transfer, suggesting that these two bands do not contain O-repeating units. Assuming two O-repeating units for the first bands detected in the transfer, we calculated that fraction 2 has 31 O-repeating units.

(Supported by AI18506.)

Meningococcal Outer Membrane Protein-Detoxified Lipopolysaccharide Vaccine

W D Zollinger; E E Moran; H Collins; R C Seid

Department of Bacterial Diseases, Walter Reed Army Institute of Research, Washington, DC 20307–5100

A vaccine for group B meningococcal disease was prepared by combining alkaline detoxified lipopolysaccharide (dLPS) and purified outer membrane proteins (OMP) in a noncovalent complex. Alkaline treatment of the LPS removed all ester-linked fatty acids and resulted in a 1000-fold reduction of toxicity as determined in five different assays. The resultant dLPS retained full antigenicity and was able to bind hydrophobically to and solubilize the OMP. Immunogenicity of the OMP in mice was equivalent to that obtained with OMP–C polysaccharide complexes. Advantages of using dLPS in place of capsular polysaccharide to solubilize the OMP include the possibility of inducing bactericidal antibodies against cross-reactive LPS determinants, increased stability of the noncovalent complex, and ability to use a single vaccine for multiple doses.

Author index

Subject index

467

human immunodeficiency virus (HIV)
  see also acquired
    immunodeficiency syndrome
  characteristics 272–3, 392–4
  genetic variability 274–5, 397–8
  immune response 273–4, 396–7
hydroxycoumarin, 21, 23, 25–6

idiotype
  network 342–3
  vaccines 323–6, 328–30, 342–9,
    352–6, 359–70, 377–80, 382–7,
    398–9, 443
    cancer 382–7
    hepatitis B 352–6
    influenza A 343–9
    parasites
      schistosomiasis 378
      trypanosomiasis 378–9
    Sendai virus 361–70
immune responses, 441, 456
  EBV 458
  HIV 273–4
  lipid A 79
  measles virus 437
  M. leprae 249
  M. tuberculosis 249
  P. falciparum 256–8
  reovirus type 3 330–31
  secretory 261, 268–9
  Sendai virus 361–8
  S. mutans 110
  suppression 457
  vaccinia melanoma oncolysate
    (VMO) therapy 437
immunoglobulin (Ig)
  chimeric molecules 221–30
  complement 172, 177–8, 184
  conjugates with antigen 6–7, 11–12,
    54–5
  isotypes 377
immunotoxin, 3, 7, 10–12
influenza A virus
  hemagglutinin 65–6, 203–4, 344–8
  neuraminidase 203, 348–9
  structure 202–3
  vaccinia virus recombinants 203–6

killer cells, 460
Klebsiella pneumoniae, 438

Leishmania major, 195, 460
lipooligosaccharide (LOS), 90, 451
  antibodies 449

lipopolysaccharide (LPS), 73–85,
    297–9, 463–4
  antibodies 439, 461
  antigenic determinants 78–9
  lipid A 75–8, 79–84
  R mutants 74–7
  structure 73–8
lysozyme, 42–6, 63–4
  antibodies 42–6

malaria, 195, 251–60, 440
measles virus, 140, 437
Moraxella nonliquifaciens, 32
mucosal immunity, 136–41
  measles virus 140
  poliovirus 139
  respiratory syncytial virus (RSV) 140
  rubella virus 138
  varicella-zoster virus (VZV) 137–8
Mycobacterium bovis, 249
Mycobacterium leprae, 194–5, 197,
    245–9
  genes 246
  proteins 246
  recombinant clones 246–9
  T-cell response 194–5, 197, 249
Mycobacterium tuberculosis, 245–9
  genes 246
  proteins 246
  recombinant clones 246–9
myoglobin, 58, 60–3
myohemerythrin, 30, 33–8

natural killer cells, 460
Neisseria gonorrhoeae, 29, 31, 177, 439,
    451
  complement 177–8
  pili
    antigenic variation 31
    structure 30–1
Neisseria lactamica, 456
Neisseria meningitidis, 32, 170–3, 449,
    464
  capsular epitopes 170–1
  complement 173
  immune response 172–3

parainfluenza virus, 453
peptides *see* vaccines, synthetic peptides
Plasmodium falciparum, 195, 251, 259,
    440
poliovirus, 139
Pseudomonas aeruginosa, 32, 455
pseudorabies virus, 440